Medical Radiology

Radiation Oncology

Series Editors
Nancy Y. Lee
Jiade J. Lu

Medical Radiology - Radiation Oncology is a unique series that aims to document the most innovative technologies in all fields within radiology, thereby informing the physician in practice of the latest advances in diagnostic and treatment techniques.

The contents range from contemporary statements relating to management for various disease sites to explanations of the newest techniques for tumor identification and of mechanisms for the enhancement of radiation effects, with the emphasis on maximizing cure and minimizing complications.

Each volume is a comprehensive reference book on a topical theme, and the editors are always experts of high international standing. Contributions are included from both clinicians and researchers, ensuring wide appeal.

Branislav Jeremić
Editor

Advances in Radiation Oncology in Lung Cancer

Third Edition

Volume II

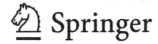

Editor
Branislav Jeremić
School of Medicine
University of Kragujevac
Kragujevac, Serbia

ISSN 0942-5373 ISSN 2197-4187 (electronic)
Medical Radiology
ISSN 2731-4715 ISSN 2731-4723 (electronic)
Radiation Oncology
ISBN 978-3-031-34846-4   ISBN 978-3-031-34847-1   (eBook)
https://doi.org/10.1007/978-3-031-34847-1

© The Editor(s) (if applicable) and The Author(s), under exclusive license to Springer Nature Switzerland AG 2005, 2011, 2023
This work is subject to copyright. All rights are solely and exclusively licensed by the Publisher, whether the whole or part of the material is concerned, specifically the rights of translation, reprinting, reuse of illustrations, recitation, broadcasting, reproduction on microfilms or in any other physical way, and transmission or information storage and retrieval, electronic adaptation, computer software, or by similar or dissimilar methodology now known or hereafter developed.
The use of general descriptive names, registered names, trademarks, service marks, etc. in this publication does not imply, even in the absence of a specific statement, that such names are exempt from the relevant protective laws and regulations and therefore free for general use.
The publisher, the authors, and the editors are safe to assume that the advice and information in this book are believed to be true and accurate at the date of publication. Neither the publisher nor the authors or the editors give a warranty, expressed or implied, with respect to the material contained herein or for any errors or omissions that may have been made. The publisher remains neutral with regard to jurisdictional claims in published maps and institutional affiliations.

This Springer imprint is published by the registered company Springer Nature Switzerland AG
The registered company address is: Gewerbestrasse 11, 6330 Cham, Switzerland

For
Aleksandra and Marta.

Preface

Worldwide, there is an estimated 19.3 million new cancer cases with almost 10.0 million cancer deaths occurred in 2020. Lung cancer is now the second most commonly diagnosed cancer, with an estimated 2,206,771 new cases annually occurring. It, however, remains the leading cause of cancer death, with an estimated 1.8 million deaths (18%). Due to continuing efforts of the tobacco industry shifting its focus from developed to a developing world, more than 50% of new cases continue to occur in the latter one in the past decade. It is, therefore, not unexpectedly a big burden to national health care systems worldwide with hundreds of thousands of patients succumbing to it every year.

Radiation therapy remains the cornerstone of modern treatment approaches, regardless of histology and stage of the disease. It is used in both curative and palliative setting, being the most cost-effective treatment option in lung cancer. Recent decades witnessed important technological and biological developments which enabled continuous and efficient adaptation to the growing demands to offer precision medicine in the twenty-first century. Together with other two treatment modalities, surgery and systemic therapy, it successfully evolves focusing on both patient and society needs. Indeed, there seems to be very few competitors among medical disciplines that have so broadly embraced scientific novelties such as computer-driven technological aspects as is the case with radiation therapy.

This, updated and third edition of the book initially published in 2004 and 2011, respectively, remains focused upon constant research and development in the field of radiation oncology as the indispensable part of our comprehensive and hopefully orchestrated approach in the diagnosis and treatment of lung cancer. While the intervening 10 years may deem too short for any major leaps in this field, I am sure this third edition will stand the test of time as the necessary checkpoint in the global development in this field.

To demonstrate this premise, while many chapters of the first and the second edition respectively remained, many are updated and, furthermore, many are completely new additions, bringing more substance to keep the pace with the most recent scientific achievements in the field, becoming new standards of care almost daily. Various, non-radiation oncology aspects are again included in the book with the same goal. Ultimately, the book is composed in such a way to enable both radiation oncologists and other lung cancer specialists benefit from reading it.

As with the previous two efforts, I have had great pleasure and very much privilege of having a distinguished faculty joining me. They dedicated their professional lives to the fight against lung cancer, having continuously provided substantial contribution in this field. They painstakingly focused on more comprehensive understanding of basic premises of biology and technology, its successful incorporation in the diagnosis and treatment of the disease and finally ending up in state-of-the-art approaches in the third decade of the new millennium.

I would also like to thank my former and current staff colleagues with whom I have collaborated around the world, especially those still living and working in developing countries. From such collaboration, I grew up not only as a better and more mature medical professional but also a better human being. I would also like to express my gratitude to Alexander von Humboldt Foundation, Bonn, Germany, for their continuous support since 1998. Without them all it would simply be impossible to imagine both the final shape of the book and its timely delivery.

Belgrade, Serbia   Branislav Jeremić

Contents

Volume I

Part I Basic Science of Lung Cancer

Genomic Alterations in Lung Cancer 3
Daniel Morgensztern

Epigenetic Events in Lung Cancer 17
Octavio A. Romero and Montse Sanchez-Cespedes

Part II Clinical Investigations

Interventional Pulmonology. 35
Branislav Perin and Bojan Zarić

Pathology of Lung Cancer 45
Mari Mino-Kenudson

Role of Radiologic Imaging in Lung Cancer 67
Salome Kukava and George Tsivtsivadze

**Place and Role of PET/CT in the Diagnosis and Staging
of Lung Cancer** 85
Salome Kukava and Michael Baramia

Surgical Staging of Lung Cancer. 113
Jarrod Predina, Douglas J. Mathisen, and Michael Lanuti

Part III Basic Treatment Considerations

**Surgical Workup and Management of Early-Stage
Lung Cancer** 131
Stephanie H. Chang, Joshua Scheinerman, Jeffrey Jiang,
Darian Paone, and Harvey Pass

Radiation Biology of Lung Cancer 151
Jose G. Bazan

**Radiation Time, Dose, and Fractionation in the Treatment
of Lung Cancer** 171
David L. Billing and Andreas Rimner

Optimizing Lung Cancer Radiotherapy Treatments Using Personalized Dose-Response Curves 189
Joseph O. Deasy, Jeho Jeong, Maria Thor, Aditya Apte,
Andrew Jackson, Ishita Chen, Abraham Wu, and Andreas Rimner

Tumor Motion Control 213
Hiroki Shirato, Shinichi Shimizu, Hiroshi Taguchi,
Seishin Takao, Naoki Miyamoto, and Taeko Matsuura

PET and PET/CT in Treatment Planning 237
Michael MacManus, Sarah Everitt, and Rodney J. Hicks

Target Volume Delineation in Non-small Cell Lung Cancer 255
Jessica W. Lee, Haijun Song, Matthew J. Boyer,
and Joseph K. Salama

The Radiation Target in Small Cell Lung 271
Gregory M. M. Videtic

Radiation Sensitizers 285
Mansi K. Aparnathi, Sami Ul Haq, Zishan Allibhai,
Benjamin H. Lok, and Anthony M. Brade

Radioprotectors in the Management of Lung Cancer 303
Zhongxing Liao, Ting Xu, and Ritsuko Komaki

Chemotherapy for Lung Cancer 321
Mariam Alexander, Elaine Shum, Aditi Singh,
and Balazs Halmos

Targeted Therapies in Non-small Cell Lung Cancer 347
Jessica R. Bauman and Martin J. Edelman

Immunotherapy of Lung Cancer 371
Igor Rybkin and Shirish M. Gadgeel

Combined Radiotherapy and Chemotherapy:
Theoretical Considerations and Biological Premises 385
Michael K. Farris, Cole Steber, Corbin Helis,
and William Blackstock

Mechanisms of Action of Radiotherapy and Immunotherapy
in Lung Cancer: Implications for Clinical Practice 399
Kewen He, Ugur Selek, Hampartsoum B. Barsoumian,
Duygu Sezen, Matthew S. Ning, Nahum Puebla-Osorio,
Jonathan E. Schoenhals, Dawei Chen, Carola Leuschner,
Maria Angelica Cortez, and James W. Welsh

Part IV   Current Treatment Strategies in Early-Stage Non-small Cell Lung Cancer

Early Non-small Cell Lung Cancer: The Place of Radical
Non-SABR Radiation Therapy 417
Tathagata Das and Matthew Hatton

**Never-Ending Story: Surgery Versus SBRT in
Early-Stage NSCLC** 433
James Taylor, Pamela Samson, William Stokes,
and Drew Moghanaki

**Stereotactic Ablative Radiotherapy for Early-Stage
Lung Cancer** 445
Dat T. Vo, John H. Heinzerling, and Robert D. Timmerman

**Role of Postoperative Radiation Therapy in Non-Small
Cell Lung Cancer** 471
Alexander K. Diaz and Chris R. Kelsey

**The Role of Thermal Ablation in the Treatment of Stage
I Non-small Cell Lung Cancer** 483
Roberto B. Kutcher-Diaz, Aaron Harman, and John Varlotto

Part V Current Treatment Strategies in Locally Advanced and Metastatic Non-small Cell Lung Cancer

Lung Dose Escalation 507
Kenneth E. Rosenzweig

**Multimodality Treatment of Stage IIIA/N2 NSCLC:
Why Always NO to Surgery?** 517
Branislav Jeremić, Ivane Kiladze, and Slobodan Milisavljevic

**Multimodality Treatment of Stage IIIA/N2 Non-Small
Cell Lung Cancer: When YES to Surgery** 533
Sean All and David J. Sher

**Combined Radiation Therapy and Chemotherapy as an
Exclusive Treatment Option in Locally Advanced Inoperable
Non-small Cell Lung Cancer** 547
Branislav Jeremić, Pavol Dubinsky, Slobodan Milisavljević,
and Ivane Kiladze

**Optimizing Drug Therapies in the Maintenance Setting After
Radiochemotherapy in Non-small Cell Lung Cancer** 571
Steven H. Lin and David Raben

**Prophylactic Cranial Irradiation in Non-small Cell
Lung Cancer** 581
Hina Saeed, Monica E. Shukla, and Elizabeth M. Gore

**Palliative External Beam Thoracic Radiation Therapy
of Non-small Cell Lung Cancer** 597
Stein Sundstrøm

**Intraoperative Radiotherapy in Lung Cancer: Methodology
(Electrons or Brachytherapy), Clinical Experiences, and
Long-Term Institutional Results** 605
Felipe A. Calvo, Javier Aristu, Javier Serrano, Mauricio Cambeiro,
Rafael Martinez-Monge, and Rosa Cañón

Brachytherapy for Lung Cancer 623
Raul Hernanz de Lucas, Teresa Muñoz Miguelañez,
Alfredo Polo, Paola Lucia Arrieta Narvaez,
and Deisy Barrios Barreto

**Oligometastatic Disease: Basic Aspects and Clinical
Results in NSCLC** 637
Gukan Sakthivel, Deepinder P. Singh, Haoming Qiu,
and Michael T. Milano

Part VI   Current Treatment Strategies in Small Cell Lung Cancer

**Radiation Therapy in Limited Disease Small Cell
Lung Cancer** 651
Branislav Jeremić, Ivane Kiladze, Pavol Dubinsky,
and Slobodan Milisavljević

**Role of Thoracic Radiation Therapy in Extensive Disease
Small Cell Lung Cancer** 667
Branislav Jeremić, Mohamed El-Bassiouny, Ramy Ghali,
Ivane Kiladze, and Sherif Abdel-Wahab

Prophylactic Cranial Irradiation in Small Cell Lung Cancer 677
William G. Breen and Yolanda I. Garces

Volume II

Part VII   Treatment in Specific Patient Groups and Other Settings

Radiation Therapy for Lung Cancer in Elderly 691
Erkan Topkan, Ugur Selek, Berrin Pehlivan, Ahmet Kucuk,
and Yasemin Bolukbasi

Radiation Therapy for Intrathoracic Recurrence of Lung Cancer . 717
Yukinori Matsuo, Hideki Hanazawa, Noriko Kishi,
Kazuhito Ueki, and Takashi Mizowaki

Treatment of Second Lung Cancers 739
Reshad Rzazade and Hale Basak Caglar

Radiation Therapy for Brain Metastases 755
Dirk Rades, Sabine Bohnet, and Steven E. Schild

**Radiation Therapy for Metastatic Lung Cancer: Bone
Metastasis and Metastatic Spinal Cord Compression** 779
Begoña Taboada-Valladares, Patricia Calvo-Crespo, and Antonio
Gómez-Caamaño

Radiation Therapy for Metastatic Lung Cancer: Liver Metastasis . 795
Fiori Alite and Anand Mahadevan

**Advances in Supportive and Palliative Care for
Lung Cancer Patients** 809
Michael J. Simoff, Javier Diaz-Mendoza, A. Rolando Peralta,
Labib G. Debiane, and Avi Cohen

Part VIII Other Intrathoracic Malignancies

Thymic Cancer 833
Gokhan Ozyigit and Pervin Hurmuz

Advances in Radiation Therapy for Malignant Pleural Mesothelioma.. 849
Gwendolyn M. Cramer, Charles B. Simone II, Theresa M. Busch, and Keith A. Cengel

Primary Tracheal Tumors 863
Shrinivas Rathod

Pulmonary Carcinoid 879
Roshal R. Patel, Brian De, and Vivek Verma

Part IX Treatment-Related Toxicity

Hematological Toxicity in Lung Cancer 907
Francesc Casas, Diego Muñoz-Guglielmetti, Gabriela Oses, Carla Cases, and Meritxell Mollà

Radiation Therapy-Induced Lung and Heart Toxicity 925
Soheila F. Azghadi and Megan E. Daly

Spinal Cord 941
Timothy E. Schultheiss

Radiation Therapy-Related Toxicity: Esophagus 955
Srinivas Raman and Meredith Giuliani

Brain Toxicity 969
C. Nieder

Part X Quality of Life Studies and Prognostic Factors

Patient-Reported Outcomes in Lung Cancer................... 987
Newton J. Hurst Jr, Farzan Siddiqui, and Benjamin Movsas

Importance of Prognostic Factors in Lung Cancer 1001
Lukas Käsmann

Part XI Technological Advances in Lung Cancer

Intensity-Modulated Radiation Therapy and Volumetric Modulated Arc Therapy for Lung Cancer 1021
Jacob S. Parzen and Inga S. Grills

Image-Guided Radiotherapy in Lung Cancer 1049
Julius Weng, Patrick Kupelian, and Percy Lee

Heavy Particles in Non-small Cell Lung Cancer: Protons 1059
Charles B. Simone II

Heavy Particles in Non-small Cell Lung Cancer: Carbon Ions 1075
S. Tubin, P. Fossati, S. Mori, E. Hug, and T. Kamada

**The Role of Nanotechnology for Diagnostic and Therapy
Strategies in Lung Cancer** 1093
Jessica E. Holder, Minnatallah Al-Yozbaki,
and Cornelia M. Wilson

Part XII Clinical Research in Lung Cancer

Translational Research in Lung Cancer 1113
Haoming Qiu, Michael A. Cummings, and Yuhchyau Chen

**Radiation Oncology of Lung Cancer: Why We Fail(ed)
in Clinical Research?** 1135
Branislav Jeremić, Nenad Filipović, Slobodan Milisavljević,
and Ivane Kiladze

**Randomized Clinical Trials: Pitfalls in Design, Analysis,
Presentation, and Interpretation** 1147
Lawrence Kasherman, S. C. M. Lau, K. Karakasis, N. B. Leighl,
and A. M. Oza

Part VII

Treatment in Specific Patient Groups and Other Settings

Radiation Therapy for Lung Cancer in Elderly

Erkan Topkan, Ugur Selek, Berrin Pehlivan, Ahmet Kucuk, and Yasemin Bolukbasi

Contents

1 Introduction 691
2 **Non-small Cell Lung Cancer (NSCLC)** 693
2.1 Early-Stage NSCLC 693
2.2 Stereotactic Body Radiotherapy (SBRT) 696
2.3 Locally Advanced NSCLC 699
2.4 Stage 4 NSCLC 702
3 **Small Cell Lung Cancer (SCLC)** 703
3.1 Limited-Stage SCLC 704
3.2 SBRT for Stage I or II Node-Negative SCLC 706
3.3 Extensive-Stage SCLC 707
3.4 Prophylactic Cranial RT for LS-SCLC and ES-SCLC 707
4 Conclusion 708
References 708

E. Topkan (✉)
Department of Radiation Oncology, Baskent University Medical Faculty, Adana, Turkey
e-mail: docdretopkan@hotmail.com

U. Selek · Y. Bolukbasi
Department of Radiation Oncology, School of Medicine, Koc University, Istanbul, Turkey

Department of Radiation Oncology, University of Texas, MD Anderson Cancer Center, Houston, TX, USA

B. Pehlivan
Department of Radiation Oncology, Bahcesehir University, Istanbul, Turkey

A. Kucuk
Mersin City Education and Research Hospital, Clinic of Radiation Oncology, Mersin, Turkey

Abstract

Elderly cancer patients with non-small and small cell lung cancer are altogether underrepresented nearly in all benchmark clinical trials; however, the embodiment of elderly patients in clinical studies should be emphatically encouraged to construct a proof-based optimal treatment of this specific age group. As most retrospective studies reveal similar oncologic results in elderly lung cancer patients compared to younger counterparts when treated with stage-specific recommendations, concerted efforts to accurately identify qualified patients to be prescribed standard treatments should be motivated. Therefore, we counsel a baseline and continuing guidance of geriatric assessment to promote individualized care, support, and tailored treatment protocols to avoid under- and overtreatments in elderly lung cancer patients.

1 Introduction

Lung cancer (LC) represents a globally prominent cause of cancer-related deaths, with an unfortunate continued incidence rising in aging populations (Malvezzi et al. 2015). According to the population-based studies, LCs are most frequently diagnosed among people aged 65–74 (median age 71) years of age with higher death rates among the middle-aged and elderly (aged

55–64: 20.3%, 65–74: 32.4%, 75–84: 28.3%) populations (Cancer Stat Facts: Lung and Bronchus Cancer 2021). Age-adjusted incidence and death rates for the leading cancers were examined by point analysis through linkage with Medicare claims, and the prevalence of comorbid conditions was documented to be commonest in LC patients (Edwards et al. 2014). Consequently, research on the elderly population has increased over the years to overcome the difficulties in management, mostly with an age cutoff threshold between 65 and 75 years in the absence of a customarily affirmed elderly definition. Elderly LCs have been traditionally managed with so-called standard therapies based on the results of selected populations underrepresenting such patients, while only a few clinical trials specifically targeted elderly patients. The elderly definition most suitably correlates with the fragility that interferes with the decision algorithm in geriatric oncology (Extermann 2000). Therefore, biological fitness relying upon the performance status and comorbidities seems to prevail as the principal guide in selecting the best-fit treatment decisions per patient, manifesting disease stage and tumor histology bases (Wang et al. 2012). On the other hand, aging, not directly reflected by chronological age, is a multidimensional process with individualized changes of physiologic, medical, immune, social, behavioral, emotional, and cognitive changes along with gradual declines in the functional reserves of organ systems and stress tolerance (Montella et al. 2002). Hence, efforts to use geriatric screening tools and comprehensive geriatric assessment (CGA) can independently possess a prognostic value in identifying the fit-enough elderly patients for aggressive definitive treatment approaches (Antonio et al. 2018; Couderc et al. 2020). In the background of scarce robust data on the elderly, the European Organization for Research and Treatment of Cancer (EORTC, Elderly Task Force and Lung Cancer Group) and the International Society for Geriatric Oncology (SIOG) worked on opinion papers based on the consensus of the expert panels (Dubianski et al. 2019).

Screening for the potential vulnerability has been recommended by the SIOG Taskforce (Decoster et al. 2015), including the G8 (Fig. 1) (Kenis et al. 2014), Triage Risk Screening Tool (TRST, Fig. 2) (Kenis et al. 2014), and Vulnerable Elders-13 Survey (VES-13, Fig. 3) (Mohile et al. 2007). The G8 survey comprises eight items to be completed typically in less than 10 min per patient, and impaired G8 scoring was associated with overall survival (OS) in curatively irradiated elderly cancer patients (Middelburg et al. 2020). The TRST deals particularly with the patients ≥75 years, including five yes/no items estimated to be finished typically in <2 min, and VES-13 tool is a self-performed survey completed substantially in <10 min, endeavoring to identify ≥65-year-old population with increased risk of death or functional deterioration. The CGA is recommended in case of anticipated frailties to determine hazards for the chosen treatment (Wildiers et al. 2014) by assessing the patient's functional status, fatigue, comorbidity, cognition, mental health, social support, nutrition, and geriatric syndromes like dementia, delirium, falls, and sarcopenia.

The functional lung capacity of senior patients would likewise serve useful in the wise decision whether these patients would be qualified for the intended treatment or not. However, pulmonary function tests (PFTs) assessing the lung functions via the measured lung volume, capacity, flow rates, and gas exchange should be executed noninvasively in the elderly (Sezen et al. 2019).

In this chapter, we focus on the current significant issues in radiation therapy (RT) of elderly LCs, covering both non-small cell (NSCLC) and small cell LC (SCLC) to guide physicians in the decision-making of appropriate treatment, but will leave details of systemic treatment and tumor, and RT-related general issues aside from being elderly, such as the treatment duration (Topkan et al. 2019b), treatment technique (Selek et al. 2014), impact of tumor cavitation (Topkan et al. 2018b), or risk of fatal pulmonary hemorrhage (Topkan et al. 2018a), are left to be discussed by other experts in this book. Besides, as space is limited, emerging prognostic influences in immunotherapy and inflammation landscape on the

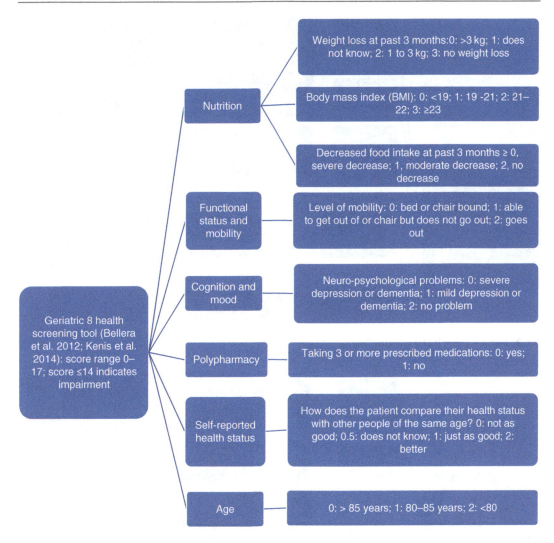

Fig. 1 Geriatric 8 health screening tool

outcomes of lung cancer patients also need to be addressed in the elderly in the future because of their established role in nonelderly counterparts, like the systemic inflammation response index (Topkan et al. 2021; Kucuk et al. 2020), prognostic nutritional index (Ozdemir et al. 2020), influence of anemia (Topkan et al. 2018c), specific prognostic scores (Topkan et al. 2019a), and impact of weight change (Topkan et al. 2013a) to stratify patients treated with chemoradiotherapy into fundamentally distinct prognostic groups.

2 Non-small Cell Lung Cancer (NSCLC)

2.1 Early-Stage NSCLC

Long-term survival with untreated NSCLC is uncommon even for stage I disease, with most patients succumbing due to progressive LC. Raz et al. examined the natural history of 1432 stage I NSCLC patients without any definitive therapy between 1989 and 2003 (Raz et al. 2007). The investigators announced median and 5-year

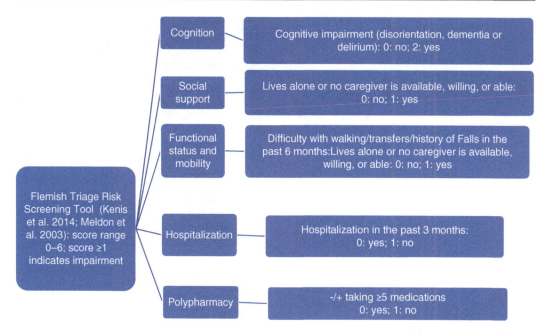

Fig. 2 Flemish Triage Risk Screening Tool

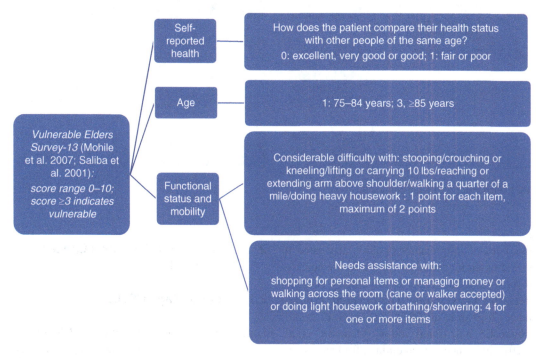

Fig. 3 Vulnerable Elders Survey-13

overall survival (OS) rates of only 13 months and 9%, respectively, even for patients with T1 tumors. Nearly one-fourth of all early-stage elderly NSCLC patients cannot undergo surgery due to advanced age and accompanying comorbid conditions. However, obstinate unwillingness to undergo recommended treatment is only occasionally reported (Bach et al. 1999).

Wisnivesky et al. analyzed the Surveillance, Epidemiology, and End Results (SEER) registry to identify histologically confirmed stage I–II NSCLC patients who underwent radiotherapy (RT) (Wisnivesky et al. 2005). The authors documented significantly better median OS times for stages I (21 months vs. 14 months; $P = 0.001$) and II (14 months vs. 9 months; $P = 0.001$) with RT as opposed to no treatment, respectively. To minimize biases for patients with multiple comorbidities who were less likely to receive RT and/or chemotherapy (CT), Wisnivesky et al., using the propensity score matching methodology, published a similar analysis of 6065 histologically confirmed but unresected stage I–II NSCLC patients of whom 59% received RT (Wisnivesky et al. 2010). The OS ($P < 0.0001$) and LC-specific survival ($P < 0.0001$) were significantly superior with RT compared to no treatment. In order to examine outcomes for the elderly after radical RT or surgery, Palma et al. analyzed the British Columbia prospective databases for curatively treated 558 stage I NSCLC patients (surgery: 56%; RT: 44%) (Palma et al. 2010b). Albeit elderly patients (≥ 75 years) appeared to be less likely to undergo curative resection than younger patients (43% vs. 72%; $P < 0.0001$), the results of the multivariate analyses could not yield a critical incentive for age concerning the OS outcomes after the surgery ($P = 0.87$) or RT ($P = 0.43$). Since the respective 5-year OS rates were 69% and 23% after surgery and RT, Palma et al. emphasized that medically fit elderly patients should not be excluded from radical treatments just relying upon their chronologic age.

Numerous small retrospective series documented significant trends toward superior survival times in elderly patients with RT (Coy and Kennelly 1980; Newaishy and Kerr 1989) without notable contrasts in the results after RT alone or surgery (Noordijk et al. 1988) concerning the OS, disease-specific survival, or local progression-free survival (PFS) when confronted with those of younger adults (Slotman et al. 1994; Gauden et al. 1995; Krol et al. 1996). Jeremic et al. also underlined no notable distinction between the younger and elderly patients for stage I–II NSCLCs in either OS or relapse-free survival with hyperfractionated RT of 69.6 Gy (Jeremic et al. 1997, 1999a). Hayakawa et al. published a retrospective series of 97 patients (>75 years) with inoperable or unresectable NSCLC compared to 206 younger patients, most treated with a total dose of conventionally fractionated >60 Gy (Hayakawa et al. 2001). The authors classified the elderly patients into two groups: group A = 75–79 years and group B ≥ 80 years. The 5-year OS rates were 13% and 4% for groups A and B, which were not statistically distinct from the 12% OS rate observed in the younger patients. Importantly, indicating the definitive RT as an efficient and safe treatment option for ≥ 75-year-old NSCLC patients, the decline in the general performance status was comparable between the senior and younger patients (8% vs. 5%; $P > 0.05$). Gauden and Tripcony ratified these results with a retrospective cohort analysis incorporating 347 T1-2N0M0 NSCLC patients who underwent 50 Gy RT given in 20 fractions due to weak performance status, old age, or refusal to undergo surgery (Gauden and Tripcony 2001). The 5-year OS and recurrence-free survival rates in <70- vs. ≥ 70-year groups were 22% vs. 34% and 18% and 30%, respectively, with no outstanding factual distinction. Therefore, the speculation that older age groups might experience more unfortunate outcomes may have failed as the 75–79-year group showed better survival than other age groups in this investigation. Likewise, San Jose et al. reported that RT alone was an effective and relatively low toxic treatment option for stages I–II NSCLCs patients aged between 71 and 97 years (San Jose et al. 2006). Ahmad et al. retrospectively analyzed 75 patients (≥ 60 years) with stage I inoperable NSCLCs treated with a definitive hypofractionated RT schedule (65 Gy given in 2.5 Gy per day) (Ahmad et al. 2011). The authors announced grade ≥ 3 radiation-related toxicity only in three patients with no treatment-related deaths. The median local failure-free survival and OS were reported as 19.6 and 21.2 months, respectively. Basing on these results, the researchers called attention to hypofractionated RT as an effective and safe treatment strategy for stage I elderly NSCLCs. Therefore, abovementioned RT results in early-stage elderly NSCLCs do not suggest age-related excessive severe acute or late toxicity incidences but assert reasonable median and 5-year OS rates of 20–27 months and 15–34%, respectively.

As modern RT kicked in, studies aimed to improve patient outcomes with more complex RT techniques. In one such work, Park et al. questioned whether complex RT planning was linked to enhanced results in unresected stage I–II elderly NSCLCs using the SEER database and identified 1998 patients aged >65 years, 25% of whom received complexly planned RT (Park et al. 2011). The results of this study unveiled that more complex RT plans were associated with the superior OS (HR: 0.84) and LC-specific survival (HR: 0.81) rates after controlling for propensity scores. Moreover, Yu et al. reported their multicenter prospective results in 80 elderly stage I–II NSCLC patients treated with intensity-modulated RT (IMRT) of 66.6 Gy targeting only the primary tumor (Yu et al. 2008). The authors reported no grade 4–5 toxicity with the respective median and 5-year OS rates of 38 months and 25.3%. Therefore, Yu and colleagues exhibited that involved-field RT using IMRT improved the treatment tolerability and outcomes in elderly patients without any increments in regional failures (Fig. 4).

2.2 Stereotactic Body Radiotherapy (SBRT)

The 30- and 90-day postoperative mortality rates, by all accounts, are unacceptably high in the elderly NSCLC population (Powell et al. 2013). A recent post hoc analysis of 15,554 surgical patients revealed that increased 30- and 90-day mortality risks were unequivocally connected with weaker performance status and advancing age regardless of the surgical procedure (O'Dowd et al. 2016). Denoting the intolerability of extensive surgical procedures in elderly NSCLCs, the authors declared that postoperative mortality rates were notably higher with pneumonectomy than lobectomy in this age group. Accordingly, with its toxicity-reducing and survival-enhancing qualities, SBRT has grounded soundly in the management of early-stage elderly NSCLCs, particularly in cases presenting with severe comorbid conditions (Nanda et al. 2015). SBRT is the focused delivery of one or several fractions of high doses of RT by utilizing exceptionally quality-guaranteed techniques. Following the initial endeavors describing the stereotactic RT to extracranial targets in a similar fashion accomplished for intracranial targets from the Karolinska Hospital in 1995 (Blomgren et al. 1995), many institutions followed the same pathway to deliver high-precision RT stereotactically to a dedicated extracranial site. The initial studies almost invariably included the medically inoperable patients or those declining the surgery and presenting with clinical T1-2N0M0 tumors (McGarry et al. 2005; Le et al. 2006).

The amended definition of likely toxicities and their tolerance limits brought a more secure predictivity of the SBRT conveyance (Timmerman et al. 2006; Lagerwaard et al. 2008; Chang et al. 2014). Medically inoperable early-stage NSCLC patients with limited lung capacities found a conclusive treatment opportunity as their pulmonary function tests (PFTs) after SBRT appeared to be preserved to a large extent, even in severe chronic obstructive pulmonary disease (COPD) conditions (Palma et al. 2012). To date, SBRT has been delivered in various ways, including the three-dimensional conformal RT, IMRT, volumetric modulated arc therapy (VMAT), and proton RT. The precise dose gradients achieved with optional target coverage and superior critical structure doses may minimize the long-term toxicity rates without forfeiting the tumor control rates.

The Amsterdam Cancer Registry population-based time-trend analysis examined the influence of introducing SBRT in three eras as pre-SBRT (A: 1999–2001), some availability of SBRT (B: 2002–2004), and full access to SBRT (C: 2005–2007) in 875 elderly (≥75 years) patients with stage I NSCLC (Palma et al. 2010a). The authors reported a decline in the proportion of untreated elderly patients with the SBRT influence (0%, 23%, and 55% for eras A to C, respectively),

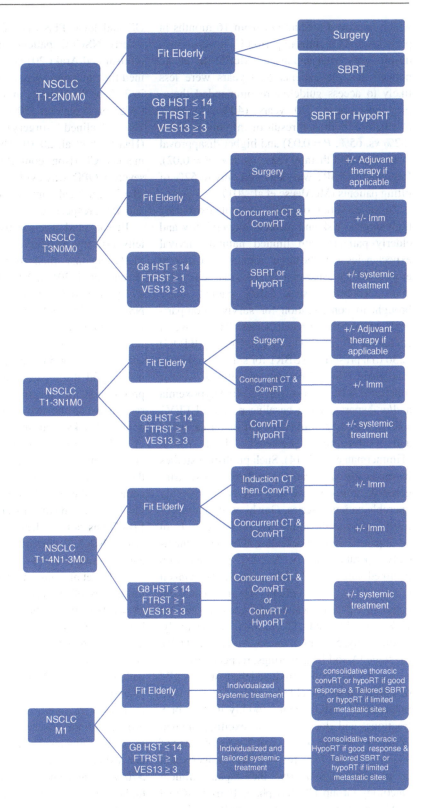

Fig. 4 Simple management algorithm for elderly patients with non-small cell lung cancer. *NSCLC* non-small cell lung cancer, *CT* chemotherapy, *Imm* immunotherapy (durvalumab), *ConvRT* conventionally fractionated RT (60–66 Gy, 2 Gy/fraction/day, in 30–33 fractions in 30–33 weekdays), *G8 HST* Geriatric 8 health screening tool (total score: 0–17), *FTRST* Flemish Triage Risk Screening Tool (total score: 0–6), *VES-13* Vulnerable Elders Survey-13 (total score: 0–10), *SBRT* stereotactic body RT (50–70 Gy, 7–12.5 Gy/fraction, in 3–10 fractions), *HypoRT* hypofractionated radiotherapy (30–45 Gy, 3 Gy/fraction, in 10–15 fractions in 10–15 weekdays, or 55 Gy, 2.75 Gy/fraction, in 20 fractions in 20 weekdays)

which improved median OS from 16 months in period A to 21 months in period C. Nevertheless, despite this vital evidence, McAleese et al. noticed that the patients ≥70 years were less likely to access guideline-recommended therapies than those <70 years (40% vs. 60%, $P = 0.001$), both as a result of infrequent offers (52% vs. 65%, $P = 0.03$) and higher disapproval of the intended therapy (22% vs. 8%, $P = 0.02$). Regrettably, SBRT was delivered only to 52% of fitting patients (McAleese et al. 2017).

In the evolution of SBRT, patients exhibiting high surgical risk and medical inoperability and elderly patients with limited natural survival expectancies were the target population (Crabtree et al. 2010; Parashar et al. 2010; Haasbeek et al. 2008). Therefore, such SBRT patients were brought to consideration for survival comparisons against the surgical series. The phase II Radiation Therapy Oncology Group (RTOG) 0236 trial prescribing SBRT for stage I medically inoperable NSCLC patients enrolled a weaker functional status cohort with baseline hypoxemia and/or hypercapnia, a baseline predicted FEV1 <40%, seriously diminished diffusion capacity, and postoperative predicted FEV1 <30% (Timmerman et al. 2014). Such published studies in medically inoperable populations also triggered the retrospective analysis of conceivably operable patients' series. Onishi et al. retrospectively analyzed the multi-institutional data from 14 Japanese centers revealing 87 stage I medically operable elderly NSCLC patients who declined surgery and underwent SBRT (Onishi et al. 2011). The authors reported excellent cumulative 5-year local control rates of 92% and 73% for T1 and T2 tumors, respectively. Additionally, 5-year OS rates were 72% and 62% for stage IA and IB gatherings, respectively.

Lagerwaard et al. introduced the results of 177 potentially operable elderly patients treated with risk-adapted SBRT scheme (60 Gy in 3, 5, or 8 fractions) and documented an exciting median OS of 61.5 months with 1- and 3-year OS rates of 94.7% and 84.7%, respectively (Lagerwaard et al. 2012). Similarly, the Japan Clinical Oncology Group (JCOG) phase II trial (JCOG 0403) researchers reported 3-year 69% and 76% OS and local PFS rates for operable stage IA elderly NSCLC patients managed with SBRT (Onishi and Araki 2013). Haasbeek et al. examined the outcomes of risk-adapted SBRT (60 Gy in 3, 5, or 8 fractions) in a group of 193 elderly (≥75 years) patients (80% medically inoperable, 20% declined surgery) with 203 tumors (Haasbeek et al. 2010). The study cohort had a median Charlson comorbidity score of 4, as severe COPD was evident in 25% of all cases. The 3-year local control and OS rates were 89% and 45%, respectively.

Brooks et al. comparatively assessed the toxicity, efficacy, and survival outcomes of the lung SBRT against their historic surgical results (Brooks et al. 2017). A total of 772 (442 patients <75 years and 330 patients ≥75 years) stage I–II NSCLC patients who underwent SBRT of 50 Gy in 4 fractions or 70 Gy in 10 fractions were analyzed. None of the ≥75-year-old patients experienced grade 4 or 5 toxicities, with no statistically meaningful discrepancy in the toxicity, time to progression, LC-specific survival, or 2-year OS rates between the two groups. Given these outcomes, Brooks et al. intimated that the viability of SBRT is fundamentally the same as for the elderly and average-age population. Moreover, the investigators expressed that the survival outcomes of the SBRT were not just practically identical with the historic surgical results, but the SBRT was notably less toxic in the early-stage senior NSCLC patients with respective <10% and 0% grade 3 and 4–5 toxicity rates.

Stokes et al. confronted the postinterventional mortalities of surgery ($N = 76,623$) and SBRT ($N = 8216$) utilizing the National Cancer Database between 2004 and 2013 for the early-stage (cT1-2AN0M0) NSCLC patients (Stokes et al. 2018). Among the propensity score-matched 27,200 patients, the 30- (2.41% vs. 0.79%; $P < 0.001$) and 90-day (4.23% vs. 2.82%; $P < 0.001$) mortality rates were significantly higher in the surgery group, with the observation that the surgery was steadily getting less secure as the functions of age and extent of resection while the blend of age >70 years and pneumonectomy embodying the highest-risk group for treatment-related mortality. Li et al. compared the survival and safety data of SBRT conventional RT with a meta-analysis primarily involving inoperable elderly early-stage NSCLC patients (Li et al. 2020). Results of the 17,973 patients (SBRT: 7395; conventional RT: 10,578) from 17 studies uncovered that the SBRT bunch had superior OS ($P < 0.00001$), LC-specific survival ($P < 0.00001$), and PFS ($P < 0.00001$) rates opposed with the conventional RT. Further, reassuringly, the SBRT gather had essentially lower rates of dyspnea, esophagitis, and radiation pneumonitis with no notable distinction in grade 3–5 adverse events ($P = 0.35$).

2.3 Locally Advanced NSCLC

Indeed, even the medically fit elderly patients have been commonly deemed to be more vulnerable to toxic events than their younger counterparts: an irrational tendency to be resistant to offer intense radiochemotherapy protocols for these patients. As an unfortunate result, elderly patients constituted less than 25% of the study population in the benchmark randomized controlled studies of concurrent chemoradiotherapy (CCRT) in locally advanced NSCLCs (LA-NSCLCs) (Furuse et al. 1999; Curran Jr. et al. 2011) despite more than 40% of all NSCLCs manifest in this age group. In any case, it is clear that the results of randomized controlled investigations of CCRT consistently pointed out that elderly patients (>70 years) with LA-NSCLC and their younger counterparts had nearly equivalent survival and late toxicity rates, which comes at the expense of modestly increased grade ≥3 acute toxicity rates (Rocha Lima et al. 2002).

Kusumoto et al. presented comparable median survival times for patients with LA-NSCLC in 64 elderly and 36 younger patients (Kusumoto et al. 1986). Zachariah et al. observed 43% response in their patients aged 80 and older after conventionally fractionated 59–66 Gy RT without details on survival results (Zachariah et al. 1997), while Gava et al. reported a 1-year survival rate of 44% in a similar group of 38 patients (Gava et al. 1997). However, Nakano et al. reported inferior median OS times with RT alone in the elderly than the younger stage III NSCLC patients (6.3 months vs. 11.5 months; $P = 0.0043$) (Nakano et al. 1999). More deaths in elderly patients were credited mainly to more frequent respiratory infections and lower prognostic nutritional indexes. Conversely, Pignon et al. presented the results of 1208 NSCLC patients registered in EORTC trials for the influence of age on treatment results, as well as acute and late toxicity of curative thoracic RT (TRT) via six age ranges from 50 to ≥70 years (Pignon et al. 1998). The researchers indicated that adjusted survival and acute and late toxicity rates were comparable between the age bunches. Therefore, Pignon et al. bolstered the confidence that age per se is not alone sufficient to omit definitive RT whenever indicated.

Lonardi et al. evaluated a single-center Italian data of 48 symptomatic patients aged ≥75 years treated with up to 50 Gy conventionally fractionated RT for the inoperable stage IIIA–B NSCLCs, revealing successful palliation besides partial remission and disease stabilization in 21 (43.8%) and 17 (35.4%) patients, respectively (Lonardi et al. 2000). The toxicity was negligible with mostly grade 1–2 esophagitis. Encouraging the need to deliver definitive RT for achieving better local control and survival outcomes in elderly patients like their more youthful equivalents, the total dose appeared to straightforwardly relate with survival (20% for ≥50 Gy vs. 4% for <50 Gy at 24 months; $P = 0.03$). Tombolini et al. analyzed their medically inoperable stage IIIA–B NSCLC patients aged ≥70 years who underwent RT alone (conventional 50–60 Gy) and reported respective 27% and 14.6% OS and PFS rates at 2 years (Tombolini et al. 2000). Hayakawa et al. compared the results after ≥60 Gy definitive RT in inoperable or unresectable 97 elderly NSCLCs (≥75 years) against 206 patients <75 years (Hayakawa et al. 2001). The authors arranged the elderly patients into two groups, group A (75–79 years) and group B (≥80 years), and posted the OS rates in 2 and 5 years as 32% and 13% for group A, 28% and 4% for group B, and 36% and 12% for the younger group, respectively, without statistically significant differences among the groups. Additionally, the acute and late toxicity rates were indistinctive among the three groups.

Pergolizzi et al. initially reported the results of a prospective phase II study utilizing limited-field RT (median 60 Gy, 2 Gy/fraction/day) in 16 stage IIIA elderly patients (≥ 75 years), where the authors achieved better OS times with ≥ 60 Gy (34 months vs. 14 months, $P = 0.017$) and KPS ≥ 80 (34 months vs. 12 months, $P = 0.002$) in the absence of severe acute or late significant toxicity (Pergolizzi et al. 1997).

As CCRT has remained the norm of care in medically fit, locally advanced nonresectable NSCLC (Furuse et al. 1999; Curran Jr. et al. 2011), the inquiry was whether the elderly patients would be dealt with equivalent as well. Though initial retrospective series featured the appropriateness of CCRT in the elderly without any overriding concerns in subgroup examinations (Furuse et al. 1999; Schaake-Koning et al. 1992; Jeremic et al. 1998b; Clamon et al. 1999), Werner-Wasik et al. identified 1999 LA-NSCLC patients treated with RT in 9 RTOG trials between 1983 and 1994 with/without CT (Werner-Wasik et al. 2000). This recursive partitioning analysis (RPA) provided five subgroups with significantly different median OS times: group I: KPS of ≥ 90 and received CT (16.2 months); group II: KPS of ≥ 90 but no CT and PE (11.9 months); group III: KPS <90, <70 years, with nonlarge cell histology (9.6 months); group IV: KPS ≥ 90 but with malignant pleural effusion (MPE), or KPS <90, <70 years, but with large cell histology, or >70 years but without MPE (5.6–6.4 months); and group V: >70 years and with MPE (2.9 months). As age ≥ 70 years was found to negatively impact survival in the recursive partitioning analysis, Movsas et al. published a quality-adjusted survival analysis examining 979 patients enrolled into six prospective RTOG trials with inoperable stage II–IIIB NSCLC patients treated with RT with/without CT and proposed the benefit of treatment intensification to be age and histology dependent, wherein specifically the elderly had the best quality-adjusted survival with RT alone, but not with CCRT (Movsas et al. 1999). However, conversely, Langer et al. reported that medically fit >70-year-old patients who enrolled on RTOG 9410 benefited from CCRT as their more youthful counterparts (Langer et al. 2001). Rocha Lima et al. also recognized that patients >70 years could complete the treatment and attained clinical outcomes comparable to younger patients in the randomized Cancer and Leukemia Group B (CALGB) trial of induction CT followed by either RT alone or CCRT for locally advanced (LA) NSCLCs (Rocha Lima et al. 2002).

Schild et al. presented an age-based reanalysis of a phase III North Central Cancer Treatment Group (NCCTG) trial for stage III NSCLC patients: to decide if etoposide plus cisplatin CT in addition to either hyperfractionated RT or everyday RT results in superior outcomes (Schild et al. 2003). Elderly and younger patients exhibited comparable 5-year OS rates (18% vs. 13% for elderly patients; $P = 0.4$). However, particularly grade 4 myelosuppression ($P = 0.003$) and pneumonitis ($P = 0.02$) were more common in the elderly group. Enlighted with these results, Schild et al. encouraged the enrollment of the medically fit elderly patients into standard CCRT protocols with close monitoring. Schild et al. then reported two recent phase III trials (NCCTG 90-24-51, with three arms: once-daily RT alone, twice-daily RT alone, and concurrent etoposide and cisplatin plus twice-daily RT; NCCTG 94-24-52, with two arms: concurrent etoposide and cisplatin with either once- or twice-daily RT) for stage III NSCLC, with only 166 patients ≥ 65 years (Schild et al. 2007). The median and 5-year survival rates in RT alone vs. CCRT were 10.5 months and 5.4% vs. 13.7 months and 14.7%, respectively ($P < 0.5$, for each), despite greater toxicity (grade ≥ 3) for patients receiving CCRT (89.9% vs. 32.4%; $P < 0.01$). This examination likewise underlined that older patients may enjoy a survival advantage with CCRT as opposed to RT alone.

Firat et al. contemplated their retrospective cohort of 102 patients (56% with sequential and/or concurrent CT) to determine the influence of age and comorbidity on the combined modality therapy of stage III NSCLC and indicated that ≥ 70 years was not a critical factor in results (Firat et al. 2006). Consequently, the authors concluded that physicians' biases regarding the tolerability of CCRT might explain the underrepresentation of the elderly in NSCLC trials. Semrau et al. retrospectively examined the correlation between impaired organ functions, age, tumor-associated symptoms, social factors, and acute toxicity and survival outcomes after CCRT (Semrau et al. 2008). As multivariate analyses uncovered significantly inferior survival in patients suffering from cardiac or pulmonary dysfunction ($P = 0.039$), Semrau et al. suggested that cardiac and pulmonary dysfunction might be related to diminished survival in elderly or poor-risk patients with inoperable NSCLC after CCRT. Coate et al. retrospectively analyzed a cohort of 740 stage III NSCLC patients receiving palliative CT or RT (≤ 40 Gy), nonsurgical multimodality (>40 Gy RT $\pm$ CT), or surgical multimodality (CT, RT, and surgery) (Coate et al. 2011). Though patients >65 years were more prone to have poor performance status ($P < 0.0001$), multiple comorbidities ($P < 0.0001$), and higher rates of grade 3–4 toxicity ($P = 0.18$) and toxic deaths ($P = 0.76$) and to receive palliative therapy only ($P < 0.0001$), the survival outcomes were comparable between all age groups ($P > 0.05$). Topkan et al. retrospectively assessed the toxicity and efficacy of CCRT in medically fit 89 septuagenarians with stage IIIB NSCLCs (Topkan et al. 2013b). Definitive RT (66 Gy, 2 Gy/fraction/day) with concurrent cisplatin-based doublet CT was relatively well tolerated with no grade 4–5 acute toxicity. Median overall, local-regional PFS, and PFS were 17.7, 10.5, and 7.8 months, respectively. Uniquely, the number of CT cycles ($P < 0.001$) and weight loss ($P < 0.001$) stayed as critical factors to influence the survival results in multivariate analyses. Franceschini et al. retrospectively analyzed the feasibility and acute toxicity of radical hypofractionated RT with VMAT for 41 elderly stage III inoperable NSCLC patients (Franceschini et al. 2017). As a promising strategy, the 18-month OS rate was 35.1% in the absence of grade 3–4 toxicity records. Stinchcombe et al. announced the pooled analysis of 832 elderly (age ≥ 70) patients treated with CCRT for stage III NSCLC in comparison to 2768 younger patients in 16 phase II or III trials conducted by the US National Cancer Institute-supported cooperative groups (Stinchcombe et al. 2017). In unadjusted and multivariable models, elderly patients had worse OS (HR 1.20 and HR 1.17, respectively), while PFS was similar (HR 1.01 and HR 1.00, respectively), with higher rates of grade ≥ 3 complications (OR 1.35 and OR 1.38, respectively). Kim et al. examined the outcomes of CCRT vs. RT alone following induction CT in 82 elderly (≥ 70 years) patients with stage III NSCLCs (Kim et al. 2019). After induction CT, treatment tolerance was significantly worse with CCRT ($P = 0.046$), yet the median survival was indistinctive (21.1 months vs. 18.1 months for RT; $P > 0.05$).

Jeremic et al. prospectively surveyed the toxicity and efficacy of accelerated hyperfractionated RT of 51 Gy in 34 fractions over 3.5 weeks with concurrent carboplatin/oral etoposide in 55 elderly stage III (>70 years) NSCLC patients and have reported respective 2- and 5-year OS rates of 24% and 9.1% in the absence of grade ≥ 5 toxicity (Jeremic et al. 1999b). Atagi et al. prospectively exhibited the practicability of CCRT (50–60 Gy, 2 Gy/fraction/day) with daily low-dose carboplatin in 38 elderly patients with locally advanced or medically inoperable NSCLCs (Atagi et al. 2000). The respective median and 2-year OS rates were 15.1 months and 20.5% for stage III patients. Nakano et al. performed a prospective CCRT study with low-dose cisplatin with the Atagi's RT scheme in 11 elderly unresectable LA-NSCLC patients where the treatment protocol was well tolerated with promising 82%, 23 months, and 53% rates of overall response, median, and 2-year survival, individually (Nakano et al. 2003).

Following all these phase II endeavors, Atagi et al. published the results of the phase III trial (JCOG9812), assessing RT alone or simultaneously with carboplatin in unresectable stage III NSCLC patients (Atagi et al. 2005). The study was terminated prematurely due to unexpected treatment-related death records. However, cautious assessments uncovered that the treatment protocol has deviated in 60% of cases with 7% protocol violations in lung dose constraints, where two of four deaths were ascribed to radiation pneumonitis. Overall, the median OS for RT alone vs. CCRT remained 428 days vs. 554 days, exclusively. Jatoi et al. tested the CCRT with conventionally fractionated 60 Gy RT plus cetuximab in 57 elderly and/or poor-performance-status LA-NSCLC patients (Jatoi et al. 2010). The respective 15.1 and 7.2 months of median OS and time-to-progression rates were encouraging in the absence of treatment-related deaths. Aoe et al. reported their phase II trial comprising 30 LA-NSCLC patients aged ≥76 years who received conventionally fractionated 60 Gy RT and concurrent S-1 (Aoe et al. 2014). Albeit the primary endpoint was not met, concurrent S-1-based CCRT yielded favorable survival with median PFS and OS of 13.0 and 27.9 months, respectively. Strom et al. documented an elderly (≥70 years) unresectable stage III NSCLC subgroup analysis in their phase III trial, where palliative CCRT (42 Gy in 15 fractions) provided a significantly superior outcome than CT alone, except those with weaker performance status (Strom et al. 2015). They revealed that the median OS was improved in both age gatherings. Consequently, the authors inferred that elderly patients could tolerate and profit from CCRT with the doses adjusted to age and palliative intent, except for those with weaker performance scores. Tamiya et al. in their phase I–II study evaluated the combination of pemetrexed plus 60 Gy RT (2 Gy/day) in 41 elderly IIIA–B NSCLCs (Tamiya et al. 2018). Although the respective median OS and PFS rates of 24.9 and 6.9 months were promising, the authors acknowledged caution to prescribe this treatment in elderly patients as two treatment-related deaths were ascribed to radiation pneumonitis. Chen et al. conducted a comparative study for the efficacy and toxicity of IMRT with concurrent weekly nedaplatin vs. IMRT alone (2 Gy/fraction/day, 52–66 Gy) in 117 nonsurgical stage III–IV elderlies (Chen et al. 2018). The median (11.0 months vs. 7.0 months; $P < 0.001$) and 3-year (14.7% vs. 8.0%; $P < 0.001$) OS rates were significantly superior with the nedaplatin-based CCRT than the RT alone, which came at the expense of moderately increased hematologic toxicity rates. Recently, Niho et al. conducted a phase I–II study of carboplatin and S-1 plus concurrent 60 Gy (2.0 Gy/day) RT for the elderly stage III NSCLC patients (≥71 years) (Niho et al. 2019). The researchers documented promising efficacy of this novel combination for elderly patients, with the hopeful 1-year PFS of 16.8 months and overall grade 3 radiation pneumonitis rate of 18%. And finally, Yamaguchi et al. assessed the efficacy of concurrent carboplatin plus vinorelbine administered during the RT (60 Gy; 2.0 Gy/day) course with a multicenter phase II study incorporating 50 elderly (≥70 years) LA-NSCLC patients (Yamaguchi et al. 2020). This novel CCRT blend displayed an acceptable objective response rate (70%) and relative safety without treatment-related deaths in this patient group and provided 2-year PFS and OS rates of 21.1% and 41.1%, respectively.

Overall, though the literature is yet unsettled for choosing the elderly nonmetastatic patients for definitive treatments, appropriately selected medically fit elderly stage III NSCLC patients may sensibly be endorsed to carefully decided combined modality therapies for an expected survival similar to that of more youthful patients. There are also ongoing efforts to combining targeted therapies and immunotherapy with RT in elderly and frail unresectable stage III NSCLC patients who are unfit for CCRT.

2.4 Stage 4 NSCLC

The current standard of care for metastatic NSCLCs incorporates systemic CT, targeted therapies, and nowadays immunotherapies. In any case, RT remains a vital palliative measure for many depreciating symptoms in such patients independent of their chronologic age. But tragically, the results of a retrospective population-based cohort study using SEER-Medicare data of 11,084 elderly (≥65 years) metastatic NSCLC patients proved that only 58% of these patients were offered and received RT (Hayman et al. 2007). Palliative RT usually aims for pure symptom improvement, but it may additionally provide lengthened survival in cases with a limited metastatic burden, even if curative treatment does not represent a genuine prospect in most.

Regrettably, research on results of palliative RT and related prognosticators is scant in geriatric patients. In one such study, Jeremic et al. evaluated the concurrent short-term CT and palliative RT in 47 evaluable elderly patients, who underwent two cycles of carboplatin and oral etoposide concurrently with a total of 14 Gy palliative RT administered on days 1 and 8 (Jeremic et al. 1999c). Declaring the efficacy and safety of short-course CT and palliative RT in this particular age gathering, the authors have noticed an overall objective response rate of 28%, with a median response duration of 5 months in the absence of any grade 4–5 toxic events owing to the treatment convention.

As comparable treatments used for the more youthful patients have been attested to be almost similarly tolerated in more elderly patients, it is comprehensible from the accessible evidence that chronologic age alone should not be valued as a critical factor precluding an elderly patient from palliative RT (O'Donovan and Morris 2020). However, the use of single-fraction or hypofractionated regimes might be more appropriate, where feasible. For example, for brain metastases, longer fractionation schedules have demonstrated no OS advantage in poor-prognosis patients (Sarin and Dinshaw 1997). Similarly, the efficacy of single-fraction palliative RT schedules seems to be comparable to the more protracted multifractionated ones (Lee et al. 2018). Nonetheless, a baseline frailty assessment is of paramount importance in selecting suitable patients who may unquestionably benefit from the prescribed palliative RT.

3 Small Cell Lung Cancer (SCLC)

SCLC is a highly aggressive and principally lethal LC with a dismal 14–15% survival rate at 2 years (Siegel et al. 2021). Although the staging is encouraged to base on the American Joint Committee on Cancer (AJCC) 8th ed., practically all treatment decisions are usually outlined relying upon either limited- (LS-SCLC) or extensive-stage (ES-SCLC) disease as described in the framework of the Veterans Administration Lung Group staging system (Micke et al. 2002). This system stratifies the disease burden as LS-SCLC if amenable to definitive-intent TRT within a reasonable treatment volume (localized or locoregional disease of AJCC stage I–III, disease limited to one hemithorax and regional nodes without the presence of extrathoracic disease) and as ES-SCLC (AJCC stage IV) stage encompassing the rest. However, RT plays indispensable roles in both stages: as a curative-intent RT for the intrathoracic primary followed by the prophylactic cranial irradiation (PCI) in LS (Auperin et al. 1999; Faivre-Finn et al. 2017), as a consolidative measure for thoracic plus/minus extrathoracic disease after the completion of the frontline systemic therapy along with the individualized consideration of PCI in ES-SCLC, or as a palliative measure in widespread disease conditions (Simone 2nd et al. 2020; Takahashi et al. 2017; Slotman et al. 2015). However, areas of contention continue in the treatment of the elderly population as in the NSCLCs.

Initial data which evaluated age as a prognostic factor was inconsistent. The CALGB researchers reviewed the data of 1745 LS- or ES-SCLC patients enrolled in five separate trials to determine the pretreatment prognostic factors and noted that >60-year-old LD patients had higher mortality rates than younger patients ($P = 0.008$), but age was not predictive of survival duration among patients with ED (Spiegelman et al. 1989). The Southwest Oncology Group (SWOG) investigators analyzed 2580 SCLC patients (1363 LS and 1217 ES) and showed that the most vital prognostic split was LS vs. ES, while younger age (<70 years) was important only in LS but not in ES (Albain et al. 1990). On the other hand, Osterlind and Anderson investigated 874 Danish patients (443 LS, 431 ES) managed with combination CT with/without RT and uncovered no significant difference in survival results at an age cutoff of 60 years (Osterlind and Andersen 1986). Likewise, Sagman et al. evaluated a cohort of 288 LS- and ES-SCLC patients treated with combination CT as part of four clinical trials and did not define age as an independent prognostic factor for survival (Sagman et al. 1991). Shepherd et al.

retrospectively reviewed 123 elderly LS- and ES-SCLC patients (≥70 years) and found no notable survival contrasts between the 70–74, 75–80, and >80 years of age gatherings ($P = 0.4$) (Shepherd et al. 1994). In either stage, the more intensive therapy was linked to superior OS rates, with 4–6 cycles of CT representing the best outcome group. Noguchi et al. retrospectively compared the outcomes of 45 SCLC patients of ≥80 years with those of 38 patients aged 70–79 years (Noguchi et al. 2010). The authors demonstrated that 53% of the ≥80 years of age cohort enjoyed significant survival advantage with combination CT and TRT as median and 1-year OS appeared significantly better contrasted with the rest left untreated due to advanced age (>85 years), weaker performance status (PS), and/or severe comorbidities ($P < 0.01$). Remarkably, the OS benefit was evident even in the treated patients with PS 2–3 or with a moderate degree of comorbidity compared with those left untreated. Furthermore, the OS result was practically identical to those of patients aged 70–79 years regardless of comparably lower CT doses in this group (Fig. 5).

3.1 Limited-Stage SCLC

Any curative treatment approach for LS-SCLC patients could not be wise without appropriately planned RT due to well-defined survival benefits (Gaspar et al. 2012; Lally et al. 2009), and therefore, CCRT is considered as the current standard of care for thorough selected medically fit young and elderly patients (Christodoulou et al. 2019; Stinchcombe et al. 2019). Age seems not to be a significant adverse prognostic variable in LS-SCLC patients. Siu et al. retrospectively evaluated the prognostic worth of age in 608 LS-SCLCs patients treated with combination CT plus TRT trailed by PCI (Siu et al. 1996). The authors declared that overall response rates (78% vs. 82%; $P = 0.50$), 5-year OS rates (11% vs. 8%; $P = 0.14$), and incidence of either hematologic or nonhematologic toxicity rates were comparable in young and elderly patient groups. Dajczman et al. analyzed the age-based management of SCLC patients and found no significant outcome differences between the <60, 60–69, and ≥70 years of age groups per stage and weight loss variables, despite weaker performance status and more common comorbidities noted in ≥70 years of age group (Dajczman et al. 1996). The researchers uncovered that elderly patients were treated less intensely with regrettably the highest supportive care alone rates. In support, Jara et al. reported that the elderly patients (>70 years) were offered fewer cycles of CT (≤4 cycles), lesser per cycle CT doses, and lesser total RT doses more frequently than their more youthful accomplices (Jara et al. 1999).

Ludbrook et al. surveyed the data of 174 LS-SCLC patients treated at the British Columbia Cancer Agency (Ludbrook et al. 2003). Prescription of CCRT seemed to be age dependent (<65: 86% vs. 65–74: 66% vs. ≥75 years: 40%; $P < 0.0001$). TRT use was similar among all age groups ($P > 0.05$), while CT was tailored significantly with less intensive regimes, fewer cycles, and lower total doses with advancing age ($P < 0.05$). In the context of standard treatments being unadministered properly with the advancing age, overall response rates to primary treatment (<65: 91% vs. 65–74: 79% vs. ≥75 years: 74%; $P = 0.014$) and median OS rates (<65: 17 vs. 5–74: 12 vs. ≥75 years: 7 months; $P = 0.003$) were found decreasing with advancing age. However, the authors revealed that age and Charlson comorbidity scores were not meaningfully associated with treatment response and OS in the multivariate analysis. Consequently, it is prudent to assume that the adverse treatment response and OS rates confronted in the more elderly groups were possibly related to their more flaccid performance status and suboptimal treatments rather than the chronologic age.

The phase III North Central Cancer Group (NCCG) LS-SCLC trial administered initial three cycles of cisplatin and etoposide to all patients trailed by randomization of 262 patients to split-course twice-daily TRT (TDTRT: 48 Gy) vs. continuous once-daily TRT (ODTRT: 50.4 Gy) concurrent with two other cycles of cisplatin and etoposide, followed by PCI (30 Gy in 15 fractions) if they sustained a complete response

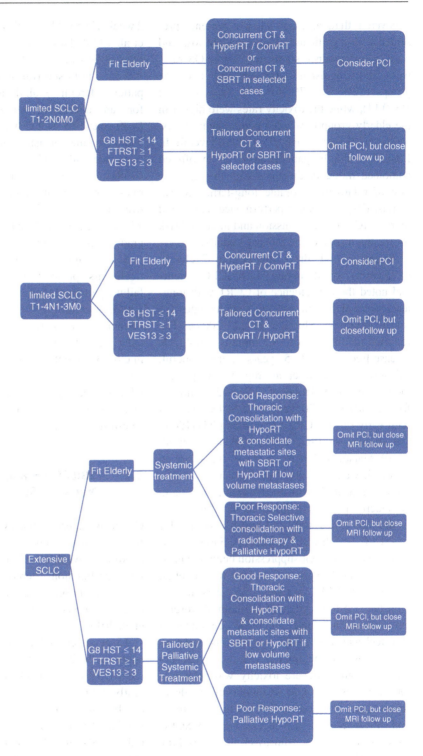

Fig. 5 Simple algorithm for elderly patients with small cell lung cancer. *SCLC* small cell lung cancer, *G8 HST* Geriatric 8 health screening tool (total score: 0–17), *FTRST* Flemish Triage Risk Screening Tool (total score: 0–6), *VES-13* Vulnerable Elders Survey-13 (total score: 0–10), *SBRT* stereotactic body radiotherapy (50–70 Gy, 7–12.5 Gy/fraction, in 3–10 fractions), *PCI* prophylactic cranial radiotherapy (25 Gy, 2.5 Gy/fraction, in 10 fractions in 10 weekdays), *HypoRT* hypofractionated radiotherapy (30–45 Gy, 3 Gy/fraction, in 10–15 fractions in 10–15 weekdays, or 55 Gy, 2.75 Gy/fraction, in 20 fractions in 20 weekdays), *HyperRT* hyperfractionated radiotherapy (45 Gy, 1.5 Gy/fraction BID, in 30 fractions in 15 weekdays), *RT* conventional fractionated radiotherapy (66–70 Gy, 2 Gy/fraction/day, in 33–35 fractions in 33–35 weekdays)

(Bonner et al. 1999). The authors disclosed that the TDTRT did not improve local control or survival rates over the ODTRT if TRT was deferred until the fourth cycle of CT. Schild et al. analyzed this prospective data for the link between age and outcomes (Schild et al. 2005). The authors uncovered that, although elderly patients presented with significantly higher weight loss and weaker performance status, the 5-year OS rates were undistinguishable between the two age groups (22% vs. 17% for >70 years of age; $P = 0.14$), while the toxicity rates were higher in the elderly group (grade ≥ 4 pneumonia: 0% vs. 6% for >70 years of age; $P = 0.008$). Overall, fit LS-SCLC elderly patients need to be offered combined modality therapies with the expectation of relatively favorable long-term survival results, despite weaker performance status and more weight loss at admission and increased risk for treatment-related pulmonary toxicity.

Shimizu et al. drew attention to 7 elderly (≥ 75 years) patients among 94 LS-SCLC patients and noted the convenience of CCRT with long-term survival benefit and fair toxicity rates for select elderlies (Shimizu et al. 2007). The reported median OS of 24.7 months and 42.9% disease-free rate at 5 years were hopeful. Likewise, Okamoto et al. reported respective median PFS and OS times of 14.2 and 24.1 months for 12 elderly (≥ 70 years) LS-SCLC patients with early-onset CCRT via utilizing TDTRT in the absence of toxic deaths (Okamoto et al. 2010). Matsui et al. performed a phase II trial on the efficacy and toxicity of the Egorin's carboplatin dosing formula with 14-day oral etoposide in 38 elderly patients (Matsui et al. 1998). The median OS times were 15.1 and 8.6 months for LS-SCLC and ES-SCLC patients, individually, with grade 3–4 myelosuppression being the principal toxicity. The phase II trial by Westeel et al. assessed 66 SCLC patients >65 years treated with tailored four cycles of cisplatin, doxorubicin, vincristine, and etoposide combination (Westeel et al. 1998). TRT was administered concurrently with cisplatin/etoposide during the second CT course. Severe toxicity was relatively rare with just a single treatment-related death report. The estimated median OS times were 70 and 46 weeks for LS-SCLC and ES-SCLC patients, respectively. Murray et al. assessed the efficacy of an abbreviated treatment plan consisting of two cycles of CT (cyclophosphamide, doxorubicin, and vincristine) plus TRT (20 Gy in 5 fractions in a week and 30 Gy in 10 fractions in 2 weeks) in 55 elderly LS-SCLC patients (Murray et al. 1998). This study's median and 5-year OS rates of 54 weeks and 18%, respectively, suggest that long-term survival may be possible in such patients. Jeremic et al. designed a phase II study for an alternative strategy in 72 elderly (≥ 70 years) LS-SCLC with a short-term combination regime consisting of carboplatin and oral etoposide with TDTRT of 45 Gy (Jeremic et al. 1998a). The respective median and 5-year OS rates were 15 months and 13% in this study. The overall acute grade 3 toxicity was encountered in <10% of cases, with only one reported case of grade 4 acute thrombocytopenia.

Interestingly, less compliance with concurrent treatments appears to not end up with expanded failure patterns (McKenna Sr. 1994; Joss et al. 1995). Accordingly, lower doses of various chemotherapeutics merit strong consideration in the elderly SCLCs. Overall, many LS-SCLC series in elderly patients outlined comparable response rates and outcomes with younger counterparts, while the elderly mostly received tailored, abbreviated, less intensive CT and/or TRT mainly for an effort to reduce hematological toxicities.

3.2 SBRT for Stage I or II Node-Negative SCLC

Given its superior efficacy and toxicity profiles for inoperable candidates with severe comorbid conditions, weaker performance status, and limited lung functions, stereotactic body RT (SBRT) has gained progressive utilization as an ablative treatment modality for stage I–II SCLCs (Videtic et al. 2017).

Li et al. carried out a prospective phase II study with 29 LS-SCLC patients assigned to receive SBRT (40–45 Gy in 10 fractions) concurrently with 4–6 cycles of cisplatin/etoposide combination (Li et al. 2014). The respective median PFS and OS were 12 and 27 months, with only 13.8% and 0% grade 3 and 4–5 toxicity records, respectively. This phase II trial was an inspiring dataset demonstrating the feasibility of combination CT and early concurrent SBRT as a safe and compelling treatment for LS-SCLC patients. Verma et al. assessed the role of SBRT for the inoperable stage I SCLCs with a multi-institutional cohort study comprising 74 elderly patients with 76 lesions (Verma et al. 2017). Even though CT and PCI were prescribed to 56% and 23% of patients, the respective 3-year local control and median OS rates of 96.1% and 34.0% were encouraging with a median SBRT dose of 50 Gy (10 Gy per fraction). Toxicities were uncommon; 5.2% experienced grade ≥2 pneumonitis. Multivariate analysis results revealed the CT as an independent predictor of superior OS (31.4 months vs. 14.3 months without CT; $P = 0.02$). The post-SBRT failures were mostly distant (45.8%), followed by nodal (25.0%), and "elsewhere lung" (20.8%) failures. Accordingly, Verma et al. concluded that SBRT (≥50 Gy) with CT should be viewed as a standard treatment choice for stage T1-2N0 SCLC patients. In the impressive background from NSCLCs and such proof from SCLCs, SBRT has been a viable option, particularly for the elderly patients who have histologically confirmed T1-2N0M0 and peripherally located SCLCs.

3.3 Extensive-Stage SCLC

ES-SCLC is composed of both regional and distant metastatic and nonmetastatic local tumor burden outsized for the locoregional-only approach. The standard management of ES-SCLC had long been CT alone, and the role of RT had remained for palliation at all. The TRT in ES-SCLC given as definitive intent, rather than palliative approach, has continuously been studied with constructive feedback of Jeremic et al. (1999d). The TRT gained significant consideration due to the high rates of locoregional failures with CT alone in the lack of effective rescue treatment with second-line chemotherapies. The premise that TRT will control intrathoracic tumor burden may result in improved disease control, and hopefully OS results, if succeeded.

Jeremic and colleagues' pivotal investigation examined the usefulness and toxicity of up-front cisplatin/etoposide with/without accelerated hyperfractionated RT and concurrent daily carboplatin/etoposide in 210 ES-SCLC patients (Jeremic et al. 1999d). Following three cycles of CT, overall complete responders or partial responders at the locoregional primary with a complete response at distant sites were randomized to either TRT (twice daily, 54 Gy in 36 fractions) in combination with CT followed by two cycles of CT (CCRT: $N = 55$) or an additional four cycles of CT (CT alone: $N = 54$). Importantly, PCI (25 Gy in 10 fractions) was prescribed to all patients with complete responses at distant sites. The investigators presented encouragingly superior median (17 months vs. 11 months; $P < 0.05$) and 5-year (9.1% vs. 3.7%; $P < 0.05$) OS rates with CCRT over the CT-alone arm, which came at the cost of moderately increased acute high-grade toxicity rates.

Following this breakthrough in ES-SCLC, Slotman et al. concluded the discussion with an EORTC phase III trial, which randomized 498 ES-SCLC patients to either TRT (30 Gy in 10 fractions) or no TRT, while all CT responders underwent PCI (Slotman et al. 2015). The 2-year OS (13% vs. 3%, $P = 0.004$) rate was significantly improved with the consolidative RT in this study. The NRG Oncology RTOG 0937 phase II trial randomized ES-SCLC patients with 1–4 extracranial metastases after a complete/partial response to CT to one of the PCI (42 patients, 25 Gy in 10 fractions) alone or PCI plus consolidative RT (44 patients, 45 Gy in 15 fractions) to intrathoracic disease and extracranial metastases (Gore et al. 2017). This study was closed before meeting the accrual target, as the time-to-progression results favored the PCI plus consolidative RT arm (HR = 0.53; $P = 0.01$) over no-consolidation arm in the planned interim analysis though the 1-year OS rates were indistinct.

3.4 Prophylactic Cranial RT for LS-SCLC and ES-SCLC

There is an ongoing debate on subgroups that are less likely to profit from PCI. Unfortunately, most of the randomized data with a benefit from PCI prohibited elderly patients to date, and there is additionally a contention that patients over

70 years or at stage I might be unlikely to derive an OS advantage from the PCI (Yang et al. 2018; Xu et al. 2017; Rule et al. 2015). The risk-benefit ratio of PCI ought to be carefully weighed in such patients considering the PCI-related neurotoxicity and negative impacts on quality-of-life measures.

Wolfson et al. examined the impact of three different doses and fractionation schedule of PCI on the incidence of chronic neurotoxicity in LS-SCLC patients who achieved a complete response after CT and TRT: arm 1: 25 Gy in 10 daily fractions ($N = 131$), arm 2: 36 Gy in 18 daily fractions ($N = 67$), and arm 3: 36 Gy in 24 twice-daily fractions ($N = 66$) (Wolfson et al. 2011). The authors reported significantly increased chronic neurotoxicity incidence in the 36 Gy PCI cohorts at 12-month evaluations ($P = 0.02$), with advancing age distinguished as the principal indicator of chronic neurotoxicity in the logistic regression analysis ($P = 0.005$). Rule et al. examined the worth of PCI in 155 elderly (≥ 70 years) SCLC patients enrolled on four prospective phase II or III trials of the NCCTG, where 91 received PCI (30 Gy in 15 or 25 Gy in 10 fractions) while 64 did not (Rule et al. 2015). The authors called attention to altogether significantly superior better median (12.0 months vs. 7.6 months; $P = 0.001$) and 3-year (13.2% vs. 3.1%; $P = 0.001$) OS rates with PCI. The results of the multivariate analysis uncovered the early disease stage (LS vs. ES; $P = 0.0072$) as the unique variable to connect with significantly superior OS times in the entire investigation associate, while PCI utilization was the sole factor linking to a survival advantage in ES-SCLC accomplice ($P = 0.03$). However, grade ≥ 3 or higher adverse events were significantly more frequent in the PCI cohort (71.4% vs. 47.5%; $P = 0.0031$). Farooqi et al. reviewed the results of a cohort of 658 LS-SCLC (151 of them ≥ 70 years) patients after a complete response with CCRT to weigh whether PCI can improve OS results and suppress the brain metastasis advancement or not, where 364 patients received PCI (Farooqi et al. 2017). Albeit the authors discovered the PCI to reduce the risks of death [HR: 0.73; $P = 0.001$] and the emergence of brain metastasis (HR 0.54, $P < 0.001$), interestingly OS was not enhanced with PCI in the subgroup of patients ≥ 70 years presenting with ≥ 5 cm tumors ($P = 0.739$).

A recent modern Japanese randomized phase III trial compared the observation with MRI surveillance (at 3-month intervals up to 12, 18, and 24 months after enrollment) vs. PCI (25 Gy in 10 fractions) in ES-SCLC patients (Takahashi et al. 2017). Although PCI reduced the incidence of brain metastasis to 48% from the 69% of MRI surveillance, this superiority did not prove improved OS results. Accordingly, the authors recommended the MRI surveillance as a valuable alternative to PCI for patients who can adhere to MRI follow-up schedule. On that account, given the commonness of severe PCI toxicity in the elderly population, MRI surveillance should be encouraged in suitable patients, rather than the standard recommendation of PCI to all patients.

4 Conclusion

Elderly cancer patients with NSCLC and SCLC are significantly underrepresented in all clinical trials, while the physiological fitness to be eligible for radical treatments is not routinely implemented. Therefore, the inclusion of appropriately selected elderly patients in clinical studies needs to be strongly encouraged to construct an evidence base for this age group. Additionally, we recommend baseline and continuing guidance of geriatric assessments to promote individualized care, support, and tailored treatment protocols, as well as avoid under- or overtreatments in elderly cancer patients, where bespoke RT should be in mind in all stages.

References

Ahmad E, Sandhu AP, Fuster MM, Messer K, Pu M, Nobiensky P, Bazhenova L, Seagren S (2011) Hypofractionated radiotherapy as definitive treatment of stage I non-small cell lung cancer in older patients. Am J Clin Oncol 34(3):254–258

Albain KS, Crowley JJ, LeBlanc M, Livingston RB (1990) Determinants of improved outcome in small-cell lung cancer: an analysis of the 2,580-patient Southwest Oncology Group data base. J Clin Oncol 8(9):1563–1574

Antonio M, Saldana J, Linares J, Ruffinelli JC, Palmero R, Navarro A, Arnaiz MD, Brao I, Aso S, Padrones S, Navarro V, Gonzalez-Barboteo J, Borras JM, Cardenal F, Nadal E (2018) Geriatric assessment may help decision-making in elderly patients with inoperable, locally advanced non-small-cell lung cancer. Br J Cancer 118(5):639–647

Aoe K, Takigawa N, Hotta K, Maeda T, Kishino D, Nogami N, Tabata M, Harita S, Okada T, Kubo T, Hosokawa S, Fujiwara K, Gemba K, Yasugi M, Kozuki T, Kato Y, Katsui K, Kanazawa S, Ueoka H, Tanimoto M, Kiura K (2014) A phase II study of S-1 chemotherapy with concurrent thoracic radiotherapy in elderly patients with locally advanced non-small-cell lung cancer: the Okayama Lung Cancer Study Group Trial 0801. Eur J Cancer 50(16):2783–2790

Atagi S, Kawahara M, Ogawara M, Matsui K, Masuda N, Kudoh S, Negoro S, Furuse K (2000) Phase II trial of daily low-dose carboplatin and thoracic radiotherapy in elderly patients with locally advanced non-small cell lung cancer. Jpn J Clin Oncol 30(2):59–64

Atagi S, Kawahara M, Tamura T, Noda K, Watanabe K, Yokoyama A, Sugiura T, Senba H, Ishikura S, Ikeda H, Ishizuka N, Saijo N, Japan Clinical Oncology G (2005) Standard thoracic radiotherapy with or without concurrent daily low-dose carboplatin in elderly patients with locally advanced non-small cell lung cancer: a phase III trial of the Japan Clinical Oncology Group (JCOG9812). Jpn J Clin Oncol 35(4):195–201

Auperin A, Arriagada R, Pignon JP, Le Pechoux C, Gregor A, Stephens RJ, Kristjansen PE, Johnson BE, Ueoka H, Wagner H, Aisner J (1999) Prophylactic cranial irradiation for patients with small-cell lung cancer in complete remission. Prophylactic Cranial Irradiation Overview Collaborative Group. N Engl J Med 341(7):476–484

Bach PB, Cramer LD, Warren JL, Begg CB (1999) Racial differences in the treatment of early-stage lung cancer. N Engl J Med 341(16):1198–1205

Blomgren H, Lax I, Naslund I, Svanstrom R (1995) Stereotactic high dose fraction radiation therapy of extracranial tumors using an accelerator. Clinical experience of the first thirty-one patients. Acta Oncol 34(6):861–870

Bonner JA, Sloan JA, Shanahan TG, Brooks BJ, Marks RS, Krook JE, Gerstner JB, Maksymiuk A, Levitt R, Mailliard JA, Tazelaar HD, Hillman S, Jett JR (1999) Phase III comparison of twice-daily split-course irradiation versus once-daily irradiation for patients with limited stage small-cell lung carcinoma. J Clin Oncol 17(9):2681–2691

Brooks ED, Sun B, Zhao L, Komaki R, Liao Z, Jeter M, Welsh JW, O'Reilly MS, Gomez DR, Hahn SM, Heymach JV, Rice DC, Chang JY (2017) Stereotactic ablative radiation therapy is highly safe and effective for elderly patients with early-stage non-small cell lung cancer. Int J Radiat Oncol Biol Phys 98(4):900–907

Cancer Stat Facts: Lung and Bronchus Cancer (2021). https://seer.cancer.gov/statfacts/html/lungb.html. Accessed 1 Oct 2021

Chang JY, Li QQ, Xu QY, Allen PK, Rebueno N, Gomez DR, Balter P, Komaki R, Mehran R, Swisher SG, Roth JA (2014) Stereotactic ablative radiation therapy for centrally located early stage or isolated parenchymal recurrences of non-small cell lung cancer: how to fly in a "no fly zone". Int J Radiat Oncol Biol Phys 88(5):1120–1128

Chen F, Hu P, Liang N, Xie J, Yu S, Tian T, Zhang J, Deng G, Zhang J (2018) Concurrent chemoradiotherapy with weekly nedaplatin versus radiotherapy alone in elderly patients with non-small-cell lung cancer. Clin Transl Oncol 20(3):294–301

Christodoulou M, Blackhall F, Mistry H, Leylek A, Knegjens J, Remouchamps V, Martel-Lafay I, Farre N, Zwitter M, Lerouge D, Pourel N, Janicot H, Scherpereel A, Tissing-Tan C, Peignaux K, Geets X, Konopa K, Faivre-Finn C (2019) Compliance and outcome of elderly patients treated in the concurrent once-daily versus twice-daily radiotherapy (CONVERT) trial. J Thorac Oncol 14(1):63–71

Clamon G, Herndon J, Cooper R et al (1999) Radiosensitization with carboplatin for patients with unresectable stage III non-small-cell lung cancer: a phase III trial of the Cancer and Leukemia Group B and the Eastern Cooperative Oncology Group. J Clin Oncol 17:4–11

Coate LE, Massey C, Hope A, Sacher A, Barrett K, Pierre A, Leighl N, Brade A, de Perrot M, Waddell T, Liu G, Feld R, Burkes R, Cho BC, Darling G, Sun A, Keshavjee S, Bezjak A, Shepherd FA (2011) Treatment of the elderly when cure is the goal: the influence of age on treatment selection and efficacy for stage III non-small cell lung cancer. J Thorac Oncol 6(3):537–544

Couderc AL, Tomasini P, Rey D, Nouguerede E, Correard F, Barlesi F, Thomas P, Villani P, Greillier L (2020) Octogenarians treated for thoracic and lung cancers: impact of comprehensive geriatric assessment. J Geriatr Oncol 12(3):402–409

Coy P, Kennelly GM (1980) The role of curative radiotherapy in the treatment of lung cancer. Cancer 45(4):698–702

Crabtree TD, Denlinger CE, Meyers BF, El Naqa I, Zoole J, Krupnick AS, Kreisel D, Patterson GA, Bradley JD (2010) Stereotactic body radiation therapy versus surgical resection for stage I non-small cell lung cancer. J Thorac Cardiovasc Surg 140(2):377–386

Curran WJ Jr, Paulus R, Langer CJ, Komaki R, Lee JS, Hauser S, Movsas B, Wasserman T, Rosenthal SA, Gore E, Machtay M, Sause W, Cox JD (2011) Sequential vs. concurrent chemoradiation for stage III non-small cell lung cancer: randomized phase III trial RTOG 9410. J Natl Cancer Inst 103(19): 1452–1460

Dajczman E, Fu LY, Small D, Wolkove N, Kreisman H (1996) Treatment of small cell lung carcinoma in the elderly. Cancer 77(10):2032–2038

Decoster L, Van Puyvelde K, Mohile S, Wedding U, Basso U, Colloca G, Rostoft S, Overcash J, Wildiers H, Steer C, Kimmick G, Kanesvaran R, Luciani A, Terret C, Hurria A, Kenis C, Audisio R, Extermann M (2015) Screening tools for multidimensional health problems warranting a geriatric assessment in older cancer patients: an update on SIOG recommendations. Ann Oncol 26(2):288–300

Dubianski R, Wildes TM, Wildiers H (2019) SIOG guidelines—essential for good clinical practice in geriatric oncology. J Geriat Oncol 10(2):196–198

Edwards BK, Noone AM, Mariotto AB, Simard EP, Boscoe FP, Henley SJ, Jemal A, Cho H, Anderson RN, Kohler BA, Eheman CR, Ward EM (2014) Annual Report to the Nation on the status of cancer, 1975-2010, featuring prevalence of comorbidity and impact on survival among persons with lung, colorectal, breast, or prostate cancer. Cancer 120(9):1290–1314

Extermann M (2000) Measurement and impact of comorbidity in older cancer patients. Crit Rev Oncol Hematol. 35(3):181–200

Faivre-Finn C, Snee M, Ashcroft L, Appel W, Barlesi F, Bhatnagar A, Bezjak A, Cardenal F, Fournel P, Harden S, Le Pechoux C, McMenemin R, Mohammed N, O'Brien M, Pantarotto J, Surmont V, Van Meerbeeck JP, Woll PJ, Lorigan P, Blackhall F (2017) Concurrent once-daily versus twice-daily chemoradiotherapy in patients with limited-stage small-cell lung cancer (CONVERT): an open-label, phase 3, randomised, superiority trial. Lancet Oncol 18(8):1116–1125

Farooqi AS, Holliday EB, Allen PK, Wei X, Cox JD, Komaki R (2017) Prophylactic cranial irradiation after definitive chemoradiotherapy for limited-stage small cell lung cancer: do all patients benefit? Radiother Oncol 122(2):307–312

Firat S, Pleister A, Byhardt RW, Gore E (2006) Age is independent of comorbidity influencing patient selection for combined modality therapy for treatment of stage III nonsmall cell lung cancer (NSCLC). Am J Clin Oncol 29(3):252–257

Franceschini D, De Rose F, Cozzi L, Navarria P, Clerici E, Franzese C, Comito T, Tozzi A, Iftode C, D'Agostino G, Sorsetti M (2017) Radical hypo-fractionated radiotherapy with volumetric modulated arc therapy in lung cancer: a retrospective study of elderly patients with stage III disease. Strahlenther Onkol 193(5):385–391

Furuse K, Fukuoka M, Kawahara M, Nishikawa H, Takada Y, Kudoh S, Katagami N, Ariyoshi Y (1999) Phase III study of concurrent versus sequential thoracic radiotherapy in combination with mitomycin, vindesine, and cisplatin in unresectable stage III non-small-cell lung cancer. J Clin Oncol 17(9):2692–2699

Gaspar LE, McNamara EJ, Gay EG, Putnam JB, Crawford J, Herbst RS, Bonner JA (2012) Small-cell lung cancer: prognostic factors and changing treatment over 15 years. Clin Lung Cancer 13(2):115–122

Gauden SJ, Tripcony L (2001) The curative treatment by radiation therapy alone of stage I non-small cell lung cancer in a geriatric population. Lung Cancer 32(1):71–79

Gauden S, Ramsay J, Tripcony L (1995) The curative treatment by radiotherapy alone of stage I non-small cell carcinoma of the lung. Chest 108(5):1278–1282

Gava A, Bertossi L, Zorat PL, Ausili-Cefaro G, Olmi P, Pavanato G, Mandoliti G, Polico C (1997) Radiotherapy in the elderly with lung carcinoma: the experience of the Italian "Geriatric Radiation Oncology Group". Rays 22(1 Suppl):61–65

Gore EM, Hu C, Sun AY, Grimm DF, Ramalingam SS, Dunlap NE, Higgins KA, Werner-Wasik M, Allen AM, Iyengar P, Videtic GMM, Hales RK, McGarry RC, Urbanic JJ, Pu AT, Johnstone CA, Stieber VW, Paulus R, Bradley JD (2017) Randomized phase II study comparing prophylactic cranial irradiation alone to prophylactic cranial irradiation and consolidative extracranial irradiation for extensive-disease small cell lung cancer (ED SCLC): NRG Oncology RTOG 0937. J Thorac Oncol 12(10):1561–1570

Haasbeek CJ, Senan S, Smit EF, Paul MA, Slotman BJ, Lagerwaard FJ (2008) Critical review of nonsurgical treatment options for stage I non-small cell lung cancer. Oncologist 13(3):309–319

Haasbeek CJ, Lagerwaard FJ, Antonisse ME, Slotman BJ, Senan S (2010) Stage I nonsmall cell lung cancer in patients aged > or =75 years: outcomes after stereotactic radiotherapy. Cancer 116(2):406–414

Hayakawa K, Mitsuhashi N, Katano S, Saito Y, Nakayama Y, Sakurai H, Akimoto T, Hasegawa M, Yamakawa M, Niibe H (2001) High-dose radiation therapy for elderly patients with inoperable or unresectable non-small cell lung cancer. Lung Cancer 32(1):81–88

Hayman JA, Abrahamse PH, Lakhani I, Earle CC, Katz SJ (2007) Use of palliative radiotherapy among patients with metastatic non-small-cell lung cancer. Int J Radiat Oncol Biol Phys 69(4):1001–1007

Jara C, Gomez-Aldaravi JL, Tirado R, Meseguer VA, Alonso C, Fernandez A (1999) Small-cell lung cancer in the elderly—is age of patient a relevant factor? Acta Oncol 38(6):781–786

Jatoi A, Schild SE, Foster N, Henning GT, Dornfeld KJ, Flynn PJ, Fitch TR, Dakhil SR, Rowland KM, Stella PJ, Soori GS, Adjei AA (2010) A phase II study of cetuximab and radiation in elderly and/or poor performance status patients with locally advanced non-small-cell lung cancer (N0422). Ann Oncol 21(10):2040–2044

Jeremic B, Shibamoto Y, Acimovic L, Milisavljevic S (1997) Hyperfractionated radiotherapy alone for clinical stage I nonsmall cell lung cancer. Int J Radiat Oncol Biol Phys 38(3):521–525

Jeremic B, Shibamoto Y, Acimovic L, Milisavljevic S (1998a) Carboplatin, etoposide, and accelerated hyperfractionated radiotherapy for elderly patients with limited small cell lung carcinoma: a phase II study. Cancer 82(5):836–841

Jeremic B, Shibamoto Y, Milicic B, Nikolic N, Dagovic A, Milisavljevic S (1998b) Concurrent radiochemotherapy for patients with stage III non-small-cell lung cancer (NSCLC): long-term results of a phase II study. Int J Radiat Oncol Biol Phys 42(5):1091–1096

Jeremic B, Shibamoto Y, Acimovic L, Milisavljevic S (1999a) Hyperfractionated radiotherapy for clinical stage II non-small cell lung cancer. Radiother Oncol 51(2):141–145

Jeremic B, Shibamoto Y, Milicic B, Milisavljevic S, Nikolic N, Dagovic A, Aleksandrovic J, Radosavljevic-Asic G (1999b) A phase II study of concurrent accelerated hyperfractionated radiotherapy and carboplatin/oral etoposide for elderly patients with stage III non-small-cell lung cancer. Int J Radiat Oncol Biol Phys 44(2):343–348

Jeremic B, Shibamoto Y, Milicic B, Milisavljevic S, Nikolic N, Dagovic A, Radosavljevic-Asic G (1999c) Short-term chemotherapy and palliative radiotherapy for elderly patients with stage IV non-small cell lung cancer: a phase II study. Lung Cancer 24(1):1–9

Jeremic B, Shibamoto Y, Nikolic N, Milicic B, Milisavljevic S, Dagovic A, Aleksandrovic J, Radosavljevic-Asic G (1999d) Role of radiation therapy in the combined-modality treatment of patients with extensive disease small-cell lung cancer: a randomized study. J Clin Oncol 17(7):2092–2099

Joss RA, Bacchi M, Hurny C, Bernhard J, Cerny T, Martinelli G, Leyvraz S, Senn HJ, Stahel R, Siegenthaler P et al (1995) Early versus late alternating chemotherapy in small-cell lung cancer. Swiss Group for Clinical Cancer Research (SAKK). Ann Oncol 6(2):157–166

Kenis C, Decoster L, Van Puyvelde K, De Greve J, Conings G, Milisen K, Flamaing J, Lobelle JP, Wildiers H (2014) Performance of two geriatric screening tools in older patients with cancer. J Clin Oncol 32(1):19–26

Kim DY, Song C, Kim SH, Kim YJ, Lee JS, Kim JS (2019) Chemoradiotherapy versus radiotherapy alone following induction chemotherapy for elderly patients with stage III lung cancer. Radiat Oncol J 37(3):176–184

Krol AD, Aussems P, Noordijk EM, Hermans J, Leer JW (1996) Local irradiation alone for peripheral stage I lung cancer: could we omit the elective regional nodal irradiation? Int J Radiat Oncol Biol Phys 34(2):297–302

Kucuk A, Ozkan EE, Eskici Oztep S, Mertsoylu H, Pehlivan B, Selek U, Topkan E (2020) The influence of systemic inflammation response index on survival outcomes of limited-stage small-cell lung cancer patients treated with concurrent chemoradiotherapy. J Oncol 2020:8832145

Kusumoto S, Koga K, Tsukino H, Nagamachi S, Nishikawa K, Watanabe K (1986) Comparison of survival of patients with lung cancer between elderly (greater than or equal to 70) and younger (70 greater than) age groups. Jpn J Clin Oncol 16(4):319–323

Lagerwaard FJ, Haasbeek CJ, Smit EF, Slotman BJ, Senan S (2008) Outcomes of risk-adapted fractionated stereotactic radiotherapy for stage I non-small-cell lung cancer. Int J Radiat Oncol Biol Phys 70(3):685–692

Lagerwaard FJ, Verstegen NE, Haasbeek CJ, Slotman BJ, Paul MA, Smit EF, Senan S (2012) Outcomes of stereotactic ablative radiotherapy in patients with potentially operable stage I non-small cell lung cancer. Int J Radiat Oncol Biol Phys 83(1):348–353

Lally BE, Geiger AM, Urbanic JJ, Butler JM, Wentworth S, Perry MC, Wilson LD, Horton JK, Detterbeck FC, Miller AA, Thomas CR Jr, Blackstock AW (2009) Trends in the outcomes for patients with limited stage small cell lung cancer: an analysis of the Surveillance, Epidemiology, and End Results database. Lung Cancer 64(2):226–231

Langer CJ, Hsu C, Curran W, Komaki R, Lee JS, Byhardt R, Sause W (2001) Do elderly patients (pts) with locally advanced non-small cell lung cancer (NSCLC) benefit from combined modality therapy? A secondary analysis of RTOG 94-10. Int J Radiat Oncol Biol Phys 51(3 Suppl 1):20–21

Le QT, Loo BW, Ho A, Cotrutz C, Koong AC, Wakelee H, Kee ST, Constantinescu D, Whyte RI, Donington J (2006) Results of a phase I dose-escalation study using single-fraction stereotactic radiotherapy for lung tumors. J Thorac Oncol 1(8):802–809

Lee KA, Dunne M, Small C, Kelly PJ, McArdle O, O'Sullivan J, Hacking D, Pomeroy M, Armstrong J, Moriarty M, Clayton-Lea A, Parker I, Collins CD, Thirion P (2018) (ICORG 05-03): prospective randomized non-inferiority phase III trial comparing two radiation schedules in malignant spinal cord compression (not proceeding with surgical decompression); the quality of life analysis. Acta Oncol 57(7):965–972

Li C, Xiong Y, Zhou Z, Peng Y, Huang H, Xu M, Kang H, Peng B, Wang D, Yang X (2014) Stereotactic body radiotherapy with concurrent chemotherapy extends survival of patients with limited stage small cell lung cancer: a single-center prospective phase II study. Med Oncol 31(12):369

Li C, Wang L, Wu Q, Zhao J, Yi F, Xu J, Wei Y, Zhang W (2020) A meta-analysis comparing stereotactic body radiotherapy vs conventional radiotherapy in inoperable stage I non-small cell lung cancer. Medicine 99(34):e21715

Lonardi F, Coeli M, Pavanato G, Adami F, Gioga G, Campostrini F (2000) Radiotherapy for non-small cell lung cancer in patients aged 75 and over: safety, effectiveness and possible impact on survival. Lung Cancer 28(1):43–50

Ludbrook JJ, Truong PT, MacNeil MV, Lesperance M, Webber A, Joe H, Martins H, Lim J (2003) Do age and comorbidity impact treatment allocation and outcomes in limited stage small-cell lung cancer? a community-based population analysis. Int J Radiat Oncol Biol Phys 55(5):1321–1330

Malvezzi M, Bertuccio P, Rosso T, Rota M, Levi F, La Vecchia C, Negri E (2015) European cancer mortality predictions for the year 2015: does lung cancer have the highest death rate in EU women? Ann Oncol 26(4):779–786

Matsui K, Masuda N, Fukuoka M, Yana T, Hirashima T, Komiya T, Kobayashi M, Kawahara M, Atagi S, Ogawara M, Negoro S, Kudoh S, Furuse K (1998) Phase II trial of carboplatin plus oral etoposide for elderly patients with small-cell lung cancer. Br J Cancer 77(11):1961–1965

McAleese J, Baluch S, Drinkwater K, Bassett P, Hanna GG (2017) The elderly are less likely to receive recommended radical radiotherapy for non-small cell lung cancer. Clin Oncol (R Coll Radiol) 29(9):593–600

McGarry RC, Papiez L, Williams M, Whitford T, Timmerman RD (2005) Stereotactic body radiation therapy of early-stage non-small-cell lung carcinoma: phase I study. Int J Radiat Oncol Biol Phys 63(4):1010–1015

McKenna RJ Sr (1994) Clinical aspects of cancer in the elderly. Treatment decisions, treatment choices, and follow-up. Cancer 74(7 Suppl):2107–2117

Micke P, Faldum A, Metz T, Beeh KM, Bittinger F, Hengstler JG, Buhl R (2002) Staging small cell lung cancer: Veterans Administration Lung Study Group versus International Association for the Study of Lung Cancer—what limits limited disease? Lung Cancer 37(3):271–276

Middelburg JG, Middelburg RA, van Zwienen M, Mast ME, Bhawanie A, Jobsen JJ, Rozema T, Maas H, Geijsen ED, van der Leest AH, van den Bongard D, van Loon J, Budiharto T, Aarts MJ, Terhaard CHJ, Struikmans H, Lpro (2020). Impaired geriatric 8 score is associated with worse survival after radiotherapy in older patients with cancer. Clin Oncol (R Coll Radiol). 33(4): E203-E210.

Mohile SG, Bylow K, Dale W, Dignam J, Martin K, Petrylak DP, Stadler WM, Rodin M (2007) A pilot study of the vulnerable elders survey-13 compared with the comprehensive geriatric assessment for identifying disability in older patients with prostate cancer who receive androgen ablation. Cancer 109(4):802–810

Montella M, Gridelli C, Crispo A, Scognamiglio F, Ruffolo P, Gatani T, Boccia V, Maione P, Fabbrocini G (2002) Has lung cancer in the elderly different characteristics at presentation? Oncol Rep 9(5):1093–1096

Movsas B, Scott C, Sause W, Byhardt R, Komaki R, Cox J, Johnson D, Lawton C, Dar AR, Wasserman T, Roach M, Lee JS, Andras E (1999) The benefit of treatment intensification is age and histology-dependent in patients with locally advanced non-small cell lung cancer (NSCLC): a quality-adjusted survival analysis of radiation therapy oncology group (RTOG) chemoradiation studies. Int J Radiat Oncol Biol Phys 45(5):1143–1149

Murray N, Grafton C, Shah A, Gelmon K, Kostashuk E, Brown E, Coppin C, Coldman A, Page R (1998) Abbreviated treatment for elderly, infirm, or noncompliant patients with limited-stage small-cell lung cancer. J Clin Oncol 16(10):3323–3328

Nakano K, Hiramoto T, Kanehara M, Doi M, Furonaka O, Miyazu Y, Hada Y (1999) [Radiotherapy alone for elderly patients with stage III non-small cell lung cancer]. Nihon Kokyuki Gakkai Zzasshi 37(4):276–281

Nakano K, Yamamoto M, Iwamoto H, Hiramoto T (2003) [Daily low-dose cisplatin plus concurrent high-dose thoracic radiotherapy in elderly patients with locally advanced unresectable non-small cell lung cancer]. Gan To Kagaku Ryoho 30(9):1283–1287

Nanda RH, Liu Y, Gillespie TW, Mikell JL, Ramalingam SS, Fernandez FG, Curran WJ, Lipscomb J, Higgins KA (2015) Stereotactic body radiation therapy versus no treatment for early stage non-small cell lung cancer in medically inoperable elderly patients: a National Cancer Data Base analysis. Cancer 121(23):4222–4230

Newaishy GA, Kerr GR (1989) Radical radiotherapy for bronchogenic carcinoma: five year survival rates. Clin Oncol (R Coll Radiol) 1(2):80–85

Niho S, Hosomi Y, Okamoto H, Nihei K, Tanaka H, Hida T, Umemura S, Goto K, Akimoto T, Ohe Y (2019) Carboplatin, S-1 and concurrent thoracic radiotherapy for elderly patients with locally advanced non-small cell lung cancer: a multicenter Phase I/II study. Jpn J Clin Oncol 49(7):614–619

Noguchi T, Mochizuki H, Yamazaki M, Kawate E, Suzuki Y, Sato T, Takahashi H (2010) A retrospective analysis of clinical outcomes of patients older than or equal to 80 years with small cell lung cancer. J Thorac Oncol 5(7):1081–1087

Noordijk EM, vd Poest Clement E, Hermans J, Wever AM, Leer JW (1988) Radiotherapy as an alternative to surgery in elderly patients with resectable lung cancer. Radiother Oncol 13(2):83–89

O'Donovan A, Morris L (2020) Palliative radiation therapy in older adults with cancer: age-related considerations. Clin Oncol (R Coll Radiol) 32(11):766–774

O'Dowd EL, Luchtenborg M, Baldwin DR, McKeever TM, Powell HA, Moller H, Jakobsen E, Hubbard RB (2016) Predicting death from surgery for lung cancer: a comparison of two scoring systems in two European countries. Lung Cancer 95:88–93

Okamoto K, Okamoto I, Takezawa K, Tachibana I, Fukuoka M, Nishimura Y, Nakagawa K (2010) Cisplatin and etoposide chemotherapy combined with early concurrent twice-daily thoracic radiotherapy for limited-disease small cell lung cancer in elderly patients. Jpn J Clin Oncol 40(1):54–59

Onishi H, Araki T (2013) Stereotactic body radiation therapy for stage I non-small-cell lung cancer: a historical overview of clinical studies. Jpn J Clin Oncol 43(4):345–350

Onishi H, Shirato H, Nagata Y, Hiraoka M, Fujino M, Gomi K, Karasawa K, Hayakawa K, Niibe Y, Takai Y, Kimura T, Takeda A, Ouchi A, Hareyama M, Kokubo M, Kozuka T, Arimoto T, Hara R, Itami J, Araki T (2011) Stereotactic body radiotherapy (SBRT) for operable stage I non-small-cell lung cancer: can SBRT be comparable to surgery? Int J Radiat Oncol Biol Phys 81(5):1352–1358

Osterlind K, Andersen PK (1986) Prognostic factors in small cell lung cancer: multivariate model based on 778 patients treated with chemotherapy with or without irradiation. Cancer Res 46(8):4189–4194

Ozdemir Y, Topkan E, Mertsoylu H, Selek U (2020) Low prognostic nutritional index predicts poor clinical outcomes in patients with stage IIIB non-small-cell lung carcinoma undergoing chemoradiotherapy. Cancer Manag Res 12:1959–1967

Palma D, Visser O, Lagerwaard FJ, Belderbos J, Slotman BJ, Senan S (2010a) Impact of introducing stereotactic lung radiotherapy for elderly patients with stage I non-small-cell lung cancer: a population-based time-trend analysis. J Clin Oncol 28(35):5153–5159

Palma DA, Tyldesley S, Sheehan F, Mohamed IG, Smith S, Wai E, Murray N, Senan S (2010b) Stage I non-small cell lung cancer (NSCLC) in patients aged 75 years and older: does age determine survival after radical treatment? J Thorac Oncol 5(6):818–824

Palma D, Lagerwaard F, Rodrigues G, Haasbeek C, Senan S (2012) Curative treatment of stage I non-small-cell lung cancer in patients with severe COPD: stereotactic radiotherapy outcomes and systematic review. Int J Radiat Oncol Biol Phys 82(3):1149–1156

Parashar B, Patel P, Monni S, Singh P, Sood N, Trichter S, Sabbas A, Wernicke AG, Nori D, Chao KS (2010) Limited resection followed by intraoperative seed implantation is comparable to stereotactic body radiotherapy for solitary lung cancer. Cancer 116(21):5047–5053

Park CH, Bonomi M, Cesaretti J, Neugut AI, Wisnivesky JP (2011) Effect of radiotherapy planning complexity on survival of elderly patients with unresected localized lung cancer. Int J Radiat Oncol Biol Phys 81(3):706–711

Pergolizzi S, Settineri N, Maisano R, Santacaterina A, Faranda C, Russi E, Raffaele L, Adamo V (1997) Curative radiotherapy (RT) using limited RT treatment fields in elderly patients with non-small cell lung cancer in clinical stage IIIA. Oncol Rep 4(5): 961–965

Pignon T, Gregor A, Schaake Koning C, Roussel A, Van Glabbeke M, Scalliet P (1998) Age has no impact on acute and late toxicity of curative thoracic radiotherapy. Radiother Oncol 46(3):239–248

Powell HA, Tata LJ, Baldwin DR, Stanley RA, Khakwani A, Hubbard RB (2013) Early mortality after surgical resection for lung cancer: an analysis of the English National Lung cancer audit. Thorax 68(9):826–834

Raz DJ, Zell JA, Ou SH, Gandara DR, Anton-Culver H, Jablons DM (2007) Natural history of stage I non-small cell lung cancer: implications for early detection. Chest 132(1):193–199

Rocha Lima CM, Herndon JE 2nd, Kosty M, Clamon G, Green MR (2002) Therapy choices among older patients with lung carcinoma: an evaluation of two trials of the Cancer and Leukemia Group B. Cancer 94(1):181–187

Rule WG, Foster NR, Meyers JP, Ashman JB, Vora SA, Kozelsky TF, Garces YI, Urbanic JJ, Salama JK, Schild SE (2015) Prophylactic cranial irradiation in elderly patients with small cell lung cancer: findings from a North Central Cancer Treatment Group pooled analysis. J Geriatr Oncol 6(2):119–126

Sagman U, Feld R, Evans WK, Warr D, Shepherd FA, Payne D, Pringle J, Yeoh J, DeBoer G, Malkin A et al (1991) The prognostic significance of pretreatment serum lactate dehydrogenase in patients with small-cell lung cancer. J Clin Oncol 9(6):954–961

San Jose S, Arnaiz MD, Lucas A, Navarro V, Serrano G, Zaderazjko M, Jeremic B, Guedea F (2006) Radiation therapy alone in elderly with early stage non-small cell lung cancer. Lung Cancer 52(2):149–154

Sarin R, Dinshaw KA (1997) Final results of the Royal College of Radiologists' trial comparing two different radiotherapy schedules in the treatment of cerebral metastases. Clin Oncol (R Coll Radiol) 9(4):272

Schaake-Koning C, van den Bogaert W, Dalesio O, Festen J, Hoogenhout J, van Houtte P, Kirkpatrick A, Koolen M, Maat B, Nijs A et al (1992) Effects of concomitant cisplatin and radiotherapy on inoperable non-small-cell lung cancer. N Engl J Med 326(8):524–530

Schild SE, Stella PJ, Geyer SM, Bonner JA, McGinnis WL, Mailliard JA, Brindle J, Jatoi A, Jett JR, North Central Cancer Treatment G (2003) The outcome of combined-modality therapy for stage III non-small-cell lung cancer in the elderly. J Clin Oncol 21(17):3201–3206

Schild SE, Stella PJ, Brooks BJ, Mandrekar S, Bonner JA, McGinnis WL, Mailliard JA, Krook JE, Deming RL, Adjei AA, Jatoi A, Jett JR (2005) Results of combined-modality therapy for limited-stage small cell lung carcinoma in the elderly. Cancer 103(11):2349–2354

Schild SE, Mandrekar SJ, Jatoi A, McGinnis WL, Stella PJ, Deming RL, Jett JR, Garces YI, Allen KL, Adjei AA, North Central Cancer Treatment Group (2007) The value of combined-modality therapy in elderly patients with stage III nonsmall cell lung cancer. Cancer 110(2):363–368

Selek U, Bolukbasi Y, Welsh JW, Topkan E (2014) Intensity-modulated radiotherapy versus 3-dimensional conformal radiotherapy strategies for locally advanced non-small-cell lung cancer. Balkan Med J 31(4):286–294

Semrau S, Klautke G, Virchow JC, Kundt G, Fietkau R (2008) Impact of comorbidity and age on the outcome of patients with inoperable NSCLC treated with concurrent chemoradiotherapy. Respir Med 102(2):210–218

Sezen CB, Gokce A, Kalafat CE, Aker C, Tastepe AI (2019) Risk factors for postoperative complications and long-term survival in elderly lung cancer patients: a single institutional experience in Turkey. Gen Thorac Cardiovasc Surg 67(5):442–449

Shepherd FA, Amdemichael E, Evans WK, Chalvardjian P, Hogg-Johnson S, Coates R, Paul K (1994) Treatment of small cell lung cancer in the elderly. J Am Geriatr Soc 42(1):64–70

Shimizu T, Sekine I, Sumi M, Ito Y, Yamada K, Nokihara H, Yamamoto N, Kunitoh H, Ohe Y, Tamura T (2007) Concurrent chemoradiotherapy for limited-disease small cell lung cancer in elderly patients aged 75 years or older. Jpn J Clin Oncol 37(3):181–185

Siegel RL, Miller KD, Fuchs HE, Jemal A (2021) Cancer statistics, 2021. CA Cancer J Clin 71(1):7–33

Simone CB 2nd, Bogart JA, Cabrera AR, Daly ME, DeNunzio NJ, Detterbeck F, Faivre-Finn C, Gatschet

N, Gore E, Jabbour SK, Kruser TJ, Schneider BJ, Slotman B, Turrisi A, Wu AJ, Zeng J, Rosenzweig KE (2020) Radiation therapy for small cell lung cancer: an ASTRO clinical practice guideline. Pract Radiat Oncol 10(3):158–173

Siu LL, Shepherd FA, Murray N, Feld R, Pater J, Zee B (1996) Influence of age on the treatment of limited-stage small-cell lung cancer. J Clin Oncol 14(3):821–828

Slotman BJ, Njo KH, Karim AB (1994) Curative radiotherapy for technically operable stage I nonsmall cell lung cancer. Int J Radiat Oncol Biol Phys 29(1):33–37

Slotman BJ, van Tinteren H, Praag JO, Knegjens JL, El Sharouni SY, Hatton M, Keijser A, Faivre-Finn C, Senan S (2015) Use of thoracic radiotherapy for extensive stage small-cell lung cancer: a phase 3 randomised controlled trial. Lancet 385(9962):36–42

Spiegelman D, Maurer LH, Ware JH, Perry MC, Chahinian AP, Comis R, Eaton W, Zimmer B, Green M (1989) Prognostic factors in small-cell carcinoma of the lung: an analysis of 1,521 patients. J Clin Oncol. 7(3):344–354

Stinchcombe TE, Zhang Y, Vokes EE, Schiller JH, Bradley JD, Kelly K, Curran WJ Jr, Schild SE, Movsas B, Clamon G, Govindan R, Blumenschein GR, Socinski MA, Ready NE, Akerley WL, Cohen HJ, Pang HH, Wang X (2017) Pooled analysis of individual patient data on concurrent chemoradiotherapy for stage III non-small-cell lung cancer in elderly patients compared with younger patients who participated in US National Cancer Institute Cooperative Group studies. J Clin Oncol 35(25):2885–2892

Stinchcombe TE, Fan W, Schild SE, Vokes EE, Bogart J, Le QT, Thomas CR, Edelman MJ, Horn L, Komaki R, Cohen HJ, Kishor Ganti A, Pang H, Wang X (2019) A pooled analysis of individual patient data from National Clinical Trials Network clinical trials of concurrent chemoradiotherapy for limited-stage small cell lung cancer in elderly patients versus younger patients. Cancer 125(3):382–390

Stokes WA, Bronsert MR, Meguid RA, Blum MG, Jones BL, Koshy M, Sher DJ, Louie AV, Palma DA, Senan S, Gaspar LE, Kavanagh BD, Rusthoven CG (2018) Post-treatment mortality after surgery and stereotactic body radiotherapy for early-stage non-small-cell lung cancer. J Clin Oncol 36(7):642–651

Strom HH, Bremnes RM, Sundstrom SH, Helbekkmo N, Aasebo U (2015) How do elderly poor prognosis patients tolerate palliative concurrent chemoradiotherapy for locally advanced non-small-cell lung cancer stage III? A Subset Analysis From a Clinical Phase III Trial. Clin Lung Cancer 16(3):183–192

Takahashi T, Yamanaka T, Seto T, Harada H, Nokihara H, Saka H, Nishio M, Kaneda H, Takayama K, Ishimoto O, Takeda K, Yoshioka H, Tachihara M, Sakai H, Goto K, Yamamoto N (2017) Prophylactic cranial irradiation versus observation in patients with extensive-disease small-cell lung cancer: a multicentre, randomised, open-label, phase 3 trial. Lancet Oncol 18(5):663–671

Tamiya A, Morimoto M, Fukuda S, Naoki Y, Ibe T, Okishio K, Goto H, Yoshii A, Kita T, Nogami N, Fujita Y, Atagi S (2018) A phase I/II trial of pemetrexed plus radiotherapy in elderly patients with locally advanced non-small cell lung cancer. Invest New Drugs 36(4):667–673

Timmerman R, McGarry R, Yiannoutsos C, Papiez L, Tudor K, DeLuca J, Ewing M, Abdulrahman R, DesRosiers C, Williams M, Fletcher J (2006) Excessive toxicity when treating central tumors in a phase II study of stereotactic body radiation therapy for medically inoperable early-stage lung cancer. J Clin Oncol 24(30):4833–4839

Timmerman RD, Hu C, Michalski J, Straube W, Galvin J, Johnstone D, Bradley J, Barriger R, Bezjak A, Videtic GM, Nedzi L, Werner-Wasik M, Chen Y, Komaki R, Choy H (2014) Long-term results of RTOG 0236: a phase II trial of stereotactic body radiation therapy (SBRT) in the treatment of patients with medically inoperable stage I non-small cell lung cancer. Int J Radiat Oncol Biol Phys 90(1):S30

Tombolini V, Bonanni A, Donato V, Raffetto N, Santarelli M, Valeriani M, Enrici RM (2000) Radiotherapy alone in elderly patients with medically inoperable stage IIIA and IIIB non-small cell lung cancer. Anticancer Res 20(6C):4829–4833

Topkan E, Parlak C, Selek U (2013a) Impact of weight change during the course of concurrent chemoradiation therapy on outcomes in stage IIIB non-small cell lung cancer patients: retrospective analysis of 425 patients. Int J Radiat Oncol Biol Phys 87(4):697–704

Topkan E, Parlak C, Topuk S, Guler OC, Selek U (2013b) Outcomes of aggressive concurrent radiochemotherapy in highly selected septuagenarians with stage IIIB non-small cell lung carcinoma: retrospective analysis of 89 patients. Lung Cancer 81(2):226–230

Topkan E, Selek U, Ozdemir Y, Besen AA, Guler OC, Yildirim BA, Mertsoylu H, Findikcioglu A, Ozyilkan O, Pehlivan B (2018a) Risk factors for fatal pulmonary hemorrhage following concurrent chemoradiotherapy in stage 3B/C squamous-cell lung carcinoma patients. J Oncol 2018:4518935

Topkan E, Selek U, Ozdemir Y, Yildirim BA, Guler OC, Ciner F, Besen AA, Findikcioglu A, Ozyilkan O (2018b) Incidence and impact of pretreatment tumor cavitation on survival outcomes of stage III squamous cell lung cancer patients treated with radical concurrent chemoradiation therapy. Int J Radiat Oncol Biol Phys 101(5):1123–1132

Topkan E, Selek U, Ozdemir Y, Yildirim BA, Guler OC, Mertsoylu H, Hahn SM (2018c) Chemoradiotherapy-induced hemoglobin nadir values and survival in patients with stage III non-small cell lung cancer. Lung Cancer. 121:30–36

Topkan E, Bolukbasi Y, Ozdemir Y, Besen AA, Mertsoylu H, Selek U (2019a) Prognostic value of pretreatment Glasgow prognostic score in stage IIIB geriatric non-small cell lung cancer patients undergoing radical chemoradiotherapy. J Geriatr Oncol 10(4):567–572

Topkan E, Ozdemir Y, Kucuk A, Besen AA, Mertsoylu H, Sezer A, Selek U (2019b) Significance of overall concurrent chemoradiotherapy duration on survival outcomes of stage IIIB/C non-small-cell lung carcinoma patients: analysis of 956 patients. PLoS One 14(7):e0218627

Topkan E, Selek U, Kucuk A, Haksoyler V, Ozdemir Y, Sezen D, Mertsoylu H, Besen AA, Bolukbasi Y, Ozyilkan O, Pehlivan B (2021) Prechemoradiotherapy systemic inflammation response index stratifies stage IIIB/C non-small-cell lung cancer patients into three prognostic groups: a propensity score-matching analysis. J Oncol 2021:6688138

Verma V, Simone CB 2nd, Allen PK, Gajjar SR, Shah C, Zhen W, Harkenrider MM, Hallemeier CL, Jabbour SK, Matthiesen CL, Braunstein SE, Lee P, Dilling TJ, Allen BG, Nichols EM, Attia A, Zeng J, Biswas T, Paximadis P, Wang F, Walker JM, Stahl JM, Daly ME, Decker RH, Hales RK, Willers H, Videtic GM, Mehta MP, Lin SH (2017) Multi-institutional experience of stereotactic ablative radiation therapy for stage I small cell lung cancer. Int J Radiat Oncol Biol Phys 97(2):362–371

Videtic GMM, Donington J, Giuliani M, Heinzerling J, Karas TZ, Kelsey CR, Lally BE, Latzka K, Lo SS, Moghanaki D, Movsas B, Rimner A, Roach M, Rodrigues G, Shirvani SM, Simone CB 2nd, Timmerman R, Daly ME (2017) Stereotactic body radiation therapy for early-stage non-small cell lung cancer: Executive Summary of an ASTRO Evidence-Based Guideline. Pract Radiat Oncol 7(5):295–301

Wang S, Wong ML, Hamilton N, Davoren JB, Jahan TM, Walter LC (2012) Impact of age and comorbidity on non-small-cell lung cancer treatment in older veterans. J Clin Oncol 30(13):1447–1455

Werner-Wasik M, Scott C, Cox JD, Sause WT, Byhardt RW, Asbell S, Russell A, Komaki R, Lee JS (2000) Recursive partitioning analysis of 1999 Radiation Therapy Oncology Group (RTOG) patients with locally-advanced non-small-cell lung cancer (LA-NSCLC): identification of five groups with different survival. Int J Radiat Oncol Biol Phys 48(5):1475–1482

Westeel V, Murray N, Gelmon K, Shah A, Sheehan F, McKenzie M, Wong F, Morris J, Grafton C, Tsang V, Goddard K, Murphy K, Parsons C, Amy R, Page R (1998) New combination of the old drugs for elderly patients with small-cell lung cancer: a phase II study of the PAVE regimen. J Clin Oncol 16(5):1940–1947

Wildiers H, Heeren P, Puts M, Topinkova E, Janssen-Heijnen ML, Extermann M, Falandry C, Artz A, Brain E, Colloca G, Flamaing J, Karnakis T, Kenis C, Audisio RA, Mohile S, Repetto L, Van Leeuwen B, Milisen K, Hurria A (2014) International Society of Geriatric Oncology consensus on geriatric assessment in older patients with cancer. J Clin Oncol 32(24):2595–2603

Wisnivesky JP, Bonomi M, Henschke C, Iannuzzi M, McGinn T (2005) Radiation therapy for the treatment of unresected stage I-II non-small cell lung cancer. Chest 128(3):1461–1467

Wisnivesky JP, Halm E, Bonomi M, Powell C, Bagiella E (2010) Effectiveness of radiation therapy for elderly patients with unresected stage I and II non-small cell lung cancer. Am J Respir Crit Care Med 181(3):264–269

Wolfson AH, Bae K, Komaki R, Meyers C, Movsas B, Le Pechoux C, Werner-Wasik M, Videtic GM, Garces YI, Choy H (2011) Primary analysis of a phase II randomized trial Radiation Therapy Oncology Group (RTOG) 0212: impact of different total doses and schedules of prophylactic cranial irradiation on chronic neurotoxicity and quality of life for patients with limited-disease small-cell lung cancer. Int J Radiat Oncol Biol Phys 81(1):77–84

Xu J, Yang H, Fu X, Jin B, Lou Y, Zhang Y, Zhang X, Zhong H, Wang H, Wu D, Han B (2017) Prophylactic cranial irradiation for patients with surgically resected small cell lung cancer. J Thorac Oncol 12(2):347–353

Yamaguchi M, Hirata H, Ebi N, Araki J, Seto T, Maruyama R, Akamine S, Inoue Y, Semba H, Sasaki J, Okamoto T (2020) Phase II study of vinorelbine plus carboplatin with concurrent radiotherapy in elderly patients with non-small-cell lung cancer. Jpn J Clin Oncol 50(3):318–324

Yang Y, Zhang D, Zhou X, Bao W, Ji Y, Sheng L, Cheng L, Chen Y, Du X, Qiu G (2018) Prophylactic cranial irradiation in resected small cell lung cancer: a systematic review with meta-analysis. J Cancer 9(2):433–439

Yu HM, Liu YF, Yu JM, Liu J, Zhao Y, Hou M (2008) Involved-field radiotherapy is effective for patients 70 years old or more with early stage non-small cell lung cancer. Radiother Oncol 87(1):29–34

Zachariah B, Balducci L, Venkattaramanabalaji GV, Casey L, Greenberg HM, DelRegato JA (1997) Radiotherapy for cancer patients aged 80 and older: a study of effectiveness and side effects. Int J Radiat Oncol Biol Phys 39(5):1125–1129

Radiation Therapy for Intrathoracic Recurrence of Lung Cancer

Yukinori Matsuo, Hideki Hanazawa, Noriko Kishi, Kazuhito Ueki, and Takashi Mizowaki

Contents

1 Introduction 718
2 Postsurgical Locoregional Recurrence 718
2.1 Bronchial Stump Recurrence 719
2.2 Isolated LN Recurrence 721
3 Definitive Reirradiation for Locoregional Recurrence 721
3.1 Definitive Reirradiation with CFRT 722
3.2 Reirradiation Using SBRT 724
3.3 Reirradiation with Particle Therapy 726
3.4 Dose Constraints for Organs at Risk 727
4 Definitive Treatment for Recurrent Small Cell Lung Cancer 728
5 Palliative Reirradiation 729
5.1 Reirradiation with EBRT 729
5.2 Endobronchial Brachytherapy for Reirradiation 731
References 732

Y. Matsuo (✉) · H. Hanazawa · N. Kishi · K. Ueki · T. Mizowaki
Department of Radiation Oncology and Image-applied Therapy, Graduate School of Medicine, Kyoto University, Kyoto, Japan
e-mail: ymatsuo@kuhp.kyoto-u.ac.jp

Abstract

Radiation therapy (RT) plays an important role in the management of recurrent lung cancer after surgery or definitive RT, not only for palliative but also for curative purposes. Definitive RT for locoregional recurrence after surgical resection facilitates comparative survival for de novo stage III lung cancer with acceptable toxicities. Recent technological advances in beam delivery for highly conformal RT (SBRT, IMRT, proton, etc.) and imaging modalities (FDG PET for early detection of tumor recurrence, 4D CT for precise target delineation in treatment planning, cone beam CT for daily patient positioning, etc.) have permitted reirradiation of patients for curative purposes, which had been previously considered difficult. A better performance status with good pulmonary function, a longer period after previous RT, and a smaller volume of the recurrent tumor may facilitate better survival. However, reirradiation is associated with a potential risk of severe toxicities. When applying reirradiation, careful attention to the proximity of the recurrent tumor to organs at risk and evaluation of cumulative dose distributions are needed. In palliative settings, thoracic RT offers quick and efficient palliation of symptoms.

1 Introduction

Radiation therapy (RT) is an essential treatment modality for the initial management of various stages of lung cancer as well as surgery and chemotherapy. RT also plays an important role in the management of recurrent lung cancer, not only for palliative but also for curative purposes.

The standard treatment for clinical stage I–II non-small cell lung cancer (NSCLC) is surgical resection, followed by adjuvant chemotherapy if needed (National Comprehensive Cancer Network 2021a). Approximately, a quarter of patients with NSCLC who undergo complete resection develop tumor recurrence (Sonobe et al. 2014). Among them, patients with isolated local recurrence, which accounts for 20% of the postsurgical recurrence (Yano 2014), are supposed to be provided curative treatment with salvage local treatment, where radiotherapy contributes.

Concurrent chemoradiotherapy is the standard treatment for unresectable stage III NSCLC. Locoregional recurrence is a dominant pattern of recurrence after concurrent chemo-RT, with an incidence of 30–35% (Mitsuyoshi et al. 2017). Salvage surgery is only applied to selected patients with locoregional recurrence after chemo-RT (Dickhoff et al. 2018). The recent development of highly conformal radiotherapy (stereotactic body radiotherapy [SBRT] and intensity-modulated radiotherapy [IMRT]) and various imaging techniques (18F-fluorodeoxyglucose positron emission tomography [FDG PET] for recurrent tumor localization, four-dimensional computed tomography [4D CT] for treatment planning, cone beam CT for patient positioning, etc.) has permitted easier patient reirradiation, which was previously considered difficult.

As the population ages, the number of SBRT applications for early-stage NSCLC is increasing (Okami 2019). SBRT offers 80–90% of local tumor control (Nagata et al. 2015), which leads to better survival than conventionally fractionated RT (CFRT) (Ball et al. 2019). SBRT is now considered the standard treatment for medically inoperable cases of early-stage NSCLC. A few patients develop isolated local (4–8%) or regional recurrence (4–5%) after SBRT. Although salvage surgery may lead to longer survival in patients with isolated local tumor recurrence (Hamaji et al. 2015), the indication of salvage surgery is limited by the conditions of the patients that require SBRT as initial treatment. Repeat SBRT or CFRT is an option for locoregional recurrence after initial SBRT (Brooks et al. 2020).

Similar to curative-intent treatment, thoracic RT plays an essential role in the palliative setting of lung cancer. Locoregional regrowth of lung cancer causes symptoms of hemoptysis, cough, chest pain, dyspnea, obstructive pneumonia, dysphagia, superior vena cava occlusion (SVCO), and hoarseness (Kepka and Olszyna-Serementa 2010). Thoracic RT offers quick and efficient palliation of symptoms, with a symptom control rate of 60–70% (Fairchild et al. 2008).

In this chapter, we review the literature and summarize the available evidence on RT for intrathoracic recurrence for curative or palliative purposes. RT for second primary lung cancer or oligometastatic tumors will be discussed in other chapters.

2 Postsurgical Locoregional Recurrence

Postsurgical recurrences are usually divided into chest wall/pleural, lung parenchymal, bronchial stump, and mediastinal lymph node (LN) recurrences and their combinations. The NCCN Guidelines for NSCLC recommend surgical resection (as a preferred therapy) and external beam RT (EBRT) for resectable locoregional recurrence (National Comprehensive Cancer Network 2021a). However, the indications for repeat surgical resection are very limited (Hung et al. 2009). Stojiljkovic et al. reported their experiences in 51 patients with local recurrence after the initial resection for stage I–IV NSCLC (Stojiljkovic et al. 2013). The most frequent site of recurrence that was surgically retreated was the chest wall. Surgery has rarely been applied to bronchial stump or mediastinal LN recurrence.

Definitive local treatment for locoregional recurrence of NSCLC may facilitate survival outcomes similar to those in patients with de novo locally advanced NSCLC who are treated with definitive chemo-RT (Cai et al. 2010; Friedes et al. 2020). Cai et al. (2010) compared the survivals in patients with postsurgical recurrence and newly diagnosed NSCLC, both of which were treated with RT. The 5-year overall survival (OS) was 14.8% in the patients with postsurgical recurrence and 11.0% in newly diagnosed patients, respectively, favoring those with recurrence. From published data during the past decade (Table 1), it can be assumed that when postsurgical locoregional recurrent patients are treated with definitive RT, the 5-year OS rate is 30–40% and the median survival time (MST) is 20–40 months (Bae et al. 2012; Ma et al. 2017; Wu et al. 2017; Nakamichi et al. 2017; Lee et al. 2019). There is no concrete evidence of an appropriate RT technique or the validity of elective regional irradiation. The proportion of patients who receive concurrent chemotherapy with salvage RT varies significantly from 20 to 100% in the reports. Platinum doublet regimens are commonly used. Two studies have found that the concurrent use of chemotherapy and radiotherapy facilitates better prognosis (Kim et al. 2017; Nakamichi et al. 2017).

Recent findings on the treatment strategy include the application of SBRT for postsurgical locoregional recurrence. Takeda et al. reported 23 locally recurrent cases, including stump, staple line, and thoracic wall recurrences, with a prescribed dose of 40–60 Gy in 5–10 fractions (Takeda et al. 2013). Twelve patients had centrally located recurrent lesions, including one invading the aorta. The 2-year local control (LC) rate and OS rate were 87% and 76.4%, respectively. They reported two cases of bronchial stenosis within the planning target volume (PTV) as late toxicity. Agoli et al. also indicated the possibility of SBRT in 28 patients with postoperative locally recurrent NSCLC (Agolli et al. 2015). The treated sites included stump (3%), thoracic wall (7%), ipsilateral lung lesion (60%), and mediastinal LN (30%) recurrences. The prescribed doses were 23 Gy in one fraction for mediastinal LNs, 30 Gy in one fraction for peripheral tumors, and 45 Gy in three fractions for central tumors. The OS rate at 2 years was 57.5%. No severe esophageal or tracheal fistula or bleeding was reported as late toxicity. According to a more recent study by Sittenfeld et al., 48 patients received SBRT for isolated local recurrence after surgery (Sittenfeld et al. 2020). Half of the cases had a peripheral tumor, and a quarter had central and ultra-central tumors. With approximately 70% of OS rate at 2 years, severe late toxicity of grade 3 was observed in three patients: cough, atelectasis, and soft tissue necrosis leading to a broncho-cutaneous fistula. The incidence of severe toxicities was slightly higher than that of CFRT. Thus, SBRT may be an option for selected patients: those with a peripherally located lesion and sufficient pulmonary function. However, intensive hypofractionated SBRT to a central lesion requires careful consideration of toxicities.

2.1 Bronchial Stump Recurrence

Recurrence confined to the bronchial stumps seems to have a better prognosis than combined stump and node recurrences according to the reports of several studies published in the late 1990s (Jeremic and Bamberg 2002). With the prescribed dose of more than 50 Gy with radical intent, MST was approximately 30 months, and the 2- and 5-year survival rates were approximately 55% and 30%, respectively (Kagami et al. 1998; Jeremic and Bamberg 2002; Kono et al. 1998). Combined stump and node recurrences resulted in a shorter MST of approximately 1 year. Although there seems to be a dose-response effect on bronchial stump-only recurrences, the optimal dose is unclear. As in locally advanced NSCLC, CFRT with 60–66 Gy is recommended for isolated bronchial stump recurrence. The benefits of concurrent chemotherapy have not been sufficiently proven.

Table 1 Selected series on salvage radiotherapy for locoregional recurrence after surgery for lung cancer

Author	N	Recurrent site or stage	Total dose (median) (Gy)	Concurrent chemo (%)	5-year in-field LC (%)	5-year PFS (%)	5-year OS (%)	MST (months)	Toxicities
Locoregional recurrence									
Bae et al. (2012)	64	Stump or chest wall 45.3%, LN 40.6%, Combined 14.1%	40–66	22	52.3 (2 years)	–	47.9 (2 years)	18.5	Pneumonitis 11% (G3~) Esophagitis 0 (G3~)
Ma et al. (2017)	74	Stump 10.8%, LN 75.7%, Ipsilateral lung 8.1%, combined 5.4%	66	60	–	42.5 (2 years)	84.2 (2 years)	–	Pneumonitis 1.4% (G3~) Esophagitis 9.5% (G3~)
Wu et al. (2017)	152	rI-II-III = 22.3–20.4–57.2%	CFRT: 45–90 (60) SBRT: 30–60 (45)	94	–	–	28	23	–
Nakamichi et al. (2017)	74	rT: 0/1-2 = 72–28% rN: 0–2/3 = 69–31%	50–70 (60)	24	–	31 (2 years)	37	34.4	Pneumonitis 7% (G3~) Esophagitis 7% (G2~)
Lee et al. (2019)	127	rI-II-IIIa-IIIb-c = 7.1–9.4–44.9–38.6%	37–70 (60)	100	73.8	22.3	43.9	49	Pneumonitis 4.7% (G3~) Esophagitis 45% (G2~)
Stump recurrence									
Kagami et al. (1998)	10	Stump	47.5–65		–	–	30	18	Acute toxicity none (G3~) Late toxicity none (severe)
Jeremic (1999)	15	Stump	55–60		–	–	33	36	–
Isolated regional LN									
Okami et al. (2013)	50	N1-2-3 = 20–56–24%	50–84	12	61.1	22.2	36.1	37.3	Pneumonitis 2% (G3~) Acute toxicity 14% (G2~)
Seol et al. (2017)	31	Single LN: 48.4% Multiple LNs: 51.6%	51–66	23	75.8 (2 years)	50.9 (2 years)	58.4 (2 years)	–	Pneumonitis 3.2% (G3~)
Manabe et al. (2018)	27[a]	–	54–66 (64)	11.1	81	30	24	–	Pneumonitis 4% (G3~) Esophagitis 7% (G2~)

LC local control, *PFS* progression-free survival, *OS* overall survival, *MST* median survival time, *LN* lymph node, *G* grade, *CFRT* conventionally fractionated radiotherapy, *SBRT* stereotactic body radiotherapy

[a] Includes 13 post-SBRT recurrent patients

2.2 Isolated LN Recurrence

Okami et al. reported 50 cases in which high-dose RT was delivered after the diagnosis of isolated regional LN recurrence (Okami et al. 2013). In approximately half of the cases, the elective LN area was included in the irradiation field. Progression-free survival (PFS) and OS rates at 5 years were 22% and 36%, respectively. Only one patient (2%) developed grade 3 pneumonitis. The absence of symptoms and a single LN station were prognostic factors for better survival. Another study by Seol et al. reviewed 31 cases of regional LN recurrence (Seol et al. 2017). Definitive RT with a total dose of 66 Gy was administered for curative purposes. In this study, the clinical target volume (CTV) included nodal areas adjacent to the involved LNs, which were assumed to have a high risk. The PFS at 2 years was 50.9%. One patient (3.2%) experienced grade 3 pneumonitis as late toxicity. An LN size of <3 cm was a marginally significant factor for better OS. Data from the SBRT series also help in the treatment decisions for isolated LN recurrence. Manabe et al. reported 27 patients who developed isolated regional LN recurrence after SBRT or surgery and underwent salvage RT for recurrence (Manabe et al. 2018). The median dose of salvage RT was 60 Gy for post-SBRT patients and 66 Gy for post-surgery patients. The local control rates at 5 years were 58% and 92% for the post-SBRT and post-surgery groups, respectively. Severe toxicities were observed in three patients (grade 5 pneumonitis, grade 3 esophagitis, and grade 3 dermatitis in one patient each). Ward et al. evaluated salvage RT for isolated nodal failure after SBRT (Ward et al. 2016). The most common regimen was 45 Gy in 15 fractions (for 53% of the patients), although various dose regimens ranging from 17 Gy in 2 fractions to 60.4 Gy in 33 fractions were also used. No patients experienced grade 3 events due to radiation. The authors suggested that 45 Gy in 15 fractions is ideal for several medically inoperable patients, but 60 Gy in 30 fractions with chemotherapy would be an option for selected patients.

3 Definitive Reirradiation for Locoregional Recurrence

Reirradiation is a double-edged sword for the management of recurrent cancer. It can provide excellent local control of the tumor, leading to symptom relief and/or potential cure, while increasing the risk of severe toxicities, such as radiation pneumonitis, bronchial fistula, and radiation myelitis. We need to balance the benefits and risks when considering reirradiation. There is no strong consensus on reirradiation for recurrent lung cancer. Expert opinions may be helpful in this situation. Hunter et al. proposed a seven-step process for reirradiation of recurrent NSCLC in their review paper (Hunter et al. 2021). The process consists of disease assessment (restaging with PET and brain MRI, histological confirmation, and review of other treatment options), patient assessment (performance status, pulmonary function, comorbidities, etc.), initial RT plan review (doses to the organs at risk [OARs], and time from previous RT), consent process (discussion of benefit vs. risks including severe and fatal toxicities), RT planning (assessment of field overlap, CTV margin reduction, highly conformal techniques, etc.), radiosensitization (concurrent chemotherapy), and ongoing care/follow-up. Rulach et al. conducted an international expert survey on radical thoracic reirradiation for NSCLC (Rulach et al. 2021). The experts agreed to 33 statements including the following key recommendations: appropriate patients should have a good performance status and can have locally relapsed disease or second primary cancers, and there are no absolute values for pulmonary function that precludes reirradiation; a full diagnostic workup should be performed in patients with suspected local recurrence; any reirradiation should be delivered using optimal image guidance and highly conformal techniques. No consensus was reached on the minimal interval between the initial treatment and reirradiation. The American Radium Society and the American College of Radiology have recently compiled the appropriate use criteria systematic review and guidelines on reirradiation for NSCLC (Simone et al. 2020). IMRT in CFRT is recommended over three-dimensional conformal RT (3D CRT). Furthermore, particle therapy is referred to as a method to reduce toxicity and/or enable safer dose escalation compared with 3D CRT or IMRT. The concurrent use of chemotherapy and RT has been suggested, but the decision should be based on individual patient/tumor characteristics. However, the concurrent use of targeted therapy or immunotherapy and reirradiation is not recommended outside of a clinical trial. SBRT can be an optimal option for reirradiation for primary tumor recurrence in the peripheral lungs. During treatment planning for reirradiation, the evaluation of the composite dose distribution is vital to assess the risk of severe toxicities, as discussed below. Deformable image registration will improve correlative toxicity data, which may lead to a reduction in toxicity for patients undergoing reirradiation (Senthi et al. 2013; Ren et al. 2018).

3.1 Definitive Reirradiation with CFRT

Selected reports on definitive reirradiation with CFRT are shown in Table 2 (Okamoto et al. 2002; Wu et al. 2003; Tada et al. 2005; Ohguri et al. 2012; Griffioen et al. 2014; Kruser et al. 2014; Huh et al. 2014; Sumita et al. 2016; Hong et al. 2019; Schlampp et al. 2019; Yang et al. 2020; McAvoy et al. 2014). There are variations in the initial treatment (RT/chemo-RT with or without surgery), initial stage (early stage, locally advanced, or metastatic), recurrence pattern, histology, and irradiation technique (2D/3D CRT, IMRT, or SBRT). Therefore, the reported outcomes vary widely; MST, 1-year OS, and 2-year OS were 3–31 months, 47–77%, and 33–64%, respectively. The median local control (LC) time and 1-year LC were 7–13 months and 50–60%, respectively.

A prospective phase I–II study was conducted by Wu et al. (2003). They investigated the efficacy and tolerance of reirradiation with 3D CRT in 23 patients with locoregional recurrence. The median dose of initial radiotherapy was 66 Gy and that of reirradiation was 51 Gy in 2 Gy fractions. The 1- and 2-year OS rates were 59% and 21%, respectively, and the 1- and 2-year locoregional progression-free rates were 51% and 42%, respectively. No acute toxicities of ≥grade 3 were observed. Two patients (8.7%) presented with grade 3 pulmonary fibrosis as late toxicities.

McAvoy et al. reported the experiences of 102 patients with NSCLC who underwent reirradiation for intrathoracic recurrence (McAvoy et al. 2014). The median duration from the initial RT to reirradiation was 17 months. Reirradiation was delivered using IMRT with a median prescribed dose of 60.5 Gy in equivalent dose in 2 Gy fraction (EQD2). Thirty-three percent of patients received concurrent chemotherapy. The MST was 14.7 months, and the 1- and 2-year OS rates were 52.8% and 36.6%, respectively. The 1- and 2-year local failure-free survival rates were 49.2% and 34.2%, respectively. The observed severe late toxicities were grade 3 esophageal toxicities (7%) and grade 3 pulmonary toxicities (10%). No toxicities of ≥grade 4 were observed.

Schlampp et al. reported 62 patients who underwent reirradiation for locally recurrent lung cancer using 3D CRT or IMRT (Schlampp et al. 2019). The median duration from initial RT to reirradiation was 14 months. Reirradiation was delivered using 3D CRT or IMRT with a median dose of 38.5 Gy in 1.8–3 Gy per fraction. Locoregional failure was 6.5% with an MST of 9.3 months. Toxicities of ≥grade 3 were observed in five patients (9.2%). The median forced expiratory volume in 1 s (FEV_1) and vital capacity decreased slightly after reirradiation in patients for whom spirometry data were available (68% of the enrolled patients). An FEV_1 of more than 1.4 L was significantly associated with better survival after reirradiation.

3.1.1 Prognostic Factors for Treatment Outcomes and Toxicities

Several prognostic factors for treatment outcomes and toxicities in patients treated with reirradiation have been reported. A favorable prognosis was observed in patients with non-squamous cell carcinoma, preserved performance status, a small size of recurrent tumor, and a long

Table 2 Selected reports on definitive reirradiation with conventionally fractionated radiotherapy

Author	No. of pt.	Interval (months)	Re-RT dose (Gy)	PTV (cm³)	Systemic chemo	Local control	2-year OS (MST)	Toxicity G3-4	Fatal toxicity
Okamoto et al. (2002)	34	23 (5–87)	50 (10–70)	n/a	C: 15% S: 32%	n/a	51% (15 months)	7 G3 RP 2 G3 esophagitis	None
Wu et al. (2003)	23	13 (6–42)	51 (46–60)	GTV: 80 (30–138)	S: 1–3 cycles	Locoregional PFS: 51% at 1 year	21% (14 months)	2 G3 pulmonary fibrosis	None
Tada et al. (2005)	19	16 (5–60)	50 (50–60)	n/a	C: 5%	n/a	11% (7.1 months)	1 G3 RP	None
Ohguri et al. (2012)	33	7.9 (1.1–28.2)	50 (29–70)	n/a	(Hyperthermia)	12.1 months	(18.1 months)	1 G3 thrombocytopenia 1 G3 pleuritis, 1 G3 BPN	None
Griffioen et al. (2014)	24	51 (5–189)	60 (39–66)	248 (59–1140)	C: 8% S: 54%	n/a	51% at 1 year (13.5 months)	1 G3 esophagitis 1 G3 dermatitis	3 Bleeding
Kruser et al. (2014)	37	18.6	30 (12–60)	149 (26–585)	None	n/a	(5.1 months)	1 G3 dyspnea, 1 G3 RP 1 G4 bronchostenosis	None
McAvoy et al. (2014)	102	17 (0–376)	EQD2: 60.5 (25.2–155)	GTV: 27.1 (1.3–690)	C: 33%	Local PFS: 11.4 months, 49.2% at 1 year	33% (14.7 months)	7 G3 RP, 3 G4 RP; 5 G3 esophagitis, 2 G4 esophagitis	None
Huh et al. (2014)	15	12 (5–41)	36 (25.2–45.2)	GTV: 78.8 (6.8–180.4)	C: 20% S: 20%	n/a	47% at 1 year (11 months)	None	None
Sumita et al. (2016)	21	26.8 (11.4–92.3)	EQD2: NSCLC, 60 (54–87.5); SCLC, 50 (50–87.5)	57.4 (7–601.7)	C: 5%	12.9 months 57% at 1 year	64% (31.4 months)	1 G3 RP	None
Hong et al. (2019)	31	15.1 (4.4–56.3)	50 (35–65)	51.3 (13–299.3)	C: 10%	60% at 1 year	39% (20.4 months)	1 G3 pericarditis	None
Schlampp et al. (2019)	62	14 (3–103)	38.5 (20–60)	176 (n/a)	S: 35%	Locoregional PFS: 6.5 months	(9.3 months)	1 G4 trachea-esophageal fistula, 1 G3 esophageal stenosis, 2 G3 RP, 1 G3 pneumothorax	1 Pneumonia
Yang et al. (2020)	50	13 (4.3–53.3)	EQD2: 51.1 (16.2–125.0)	201.6 (12.8–1180)	C: 18% S: 42%	Time to local progression: 18 months	(25.1 months)	6 G3-4 lung	7 lung

BPN brachial plexus neuropathy, *C* concurrent, *ED* extended disease, *EQD2* equivalent dose in 2 Gy fractions, *G* grade, *LD* limited disease, *n/a* not available, *NSCLC* non-small cell lung cancer, *PFS* progression-free survival, *PTV* planning target volume, *S* sequential, *SCLC* small cell lung cancer, *RT* radiotherapy, *Re-RT* reirradiation, *RP* radiation pneumonitis duration from the initial RT (Schlampp et al. 2019; McAvoy et al. 2014). These patients can be candidates for treatment with reirradiation at high doses. High-dose reirradiation leads to better treatment outcomes of locoregionally recurrent lung cancer (Hong et al. 2019). On the other hand, the high doses used for reirradiation are associated with a higher risk of toxicity than the palliative doses (Kruser et al. 2014). Common toxicities reported after definitive reirradiation with CFRT are acute and/or late esophageal and pulmonary toxicities. Concurrent chemotherapy and high-dose reirradiation can improve the outcome, although it increases the risks of esophageal toxicities (McAvoy et al. 2014). Concurrent use of chemotherapy and high-dose reirradiation should be determined carefully, considering the risk-and-benefit balance, which can be affected by the previously mentioned factors and dose constraints for OARs. The target volume for reirradiation was an important factor. The reported relationship included a large internal gross tumor volume (GTV, ≥ 27 cm^3) with worse LC and OS, large internal target volume (≥ 94 cm^3) with worse OS (McAvoy et al. 2014), small PTV less than 300 cm^3 with improved OS (Griffioen et al. 2014), irradiation of less than two mediastinal LN stations with the better OS, and irradiation of the aorta with worse OS (Schlampp et al. 2019).

3.2 Reirradiation Using SBRT

The advantage of using SBRT for salvage therapy is its high local control. On the other hand, the disadvantage is the risk of serious adverse events. Viani et al. conducted a meta-analysis on the effectiveness and safety of reirradiation with SBRT for recurrence after thoracic RT (Viani et al. 2020). They reviewed 20 studies comprising 595 patients. LC and OS rates at 2 years in the pooled cohort were 73% and 54%, respectively. The dose for re-SBRT, tumor size, and time to recurrence were associated with survival. Grade 3 or worse toxicities were observed in 9.8% of the patients, including 1.5% of grade 5. The incidence of toxicities of grade ≥ 3 was significantly different in patients with cumulative doses of >145 Gy in EQD2 and <145 Gy (15% vs. 3%). The local control and toxicity associated with the use of high doses of SBRT present a dilemma.

In addition, when applying SBRT, it is necessary to pay attention to tumor localization. The concept of a "central" tumor was first introduced by Timmerman et al. in 2006 based on their experience of the high incidence of severe toxicity in the central lesions after SBRT (Timmerman et al. 2006). The common definition of a central tumor is provided by RTOG 0813 as a tumor within or touching the zone 2 cm around the proximal bronchial tree (the trachea, carina, and named major lobar bronchi up to their first bifurcation) or immediately adjacent to the mediastinal or pericardial pleura (i.e., the PTV touches the pleura) (Bezjak et al. 2019). In 2015, Chaudhuri et al. introduced the "ultra-central" tumor, which was defined as a tumor directly abutting the proximal bronchial tree or trachea, as an entity at higher risk for SBRT among central tumors (Chaudhuri et al. 2015). If the recurrence is limited to the peripheral lung only, SBRT can be considered for its local control potential and short-term treatment. However, for centrally located or ultra-central tumors, the application of SBRT requires special caution due to the severe toxicities in the mediastinal or hilar organs (great vessels, bronchi, trachea, etc.), especially under reirradiation conditions. CFRT is used instead in such situations.

3.2.1 Repeat SBRT

Several authors have reported on reirradiation using SBRT, but irradiation delivery techniques in the initial and salvage treatments have varied among reports. Here, we will discuss only those reports in which SBRT was used for both initial and salvage treatment (repeat SBRT) or in which CFRT was used for initial treatment and SBRT was used for salvage (SBRT after CFRT) (Table 3). Peulen et al. published the first report on the repeat SBRT in 2011 (Peulen et al. 2011). The report consisted of 29 patients with 32 lesions, including 11 centrally located lesions. Nine patients suffered from severe (grade 3 or

Table 3 Selected reports on SBRT for recurrent lung cancer after definitive radiotherapy

Author	No. of pt./lesion	Interval (months)	Location	Tumor size	Salvage SBRT dose	Local control	Survival	Toxicity G3–4	Fatal toxicity
SBRT → SBRT									
Peulen et al. (2011)	29/32	14 (5–54)	Peripheral: 21 Central: 11	PTV: 76 mL (16–355)	20–45 Gy/1–5 fr	52% at 5 months	59% at 1 year 43% at 2 years	8 patients (G3 RP, G4 SVCO, etc.)	3 Hemoptysis
Hearn et al. (2014)	10/10	14.8 (9.9–26.3)	Peripheral: 8 Central: 2	3.4 cm (1.7–4.8)	50 Gy/5 fr: 7 60 Gy/3 fr: 3	60%	n/a	None	None
Ogawa et al. (2018)	31/31	18 (4–80)	Peripheral: 22 Central: 9	3.2 cm (1.2–7.4)	48–52 Gy/4: 13 60 Gy/8 f: 13 Other: 5	53% at 3 years	36% at 3 years	None	None
CFRT → SBRT									
Kelly et al. (2000)	36	22 (0–92)	n/a	1.7 cm (0.6–3.8)	50 Gy/4 fr: 26 40 Gy/4 fr: 6 Other: 4	92%	59% at 2 years	7 G3 RP 3 G3 Esophagitis 11 CWP, etc.	None
Trovo et al. (2014)	17	18 (1–60)	Central: 17	n/a	30 Gy/5 fr: 12 30 Gy/6 fr: 5	86% at 1 year	59% at 1 year 29% at 2 years MST: 19 months	4 G3 RP	1 RP 1 Hemoptysis
Parks et al. (2016)	27/29	13.4 (2.6–112.6)	Peripheral: 11 Central lung: 1 Mediastinum: 9 Hilum: 9	PTV: 29 mL (6.5–448)	50 Gy/5 fr (30–54 Gy/3–5 fr)	Local recurrence-free survival: 72% at 2 years	79% at 2 years	6 G3 RP 1 G3 CWP 1 G4 CWP	None
Repka et al. (2017)	20	30.8 (47–90)	UC lung: 2 Mediastinum: 10 Hilum: 8	GTV: 71.4 mL, 147 mL	35 Gy/5 fr (25–45 Gy/5 fr)	30% at 1 year	45% at 1 year	1 G3 Recurrent nerve palsy	1 Hemoptysis
Sumodhee et al. (2019)	46	22.6 (6.2–101.5)	Peripheral: 22 Central: 24	3.3 cm (1–6)	60 Gy/4 fr (40–75 Gy/3–5 Fr)	44.2% at 4 years	48.9% at 2 years 30.8% at 4 years	None	1 Alveolitis 1 Hemoptysis
Sood et al. (2021)	20/21	14.6 (4–100)	Mediastinum: 4 Hilum: 12 Other UC: 5	PTV: 49.2 mL (12–181)	50 Gy/10 fr (40–70 Gy/10 fr)	83% at 1 year	68% at 1 year	1 G3 RP 1 G3 Esophagitis	2 Hemoptysis *unlikely* related

Values are expressed as median (range)
SBRT stereotactic body radiotherapy, *CFRT* conventionally fractionated radiotherapy, *pt.* patient, *UC* ultra-central, *SVCO* superior vena cava occlusion, *RP* radiation pneumonitis, *CWP* chest wall pain, *MST* median survival time

worse) toxicities, including three cases of fatal bleeding in patients with central lesions. Larger clinical target volumes and central tumor locations were associated with greater toxicity. Hearn et al. suggested appropriate patient selection for salvage SBRT (Hearn et al. 2014). They applied repeat SBRT to 10 patients after excluding 22 patients who had large tumors, tumors abutting to the mediastinum and chest wall, tumors within the zone of proximal bronchus, a history of overlapping conventional RT before initial SBRT, severe medical comorbidity, or persistent chest wall pain from initial SBRT. The treatment resulted in no grade 3–5 toxicity. Ogawa et al. reported the highest number of patients receiving salvage SBRT for "in-field" recurrence after prior SBRT for NSCLC or pulmonary metastasis (Ogawa et al. 2018). The recurrent tumor was located in the peripheral lung in 22 patients and central in 9 patients without an ultra-central location. None of the patients developed grade 3 or worse toxicities for a median follow-up period of 26 months. The local control rate was 53% at 3 years. In summary, local control by re-SBRT is approximately 60%, which is worse than that by initial SBRT but better than that for reirradiation with CFRT (Yoshitake et al. 2013). Tumor location is a key indication for repeat SBRT. Peripherally located recurrence is a candidate for definitive reirradiation with SBRT. The application of repeat SBRT to central, but not ultra-central, tumors is still controversial, but it may only be eligible if the tumor is small and image guidance and respiratory motion management are available to reduce PTV margins. Repeat SBRT for ultra-central tumors is not recommended in the currently available reports.

3.2.2 Radical SBRT After CFRT

In most of the patients with initial stage III LN involvement who were treated with initial CFRT, central or ultra-central regions were considered for salvage reirradiation. Therefore, a lower BED than that for initial SBRT was applied in several reports of salvage SBRT for this type of recurrence (Table 3). Trovo et al. delivered SBRT with 30 Gy in 5–6 fractions for 17 patients with in-field recurrence or persistence of centrally located NSCLC (Trovo et al. 2014). Two patients experienced grade 5 toxicities. Parks et al. re-treated 29 lesions in 27 patients with SBRT (Parks et al. 2016). BED for reirradiation was associated with OS and PFS. Repka et al. applied SBRT to 20 patients with ultra-central in-field recurrence, with a median dose of 35 Gy in five fractions (Repka et al. 2017). The dose was prescribed to GTV without margins, which may have resulted in balanced outcomes for LC and toxicities (LC of 83% at 1 year and grade 3 toxicities of 10%).

3.3 Reirradiation with Particle Therapy

There are only a few reports on reirradiation with particle therapy, including proton beam radiotherapy (PBT) and carbon-ion radiotherapy (CIRT). The use of particle therapy may provide dosimetric advantages, but in a retrospective analysis, there was no significant benefit of PBT over IMRT related to esophageal or pulmonary toxicities (McAvoy et al. 2014). The reported outcomes of reirradiation with PBT were MST of 11.1–18.0 months with 1-year OS and PFS rates of 47–59% and 28–59%, respectively (Chao and Berman 2018). Two multi-institutional prospective studies have reported on reirradiation with PBT. Chao et al. reported reirradiation with PBT for locoregional recurrent NSCLC in or near the previously irradiated field (Chao et al. 2017). Among the 57 enrolled patients, 52 (93%) completed the planned reirradiation. The 1-year OS and PFS rates were 59% and 58%, respectively. Fourteen patients (25%) experienced local or regional recurrences. Toxicities of grade ≥3 were observed in 24 patients (42%). Grade 5 toxicities were observed in six patients. An increase in the overlap with the central airway region, an increase in the mean dose of the esophagus and heart, and the concurrent use of chemotherapy were significantly associated with the incidence of toxicities of grade ≥3. The other was reported by Badiyan et al., which is a multi-institutional prospective registry for recurrent NSCLC (Badiyan et al. 2019). All patients ($n = 79$) completed planned reirradiation. The median OS and PFS were 15.2 months and 10.5 months, respectively. Acute and late toxicities of grade ≥3 were observed in 6% and 1% of patients, respectively. Grade 5 toxicities were observed in three patients. The multivariate analysis showed that an ECOG-PS of ≤1 was associated with OS and PFS. Retrospective studies from the MD Anderson Cancer Center were reported: 33 recurrent NSCLC patients treated with PBT between 2006 and 2011 and 27 intrathoracic cancers (81% were NSCLC) treated with intensity-modulated proton therapy (IMPT) from 2011 to 2016 (McAvoy et al. 2013, 2014; Ho et al. 2018). The 1-year OS and LC were 47% and 54% for PBT, respectively, and the corresponding rates were 54% and 78%, respectively. Among patients treated with PBT, esophageal and pulmonary toxicities of grade ≥3 were observed in 9% and 21% of patients, respectively, whereas late grade 3 toxicities were observed in 7% of patients treated with IMPT. They suggested that IMPT may allow safe reirradiation with improved outcomes.

According to two Japanese CIRT centers, 2-year OS and LC for reirradiation for lung cancer with CIRT are 54–75% and 60–92%, respectively (Hayashi et al. 2018; Karube et al. 2017; Shirai et al. 2019). Hayashi et al. reported that among patients reirradiated with CIRT for lung tumors ($n = 95$, including 73 primary lung cancer), 4% experienced severe toxicities including grade 5 bronchopleural fistula, grade 4 radiation pneumonitis, grade 3 chest pain, and grade 3 radiation pneumonitis (Hayashi et al. 2018). In another retrospective study, there were no toxicities of grade ≥3 after reirradiation with CIRT among patients with isolated LN recurrece after surgery or CIRT ($n = 15$) (Shirai et al. 2019). Further studies are warranted to evaluate the clinical benefits of CIRT for recurrent lung cancer.

3.4 Dose Constraints for Organs at Risk

To date, no established dose constraints are available. However, data on the toxicity and safety of reirradiation based on various studies are gradually being accumulated. Some of the existing literature have been introduced below. Based on these data, in an international survey, Rulach et al. and the American Radium Society have recently published their recommendations on cumulative dose constraints for OARs in the thorax (Table 4) (Rulach et al. 2021; Simone et al. 2020).

3.4.1 Lung

Liu et al. suggested predictive factors for severe pneumonitis in patients receiving SBRT after CFRT (Liu et al. 2012). Composite lung V20 of ≥30%, ECOG-PS of 2–3, FEV1 of <65%, and prior irradiation of the bilateral mediastinum were associated with severe pneumonitis. Meijneke et al. reported that none of the patients who were treated with composite median V5 of 41% (range: 8–72%) and V20 of 15% (3–47%) for the lung suffered from grade 3 or worse toxicities (Meijneke et al. 2013). According to Binkley et al., composite lung V20 ranging from 4.7% to 38.4% resulted in no grade 3 or worse pulmonary toxicities (Binkley et al. 2016).

3.4.2 Esophagus

In the report by Binkley et al., patients with grade 2–3 esophagitis had cumulative D1cc of 41–100.6 Gy for the esophagus (Binkley et al.

Table 4 Proposed constraints for cumulative doses to the organs at risk

	Rulach et al. (2021)	Simone et al. (2020)
Spinal cord	Dmax 60 Gy	Dmax <57 Gy
Esophagus	Dmax 75–100 Gy	V60 <40%, Dmax <100–110 Gy
Brachial plexus	Dmax 80–95 Gy	Dmax <85 Gy
Great vessels	Dmax 110–115 Gy	Dmax <120 Gy
Proximal bronchial tree	Dmax <80–105 Gy	Dmax <110 Gy
Skin/chest wall	ALARA	n/a
Heart	ALARA	V40 <50%
Lung	Individualized	V20 <40%

Doses are expressed as equivalent dose in 2 Gy fractions (EQD2)
Dmax maximal dose, *ALARA* as low as reasonably achievable, *n/a* not available

2016). According to Meijneke et al., among eight patients receiving a maximal accumulated dose of 70.5–123.2 Gy to the esophagus, none developed a grade 3 toxicity (Meijneke et al. 2013). Schröder et al. reported a case of grade 5 esophageal rupture with accumulated D1cc of 48.4 Gy, where a viral esophagitis was suspected to negatively affect rupture (Schröder et al. 2020).

3.4.3 Aorta

Evans et al. reported that two of eight (25%) patients receiving cumulative D1cc of >120 Gy (normalized to 1.8 Gy/fraction) in the aorta developed grade 5 aortic toxicities, which were not found in those with aorta D1cc of <120 Gy (Evans et al. 2013). Kilburn et al. reported a case of grade 5 aorto-esophageal fistula after re-SBRT of 54 Gy in three fractions for a central tumor with a cumulative EQD2 of 200 Gy to the aorta (Kilburn et al. 2014).

3.4.4 Spinal Cord

Nieder et al. summarized data on radiation myelopathy after reirradiation from their institution and published reports (Nieder et al. 2006). The risk of radiation myelitis is low after cumulative BED of <135.5 Gy_2 (=67.5 Gy in EQD2) when the treatment interval is 6 months or more and the BED of each course is <98 Gy_2 (=49 Gy in EQD2). According to a report by a study involving 19 patients who underwent re-SBRT for spinal metastasis after CFRT (Sahgal et al. 2012), the Dmax to the thecal sac should not exceed 70 Gy in EQD2 with a treatment interval of >5 months and an SBRT dose of <50% of the total dose to the cord.

3.4.5 Brachial Plexus

Chen et al. reviewed their patients who received reirradiation of the brachial plexus (Chen et al. 2017). The medians of cumulative Dmax and Dmean to the brachial plexus were 95.0 Gy (60.5–150.1 Gy) and 63.8 Gy (20.2–111.5 Gy), respectively. Six of the 13 patients (46%) with Dmax of >95 Gy and treatment interval of <2 years developed brachial plexopathy. Binkley et al. reported a case of brachial plexopathy with D0.2cc of 242.5 Gy in EQD2 (Binkley et al. 2016).

3.4.6 Proximal Bronchial Tree

Feddock et al. reported that a cumulative maximum BED_3 to the pulmonary artery of <175 Gy (=105 Gy in EQD2) appears to be safe (Feddock et al. 2013). However, two patients who developed local recurrence died of hemorrhage, and it seemed difficult to distinguish between treatment-related toxicity and local recurrence as the cause of death. In a phase I study of dose-escalated hypofractionated RT without concurrent chemotherapy, grade 4–5 toxicities were correlated with the dose to the proximal bronchial tree (Cannon et al. 2013). The EQD2 for the 5% incidence of grades 4–5 at 2 years was estimated to be 75 Gy of D3cc and 83 Gy of Dmax to the proximal bronchial tree.

4 Definitive Treatment for Recurrent Small Cell Lung Cancer

Due to the metastatic nature of small cell lung cancer (SCLC), systemic chemotherapy is recommended for recurrent SCLC (National Comprehensive Cancer Network 2021b). The chemotherapy regimen was chosen according to the duration from the completion of the initial therapy to the relapse. For patients with a relapse of >6 months, readministration of the first-line regimen is recommended. Second-line chemotherapy is considered for patients with relapse at 6 months or earlier (Gong and Salgia 2018). Very few reports are available on salvage surgery for recurrent SCLC. Survival longer than 20 months was achieved after salvage surgery in a report by Nakanishi et al. (2019). Reports on reirradiation for locoregionally recurrent SCLCs are also limited (Kruser et al. 2014; Käsmann et al. 2016). Käsmann et al. conducted a multi-institutional retrospective cohort study on thoracic reirradiation for recurrent SCLC (Käsmann et al. 2020). Thirty-three patients from four university hospitals in Germany, Japan, Turkey, and the United States were reviewed. The reirradiation was performed for a median duration of 24 months after the initial chemo-RT. The dose for reirradiation ranged from 20 to 87.5 Gy in EQD2. Grade 3 acute pulmonary toxicity was observed in one patient. The MST after reirradiation was 7 months (range: 1–54 months). For patients with a good performance status, a reirradiation dose of >40 Gy in EQD2 resulted in favorable survival (56% at 2 years). Extrathoracic disease was found to be an independent negative prognostic factor for survival of less than 6 months.

5 Palliative Reirradiation

One of the difficult clinical issues is the provision of palliative treatment for patients with lung cancer who have been previously irradiated. Systemic therapy can be considered, especially in tumors harboring gene mutations in the epidermal growth factor receptor (EGFR). If an EGFR-tyrosine kinase inhibitor (TKI) has never been administered to a patient, palliative-intent reirradiation can be postponed. EGFR-TKIs can achieve prompt symptom relief within 2–3 weeks (Xia et al. 2017). Patients who are not candidates for systemic therapy may be considered for palliative reirradiation. Drodge et al. divided the indications for reirradiation into four categories: emergent symptomatic, such as superior vena cava obstruction (SVCO); symptomatic but not emergent, such as dyspnea; asymptomatic with an impending serious event, such as airway obstruction; and asymptomatic with radiological disease progression (Drodge et al. 2014). Thus, there are several situations where reirradiation is considered to alleviate the symptoms of patients with lung cancer. The following is an overview of palliative reirradiation for lung cancer with a focus on symptom relief and a discussion of the role of brachytherapy.

5.1 Reirradiation with EBRT

Acknowledging the inherent limitations of the retrospective nature and limited size of most available studies, palliative reirradiation appears to be a feasible option for recurrent symptomatic lung cancer. Table 5 summarizes the studies on reirradiation with EBRT that reported on specific symptom relief (Green and Melbye 1982; Jackson and Ball 1987; Montebello et al. 1993; Gressen et al. 2000; Kramer et al. 2004; Cetingoz et al. 2009; Huh et al. 2014; Nieder et al. 2020). Several

Table 5 Palliative reirradiation with EBRT

Author	n	Dose[a] (median, Gy)	Hemoptysis (%)	SVCO (%)[b]	Cough (%)	Chest pain (%)	Dyspnea (%)	Total (%)	Toxicity (%)
Green and Melbye (1982)	29	53 + 35	33	n.s.	55	n.s.	44	48	Rib fracture: 3 Pneumonitis: 3
Jackson and Ball (1987)	22	55 + 30	83	0 (0/1)	50	40	67	50	Myelopathy: 5
Montebello et al. (1993)	30	60 + 30	89	75 (3/4)	64	77	53	70	Esophagitis: 20 Pneumonitis: 3
Gressen et al. (2000)	23	59 + 30	100	n.s.	60	80	73	72	G5 pneumonitis: 4
Kramer et al. (2004)	28	46–60 + 2 × 8	100	100 (4/4)	67	n.s.	35	71	G2 esophagitis 4
Cetingoz et al. (2009)	38	30 + 25	86	100 (1/1)	77	60	69	78	Esophagitis G1–2: 77 G3: 4
Huh et al. (2014)	15	63 + 36	100	n.s.	88	67	83	80	G2 pneumonitis: 7
Nieder et al. (2020)	33	39 + 30	n.s.	n.s.	n.s.	43	n.s.	38	G3 pneumonitis: 6

SVCO superior vena cava obstruction, *n.s.* not stated, *G* grade
[a] Dose of initial irradiation + reirradiation
[b] Since the number of patients is small, actual number is also shown

other reports (not in the table) that assessed general symptom improvement have also been reviewed (Okamoto et al. 2002; Poltinnikov et al. 2005; Ebara et al. 2007; Kruser et al. 2014).

The reirradiation doses in the reports varied from a hypofractionated schedule of 16 Gy/2 fractions (Kramer et al. 2004) up to 60 Gy in conventional fractionation (Okamoto et al. 2002). There is no consensus on the reirradiation dose for palliative purposes, but guidelines for general palliative irradiation may be helpful. In 2011 (updated in 2018), the American Society for Radiation Oncology (ASTRO) published clinical practice guidelines on palliative thoracic RT for lung cancer (Rodrigues et al. 2011; Moeller et al. 2018). The authors considered reserving higher dose regimens (30 Gy/10 fractions or greater) for patients with good performance status and those with sufficient life expectancy. For other patients, various shorter fractionation schedules (16–17 Gy/2 fractions, 20 Gy/5 fractions, etc.) provided similar symptomatic improvement and were preferred to reduce the treatment duration.

What makes it difficult to evaluate the effectiveness of palliative reirradiation is that there is no validated scoring system for the symptom response. Kramer et al. created their scoring system (Kramer et al. 2004), which has been used in several subsequent studies (Ebara et al. 2007; Kruser et al. 2014; Huh et al. 2014). In the series, the physician scored the relief of complaints according to the patient's statement for each symptom as follows: vanished, diminished, stabilized, or progressive. As shown in Table 5, the overall symptom improvement rates ranged from 38 to 78% of those assessable. Among the specific symptoms assessed, hemoptysis and SVCO appeared to be well palliated; the median improvement rate reported was above 80%. Reirradiation seems to be less effective for dyspnea (35–83%) and cough (50–88%), although it is difficult to assess this symptom because its causes are complex, and they may include cigarette smoking and radiation side effects (Kepka and Olszyna-Serementa 2010). Regarding the prognostic factors for symptomatic relief, the following did not appear to be significant: histology (Jackson and Ball 1987), dose (Jackson and Ball 1987; Okamoto et al. 2002), tumor size (Cetingoz et al. 2009), previous irradiation aim (radical vs. palliative) (Cetingoz et al. 2009), or specific symptom (Okamoto et al. 2002). Some patients treated palliatively received chemotherapy, but data remain insufficient to evaluate the role of chemotherapy in palliative reirradiation for lung cancer.

The median duration of symptom response reported by three series (Montebello et al. 1993; Kramer et al. 2004; Kruser et al. 2014) ranged from 0.5 to 4 months. Kruser et al. treated NSCLC patients with a median of 30 Gy in a median of 10 fractions and SCLC patients with a median of 37.5 Gy in a median of 15 fractions (Kruser et al. 2014). The percentage of assessable patients with symptom relief was high (75% and 100%, respectively), but the duration of relief was shorter in patients with SCLC than those with NSCLC at a median of 1.8 and 0.5 months, respectively. In the study by Kramer et al., the palliative effect lasted in most patients until the last month of their life (Kramer et al. 2004). However, those who lived for >6 months had recurrent complaints during their remaining life spans. In the series where all patients were palliatively treated, MST ranged from 4.9 to 11 months (median 5.6 months). Longer intervals between the initial irradiation and reirradiation (Kramer et al. 2004; Cetingoz et al. 2009) and favorable treatment response (imaging or symptoms) (Nieder et al. 2020) were associated with longer durations of survival.

The most frequent toxicities were radiation pneumonitis and esophagitis. Radiation pneumonitis tended to increase with higher doses, with the frequency of symptomatic radiation pneumonitis (grade 2 or higher) being 56% in the report by Okamoto et al. (2002) and 14% in the report by Ebara et al. (2007). In the study by Poltinnikov et al. in which hypofractionated radiotherapy was used, concurrent chemotherapy was associated with the development of acute esophagitis (Poltinnikov et al. 2005). Overall, the rate of serious complications was well tolerated considering the patient's prognosis, although the risk of late toxicity for the few long-term survivors is unknown.

5.2 Endobronchial Brachytherapy for Reirradiation

Endobronchial brachytherapy (EBB) is an attractive option for the treatment of symptomatic endobronchial disease, allowing for a highly localized dose of radiation while reducing the dose to normal tissue. Technological advances since the 1990s, such as a high dose rate (HDR) with remote afterloading and computerized dosimetry, have increased the use of EBBs (Kepka and Olszyna-Serementa 2010). The 2011 ASTRO guidelines (Rodrigues et al. 2011) and a Cochrane review published in 2012 (Reveiz et al. 2012) state that EBRT alone is more effective for palliation than EBB alone as a first-line palliative treatment for endobronchial obstruction, although EBB remains a reasonable therapeutic option for patients previously treated with EBRT who are symptomatic because of endobronchial central obstruction. Table 6 outlines some noncomparative prospective studies and several retrospective reports on HDR-EBB for recurrent lung cancer previously treated with EBRT (Gauwitz et al. 1992; Speiser and Spratling 1993; Ornadel et al. 1997; Bedwinek et al. 1992; Gollins et al. 1994; Kelly et al. 2000; Hauswald et al. 2010; Knox et al. 2018).

Various doses and fractionation schedules are used in clinical treatment, with the most common being high doses ranging from 10 to 15 Gy in one to a maximum of four fractions (at 10 mm from the source). More fractions present advantages related to reducing late toxicities, whereas a single-dose protocol is cost saving and prevents multiple bronchoscopies to the patient. The American Brachytherapy Society guidelines in 2016 recommend several dose fractionation schemes: HDR 10–15 Gy in one fraction, 14.2–

Table 6 Palliative reirradiation with HDR-EBB

Author	n (all)	Initial EBRT (Gy)	Dose/depth/fr	MST (mo)	Symptomatic response rate	Fatal toxicity (% or number of patients)
Gauwitz et al. (1992)	24	>55	15 Gy/6 mm/2 fr	8	Overall 88% Reaeration 83%	None (treatment related)
Bedwinek et al. (1992)	38	>50	6 Gy/10 mm/3 fr	6.5	Overall 76% Cough/hemoptysis 80% Fever/shortness of breath 71%	Fatal hemoptysis: 32%
Speiser and Spratling (1993)	342	n.s.	10 Gy/10 mm/3 fr 7.5 Gy/10 mm/3 fr	6.2	Hemoptysis 99% Dyspnea 86% Cough 85% (All at 1–2 mo)	Fatal hemoptysis: 7%
Gollins et al. (1994)	406	10.9–55	15–20 Gy/10 mm/1 fr	4.3	Hemoptysis 88%, stridor 75%, cough 55%, dyspnea 52%, pain 60%, collapse 7% (all at 1.5 mo)	Fatal hemoptysis: 7.9%
Ornadel et al. (1997)	117	30 (20–60)	15 Gy/10 mm/1 fr	12	Hemoptysis 89% Dyspnea 73%	Fatal hemoptysis: 11%
Kelly et al. (2000)	175	n.s.	15 Gy/6–7.5 mm/1–4 fr	6	Considerable 32% Only slight 34%	Fatal hemoptysis: 5% Tissue necrosis and fistula formation: 1 Stenosis and necrosis: 1
Hauswald et al. (2010)	41	56 (30–70)	5 Gy/10 mm/n.s. Total 15 Gy (median)	6.7	Excellent 12% Good 46%	Fatal hemorrhage: 1 Tissue necrosis: 3 Bronchomediastinal fistula: 2
Knox et al. (2018)	92	7.5–66	10 Gy/5–10 mm/1 fr	8	Hemoptysis 92% Airway obstruction 70%	None (treatment related)

EBRT external beam radiotherapy, *MST* median survival time, *mo* months, *fr* fractions, *n.s.* not stated

20 Gy in two fractions, 22.5 Gy in three fractions, 24 Gy in four fractions, and 30 Gy in six fractions (Stewart et al. 2016).

Symptom regression has been observed in 58–99% of patients. Regarding the specific symptoms reported, hemoptysis appears to be the most effective in relieving the symptoms, ranging from 88% to 99%. Improvements in other specific symptoms were reported as follows: dyspnea (52–88%), cough (55–85%), and obstruction/collapse of the airway (7–83%). The duration of relief ranged from 3.8 to 7.5 months. Regarding the factors influencing the degree of symptom relief, Bedwinek et al. reported that patients with tumors less than 5 cm were more likely to have symptomatic improvement than those with tumors greater than 5 cm (Bedwinek et al. 1992). Speiser and Spratling reported that the improvement in airway obstruction was worse in patients with recurrence than in the curative group (70% vs. 83%) (Speiser and Spratling 1993). Kelly et al. reported a significant association between the patient's subjective assessment of treatment response and objective findings from repeat bronchoscopy (Kelly et al. 2000). MST ranged from 4.3 to 12 months. Hauswald et al. reported that the prognostic factors for survival were a Karnofsky performance score of 80% or above (11.0 months vs. 4.4 months) and a total HDR-EBB dose of 15 Gy or more (8.0 months vs. 2.2 months) (Hauswald et al. 2010). In the series by Kelly et al. (2000) and Knox et al. (2018), patients who responded favorably survived significantly longer than those who did not respond.

Among the serious complications reported, fatal hemoptysis was less than 10% in most reports, with the highest rate being 32% (Bedwinek et al. 1992). However, it is somewhat difficult to discuss the frequency of side effects because fatal hemorrhage may be caused by locally progressive disease, radiation side effects, or their combination (Hauswald et al. 2010). Kelly et al. reported that the actuarial hazard rate of fatal hemoptysis as a direct result of EBB is 2% at 6 months after treatment, reaching a plateau at 5% at 14 months after treatment (Kelly et al. 2000). In the study by Gollins et al., it was implied that the doses for the first EBB treatment (20 Gy vs. 15 Gy), previous laser treatment, and repeated EBB treatments in the same location were the risk factors for extensive hemorrhage (Gollins et al. 1996).

Acknowledgment This work is partially supported by AMED under Grant Number JP20ck0106427.

References

Agolli L, Valeriani M, Carnevale A, Falco T, Bracci S, De SV et al (2015) Role of salvage stereotactic body radiation therapy in post-surgical loco-regional recurrence in a selected population of non-small cell lung cancer patients. Anticancer Res 35:1783–1789

Badiyan SN, Rutenberg MS, Hoppe BS, Mohindra P, Larson G, Hartsell WF et al (2019) Clinical outcomes of patients with recurrent lung cancer reirradiated with proton therapy on the Proton Collaborative Group and University of Florida Proton Therapy Institute Prospective Registry Studies. Pract Radiat Oncol 9(4):280–288. https://doi.org/10.1016/j.prro.2019.02.008

Bae SH, Ahn YC, Nam H, Park HC, Pyo HR, Shim YM et al (2012) High dose involved field radiation therapy as salvage for loco-regional recurrence of non-small cell lung cancer. Yonsei Med J 53(6):1120. https://doi.org/10.3349/ymj.2012.53.6.1120

Ball D, Mai GT, Vinod S, Babington S, Ruben J, Kron T et al (2019) Stereotactic ablative radiotherapy versus standard radiotherapy in stage 1 non-small-cell lung cancer (TROG 09.02 CHISEL): a phase 3 open-label, randomised controlled trial. Lancet Oncol 20(4):494–503. https://doi.org/10.1016/S1470-2045(18)30896-9

Bedwinek J, Petty A, Bruton C, Sofield J, Lee L (1992) The use of high dose rate endobronchial brachytherapy to palliate symptomatic endobronchial recurrence of previously irradiated bronchogenic carcinoma. Int J Radiat Oncol Biol Phys 22(1):23–30. http://www.ncbi.nlm.nih.gov/pubmed/1727125

Bezjak A, Paulus R, Gaspar LE, Timmerman RD, Straube WL, Ryan WF et al (2019) Safety and efficacy of a five-fraction stereotactic body radiotherapy schedule for centrally located nonsmall-cell lung cancer: NRG Oncology/RTOG 0813 trial. J Clin Oncol 37(15):1316–1325. https://doi.org/10.1200/jco.18.00622

Binkley MS, Hiniker SM, Chaudhuri A, Maxim PG, Diehn M, Loo BW et al (2016) Dosimetric factors and toxicity in highly conformal thoracic reirradiation. Int J Radiat Oncol Biol Phys 94(4):808–815. https://doi.org/10.1016/j.ijrobp.2015.12.007

Brooks ED, Verma V, Senan S, De BT, Lu S, Brunelli A et al (2020) Salvage therapy for locoregional recurrence after stereotactic ablative radiotherapy for early-stage NSCLC. J Thorac Oncol. 15:176–189

Cai X-W, Xu L-Y, Wang L, Hayman JA, Chang AC, Pickens A et al (2010) Comparative survival in patients with postresection recurrent versus newly diagnosed nonsmall-cell lung cancer treated with radiotherapy. Int J Radiat Oncol Biol Phys 76(4):1100–1105. https://doi.org/10.1016/j.ijrobp.2009.03.017

Cannon DM, Mehta MP, Adkison JB, Khuntia D, Traynor AM, Tomé WA et al (2013) Dose-limiting toxicity after hypofractionated dose-escalated radiotherapy in nonsmall-cell lung cancer. J Clin Oncol 31(34):4343–4348. https://doi.org/10.1200/jco.2013.51.5353

Cetingoz R, Arican-Alicikus Z, Nur-Demiral A, Durmak-Isman B, Bakis-Altas B, Kinay M (2009) Is re-irradiation effective in symptomatic local recurrence of non-small cell lung cancer patients? A single institution experience and review of the literature. J BUON 14(1):33–40. https://pubmed.ncbi.nlm.nih.gov/19373944/

Chao H-H, Berman AT (2018) Proton therapy for thoracic reirradiation of non-small cell lung cancer. Transl Lung Cancer Res 7(2):153–159. https://doi.org/10.21037/tlcr.2018.03.22

Chao H-H, Berman AT, Simone CB, Ciunci C, Gabriel P, Lin H et al (2017) Multi-institutional prospective study of reirradiation with proton beam radiotherapy for locoregionally recurrent nonsmall cell lung cancer. J Thorac Oncol 12(2):281–292. https://doi.org/10.1016/j.jtho.2016.10.018

Chaudhuri AA, Tang C, Binkley MS, Jin M, Wynne JF, von Eyben R et al (2015) Stereotactic ablative radiotherapy (SABR) for treatment of central and ultracentral lung tumor. Lung Cancer 89(1):50–56. https://doi.org/10.1016/j.lungcan.2015.04.014

Chen AM, Yoshizaki T, Velez MA, Mikaeilian AG, Hsu S, Cao M (2017) Tolerance of the brachial plexus to high-dose reirradiation. Int J Radiat Oncol Biol Phys 98(1):83–90. https://doi.org/10.1016/j.ijrobp.2017.01.244

Dickhoff C, Schaap PMR, Otten RHJ, Heymans MW, Heineman DJ, Dahele M (2018) Salvage surgery for local recurrence after stereotactic body radiotherapy for early stage non-small cell lung cancer: a systematic review. Ther Adv Med Oncol 10:175883591878798. https://doi.org/10.1177/1758835918787989

Drodge CS, Ghosh S, Fairchild A (2014) Thoracic reirradiation for lung cancer: a literature review and practical guide. Ann Palliat Med. 3:75–91

Ebara T, Tanio N, Etoh T, Shichi I, Honda A, Nakajima N (2007) Palliative re-irradiation for in-field recurrence after definitive radiotherapy in patients with primary lung cancer. Anticancer Res 27(1B):531–534. http://www.ncbi.nlm.nih.gov/pubmed/17348437

Evans JD, Gomez DR, Amini A, Rebueno N, Allen PK, Martel MK et al (2013) Aortic dose constraints when reirradiating thoracic tumors. Radiother Oncol 106(3):327–332. https://doi.org/10.1016/j.radonc.2013.02.002

Fairchild A, Harris K, Barnes E, Wong R, Lutz S, Bezjak A et al (2008) Palliative thoracic radiotherapy for lung cancer: a systematic review. J Clin Oncol 26(24):4001–4011. https://doi.org/10.1200/jco.2007.15.3312

Feddock J, Cleary R, Arnold S, Shelton B, Sinha P, Conrad G et al (2013) Risk for fatal pulmonary hemorrhage does not appear to be increased following dose escalation using stereotactic body radiotherapy (SBRT) in locally advanced non-small cell lung cancer (NSCLC). J Radiosurg SBRT 2:235–242

Friedes C, Mai N, Fu W, Hu C, Han P, Marrone KA et al (2020) Propensity score adjusted analysis of patients with isolated locoregional recurrence versus de novo locally advanced NSCLC treated with definitive therapy. Lung Cancer 145:119–125. https://doi.org/10.1016/j.lungcan.2020.04.035

Gauwitz M, Ellerbroek N, Komaki R, Putnam JB, Ryan MB, DeCaro L et al (1992) High dose endobronchial irradiation in recurrent bronchogenic carcinoma. Int J Radiat Oncol Biol Phys 23(2):397–400. http://www.ncbi.nlm.nih.gov/pubmed/1587762

Gollins SW, Burt PA, Barber PV, Stout R (1994) High dose rate intraluminal radiotherapy for carcinoma of the bronchus: outcome of treatment of 406 patients. Radiother Oncol 33(1):31–40

Gollins SW, Ryder WDJ, Burt PA, Barber PV, Stout R (1996) Massive haemoptysis death and other morbidity associated with high dose rate intraluminal radiotherapy for carcinoma of the bronchus. Radiother Oncol 39(2):105–116. https://doi.org/10.1016/0167-8140(96)01731-8

Gong J, Salgia R (2018) Managing patients with relapsed small-cell lung cancer. J Oncol Pract 14(6):359–366. https://doi.org/10.1200/jop.18.00204

Green N, Melbye RW (1982) Lung cancer: retreatment of local recurrence after definitive irradiation. Cancer 49:865–868

Gressen EL, Werner-Wasik M, Cohn J, Topham A, Curran WJ (2000) Thoracic reirradiation for symptomatic relief after prior radiotherapeutic management for lung cancer. Am J Clin Oncol 23(2):160–163. http://www.ncbi.nlm.nih.gov/pubmed/10776977

Griffioen GHMJ, Dahele M, de Haan PF, van de Ven PM, Slotman BJ, Senan S (2014) High-dose conventionally fractionated thoracic reirradiation for lung tumors. Lung Cancer 83(3):356–362. https://doi.org/10.1016/j.lungcan.2013.12.006

Hamaji M, Chen F, Matsuo Y, Ueki N, Hiraoka M, Date H (2015) Treatment and prognosis of isolated local relapse after stereotactic body radiotherapy for clinical stage I non-small-cell lung cancer. J Thorac Oncol 10(11):1616–1624. https://doi.org/10.1097/jto.0000000000000662

Hauswald H, Stoiber E, Rochet N, Lindel K, Grehn C, Becker HD et al (2010) Treatment of recurrent bronchial carcinoma: the role of high-dose-rate endoluminal brachytherapy. Int J Radiat Oncol Biol Phys 77(2):373–377. http://www.ncbi.nlm.nih.gov/pubmed/19836162

Hayashi K, Yamamoto N, Karube M, Nakajima M, Tsuji H, Ogawa K et al (2018) Feasibility of carbon-ion radiotherapy for re-irradiation of locoregionally recurrent, metastatic, or secondary lung tumors. Cancer Sci 109(5):1562–1569. https://doi.org/10.1111/cas.13555

Hearn JWD, Videtic GMM, Djemil T, Stephans KL (2014) Salvage stereotactic body radiation therapy (SBRT) for local failure after primary lung SBRT. Int J Radiat Oncol Biol Phys 90(2):402–406. https://doi.org/10.1016/j.ijrobp.2014.05.048

Ho JC, Nguyen QN, Li H, Allen PK, Zhang X, Liao Z et al (2018) Reirradiation of thoracic cancers with intensity modulated proton therapy. Pract Radiat Oncol 8:58–65

Hong JH, Kim Y-S, Lee S-W, Lee SJ, Kang JH, Hong SH et al (2019) High-dose thoracic re-irradiation of lung cancer using highly conformal radiotherapy is effective with acceptable toxicity. Cancer Res Treat 51(3):1156–1166. https://doi.org/10.4143/crt.2018.472

Huh GJ, Jang SS, Park SY, Seo JH, Cho EY, Park JC et al (2014) Three-dimensional conformal reirradiation for locoregionally recurrent lung cancer previously treated with radiation therapy. Thorac Cancer 5(4):281–288. https://doi.org/10.1111/1759-7714.12089

Hung J-J, Hsu W-H, Hsieh C-C, Huang B-S, Huang M-H, Liu J-S et al (2009) Post-recurrence survival in completely resected stage I non-small cell lung cancer with local recurrence. Thorax 64(3):192–196. https://doi.org/10.1136/thx.2007.094912

Hunter B, Crockett C, Faivre-Finn C, Hiley C, Salem A (2021) Re-irradiation of recurrent non-small cell lung cancer. Semin Radiat Oncol 31(2):124–132. https://doi.org/10.1016/j.semradonc.2020.11.009

Jackson MA, Ball DL (1987) Palliative retreatment of locally-recurrent lung cancer after radical radiotherapy. Med J Aust 147(8):391–394. http://www.ncbi.nlm.nih.gov/pubmed/2443823

Jeremic B, Bamberg M (2002) External beam radiation therapy for bronchial stump recurrence of non-small-cell lung cancer after complete resection. Radiother Oncol 64(3):251–257. https://doi.org/10.1016/s0167-8140(02)00023-3

Kagami Y, Nishio M, Narimatsu N, Mjoujin M, Sakurai T, Hareyama M et al (1998) Radiotherapy for locoregional recurrent tumors after resection of non-small cell lung cancer. Lung Cancer 20(1):31–35. https://doi.org/10.1016/s0169-5002(98)00008-7

Karube M, Yamamoto N, Tsuji H, Kanematsu N, Nakajima M, Yamashita H et al (2017) Carbon-ion re-irradiation for recurrences after initial treatment of stage I non-small cell lung cancer with carbon-ion radiotherapy. Radiother Oncol 125(1):31–35. https://doi.org/10.1016/j.radonc.2017.07.022

Käsmann L, Janssen S, Schild SE, Rades D (2016) Karnofsky performance score and radiation dose predict survival of patients re-irradiated for a locoregional recurrence of small cell lung cancer. Anticancer Res 36:803–805

Käsmann L, Janssen S, Baschnagel AM, Kruser TJ, Harada H, Aktan M et al (2020) Prognostic factors and outcome of reirradiation for locally recurrent small cell lung cancer—a multicenter study. Transl Lung Cancer Res 9(2):232–238. https://doi.org/10.21037/tlcr.2020.01.19

Kelly JF, Delclos ME, Morice RC, Huaringa A, Allen PK, Komaki R (2000) High-dose-rate endobronchial brachytherapy effectively palliates symptoms due to airway tumors: the 10-year M. D. Anderson cancer center experience. Int J Radiat Oncol Biol Phys 48(3):697–702. http://www.ncbi.nlm.nih.gov/pubmed/11020566

Kepka L, Olszyna-Serementa M (2010) Palliative thoracic radiotherapy for lung cancer. Expert Rev Anticancer Ther 10(4):559–569. https://doi.org/10.1586/era.10.22

Kilburn JM, Kuremsky JG, Blackstock AW, Munley MT, Kearns WT, Hinson WH et al (2014) Thoracic re-irradiation using stereotactic body radiotherapy (SBRT) techniques as first or second course of treatment. Radiother Oncol 110(3):505–510. https://doi.org/10.1016/j.radonc.2013.11.017

Kim E, Song C, Kim MY, Kim J-S (2017) Long-term outcomes after salvage radiotherapy for postoperative locoregionally recurrent non-small-cell lung cancer. Radiat Oncol J 35(1):55–64. https://doi.org/10.3857/roj.2016.01928

Knox MC, Bece A, Bucci J, Moses J, Graham PH (2018) Endobronchial brachytherapy in the management of lung malignancies: 20 years of experience in an Australian center. Brachytherapy 17(6):973–980. https://doi.org/10.1016/j.brachy.2018.07.010. http://www.ncbi.nlm.nih.gov/pubmed/30064904

Kono K, Murakami M, Sasaki R, Okamoto Y, Yodenn E, Kobayashi K et al (1998) [Radiation therapy for non-small cell lung cancer with postoperative intrathoracic recurrence]. Nihon Igaku Hoshasen Gakkai Zasshi 58:18–24

Kramer GWPM, Gans S, Ullmann E, van Meerbeeck JP, Legrand CC, Leer J-WH (2004) Hypofractionated external beam radiotherapy as retreatment for symptomatic nonsmall-cell lung carcinoma: an effective treatment? Int J Radiat Oncol Biol Phys 58(5):1388–1393. https://doi.org/10.1016/j.ijrobp.2003.09.087

Kruser TJ, McCabe BP, Mehta MP, Khuntia D, Campbell TC, Geye HM et al (2014) Reirradiation for locoregionally recurrent lung cancer. Am J Clin Oncol 37(1):70–76. https://doi.org/10.1097/coc.0b013e31826b9950

Lee KH, Ahn YC, Pyo H, Noh JM, Park SG, Kim TG et al (2019) Salvage concurrent chemo-radiation therapy for loco-regional recurrence following curative surgery of non-small cell lung cancer. Cancer Res Treat 51(2):769–776. https://doi.org/10.4143/crt.2018.366

Liu H, Zhang X, Vinogradskiy YY, Swisher SG, Komaki R, Chang JY (2012) Predicting radiation pneumonitis after stereotactic ablative radiation therapy in patients previously treated with conventional thoracic radiation therapy. Int J Radiat Oncol Biol Phys 84(4):1017–1023. https://doi.org/10.1016/j.ijrobp.2012.02.020

Ma L, Qiu B, Zhang J, Li Q-W, Wang B, Zhang X-H et al (2017) Survival and prognostic factors of non-small cell lung cancer patients with postoperative locoregional recurrence treated with radical radiotherapy. Chin J Cancer 36(1):93. https://doi.org/10.1186/s40880-017-0261-0

Manabe Y, Shibamoto Y, Baba F, Yanagi T, Iwata H, Miyakawa A et al (2018) Definitive radiotherapy for hilar and/or mediastinal lymph node metastases after stereotactic body radiotherapy or surgery for stage I non-small cell lung cancer: 5-year results. Jpn J Radiol 36(12):719–725. https://doi.org/10.1007/s11604-018-0776-6

McAvoy SA, Ciura KT, Rineer JM, Allen PK, Liao Z, Chang JY et al (2013) Feasibility of proton beam therapy for reirradiation of locoregionally recurrent non-small cell lung cancer. Radiother Oncol 109(1):38–44. https://doi.org/10.1016/j.radonc.2013.08.014

McAvoy S, Ciura K, Wei C, Rineer J, Liao Z, Chang JY et al (2014) Definitive reirradiation for locoregionally recurrent non-small cell lung cancer with proton beam therapy or intensity modulated radiation therapy: predictors of high-grade toxicity and survival outcomes. Int J Radiat Oncol Biol Phys 90(4):819–827. https://doi.org/10.1016/j.ijrobp.2014.07.030

Meijneke TR, Petit SF, Wentzler D, Hoogeman M, Nuyttens JJ (2013) Reirradiation and stereotactic radiotherapy for tumors in the lung: dose summation and toxicity. Radiother Oncol 107(3):423–427. https://doi.org/10.1016/j.radonc.2013.03.015

Mitsuyoshi T, Matsuo Y, Itou H, Shintani T, Iizuka Y, Kim YH et al (2017) Evaluation of a prognostic scoring system based on the systemic inflammatory and nutritional status of patients with locally advanced non-small-cell lung cancer treated with chemoradiotherapy. J Radiat Res 59(1):50–57. https://doi.org/10.1093/jrr/rrx060

Moeller B, Balagamwala EH, Chen A, Creach KM, Giaccone G, Koshy M et al (2018) Palliative thoracic radiation therapy for non-small cell lung cancer: 2018 update of an American Society for Radiation Oncology (ASTRO) evidence-based guideline. Pract Radiat Oncol 8(4):245–250. https://pubmed.ncbi.nlm.nih.gov/29625898/

Montebello JF, Aron BS, Manatunga AK, Horvath JL, Peyton FW (1993) The reirradiation of recurrent bronchogenic carcinoma with external beam irradiation. Am J Clin Oncol 16(6):482–488. https://doi.org/10.1097/00000421-199312000-00004. https://pubmed.ncbi.nlm.nih.gov/8256761/

Nagata Y, Hiraoka M, Shibata T, Onishi H, Kokubo M, Karasawa K et al (2015) Prospective trial of stereotactic body radiation therapy for both operable and inoperable T1N0M0 non-small cell lung cancer: Japan Clinical Oncology Group Study JCOG0403. Int J Radiat Oncol Biol Phys 93(5):989–996. https://doi.org/10.1016/j.ijrobp.2015.07.2278

Nakamichi S, Horinouchi H, Asao T, Goto Y, Kanda S, Fujiwara Y et al (2017) Comparison of radiotherapy and chemoradiotherapy for locoregional recurrence of nonsmall-cell lung cancer developing after surgery. Clin Lung Cancer 18(6):e441–e448. https://doi.org/10.1016/j.cllc.2017.05.005

Nakanishi K, Mizuno T, Sakakura N, Kuroda H, Shimizu J, Hida T et al (2019) Salvage surgery for small cell lung cancer after chemoradiotherapy. Jpn J Clin Oncol 49(4):389–392. https://doi.org/10.1093/jjco%2Fhyz010

National Comprehensive Cancer Network (2021a) Non-small cell lung cancer (Version 2.2021). https://www.nccn.org/professionals/physician_gls/pdf/nscl.pdf

National Comprehensive Cancer Network (2021b) Small cell lung cancer (Version 2.2021). https://www.nccn.org/professionals/physician_gls/pdf/sclc.pdf

Nieder C, Grosu AL, Andratschke NH, Molls M (2006) Update of human spinal cord reirradiation tolerance based on additional data from 38 patients. Int J Radiat Oncol Biol Phys 66(5):1446–1449. https://doi.org/10.1016/j.ijrobp.2006.07.1383

Nieder C, Mannsåker B, Yobuta R, Haukland E (2020) Provider decision regret - a useful method for analysis of palliative thoracic re-irradiation for lung cancer? Strahlenther Onkol 196(4):315–324. https://doi.org/10.1007/s00066-020-01577-0

Ogawa Y, Shibamoto Y, Hashizume C, Kondo T, Iwata H, Tomita N et al (2018) Repeat stereotactic body radiotherapy (SBRT) for local recurrence of non-small cell lung cancer and lung metastasis after first SBRT. Radiat Oncol 13(1):136. https://doi.org/10.1186/s13014-018-1080-4

Ohguri T, Imada H, Yahara K, Moon SD, Yamaguchi S, Yatera K et al (2012) Re-irradiation plus regional hyperthermia for recurrent non-small cell lung cancer: a potential modality for inducing long-term survival in selected patients. Lung Cancer 77(1):140–145. https://doi.org/10.1016/j.lungcan.2012.02.018

Okami J (2019) Treatment strategy and decision-making for elderly surgical candidates with early lung cancer. J Thorac Dis 11(S7):S987–S997. https://doi.org/10.21037/jtd.2019.04.01

Okami J, Nishiyama K, Fujiwara A, Konishi K, Kanou T, Tokunaga T et al (2013) Radiotherapy for postoperative thoracic lymph node recurrence of nonsmall-cell lung cancer provides better outcomes if the disease is asymptomatic and a single-station involvement. J Thorac Oncol 8(11):1417–1424. https://doi.org/10.1097/jto.0b013e3182a5097b

Okamoto Y, Murakami M, Yoden E, Sasaki R, Okuno Y, Nakajima T et al (2002) Reirradiation for locally recurrent lung cancer previously treated with radiation therapy. Int J Radiat Oncol Biol Phys 52(2):390–396. https://doi.org/10.1016/s0360-3016(01)02644-x

Ornadel D, Duchesne G, Wall P, Ng A, Hetzel M (1997) Defining the roles of high dose rate endobronchial brachytherapy and laser resection for recurrent bronchial malignancy. Lung Cancer 16(2–3):203–213. http://www.ncbi.nlm.nih.gov/pubmed/9152951

Parks J, Kloecker G, Woo S, Dunlap NE (2016) Stereotactic body radiation therapy as salvage for intrathoracic recurrence in patients with previously irradiated locally advanced nonsmall cell lung cancer. Am J Clin Oncol 39(2):147–153. https://doi.org/10.1097/coc.0000000000000039

Peulen H, Karlsson K, Lindberg K, Tullgren O, Baumann P, Lax I et al (2011) Toxicity after reirradiation of pulmonary tumours with stereotactic body radiotherapy. Radiother Oncol 101(2):260–266. https://doi.org/10.1016/j.radonc.2011.09.012

Poltinnikov IM, Fallon K, Xiao Y, Reiff JE, Curran WJ, Werner-Wasik M (2005) Combination of longitudinal and circumferential three-dimensional esophageal dose distribution predicts acute esophagitis in hypofractionated reirradiation of patients with nonsmall-cell lung cancer treated in stereotactic body frame. Int J Radiat Oncol Biol Phys 62(3):652–658. https://doi.org/10.1016/j.ijrobp.2004.10.030

Ren C, Ji T, Liu T, Dang J, Li G (2018) The risk and predictors for severe radiation pneumonitis in lung cancer patients treated with thoracic reirradiation. Radiat Oncol 13(1):69. https://doi.org/10.1186/s13014-018-1016-z

Repka MC, Aghdam N, Kataria SK, Campbell L, Suy S, Collins SP et al (2017) Five-fraction SBRT for ultracentral NSCLC in-field recurrences following high-dose conventional radiation. Radiat Oncol 12(1):162. https://doi.org/10.1186/s13014-017-0897-6

Reveiz L, Rueda J-R, Cardona AF (2012) Palliative endobronchial brachytherapy for non-small cell lung cancer. Cochrane Database Syst Rev 12:CD004284. https://pubmed.ncbi.nlm.nih.gov/23235606/

Rodrigues G, Videtic GMM, Sur R, Bezjak A, Bradley J, Hahn CA et al (2011) Palliative thoracic radiotherapy in lung cancer: an American Society for Radiation Oncology evidence-based clinical practice guideline. Pract Radiat Oncol 1(2):60–71. https://pubmed.ncbi.nlm.nih.gov/25740118/

Rulach R, Ball D, Chua KLM, Dahele M, De Ruysscher D, Franks K et al (2021) An international expert survey on the indications and practice of radical thoracic re-irradiation for non-small cell lung cancer. Adv Radiat Oncol 6:100653. https://doi.org/10.1016/j.adro.2021.100653

Sahgal A, Ma L, Weinberg V, Gibbs IC, Chao S, Chang U-K et al (2012) Reirradiation human spinal cord tolerance for stereotactic body radiotherapy. Int J Radiat Oncol Biol Phys 82(1):107–116. https://doi.org/10.1016/j.ijrobp.2010.08.021

Schlampp I, Rieber J, Adeberg S, Bozorgmehr F, Heußel CP, Steins M et al (2019) Re-irradiation in locally recurrent lung cancer patients. Strahlenther Onkol 195(8):725–733. https://doi.org/10.1007/s00066-019-01457-2

Schröder C, Stiefel I, Tanadini-Lang S, Pytko I, Vu E, Guckenberger M et al (2020) Re-irradiation in the thorax—an analysis of efficacy and safety based on accumulated EQD2 doses. Radiother Oncol 152:56–62. https://doi.org/10.1016/j.radonc.2020.07.033

Senthi S, Griffioen GHMJ, van Sörnsen de Koste JR, Slotman BJ, Senan S (2013) Comparing rigid and deformable dose registration for high dose thoracic re-irradiation. Radiother Oncol 106(3):323–326. https://doi.org/10.1016/j.radonc.2013.01.018

Seol KH, Lee JE, Cho JY, Lee DH, Seok Y, Kang MK (2017) Salvage radiotherapy for regional lymph node oligo-recurrence after radical surgery of non-small cell lung cancer. Thorac Cancer 8(6):620–629. https://doi.org/10.1111/1759-7714.12497

Shirai K, Kubota Y, Ohno T, Saitoh J-I, Abe T, Mizukami T et al (2019) Carbon-ion radiotherapy for isolated lymph node metastasis after surgery or radiotherapy for lung cancer. Front Oncol 9:731. https://doi.org/10.3389/fonc.2019.00731

Simone C, Amini A, Chetty I, Choi JI, Chun S, Donington J et al (2020) American Radium Society (ARS) and American College of Radiology (ACR) appropriate use criteria systematic review and guidelines on reirradiation for non-small cell lung cancer (NSCLC). Int J Radiat Oncol Biol Phys 108(2):E48–E49. https://doi.org/10.1016/j.ijrobp.2020.02.583

Sittenfeld SMC, Juloori A, Reddy CA, Stephans KL, Videtic GMM (2020) Salvage stereotactic body radiation therapy for isolated local recurrence after primary surgical resection of nonsmall-cell lung cancer. Clin Lung Cancer 22(3):e360–e365. https://doi.org/10.1016/j.cllc.2020.05.025

Sonobe M, Yamada T, Sato M, Menju T, Aoyama A, Sato T et al (2014) Identification of subsets of patients with favorable prognosis after recurrence in completely resected non-small cell lung cancer. Ann Surg Oncol 21(8):2546–2554. https://doi.org/10.1245/s10434-014-3630-9

Sood S, Ganju R, Shen X, Napel MT, Wang F (2021) Ultracentral thoracic re-irradiation using 10-fraction stereotactic body radiotherapy for recurrent non-small-cell lung cancer tumors: preliminary toxicity and efficacy outcomes. Clin Lung Cancer 22:e301–312

Speiser BL, Spratling L (1993) Remote afterloading brachytherapy for the local control of endobronchial carcinoma. Int J Radiat Oncol Biol Phys 25(4):579–587. https://doi.org/10.1016/0360-3016(93)90002-d

Stewart A, Parashar B, Patel M, O'Farrell D, Biagioli M, Devlin P et al (2016) American Brachytherapy Society consensus guidelines for thoracic brachytherapy for lung cancer. Brachytherapy 15(1):1–11. https://pubmed.ncbi.nlm.nih.gov/26561277/

Stojiljkovic D, Mandaric D, Miletic N, Stojsic J, Markovic I, Gavrilovic D et al (2013) Characteristics of local recurrence of lung cancer and possibilities for surgical management. J BUON 18:169–175

Sumita K, Harada H, Asakura H, Ogawa H, Onoe T, Murayama S et al (2016) Re-irradiation for locoregionally recurrent tumors of the thorax: a single-institution retrospective study. Radiat Oncol 11(1):104. https://doi.org/10.1186/s13014-016-0673-z

Sumodhee S, Bondiau PY, Poudenx M et al (2019) Long term efficacy and toxicity after stereotactic ablative reirradiation in locally relapsed stage III non-small cell lung cancer. BMC Cancer 19(1):305. https://doi.org/10.1186/s12885-019-5542-3

Tada T, Fukuda H, Matsui K, Hirashima T, Hosono M, Takada Y et al (2005) Non-small-cell lung cancer: reirradiation for loco-regional relapse previously treated with radiation therapy. Int J Clin Oncol 10(4):247–250. https://doi.org/10.1007/s10147-005-0501-1

Takeda A, Sanuki N, Eriguchi T, Enomoto T, Yokosuka T, Kaneko T et al (2013) Salvage stereotactic ablative irradiation for isolated postsurgical local recurrence of lung cancer. Ann Thorac Surg 96(5):1776–1782. https://doi.org/10.1016/j.athoracsur.2013.06.014

Timmerman R, McGarry R, Yiannoutsos C, Papiez L, Tudor K, DeLuca J et al (2006) Excessive toxicity when treating central tumors in a phase II study of stereotactic body radiation therapy for medically inoperable early-stage lung cancer. J Clin Oncol 24(30): 4833–4839. https://doi.org/10.1200/jco.2006.07.5937

Trovo M, Minatel E, Durofil E, Polesel J, Avanzo M, Baresic T et al (2014) Stereotactic body radiation therapy for re-irradiation of persistent or recurrent non-small cell lung cancer. Int J Radiat Oncol Biol Phys 88(5):1114–1119. https://doi.org/10.1016/j.ijrobp.2014.01.012

Viani GA, Arruda CV, Fendi LID (2020) Effectiveness and safety of reirradiation with stereotactic ablative radiotherapy of lung cancer after a first course of thoracic radiation. Am J Clin Oncol 43(8):575–581. https://doi.org/10.1097/COC.0000000000000709

Ward MC, Oh SC, Pham YD, Woody NM, Marwaha G, Videtic GMM et al (2016) Isolated nodal failure after stereotactic body radiotherapy for lung cancer: the role for salvage mediastinal radiotherapy. J Thorac Oncol 11(9):1558–1564. https://doi.org/10.1016/j.jtho.2016.05.003

Wu K-L, Jiang G-L, Qian H, Wang L-J, Yang H-J, Fu X-L et al (2003) Three-dimensional conformal radiotherapy for locoregionally recurrent lung carcinoma after external beam irradiation: a prospective phase III clinical trial. Int J Radiat Oncol Biol Phys 57(5):1345–1350. https://doi.org/10.1016/s0360-3016(03)00768-5

Wu AJ, Garay E, Foster A, Hsu M, Zhang Z, Chaft JE et al (2017) Definitive radiotherapy for local recurrence of NSCLC after surgery. Clin Lung Cancer 18(3):e161–e168. https://doi.org/10.1016/j.cllc.2017.01.014

Xia B, Zhang S, Ma S (2017) Management of non-small cell lung cancer with EGFR mutation: the role of radiotherapy in the era of tyrosine kinase inhibitor therapy opportunities and challenges. J Thorac Dis 9(9):3385–3393. https://doi.org/10.21037/jtd.2017.09.67

Yang W-C, Hsu F-M, Chen Y-H, Shih J-Y, Yu C-J, Lin Z-Z et al (2020) Clinical outcomes and toxicity predictors of thoracic re-irradiation for locoregionally recurrent lung cancer. Clin Transl Radiat Oncol 22:76–82. https://doi.org/10.1016/j.ctro.2020.03.008

Yano T (2014) Therapeutic strategy for postoperative recurrence in patients with non-small cell lung cancer. World J Clin Oncol 5(5):1048. https://doi.org/10.5306/wjco.v5.i5.1048

Yoshitake T, Shioyama Y, Nakamura K, Sasaki T, Ohga S, Shinoto M et al (2013) Definitive fractionated re-irradiation for local recurrence following stereotactic body radiotherapy for primary lung cancer. Anticancer Res 33:5649–5653

Treatment of Second Lung Cancers

Reshad Rzazade and Hale Basak Caglar

Contents

1 Introduction 739
2 Molecular and Biological Features of Second Lung Cancers 740
3 Surgery for Treatment of Second Lung Cancer 741
4 Oligometastatic Disease 742
5 Retrospective Studies of SABR for Second Lung Cancer 743
6 Treatment of Synchronous/Metachronous Lung Cancer 744
7 Prospective Trials of SABR for Second Lung Cancer 745
8 Surgery Versus Stereotactic Radiotherapy for Oligometastatic Second Lung Disease 747
9 Prognostic Factors 748
9.1 Histology 748
9.2 Disease-Free Interval 749
9.3 Number of Pulmonary Metastases 749
9.4 Size of Pulmonary Metastases 749
10 Conclusion 749
References 750

R. Rzazade · H. B. Caglar (✉)
Department of Radiation Oncology, Anadolu Medical Center, Kocaeli, Turkey
e-mail: halebasakcaglar@gmail.com

Abstract

Lung metastases are commonly seen in many cancers as a result of rich blood circulation. As the concept of oligometastases arouses interest local ablative therapies of lung metastases is being applied more commonly in clinical practice. Pulmonary metastasectomy and stereotactic ablative radiation therapy are the most common forms of local ablative therapies of second lung cancers. Here we present the current evidence about the treatment of second lung cancers including metastases and second primaries.

1 Introduction

Because of blood circulation, lung is the second-most common site of distant metastasis for all types of cancers (Treasure et al. 2014). Note that ~30% of all cancer patients will develop pulmonary metastasis at some point during their disease. Breast, lung, kidney, colon carcinomas, and soft tissue sarcomas are the most common tumors that metastasize to the lung (Xu and Burke 2012). Distant organ metastases detected in the lung account for <5% of all lung cancers. In autopsy studies, lung metastases were observed in 50% of cancer deaths, and some of these cases had isolated lung metastases (Gerull et al. 2020).

Historically, the standard treatment for metastatic disease has been systemic chemotherapy and has limited benefit on survival (Gloeckler Ries et al. 2003). Although there is no randomized evidence for treating pulmonary metastases, particularly for oligometastases, the use of SABR is increasing. Evidence from retrospective series demonstrates that patients with a limited disease pattern have improved results with local aggressive treatments (Kaifi et al. 2010; Rieber et al. 2016).

In this section, we talk about the molecular and biological features of pulmonary metastases and local aggressive treatment options.

2 Molecular and Biological Features of Second Lung Cancers

Metastasis can be defined as the spread of tumor cells into another organ or tissue by biological and molecular mechanisms from the organ or tissue of origin. Many tumors tend to metastasize despite standard treatments and lead to mortality. The findings of metastasis biology were first described by Paget in 1889 with the seed-soil hypothesis. In 1928, Ewing defined that metastasis to an organ is primarily associated with the vascular system of that organ (Isaiah and Margaret 1977).

There are several different features in the lung that allow additional metastases to occur compared to anywhere else in the body. The lungs receive the entire cardiac output every minute, have the densest capillary bed in the body, and have a network of membranes that can easily trap tumor cells and draw nearby oxygen for nourishment. All these features provide an ideal situation and environment for events that cause lung metastasis (Schueller and Herold 2003).

Vascularization of pulmonary metastases is variable and complex, usually involving nourishment of bronchial and pulmonary origin. There are three possible pathways for the growth of metastases in the lung: bronchial circulation, pulmonary circulation, or both (Noonan et al. 1965; Boijsen and Zsigmond 1965). In a computer topographic angiography study on resected human lungs with pulmonary metastases of different primary origin, all metastases were reported to have a pulmonary circulatory component feeding the lateral part of the tumor (Milne and Zerhouni 1987).

The process of metastasis occurs through a series of interrelated, complex, and multistep chain of events such as angiogenesis, invasion, migration-motility, extravasation, and proliferation (Kliche and Waltenberger 2001).

Laboratory studies demonstrated that cellular factors such as vascular endothelial growth factor (VEGF), interleukin-8 (IL-8), platelet-derived endothelial cell growth factor (PD-ECGF), fibroblast growth factor-2 (FGF-2, bFGF), transforming growth factor-β (TGF-β), and angiopoietin-1 (Ang-1), which play key roles in the development and invasion of lung metastases, play important roles in the tumor microenvironment. Moreover, extremely delayed antigen 4 (VLA-4) production from hematopoietic progenitor cells that allow interaction with fibronectin in fibroblasts in pre-metastatic regions has a role in metastatic invasion (Yancopoulos et al. 2000; Kaplan et al. 2005; Duda et al. 2010).

As the steps of metastasis biology and biochemical factors are clearly defined, answers to the selection of the target organ have begun to be sought. Various theories have been proposed on this subject, and the fact that the lung forms an ideal target organ because of the excess tissue blood flow but organs with similar features such as the kidney are subject to less metastasis raised the question that other factors may have a role in this process. One of the most important factors explaining this is chemokines, which are the product of a process that initiates transendothelial migration in the area of damage and inflammation. Chemokines are activated by tumor cells through VEGF-A uptake of immune cells and tumor cells into the lungs and tumor necrosis factor-α (TNF-α) and transforming growth factor-β (TGF-β) induce expression of inflammatory chemokines used for lung invasion (Wang et al. 1998; Weigelt et al. 2005; Hiratsuka et al. 2006). Among these, CXCL12 is the most important chemokine secreted and produced by the lung. CXCR4, which is intensely expressed by the lung, is a relative receptor for CXCL12. These are highly expressed in breast cancer cells and show that the CXCL12-CXCR4 interaction has a potential significance for the lung metastasis of breast cancer. Furthermore, it has been shown in mouse experiments that the blockade of CXCL12-CXCR4 reduces metastasis to the lung (Weigelt et al. 2003). Similarly, it was observed that there is additional lung metastasis in the presence of CXCR4 expression in B-16 melanoma and osteosarcoma cells (Murakami et al. 2002; Kim et al. 2008).

3 Surgery for Treatment of Second Lung Cancer

Except for lung cancer resection, metastasectomy is the most common operation performed in thoracic surgery clinics. The high survival rate after the resection of pulmonary metastases has expanded the surgical indications for these lesions. The primary problem in pulmonary metastases is determining the patient group that will benefit most from metastasectomy. In 1958, Ehrenhaft defined the criteria for pulmonary metastasectomy, and these criteria were later reviewed by Kondo et al. in 2005.

While determining the criteria, it was aimed for the patients to benefit most from the resection to be performed. Accordingly, the criteria for the resection of pulmonary metastases are as follows (Kondo et al. 2005): primary tumor being under control, absence of extrathoracic metastases, pulmonary nodules being compatible with metastasis, lesions being potentially resectable such that all lesions compatible with metastasis can be removed, and predetermination of the appropriate pulmonary being reserved for the postoperative period.

The other indications for partial or complete resection are need for diagnosis, removal of residual nodules after chemotherapy, providing necessary tissue for tumor "markers," or immunohistochemical study or reduction of tumor burden.

In 1997, the International Lung Metastasis Registry System was divided into four subgroups according to the primary cancer type in the multicenter study conducted by the study group. These subgroups were germ cell tumor (7%), melanoma (6%), sarcoma (42%), and epithelial tumor (44%). The study revealed that, regardless of the histological type, the fewer the metastases and the longer the disease-free period were, the longer the survival time after metastasectomy was, but there were broad differences in 5-year survival depending on the type of cancer: 68% for germ cell, 37% for epithelial cancer, 31% for sarcoma, and 21% for melanoma. Postoperative mortality was 1%. In conclusion, the most important positive prognostic factors for pulmonary metastasectomy were reported to be the primary source of metastasis, cell type, ability to perform complete resection, long disease-free survival, and a small number of (preferably one) metastases (Pastorino et al. 1997).

The most common reporting is in patients with primary colorectal cancer, with a 5-year survival rate of 29–54% after pulmonary metastasectomy. Advanced age, synchronous and multiple metastases, short disease-free period, high carcino-embryogenic antigen (CEA) level (≥ 5 ng/mL), mediastinal lymph node involvement, and bilateral metastasis have been reported as negative prognostic factors (Pfannschmidt et al. 2003, 2007; Higashiyama et al. 2003; Iizasa et al. 2006; Welter et al. 2007). Patients with solitary metastases are among the group that will benefit most from metastasectomy (Koga et al. 2006).

Soft tissue sarcomas metastasize to the lungs at a rate of 20–50% during the disease. Usually, pulmonary metastases are isolated metastases and metastasectomy is appropriate because they are not sensitive to chemotherapy (Gadd et al. 1993). Histologically, leiomyosarcomas (21%), malignant fibrous histiocytomas (18%), and synovial sarcomas (14%) metastasize to the lung more frequently, and according to the location, tumors located in the lower extremities metastasize to the lung more frequently than those located in the trunk (Gadd et al. 1993). In the European Organisation for Research and

Treatment of Cancer (EORTC) Soft Tissue and Bone Sarcoma Group study evaluating 255 patients with soft tissue sarcoma who underwent metastasectomy, 3-year and 5-year survival rates after metastasectomy were reported to be 54% and 38% (Van Geel et al. 1996). In a nonrandomized comparative study in which they examined 3149 patients with soft tissue sarcoma, Billingsley et al. observed that 719 patients developed pulmonary metastasectomy during follow-up, and 3-year survival was 46% in patients who underwent metastasectomy, and 17% in those who did not undergo metastasectomy (Billingsley et al. 1999). Presence of solitary metastasis, age of the patient (age >40), complete resection, long disease-free period, long tumor doubling time, and histological grade of the tumor (grades I–II) are good prognostic factors (Billingsley et al. 1999; Canter et al. 2007).

Renal cell carcinoma most often causes pulmonary metastasis by both hematogenous and lymphatic pathways. In these cancers, a 10-year survival rate of 42% has been reported after pulmonary metastasectomy (Chen et al. 2008). Although systemic treatments with tyrosine kinase inhibitors and mTOR inhibitors contribute to progression-free survival, curative pulmonary metastasectomy is an acceptable treatment method (Karam et al. 2011). Incomplete resection, short disease-free period, size of the tumor, lymph node involvement, and pleural involvement are negative prognostic factors (Kanzaki et al. 2011; Meimarakis et al. 2011).

Although >70% of all patients with metastatic melanoma develop pulmonary metastasis, only 10% of them have solitary lung metastasis (Swetter et al. 2019). The first of the two comparative studies evaluating metastasectomy in malignant melanoma included 14,057 malignant melanoma patients diagnosed between 1970 and 2004. A total of 1720 (12.2%) pulmonary metastases were detected and a survival advantage of ~12 months (19 vs. 7 months) and 10 months (18 vs. 8 months) in the presence of isolated pulmonary metastasis was reported with metastasectomy, particularly in patients with a disease-free survival time of more than 5 years (Petersen et al. 2007). In another study, a median survival of 40 months was reported with pulmonary metastasectomy, and metastasectomy was identified as the only prognostic factor affecting survival (Neuman et al. 2007).

4 Oligometastatic Disease

The presence of patients who can achieve longer survival in metastatic disease suggests that there is a metastatic subgroup where local aggressive therapies can be beneficial. This group, which is called oligometastatic disease, is a stage defined between limited stage and common disease. Oligometastasis was first defined by Hellman and Weichselbaum. They hypothesized that these tumors have a different biology from common metastatic diseases and that some of them can be treated with curative purposes (Hellman and Weichselbaum 1995). Advances in imaging methods, less invasive surgeries, targeted therapies, better control of microscopic disease, and radiotherapy treatments with higher doses and fewer side effects have increased the interest in the concept of oligometastatic disease.

With the development of radiotherapy techniques and the accumulation of experience with new techniques, stereotactic methods have begun to be used more commonly today. These developments shifted the target of radiotherapy from palliation to cure in metastatic disease. Stereotactic ablative body radiotherapy (SABR) enables high radiation doses, defined as "ablative dose," to be delivered with high precision while preserving maximum normal tissue. SABR is a safe and effective treatment method in medical inoperable early-stage non-small cell lung cancer (NSCLC) (Timmerman et al. 2003; Verstegen et al. 2013). After these promising results, it has become an increasingly attractive option as part of local ablative therapy for lung metastases. Because of advances in imaging (fast and effective 3D computed tomography (CT) and positron emission tomography (PET)), it allows earlier detection of metastatic disease (De Pas et al. 2007).

There are differences in the definition of oligometastatic disease: clinical trial protocols use the definition of 1 to 3 or 1 to 5 metastatic lesions at most (Palma et al. 2014). Recently, a consensus was reached for defining oligometastatic disease and two separate categories were created as induced (after polymetastatic disease) and true (initially diagnosed oligometastatic) (Guckenberger et al. 2020). True oligometastatic disease was classified as recurrent oligometastatic disease (previous oligometastatic disease history) and de novo oligometastatic disease (initial diagnosis of oligometastatic disease), while de novo oligometastatic disease was divided into two further subgroups as synchronous and metachronous oligometastatic disease. Considering whether oligometastatic disease was diagnosed during nontreatment period or during active systemic therapy, and whether an oligometastatic lesion progressed on current imaging, a final subclassification was made as oligorecurrence, oligoprogression, and oligopersistence. However, despite the preclinical and clinical data supporting the presence of oligometastatic disease, identification and diagnosis of patients with oligometastatic disease are solely based on imaging results because it is not clear which patients are truly oligometastatic and which patients will benefit most from ablative therapies, and there is no consensus on the definition of total tumor volume, and there is no biomarker in clinical use to identify patients with true oligometastatic disease.

5 Retrospective Studies of SABR for Second Lung Cancer

Many previous studies investigating whether SABR is a safe and effective treatment in pulmonary metastases were retrospective and with a short follow-up period in which few patients were treated. In some of these studies, pulmonary metastases of different primary disease foci were reported, while in others there was a single primary histology (Onimaru et al. 2003; Okunieff et al. 2006; Rusthoven et al. 2009; Stragliotto et al. 2012; Mehta et al. 2013; De Rose et al. 2016; Hörner-Rieber et al. 2019; Baumann et al. 2020; König et al. 2020; Pasalic et al. 2020). In a study published by Stragliotto et al. from the Karolinska Institute, a retrospective analysis of SABR application was performed on 136 metastases (97 lung metastases) of 46 patients with a diagnosis of soft tissue sarcoma (Stragliotto et al. 2012). Note that 4–10 Gy treatment was applied in 1–5 fractions to all metastatic foci. A response rate of 88% was reported after a median follow-up of 21.8 months. Because of this study, it was stated that SABR application on soft tissue sarcoma metastases was an effective and safe treatment modality. In a retrospective study conducted by Mehta et al. investigating the safety and efficacy of SABR in 25 pulmonary metastases in 16 patients with high-grade sarcoma, 38% of the patients also underwent metastasectomy (Mehta et al. 2013). Note that 54 Gy was administered in 3–4 fractions as a treatment scheme. The 43-month local control rate was reported as 94% in the study with a median follow-up of 20 months. Grade 2 or higher toxicity was not reported in any of the patients. Baumann et al. retrospectively conducted efficacy and safety studies in 39 pulmonary metastases of 30 sarcoma patients treated with SABR (Baumann et al. 2020). Moreover, 66% of the patients included in this study had a previous history of metastasectomy, and median follow-up time was reported as 25 months with most patients receiving 50 Gy treatment in 4–5 fractions. Furthermore, 1- and 2-year local control rate was reported as 94% and 86% in treated lesions. Grade 3 and above toxicity was not observed because of treatment.

NSCLC is another primary disease whose effectiveness of SABR application in pulmonary oligometastases is investigated. In a study by De Rose et al., the results of 60 patients with NSCLC with 90 pulmonary oligometastatic targets after SABR application were evaluated (De Rose et al. 2016). SABR was applied because of metachronous metastasis in 70% of patients. The treatment scheme was determined as per tumor diameter and location. After a median follow-up of 28 months, 2-year local control rate was reported as 89%. Grade 3 and above toxicity rate was 3%. The investigators stated that SABR application in pulmonary oligometastases is a part of multidisciplinary approach.

Recently, the results of SABR application in 336 pulmonary oligometastases of 301 patients with primary NSCLC were published (König et al. 2020). Although different treatments were applied to the primary diseases of the patients, all oligometastases were treated with SABR. Moreover, ~70% of patients had solitary metastasis. The median follow-up time was 16.1 months, and 2-year local control rates were reported as 82%. In the subgroup of patients followed for a longer period (2 years), lower rates of 3- and 4-year local recurrence were reported (4% and 7.6%).

In the multicenter analysis of Hoerner-Rieber et al., SABR was applied to 67 pulmonary metastases of 46 patients with primary RCC (Hörner-Rieber et al. 2019). Median follow-up time was 28.2 months (0.8–133.8 months) and median BED_{ISO} was 117 Gy (48–189 Gy). A total of three local failures were observed, and the median local failure time was reported to be 26.1 months (10.5–27.2 months). The 1- and 3-year LC rates of all patients were 98.1% and 91.9%, respectively, while the 3-year LC was 100% in the $BED_{ISO} \geq 130$ Gy group and 83.9% in the $BED_{ISO} < 130$ Gy group ($p = 0.054$). Note that 1-year and 3-year OS was 84.3% and 43.8%, respectively. In multivariate analysis, high KPS, small tumor size, and no systemic treatment after SABR were independent prognostic factors for OS.

In the analysis published by Pasalic et al., the efficacy of SABR treatment applied to 107 pulmonary metastases (78.5% metachronous) of 82 (65.8% oligometastatic) BBC patients was examined (Pasalic et al. 2020). The most common primary histology was oropharynx (29.2%) and squamous cell carcinoma (64%). Median follow-up was 20 months (9–97.6 months) and median BED_{10} was 112.5 Gy (119–151.20 Gy). One- and 2-year LC rates were 97.8% and 94.4%, respectively. These rates were 81.5% and 72.5% for intrathoracic distant control (IDC), and 93.6% and 90.3% for LRC, respectively. In the study, which had a median OS of 43 months, 1- and 2-year OS rates were 74.8% and 61.6%, respectively. Oligometastatic disease ($p = 0.008$) and nonsquamous cell carcinoma ($p = 0.03$) were significant prognostic factors for OS.

6 Treatment of Synchronous/Metachronous Lung Cancer

Majority of the publications evaluating the outcomes of the patients with early-stage lung cancer treated with SABR included the ones with solitary pulmonary nodules although 0.5% of the patients may present with multiple nodules at the initial diagnosis (Ferguson 1993). The discrimination between two different primaries and synchronous metastases is not easy and needs advanced imaging and pathological assessment. Historically multiple nodules at presentation had relatively poor outcomes in surgical series due to various reasons (Rosengart et al. 1991).

The definition of synchronous and metachronous lung cancer depends on the time sequence of the two diagnoses. Tumors in the lung presenting >180 days apart tend to be defined as metachronous (Steber et al. 2021). For the patients who are diagnosed with early-stage NSCLC and treated with definitive radiotherapy of different schedules and modalities the rate of secondary lung cancers among the group of long-term survivors was reported to be 6% at 5 years and 14.2% at 10 years (Jeremic et al. 2001).

Agolli et al. published the outcomes of patients who were diagnosed as having non-small cell lung cancer (NSCLC) with either synchronous or metachronous lung nodules treated with SABR (Agolli et al. 2015). A total of 29 nodules from 22 patients were treated. Most of the patients had only solitary lung nodule. After a median follow-up of 18 months (4–53 months) 2-year disease-free and overall survival rates were 40% and 49%, respectively. The 1- and 2-year local control rates were reported as 93% and 64% with acceptable short- and long-term toxicities. Similarly, De Rose et al. published their series of 90 synchronous (30%) and metachronous (70%) pulmonary nodules of 60 NSCLC treated with SABR (De Rose et al. 2016). The primary tumor histology was adenocarcinoma. With a median follow-up of 28 months (5.4–104.5 months) 2-year local control rate was 88.9% and 1- and 2-year overall survival rates were 94.5% and 74.6%, respectively.

More recently publications from single-center retrospective data with synchronous and metachronous lung cancers with more patients were published. Nikitas et al. reviewed their prospective lung SABR database of patients treated with early-stage NSCLC (Nikitas et al. 2019). From a total of 374 patients receiving single-course SABR, there were 14 receiving synchronous SABR, 48 metachronous SABR, and 108 surgery plus metachronous SABR. After a median follow-up of 37 months among the surviving subgroup the survival rates were similar between all groups. The group from MD Anderson Cancer Center reported the outcomes of their synchronous patients (9%) from 912 treated lung cancer database (Ayoub et al. 2020). SABR was delivered to all sites in 69.5% of the patients. At a median follow-up of 58 months 3- and 5-year overall survival rates were 67% and 52%, respectively. Of the 142 SABR-treated sites there were 4% in-field and 3% marginal recurrences and on multivariable analysis ipsilateral synchronous disease was associated with greater regional and distant failure.

The American Society for Radiation Oncology (ASTRO) guideline for the use of SABR in early-stage NSCLC considered the use in synchronous and metachronous lung tumors (Videtic et al. 2017). It is recommended to discuss the treatment of multiple primary lung cancers and metachronous lung cancers in multidisciplinary tumor boards. The curative use of SABR in this group of patients is recommended strongly according to low-moderate quality of evidence with a high rate of consensus as the outcomes in terms of local control and survival are equivalent to single tumors with similar toxicity rates.

7 Prospective Trials of SABR for Second Lung Cancer

Table 1 summarizes perspective studies investigating the use of SABR in pulmonary metastases.

Onimaru et al. published a study investigating the efficacy of SABR and normal tissue tolerance doses in 46 patients with primary lung cancer ($n = 26$) and lung metastases ($n = 20$) (Onimaru et al. 2003). A total of 32 target lesions were identified in 20 patients treated for pulmonary metastasis. The median diameter of the lesions was 2.5 cm, and small/peripheral lesions were treated with 60 Gy in eight fractions and large/central lesions were treated with 48 Gy in eight fractions. Local recurrence was seen in two cases in the median 18-month follow-up, both of which were in the low-dose group. Local control rates were reported as 70–100% for 3 years and 2-year overall survival rate was 50%. In addition to the lung, the chest wall and esophagus were defined as risky organs.

A study conducted by Okunieff et al. from the University of Rochester evaluated the effectiveness and safety of SABR in pulmonary metastases (Okunieff et al. 2006). Moreover, 49 patients were included in the study and the patients were grouped as "curative" (<5 metastases, 30 patients)

Table 1 Outcomes of prospective trials dedicated to SBRT to lung lesions

Author	Year	No. of patients	No. of lung lesions	Tumor characteristics	Fraction/T. dose (Gy)	LC (%)	OS (%)	Toxicity ≥ grade 3 (%)
Onimaru R et al.	2003	20	32	Mixed histologies	8/48 and 60	94% crude	49% at 2 years	None
Okunieff P et al.	2006	49	125	Mixed histologies	10/50	91% at 2 years	38% at 2 years	2%
Rusthoven KE et al.	2009	38	63	Mixed histologies	3/48 and 60	96% at 2 years	39% at 2 years	7.9%
Osti MF et al.	2013	66	103	Mixed histologies	1/23 and 30	89.1% at 1 year	76.4% at 1 year	3%
Nuyttens JJ et al.	2015	30	57	Mixed histologies	1–7/30–60	79% at 1 year	63% at 2 years	10%

and "palliative" (>5 metastases, 19 patients) as per the number of metastases. Note that 2.6 lesions were treated on an average in each patient with a total of 125 target lesions. After a median follow-up of 18.7 months, the median survival was reported as 23.4 months in the curative treatment group and 12.4 months in the palliative treatment group. Three-year local control was 91%, whereas grade 3 toxicity was 2% and no higher toxicity was observed.

Rustaven et al. published a phase I/II study investigating the efficacy and tolerability of SABR in patients with 1–3 lung metastases (Rusthoven et al. 2009). A total of 63 metastases with a median tumor volume of 4.2 cc in 38 patients were treated with 48–60 Gy in three fractions. After a median follow-up of 15.4 months, 1- and 2-year local control rates were reported as 100% and 96%. Moreover, local recurrence was observed in only one patient 13 months after SABR application, and median survival was calculated as 19 months, whereas grade 3 toxicity rate was reported as 7.9%.

In a study by Osti et al. reporting the application of single-fraction SABR in pulmonary oligometastases, a total of 103 lesions of 66 patients were treated (Osti et al. 2013). The treatments applied to the patients were determined as per tumor location, and 30 Gy was applied to 54 peripherally located lesions and 23 Gy was applied to 49 centrally located lesions. In the study group with a median follow-up of 15 months, 1- and 2-year local control rates were 89.1% and 82.1%, and overall survival rates were reported as 76.4% and 31.2%. Median survival was determined as 12 months. The acceptable levels of toxicity were observed after treatment with a single fraction, whereas grade 3 pneumonia was observed in only two patients. Small volume (<10 cc) and histology of the primary tumor (lung, colon, and breast vs. melanoma, renal, sarcoma) were among the prognostic factors that increased local control.

Nuyttens et al. published the results of a prospective phase II study evaluating the efficacy of SABR in a total of 57 lesions of 30 patients with pulmonary metastases that were not suitable for surgery or chemotherapy with five metastases in two organs at most, and primary tumor under control (Nuyttens et al. 2015). Many patients included in the study had primary colorectal cancers. The treatment dose and schedule were determined as per the size and location of the lesion: 60 Gy in three fractions for >3 cm peripheral lesions ($n = 23$), 30 Gy in a single fraction for peripheral lesions ≤3 cm ($n = 23$), 50 Gy in five fractions for central lesions ($n = 4$), and 56 Gy in seven fractions for ultracentral lesions ($n = 7$). In the study with a median follow-up of 36 months, 2-year local control rates were 100% in 11 central lesions, 91% in 23 peripheral lesions, and 4% in lesions treated with a single fraction. Note that 2-year disease-free and overall survival rates were reported as 33% and 63%, respectively. Acute grade 3 toxicity was reported in five patients, and chronic grade 3 toxicity was reported in three patients. Rib fractures were observed in three patients.

The first phase 1 study investigating the efficacy and safety of SABR in oligometastatic disease was published by NRG BR001 (Al-Hallaq et al. 2017). A total of 36 patients whose primary histology was breast, non-small cell lung (NSCLC), and prostate cancer were included in the study. Moreover, 45–50 Gy treatments in 3–5 fractions were applied to median 3 metastases, all of which were extracranially located. After this study, phase II studies were planned with the decision that these doses were safe. In a prospective phase II randomized study, Iyengar et al. observed that the addition of local ablative therapy with SABR to 29 oligometastatic patients with primary diagnosis of NSCLC resulted in significant improvement in disease-free survival rates (9.7 months vs. 3.5 months) (Iyengar et al. 2018). In a randomized phase II study in which 49 oligometastatic patients with primary NSCLC were evaluated, patients were randomized into groups of maintenance systemic therapy and local ablative therapy (with surgery and SABR) to oligometastatic foci after first-line systemic therapy (Gomez et al. 2019). In the interim analysis of this study, a significant increase in the disease-free survival time was detected in the patient arm to which local ablative therapy was added (11.9 months vs. 3.9 months), and overall survival times were in favor of local treatment (41.2 months vs. 17 months). The recently published SABR-COMET phase II randomized study included 99 metachronous oligometastatic patients (≤5 metastases) with different primary foci, and the long-term results of SABR application to metastatic foci in addition to standard therapy were presented (Palma et al. 2019). Median follow-up was 51 months, and 5-year OS was 42.3% and 17.7% in the SABR and standard treatment groups, respectively. While the 5-year DFS could not be calculated in the standard treatment group, it was 17.3% in the SABR group.

8 Surgery Versus Stereotactic Radiotherapy for Oligometastatic Second Lung Disease

Although there is no prospective study comparing metastasectomy and SABR in pulmonary metastases, there are five retrospective studies (Widder et al. 2013; Filippi et al. 2016; Lodeweges et al. 2017; Yu et al. 2017; Lee et al. 2018; Kanzaki et al. 2020).

A total of 110 patients were included in the study of Widder et al. retrospectively comparing surgery and SABR procedures in pulmonary oligometastases (Widder et al. 2013). While SABR was applied to 42 patients with a 60 Gy scheme in 3–8 fractions, 68 patients underwent open or VATS resection. When evaluated in terms of local control, disease-free survival, and overall survival after a median follow-up of 43 months, no difference was reported between the two treatment modalities. The longer follow-ups of the same patient cohort were reported by Lodeweges et al. and no difference was observed between overall survival rates at 6, 7, and 8 years. Toxicity was not evaluated in either of the publications with this patient group (Lodeweges et al. 2017).

Filippi et al. retrospectively evaluated surgery and SABR in 170 patients with pulmonary oligometastases with primary colorectal carcinoma (28 SABR, 142 surgery) (Filippi et al. 2016). Doses of 26–60 Gy in 1–10 fractions were administered to a total of 43 lesions of 28 patients who underwent SABR. After a median follow-up of 27 months in SABR patients and 45.8 months in surgical patients, there was no difference in overall survival rates (1- and 2-year OS of 89% and 77% with SABR vs. 96% and 82% with surgery). Moreover, no major toxicity was seen in either treatment group.

In another retrospective analysis published by Lee et al., the data of 51 patients receiving local treatment for pulmonary oligometastases (21 patients with SABR and 30 patients with surgery) were compared (Lee et al. 2018). Patients undergoing SABR received 48–60 Gy therapy in 3–4 fractions. Although negative prognostic factors were higher in the patient group treated with SABR (large tumor volume, no systemic therapy, and synchronous tumor), no difference was observed between 1- and 2-year survival rates after 13.7 months of follow-up (79.5% and 68.2% with SABR vs. 95% and 81.8% with surgery). Disease-free survival rates were in favor of surgery (1- and 2-year DFS of 23.8% and 11.9% with SABR vs. 51% and 46% with surgery). There was no difference in local control rates (1- and 2-year LC rate of 83.5% and 75% with SABR vs. 96% and 91% with surgery). Grade 3 radiation pneumonia was reported in 4.8% of patients treated with SABR.

In the study of Yu et al., 73 patients with primary osteosarcoma histology with pulmonary oligometastasis underwent surgery or SABR and the data obtained were retrospectively compared (Yu et al. 2017). SABR was applied to 33 patients and surgery was applied to 40 patients. SABR patients received treatment doses of 30–50 Gy in ten fractions. After a median follow-up of 13 months, there was no difference in disease-free survival and overall survival rates. Complicated cases requiring medical intervention (16/46) were more common in the surgical group compared to the SABR group (34.8% vs. 10.3%).

Kanzaki et al. retrospectively examined the results of SABR and surgery as two different local ablative treatment options applied to pulmonary oligometastases of different primary cancers (Kanzaki et al. 2020). In the study, which included a total of 80 patients (21 SABR patients, 59 surgery patients), the most common primary

Table 2 Outcomes of local ablative treatments for pulmonary oligometastases

Authors	No. of patients/lesions	Tumor characteristics	Fraction/T. dose (Gy)	OS (%)	PFS (%)	LC (%)
Widder J et al.	SABR: 42 Surgery: 68	Mixed histologies	3–8/60	SABR: 77% at 2 years Surgery: 82% at 2 years	SABR: 8% at 3 years Surgery: 22% at 3 years	SABR:85% at 3 years Surgery:83% at 3 years
Filippi AR et al.	SABR: 28/43 Surgery: 142	CRC	1–3/26–45	SABR: 77% at 2 years Surgery: 82% at 2 years	SABR: ~30% at 2 years Surgery: ~60% at 2 years	SABR: NA Surgery: NA
Lee YH et al.	SABR: 21 Surgery:30	Mixed histologies	3–4/48–60	SABR: 68% at 2 years Surgery: 81% at 2 years	SABR: 12% at 2 years Surgery: 46% at 2 years	SABR:75% at 2 years Surgery:91% at 2 years
Yu W et al.	SABR: 33 Surgery: 40	Osteosarcoma	10/70	SABR: 33% at 4 years Surgery: 32% at 4 years	SABR: 21% at 4 years Surgery: 27% at 4 years	SABR:NA Surgery: NA
Kanzaki et al.	SABR: 21 Surgery: 59	Mixed histologies	4/52	SABR: 52% at 3 years Surgery: 77% at 3 years	SABR: 11% at 3 years Surgery: 42% at 3 years	SABR: 92% at 3 years Surgery: 88% at 3 years

focus was colorectal adenocarcinoma. Although patients in the surgical arm were younger and received more aggressive primary disease treatment, no statistically significant difference was found between 3-year overall survival rates (52% vs. 77%). Progression-free survival (PFS) rates were in favor of surgery (42% vs. 11% at 3 years). Local control rates were similar (88% vs. 92% in 3 years), and treatment toxicities were low for both treatments.

Based on the available retrospective evidence evaluated in detail, it is impossible to say that there is a significant difference or superiority between local ablative treatment options for pulmonary oligometastases. The studies are summarized in Table 2. Prospective controlled studies are required to answer this question. However, which oligometastatic patients require aggressive local treatment is a more important issue that requires to be investigated.

9 Prognostic Factors

Certain studies investigating the efficacy and safety of radiosurgery for pulmonary metastases have examined the prognostic factors affecting the local control of the treatment. Among these factors, the histology of the primary disease and SABR scheme are the most investigated. Studies investigating these factors are listed below.

9.1 Histology

Most researchers focused on histologies traditionally considered to be radiation resistant, including colorectal adenocarcinoma (CRCa) and soft tissue sarcoma (STS).

Since the radiosensitivity index (RSI) is between 0.5 and 5.4 α/β in sarcomas, it is assumed that they have a higher response rate with low-fraction high-dose radiation (Soyfer et al. 2010). In radiobiology and gene expression analyses performed as per the primary histological type of pulmonary metastases, pulmonary metastases originating from CRC are radioresistant and it has been concluded that high BED_{10} values are required to increase local control rates (Klement 2017; Ahmed et al. 2018; Jingu et al. 2018). Multiple clinical studies demonstrated that the type of histology affects local control, disease-free survival, and overall survival in patients with pulmonary oligometastasis.

In the study of the German Radiation Oncology Association (DEGRO) study group involving 700 patients from 20 centers, primary tumor histology is a prognostic factor affecting overall survival (Rieber et al. 2016). In another multicenter study, overall survival was longer in primary head and neck and breast cancer patients with pulmonary metastases undergoing SABR compared to colorectal and lung cancers (37 and 32 months vs. 30 and 26 months) (Ricco et al. 2017). In a retrospective analysis of 200 patients published by Franceschini et al., having primary colorectal disease was identified as a negative prognostic factor in terms of local control (Franceschini et al. 2017).

The results obtained in single-center studies have been confirmed in multicenter studies with additional patients. After SABR application to pulmonary oligometastases, the effect of local control on overall survival was investigated and a total of 1547 metastases in 1378 patients were evaluated; it was shown that local control in lesions of colorectal origin was significantly lower than other histologies after a median follow-up of 24.2 months (Yamamoto et al. 2020).

9.2 Disease-Free Interval

There are multiple studies showing that the time between primary disease and oligometastatic disease affects the prognosis in oligometastatic disease (Reyes and Pienta 2015). In the study conducted by Norihisa et al., the overall survival of patients with a disease-free interval of more than 3 years was reported to be significantly longer (Norihisa et al. 2008). Similar results were reported in a study published by Niibe et al., and a disease-free interval of ≥24 months had a positive effect on the overall survival (Niibe et al. 2015). In a study in which SABR was applied to 51 pulmonary metastases of 28 patients with soft tissue sarcoma, an increase in the overall survival rate was demonstrated in patients with a disease-free interval of >24 months (Navarria et al. 2015). In another study by Kalinauskaite et al., disease-free interval was reported as an independent prognostic factor in the patient population that underwent SABR for pulmonary metastasis (Kalinauskaite et al. 2020).

9.3 Number of Pulmonary Metastases

In addition to multiple studies confirming the prognostic importance of the number of metastases in oligometastatic patients, there are multiple studies showing the prognostic significance of the number of pulmonary metastases in patients with pulmonary oligometastasis. Hof et al. evaluated 71 pulmonary metastases in 61 patients and reported that the prognosis of patients with solitary metastases was better (Hof et al. 2007). Ricardi et al., however, demonstrated that in patients with pulmonary oligometastasis (1–3 metastases), the disease-free survival rates of patients with solitary and small (<3.3 cc) metastases following SABR were factors affecting prognosis in both univariate and multivariate analyses (Ricardi et al. 2012). In a multicenter German study, the number of pulmonary metastases (solitary vs. multiple) affected overall survival (Rieber et al. 2016). In the evaluation it was stated that during SABR application, less than three metastases with low volume (<7.7 cc) and the absence of extrathoracic disease in staging performed with PET were effective prognostic factors for all oncologic parameters (Borm et al. 2018).

9.4 Size of Pulmonary Metastases

During SABR application, target lesion volume has an effect on local control. In the study conducted it was shown that the tumor diameter (≤2.5 cm) was effective on both local control and overall survival (Oh et al. 2012). In the multicenter evaluation of the German study group, it was reported that the tumor diameter was effective on survival (Rieber et al. 2016).

10 Conclusion

Oligometastatic disease has become increasingly common, especially in recent years, with the increased effectiveness of systemic treatment. It has been shown that these patients have longer survival times than polymetastatic disease; therefore, the importance of local ablative treatments on oligometastatic foci has increased. The lung is one of the important metastasis foci in multiple types of cancer for various reasons. Historically, pulmonary oligometastasis has been a clinical image that has long been treated surgically. The development of stereotactic ablative radiotherapy has made this method at least as effective and safe as surgery for pulmonary oligometastases. The subject that requires further attention should be patient selection. For this, biological factors and clinical factors should be considered.

References

Agolli L, Valeriani M, Nicosia L et al (2015) Stereotactic ablative body radiotherapy (SABR) in pulmonary oligometastatic/oligorecurrent non-small cell lung cancer patients: a new therapeutic approach. Anticancer Res 35(11):6239–6245

Ahmed KA, Scott JG, Arrington JA et al (2018) Radiosensitivity of lung metastases by primary histology and implications for stereotactic body radiation therapy using the genomically adjusted radiation dose. J Thorac Oncol. https://doi.org/10.1016/j.jtho.2018.04.027

Al-Hallaq HA, Chmura SJ, Salama JK et al (2017) Benchmark credentialing results for NRG-BR001: the First National Cancer Institute-sponsored trial of stereotactic body radiation therapy for multiple metastases. Int J Radiat Oncol Biol Phys. https://doi.org/10.1016/j.ijrobp.2016.09.030

Ayoub Z, Ning MS, Brooks ED et al (2020) Definitive management of presumed synchronous early stage non-small cell lung cancers: outcomes and utility of stereotactic ablative radiation therapy. Int J Radiat Oncol Biol Phys 107(2):261–269. https://doi.org/10.1016/j.ijrobp.2020.02.001. Epub 2020 Feb 7

Baumann BC, Bernstein KDA, DeLaney TF et al (2020) Multi-institutional analysis of stereotactic body radiotherapy for sarcoma pulmonary metastases: high rates of local control with favorable toxicity. J Surg Oncol 122:877–883. https://doi.org/10.1002/jso.26078

Billingsley KG, Burt ME, Jara E et al (1999) Pulmonary metastases from soft tissue sarcoma: analysis of patterns of disease and postmetastasis survival. Ann Surg 229:602–612. https://doi.org/10.1097/00000658-199905000-00002

Boijsen E, Zsigmond M (1965) Selective angiography of bronchial and intercostal arteries. Acta Radiol Diagn (Stockh) 3:513–528. https://doi.org/10.1177/028418516500300606

Borm KJ, Oechsner M, Schiller K et al (2018) Prognostic factors in stereotactic body radiotherapy of lung metastases. Strahlenther Onkol 194:886–893. https://doi.org/10.1007/s00066-018-1335-x

Canter RJ, Qin LX, Downey RJ et al (2007) Perioperative chemotherapy in patients undergoing pulmonary resection for metastatic soft-tissue sarcoma of the extremity: a retrospective analysis. Cancer 110:2050–2060. https://doi.org/10.1002/cncr.23023

Chen F, Fujinaga T, Shoji T et al (2008) Pulmonary resection for metastasis from renal cell carcinoma. Interact Cardiovasc Thorac Surg 7:825–828. https://doi.org/10.1510/icvts.2008.181065

De Pas TM, de Braud F, Catalano G et al (2007) Oligometastatic non-small cell lung cancer: a multidisciplinary approach in the positron emission tomographic scan era. Ann Thorac Surg 83:231–234. https://doi.org/10.1016/j.athoracsur.2006.08.017

De Rose F, Cozzi L, Navarria P et al (2016) Clinical outcome of stereotactic ablative body radiotherapy for lung metastatic lesions in non-small cell lung cancer oligometastatic patients. Clin Oncol 28:13–20. https://doi.org/10.1016/j.clon.2015.08.011

Duda DG, Duyverman AMMJ, Kohno M et al (2010) Malignant cells facilitate lung metastasis by bringing their own soil. Proc Natl Acad Sci U S A 107:21677–21682. https://doi.org/10.1073/pnas.1016234107

Ferguson MK (1993) Synchronous primary lung cancers. Chest 103(4 Suppl):398S–400S. https://doi.org/10.1378/chest.103.4_supplement.398s

Filippi AR, Guerrera F, Badellino S et al (2016) Exploratory analysis on overall survival after either surgery or stereotactic radiotherapy for lung oligometastases from colorectal cancer. Clin Oncol 28:505–512. https://doi.org/10.1016/j.clon.2016.02.001

Franceschini D, Cozzi L, De Rose F et al (2017) Role of stereotactic body radiation therapy for lung metastases from radio-resistant primary tumours. J Cancer Res Clin Oncol 143:1293–1299. https://doi.org/10.1007/s00432-017-2373-y

Gadd MA, Casper ES, Woodruff JM et al (1993) Development and treatment of pulmonary metastases in adult patients with extremity soft tissue sarcoma. Ann Surg. https://doi.org/10.1097/00000658-199312000-00002

Gerull WD, Puri V, Kozower BD (2020) The epidemiology and biology of pulmonary metastases. J Thorac Dis 13(4):2585–2589. https://doi.org/10.21037/jtd.2020.04.28

Gloeckler Ries LA, Reichman ME, Lewis DR et al (2003) Cancer survival and incidence from the Surveillance, Epidemiology, and End Results (SEER) Program. Oncologist 8:541–552. https://doi.org/10.1634/theoncologist.8-6-541

Gomez DR, Tang C, Zhang J et al (2019) Local consolidative therapy vs. maintenance therapy or observation for patients with oligometastatic non–small-cell lung cancer: long-term results of a multi-institutional, phase II, randomized study. J Clin Oncol 37:1558–1565. https://doi.org/10.1200/JCO.19.00201

Guckenberger M, Lievens Y, Bouma AB et al (2020) Characterisation and classification of oligometastatic disease: a European Society for Radiotherapy and Oncology and European Organisation for Research and Treatment of Cancer consensus recommendation. Lancet Oncol 21:e18–e28. https://doi.org/10.1016/S1470-2045(19)30718-1

Hellman S, Weichselbaum RR (1995) Oligometastases. J Clin Oncol 13:8–10

Higashiyama M, Kodama K, Higaki N et al (2003) Surgery for pulmonary metastases from colorectal cancer: the importance of prethoracotomy serum carcinoembryonic antigen as an indicator of prognosis. Jpn J Thorac Cardiovasc Surg 51:289–296. https://doi.org/10.1007/BF02719380

Hiratsuka S, Watanabe A, Aburatani H, Maru Y (2006) Tumour-mediated upregulation of chemoattractants and recruitment of myeloid cells predetermines lung metastasis. Nat Cell Biol 8:1369–1375. https://doi.org/10.1038/ncb1507

Hof H, Hoess A, Oetzel D et al (2007) Stereotactic single-dose radiotherapy of lung metastases. Strahlenther Onkol 183:673–678. https://doi.org/10.1007/s00066-007-1724-z

Hörner-Rieber J, Bernhardt D, Blanck O et al (2019) Long-term follow-up and patterns of recurrence of patients with oligometastatic NSCLC treated with pulmonary SBRT. Clin Lung Cancer 20:e667–e677. https://doi.org/10.1016/j.cllc.2019.06.024

Iizasa T, Suzuki M, Yoshida S et al (2006) Prediction of prognosis and surgical indications for pulmonary metastasectomy from colorectal cancer. Ann Thorac Surg 82:254–260. https://doi.org/10.1016/j.athoracsur.2006.02.027

Isaiah JF, Margaret LK (1977) Metastasis results from preexisting variant cells within a malignant tumor. Science 197:893–895

Iyengar P, Wardak Z, Gerber DE et al (2018) Consolidative radiotherapy for limited metastatic non-small-cell lung cancer: a phase 2 randomized clinical trial. JAMA Oncol 4(1):e173501

Jeremic B, Shibamoto Y, Acimovic L et al (2001) Second cancers occurring in patients with early stage non-small-cell lung cancer treated with chest radiation therapy alone. J Clin Oncol 19(4):1056–1063. https://doi.org/10.1200/JCO.2001.19.4.1056

Jingu K, Matsushita H, Yamamoto T et al (2018) Stereotactic radiotherapy for pulmonary oligometastases from colorectal cancer: a systematic review and meta-analysis. Technol Cancer Res Treat 17:1–7. https://doi.org/10.1177/1533033818794936

Kaifi JT, Gusani NJ, Deshaies I et al (2010) Indications and approach to surgical resection of lung metastases. J Surg Oncol 102:187–195. https://doi.org/10.1002/jso.21596

Kalinauskaite GG, Tinhofer II, Kufeld MM et al (2020) Radiosurgery and fractionated stereotactic body radiotherapy for patients with lung oligometastases. BMC Cancer 20:1–10. https://doi.org/10.1186/s12885-020-06892-4

Kanzaki R, Higashiyama M, Fujiwara A et al (2011) Long-term results of surgical resection for pulmonary metastasis from renal cell carcinoma: a 25-year single-institution experience. Eur J Cardiothorac Surg 39:167–172. https://doi.org/10.1016/j.ejcts.2010.05.021

Kanzaki R, Suzuki O, Kanou T et al (2020) The short-term outcomes of pulmonary metastasectomy or stereotactic body radiation therapy for pulmonary metastasis from epithelial tumors. J Cardiothorac Surg 15:1–7. https://doi.org/10.1186/s13019-020-1079-4

Kaplan RN, Riba RD, Zacharoulis S et al (2005) VEGFR1-positive haematopoietic bone marrow progenitors initiate the pre-metastatic niche. Nature 438:820–827. https://doi.org/10.1038/nature04186

Karam JA, Rini BI, Varella L et al (2011) Metastasectomy after targeted therapy in patients with advanced renal cell carcinoma. J Urol. https://doi.org/10.1016/j.juro.2010.09.086

Kim SY, Lee CH, Midura BV et al (2008) Inhibition of the CXCR4/CXCL12 chemokine pathway reduces the development of murine pulmonary metastases. Clin Exp Metastasis 25:201–211. https://doi.org/10.1007/s10585-007-9133-3

Klement RJ (2017) Radiobiological parameters of liver and lung metastases derived from tumor control data of 3719 metastases. Radiother Oncol. https://doi.org/10.1016/j.radonc.2017.03.014

Kliche S, Waltenberger J (2001) VEGF receptor signaling and endothelial function. IUBMB Life 52:61–66. https://doi.org/10.1080/15216540252774784

Koga R, Yamamoto J, Saiura A et al (2006) Surgical resection of pulmonary metastases from colorectal cancer: four favourable prognostic factors. Jpn J Clin Oncol 36:643–648. https://doi.org/10.1093/jjco/hyl076

Kondo H, Okumura T, Ohde Y, Nakagawa K (2005) Surgical treatment for metastatic malignancies. Pulmonary metastasis: indications and outcomes. Int J Clin Oncol 10:81–85. https://doi.org/10.1007/s10147-004-0472-7

König L, Häfner MF, Katayama S et al (2020) Stereotactic body radiotherapy (SBRT) for adrenal metastases of oligometastatic or oligoprogressive tumor patients. Radiat Oncol 15:1–9. https://doi.org/10.1186/s13014-020-1480-0

Lee YH, Kang KM, Choi HS et al (2018) Comparison of stereotactic body radiotherapy versus metastasectomy outcomes in patients with pulmonary metastases. Thorac Cancer 9:1671–1679. https://doi.org/10.1111/1759-7714.12880

Lodeweges JE, Klinkenberg TJ, Ubbels JF et al (2017) Long-term outcome of surgery or stereotactic radiotherapy for lung oligometastases. J Thorac Oncol 12:1442–1445. https://doi.org/10.1016/j.jtho.2017.05.015

Mehta N, Selch M, Wang PC et al (2013) Safety and efficacy of stereotactic body radiation therapy in the treatment of pulmonary metastases from high grade sarcoma. Sarcoma. https://doi.org/10.1155/2013/360214

Meimarakis G, Angele M, Staehler M et al (2011) Evaluation of a new prognostic score (Munich score) to predict long-term survival after resection of pulmonary renal cell carcinoma metastases. Am J Surg 202:158–167. https://doi.org/10.1016/j.amjsurg.2010.06.029

Milne ENC, Zerhouni EA (1987) Blood supply of pulmonary metastases. J Thorac Imaging. https://doi.org/10.1097/00005382-198710000-00005

Murakami T, Maki W, Cardones AR et al (2002) Expression of CXC chemokine receptor-4 enhances the pulmonary metastatic potential of murine B16 melanoma cells. Cancer Res 62:7328–7334

Navarria P, Ascolese AM, Cozzi L et al (2015) Stereotactic body radiation therapy for lung metastases from soft tissue sarcoma. Eur J Cancer 51:668–674. https://doi.org/10.1016/j.ejca.2015.01.061

Neuman HB, Patel A, Hanlon C et al (2007) Stage-IV melanoma and pulmonary metastases: factors predictive of survival. Ann Surg Oncol 14:2847–2853. https://doi.org/10.1245/s10434-007-9448-y

Niibe Y, Yamashita H, Sekiguchi K et al (2015) Stereotactic body radiotherapy results for pulmonary oligometastases: a two-institution collaborative investigation. Anticancer Res 35:4903–4908

Nikitas J, DeWees T, Rehman S et al (2019) Stereotactic body radiotherapy for early-stage multiple primary lung cancers. Clin Lung Cancer 20(2):107–116. https://doi.org/10.1016/j.cllc.2018.10.010. Epub 2018 Nov 3

Noonan CD, Margulis AR, Wright R (1965) Bronchial arterial patterns in pulmonary metastasis. Radiology 84:1033–1042. https://doi.org/10.1148/84.6.1033

Norihisa Y, Nagata Y, Takayama K et al (2008) Stereotactic body radiotherapy for oligometastatic lung tumors. Int J Radiat Oncol Biol Phys. https://doi.org/10.1016/j.ijrobp.2008.01.002

Nuyttens JJ, Der Voort V, Van Zyp NCMG, Verhoef C et al (2015) Stereotactic body radiation therapy for oligometastases to the lung: a phase 2 study. Int J Radiat Oncol Biol Phys 91:337–343. https://doi.org/10.1016/j.ijrobp.2014.10.021

Oh D, Ahn YC, Seo JM et al (2012) Potentially curative stereotactic body radiation therapy (SBRT) for single or oligometastasis to the lung. Acta Oncol (Madr) 51:596–602. https://doi.org/10.3109/0284186X.2012.681698

Okunieff P, Petersen AL, Philip A et al (2006) Stereotactic body radiation therapy (SBRT) for lung metastases. Acta Oncol (Madr) 45:808–817. https://doi.org/10.1080/02841860600908954

Onimaru R, Shirato H, Shimizu S et al (2003) Tolerance of organs at risk in small-volume, hypofractionated, image-guided radiotherapy for primary and metastatic lung cancers. Int J Radiat Oncol Biol Phys 56:126–135. https://doi.org/10.1016/S0360-3016(03)00095-6

Osti MF, Carnevale A, Valeriani M et al (2013) Clinical outcomes of single dose stereotactic radiotherapy for lung metastases. Clin Lung Cancer. https://doi.org/10.1016/j.cllc.2013.06.006

Palma DA, Salama JK, Lo SS et al (2014) The oligometastatic state-separating truth from wishful thinking. Nat Rev Clin Oncol 11:549–557. https://doi.org/10.1038/nrclinonc.2014.96

Palma DA, Olson R, Harrow S et al (2019) Stereotactic ablative radiotherapy versus standard of care palliative treatment in patients with oligometastatic cancers (SABR-COMET): a randomised, phase 2, open-label trial. Lancet 393:2051–2058. https://doi.org/10.1016/S0140-6736(18)32487-5

Pasalic D, Lu Y, Betancourt-Cuellar SL et al (2020) Stereotactic ablative radiation therapy for pulmonary metastases: improving overall survival and identifying subgroups at high risk of local failure. Radiother Oncol 145:178–185. https://doi.org/10.1016/j.radonc.2020.01.010

Pastorino U, Buyse M, Friedel G et al (1997) Long-term results of lung metastasectomy: prognostic analyses based on 5206 cases. J Thorac Cardiovasc Surg 113:37–49. https://doi.org/10.1016/S0022-5223(97)70397-0

Petersen RP, Hanish SI, Haney JC et al (2007) Improved survival with pulmonary metastasectomy: an analysis of 1720 patients with pulmonary metastatic melanoma. J Thorac Cardiovasc Surg 133:104–110. https://doi.org/10.1016/j.jtcvs.2006.08.065

Pfannschmidt J, Muley T, Hoffmann H, Dienemann H (2003) Prognostic factors and survival after complete resection of pulmonary metastases from colorectal carcinoma: experiences in 167 patients. J Thorac Cardiovasc Surg 126:732–739. https://doi.org/10.1016/S0022-5223(03)00587-7

Pfannschmidt J, Dienemann H, Hoffmann H (2007) Surgical resection of pulmonary metastases from colorectal cancer: a systematic review of published series. Ann Thorac Surg 84:324–338. https://doi.org/10.1016/j.athoracsur.2007.02.093

Reyes DK, Pienta KJ (2015) The biology and treatment of oligometastatic cancer. Oncotarget 6:8491–8524. https://doi.org/10.18632/oncotarget.3455

Ricardi U, Filippi AR, Guarneri A et al (2012) Stereotactic body radiation therapy for lung metastases. Lung Cancer. https://doi.org/10.1016/j.lungcan.2011.04.021

Ricco A, Davis J, Rate W et al (2017) Lung metastases treated with stereotactic body radiotherapy: the RSSearch® patient Registry's experience. Radiat Oncol 12:4–11. https://doi.org/10.1186/s13014-017-0773-4

Rieber J, Streblow J, Uhlmann L et al (2016) Lung cancer stereotactic body radiotherapy (SBRT) for medically inoperable lung metastases—a pooled analysis of the German working group "stereotactic radiotherapy". Lung Cancer 97:51–58. https://doi.org/10.1016/j.lungcan.2016.04.012

Rosengart TK, Martini N, Ghosn P et al (1991) Multiple primary lung carcinomas: prognosis and treatment. Ann Thorac Surg 52(4):773–778. https://doi.org/10.1016/0003-4975(91)91209-e

Rusthoven KE, Kavanagh BD, Burri SH et al (2009) Multi-institutional phase I/II trial of stereotactic body radiation therapy for lung metastases. J Clin Oncol 27:1579–1584. https://doi.org/10.1200/jco.2008.19.6386

Schueller G, Herold CJ (2003) Lung metastases. Cancer Imaging 3:126–128. https://doi.org/10.1102/1470-7330.2003.0010

Soyfer V, Corn BW, Kollender Y et al (2010) Radiation therapy for palliation of sarcoma metastases: a unique and uniform hypofractionation experience. Sarcoma. https://doi.org/10.1155/2010/927972

Steber CR, Hughes RT, Soike MH et al (2021) Stereotactic body radiotherapy for synchronous early stage non-small cell lung cancer. Acta Oncol. https://doi.org/10.1080/0284186X.2021.1892182

Stragliotto CL, Karlsson K, Lax I et al (2012) A retrospective study of SBRT of metastases in patients with primary sarcoma. Med Oncol 29:3431–3439. https://doi.org/10.1007/s12032-012-0256-2

Swetter SM, Tsao H, Bichakjian CK et al (2019) Guidelines of care for the management of primary cutaneous melanoma. J Am Acad Dermatol 80:208–250. https://doi.org/10.1016/j.jaad.2018.08.055

Timmerman R, Papiez L, McGarry R et al (2003) Extracranial stereotactic radioablation: results of a phase I study in medically inoperable stage I non-small cell lung cancer. Chest 124:1946–1955. https://doi.org/10.1378/chest.124.5.1946

Treasure T, Miloševíc M, Fiorentino F, Macbeth F (2014) Pulmonary metastasectomy: what is the practice and where is the evidence for effectiveness? Thorax 69:946–949. https://doi.org/10.1136/thoraxjnl-2013-204528

Van Geel AN, Pastorino U, Jauch KW et al (1996) Surgical treatment of lung metastases: the European Organization for Research and Treatment of Cancer-Soft Tissue and Bone Sarcoma Group study of 255 patients. Cancer. https://doi.org/10.1002/(SICI)1097-0142(19960215)77:4<675::AID-CNCR13>3.0.CO;2-Y

Verstegen NE, Oosterhuis JWA, Palma DA et al (2013) Stage I-II non-small-cell lung cancer treated using either stereotactic ablative radiotherapy (SABR) or lobectomy by video-assisted thoracoscopic surgery (VATS): outcomes of a propensity score-matched analysis. Ann Oncol 24:1543–1548. https://doi.org/10.1093/annonc/mdt026

Videtic GMM, Donington J, Giuliani M et al (2017) Stereotactic body radiation therapy for early-stage non-small cell lung cancer: executive summary of an ASTRO evidence-based guideline. Pract Radiat Oncol 7(5):295–301. https://doi.org/10.1016/j.prro.2017.04.014. Epub 2017 Jun 5

Wang JM, Deng X, Gong W, Su S (1998) Chemokines and their role in tumor growth and metastasis. J Immunol Methods 220:1–17. https://doi.org/10.1016/S0022-1759(98)00128-8

Weigelt B, Glas AM, Wessels LFA et al (2003) Gene expression profiles of primary breast tumors maintained in distant metastases. Proc Natl Acad Sci U S A 100:15901–15905. https://doi.org/10.1073/pnas.2634067100

Weigelt B, Wessels LFA, Bosma AJ et al (2005) No common denominator for breast cancer lymph node metastasis. Br J Cancer 93:924–932. https://doi.org/10.1038/sj.bjc.6602794

Welter S, Jacobs J, Krbek T et al (2007) Prognostic impact of lymph node involvement in pulmonary metastases from colorectal cancer. Eur J Cardiothorac Surg 31:167–172. https://doi.org/10.1016/j.ejcts.2006.11.004

Widder J, Klinkenberg TJ, Ubbels JF et al (2013) Pulmonary oligometastases: metastasectomy or stereotactic ablative radiotherapy? Radiother Oncol 107:409–413. https://doi.org/10.1016/j.radonc.2013.05.024

Xu L, Burke AP (2012) Pulmonary oligometastases: histological features and difficulties in determining site of origin. Int J Surg Pathol 20:577–588. https://doi.org/10.1177/1066896912449039

Yamamoto T, Niibe Y, Matsumoto Y et al (2020) Analyses of local control and survival after stereotactic body radiotherapy for pulmonary oligometastases from colorectal adenocarcinoma. J Radiat Res 61:935–944. https://doi.org/10.1093/jrr/rraa071

Yancopoulos GD, Davis S, Gale NW et al (2000) Vascular-specific growth factors and blood vessel formation. Nature 407:242–248. https://doi.org/10.1038/35025215

Yu W, Liu Z, Tang L et al (2017) Efficacy and safety of stereotactic radiosurgery for pulmonary metastases from osteosarcoma: experience in 73 patients. Sci Rep 7:1–9. https://doi.org/10.1038/s41598-017-14521-7

Radiation Therapy for Brain Metastases

Dirk Rades, Sabine Bohnet, and Steven E. Schild

Contents

1 Background 756
2 Radiation Therapy for Multiple Brain Metastases 756
2.1 Role of Whole-Brain Radiotherapy 756
2.2 Prognostic Tools for Patients Receiving Whole-Brain Radiotherapy 757
2.3 Neuro-cognitive Decline After Whole-Brain Radiotherapy 758
3 Radiation Therapy for Single Brain Metastasis 761
4 Radiation Therapy for a Limited Number of Brain Metastases 762
5 Systemic Treatment in Addition to Radiation Therapy 764
5.1 Radiosensitizers 764
5.2 "Classic" Chemotherapy 765
5.3 Targeted Therapies/Immunotherapy 766
6 Prophylactic Cranial Irradiation 769
6.1 Prophylactic Cranial Irradiation for SCLC 769
6.2 Prophylactic Cranial Irradiation for NSCLC ... 771

References 772

D. Rades (✉)
Department of Radiation Oncology, University of Lübeck, Lübeck, Germany
e-mail: Rades.Dirk@gmx.net

S. Bohnet
Department of Pulmonology, University of Lübeck, Lübeck, Germany

S. E. Schild
Department of Radiation Oncology, Mayo Clinic, Scottsdale, AZ, USA

Abstract

Lung cancer is the most common primary tumor in patients with brain metastases. Traditional treatment for multiple (>3–4) lesions includes whole-brain radiotherapy (WBRT) plus dexamethasone. When selecting a WBRT-program, the patient's survival prognosis should be considered. For single lesions, WBRT + resection produces better outcomes than WBRT or resection alone. Results improve with a boost to the metastatic site. Stereotactic radiosurgery (SRS) and fractionated stereotactic radiotherapy appear less invasive alternatives. In patients with few lesions, randomized trials demonstrated that addition of WBRT to SRS improved local/intracranial control but not OS and increased cognitive decline. However, hippocampus-sparing and memantine, which reduce cognitive decline, were not used. In secondary analyses of randomized trials (lung cancer patients only), WBRT improved OS in patients with favorable prognoses. Radiosensitizers and classic chemotherapies have not improved outcomes of WBRT. Tyrosine kinase inhibitors and immune checkpoint inhibitors (ICIs) improve intracerebral response in lung cancer patients irradiated for brain metastases; however, results regarding OS are conflicting. After introduction of ICIs and increasing availability of routine MRI-surveillance, the role of PCI needs to be re-defined. Considering availability of modern radiation techniques and rapid development of targeted therapies, additional trials are warranted for treatment of brain metastases from lung cancer.

1 Background

Brain metastases occur in 20–40% of all cancer patients during the course of their disease (Tsao et al. 2012). Lung cancer is the most common primary tumor causing brain metastases and accounts for approximately 50%. Symptoms may include headache, seizures, vision disturbances, hearing problems, nausea, vomiting, motor deficits, and others. Treatment options include whole-brain radiotherapy (WBRT), local therapies such as neurosurgical resection, stereotactic radiosurgery (SRS), and fractionated stereotactic radiation therapy (FSRT), and best supportive care including dexamethasone (Tsao et al. 2012). Treatment recommendations are based on patient characteristics (including age, performance status, and co-morbidities), general characteristics of the malignancy (including histology and extracranial disease), and characteristics of the cerebral lesions (including location, size, and number). With respect to the number of lesions, some authors differentiate between single and multiple (more than one) lesions. However, differentiation between a single lesion, a limited number of lesions, and multiple lesions appears more appropriate. The term "limited number" is not consistent in the literature and mainly used for ≤ 3 or ≤ 4 lesions.

2 Radiation Therapy for Multiple Brain Metastases

2.1 Role of Whole-Brain Radiotherapy

Most patients with multiple (>3–4) brain metastases have poor survival prognoses. This accounts particularly for lung cancer patients. The median survival of untreated patients is about 1 month (Zimm et al. 1981). Even with WBRT, these patients have a median life expectancy of only a few months (Sundstrom et al. 1998). The traditional treatment for multiple brain metastases from lung cancer includes WBRT plus dexamethasone (Khuntia et al. 2006). For patients with poor survival prognoses, short-course WBRT such as 5×4 Gy over 1 week would be preferable, if it provided similar outcomes as longer programs such as 10×3 Gy over 2 weeks and 20×2 Gy over 4 weeks. Few studies compared short-course to longer-course WBRT for multiple brain metastases (Harwood and Simson 1977; Priestman et al. 1996; Borgelt et al. 1980; Chatani et al. 1994). Whereas most studies found no significant differences in survival, one prospective study from 1996 suggested a marginally better median survival after longer-course 10×3 Gy compared to 2×6 Gy (2.8 vs. 2.5 months, $p = 0.04$) (Priestman et al. 1996).

Only one retrospective study focused on NSCLC and compared 5×4 Gy ($n = 140$) to 10×3 Gy or 20×2 Gy ($n = 264$) (Rades et al. 2007a). Overall survival (OS) rates at 6, 12, and 24 months were 40%, 16%, and 6%, respectively, after 5×4 Gy, and 30%, 17%, and 10%, respectively, after longer-course WBRT ($p = 0.55$). Another retrospective study of 146 patients compared 5×4 Gy and 10×3 Gy in patients with brain metastases from SCLC (Bohlen et al. 2010). One-year OS rates were 15% after 5×4 Gy and 22% after 10×3 Gy ($p = 0.69$), and 1-year intracranial control rates were 34% and 25% ($p = 0.32$). Thus, many patients with multiple brain metastases from NSCLC and SCLC appear not to benefit from longer-course WBRT when compared to short-course WBRT. Selected patients with brain metastases from NSCLC and very poor prognoses do not benefit from WBRT at all. In a phase III non-inferiority trial (QUARTZ), 538 patients were randomized to receive 5×4 Gy of WBRT plus best supportive care including dexamethasone (BSC) or BSC alone (Mulvenna et al. 2016). There were no significant differences regarding OS, overall quality of life, and use of dexamethasone. The quality-adjusted life years were 46.4 days in the

BSC + WBRT group and 41.7 days in the BSC alone group.

In contrast, patients with longer expected survival may be candidates for longer-course WBRT with lower doses per fraction (e.g., 20 × 2 Gy over 4 weeks). It has been suggested that the risk of radiation-induced cognitive deficits is lower with doses per fraction of <3 Gy (De Angelis et al. 1989). Moreover, in a retrospective study of 184 patients (74 lung cancer patients) with favorable survival prognoses, 20 × 2 Gy resulted in better 1-year survival (61% vs. 40%, $p = 0.008$ in the multivariate analysis) and 1-year intracranial control (44% vs. 28%, $p = 0.047$) than 10 × 3 Gy (Rades et al. 2012a). When selecting a WBRT-program for lung cancer patients, the patient's remaining lifespan should be considered, which can be estimated with the help of diagnosis-specific prognostic scores (Sperduto et al. 2010, 2012, 2017; Rades et al. 2013a, b, 2019a, b).

2.2 Prognostic Tools for Patients Receiving Whole-Brain Radiotherapy

In 2010, Sperduto et al. presented diagnosis-specific Graded Prognostic Assessment (DS-GPA) classifications for NSCLC and SCLC (Sperduto et al. 2010). Based on Karnofsky performance score (KPS), age, extracranial metastases, and number of brain lesions, four GPA-classes (0–1.0, 1.5–2.5, 3.0, and 3-5–4.0) were designed. In an update of the DS-GPA, prognostic groups for NSCLC and SCLC were re-defined and included GPA-classes 0–1.0, 1.5–2.0, 2.5–3.0, and 3-5–4.0 (Sperduto et al. 2012). Median OS times were 3.0, 5.5, 9.4, and 14.8 months, respectively, for NSCLC ($p < 0.001$), and 2.8, 4.9, 7.7, and 17.1 months, respectively, for SCLC ($p < 0.001$). The DS-GPA scores were created in patients heterogeneously treated for brain metastases including different WBRT-programs plus/minus radiosensitizers, systemic chemotherapy, or radiosurgery, which might have led to hidden selection biases.

To reduce the risk of biases, disease-specific survival scores for NSCLC and SCLC were developed in patients treated with WBRT alone (Rades et al. 2013a, b). The NSCLC-study included 514 patients who were divided in a test group ($n = 257$) and a validation group ($n = 257$) (Rades et al. 2013a). Based on gender, KPS, and extracranial metastases, three prognostic groups were designed (5–9, 11–12, and 15 points) with 6-months OS rates of 9%, 54%, and 79% in the test group ($p < 0.001$). In the validation group, 6-month OS rates were 14%, 56%, and 78% ($p < 0.001$). Similarly, a survival score was created for SCLC patients (Rades et al. 2013b). A cohort of 172 patients was divided into a test group ($n = 86$) and a validation group ($n = 86$). Based on KPS, number of brain metastases, and extracranial metastases, three groups were designed (5–8, 9–12, and 15 points). Six-month OS rates were 3%, 40%, and 89% in the test group ($p < 0.001$), and 3%, 41%, and 89% in the validation group ($p < 0.001$). Although patients used for these analyses received WBRT alone, a risk of a hidden bias remained due to inclusion of different WBRT-programs. Therefore, additional scores were developed from patients homogeneously treated with 10 × 3 Gy of WBRT alone (Rades et al. 2019a, b). The WBRT-30-NSCLC was based on age, KPS, systemic treatment prior to WBRT, extracranial metastases, and number of brain metastases (Rades et al. 2019a). Four groups were created with 6-month OS rates of 3% (9–12 points), 26% (13–17 points), 65% (18–20 points), and 100% (22 points) ($p < 0.001$). Positive predictive values of the WBRT-30-NSCLC to identify patients dying within 6 months (97%) or living for 6 months or longer (100%) were higher than for the updated DS-GPA classification (86% and 78%) and the Rades-NSCLC score (88% and 74%) (Sperduto et al. 2010, 2012; Rades et al. 2013a).

In 2019, the WBRT-30-SCLC was developed in 157 patients receiving 10 × 3 Gy of WBRT alone and based on age, KPS, extracranial metastases, and number of lesions (Rades et al. 2019b). Three groups were designed with 6-month survival rates of 6% (6–11 points), 44% (12–14 points), and 86% (16–19 points) ($p < 0.001$). The WBRT-30-SCLC was compared three other diagnosis-specific tools. Positive predictive values were 94% (WBRT-30-SCLC), 88% (original DS-GPA), 88% (updated DS-GPA), and 100% (Rades-SCLC) to predict death within 6 months, and 86%, 75%, 76%, and 100%, respectively, to predict survival of at least 6 months (Sperduto et al. 2010, 2012; Rades et al. 2013b). The Rades-SCLC appeared most accurate followed by the WBRT-30-SCLC and both DS-GPA classifications.

Another approach to optimize treatment personalization for brain metastases from NSCLC was a sub-classification of the DS-GPA in adenocarcinoma and non-adenocarcinoma patients (Sperduto et al. 2017). Since adenocarcinoma patients with gene mutations (epidermal growth factor receptor, EGFR; anaplastic lymphoma kinase, ALK) have better survival prognoses than patients without such mutations, EGFR- and ALK mutation status were included in a classification called Lung-molGPA. Median survival times of the resulting GPA-classes were 6.9 (0–1.0), 13.7 (1-5–2.0), 26.5 (2.5–3.0), and 46.8 months (3.5–4.0). The Lung-molGPA classification was externally validated in 269 patients, who also received different treatments for brain metastases possibly leading to selection biases (Nieder et al. 2017). Since patients with adenocarcinoma had better survival prognoses than other lung cancer patients in both studies, differentiation between these groups is reasonable (Sperduto et al. 2017; Nieder et al. 2017). Scores for brain metastases from adenocarcinoma in homogeneously treated patients are warranted. Moreover, when using the survival scores discussed in this chapter, one has to be aware that all scores were developed retrospectively and prior to the introduction of immune checkpoint inhibitors in first line treatment. Nevertheless, these scores may assist one design a personalized treatment.

2.3 Neuro-cognitive Decline After Whole-Brain Radiotherapy

Patients who receive WBRT may develop neuro-cognitive deficits (Shaw and Ball 2013). The most severe neuro-cognitive complication is dementia. This was reported in 2–5% of patients after WBRT, particularly if doses per fraction of ≥3 Gy or concurrent chemotherapy were administered and if patients survived for 1 year (De Angelis et al. 1989). Longer WBRT-programs with lower doses per fraction appear preferable for those with longer expected survival. Modern approaches such as hippocampus-sparing (Fig. 1) and addition of memantine reduce neuro-cognitive decline. The rationale for hippocampus-sparing WBRT is the fact that radiation-induced damage to the neural stem-cell compartment of the hippocampal dentate gyrus leading to neuro-cognitive decline (Robin and Rusthoven 2018). In 2014, results of a single-arm phase II trial of hippocampus-sparing WBRT (RTOG 0933) were reported (Gondi et al. 2014). Primary endpoint was the Hopkins Verbal Learning Test-revised Delayed Recall at 4 months following WBRT. The mean relative decline from baseline was 7.0% compared to 30% in a historical control group ($p < 0.001$). Sparing of the hippocampi may result in a higher rate of recurrences in the hippocampal and peri-hippocampal (hippocampal subgranular zone plus 5 mm) regions. In 2020, Ly et al. presented a retrospective cohort study of 2146 patients with NSCLC (Ly et al. 2020). Of 335 patients with brain metastases and cranial imaging, 30 patients (9%) had brain metastases in the hippocampal (2.4%) or peri-hippocampal (6.6%) regions. The authors considered this a low incidence and hippocampal-sparing WBRT feasible.

Later, a randomized, placebo-controlled trial (RTOG 0614) of 554 investigated memantine to protect neuro-cognitive function after WBRT (Brown et al. 2013). Memantine is used in patients with vascular dementia, where ischemia is associated with activation of the NMDA (N-methyl-D-aspartate) receptor and excitotoxicity (Robin and Rusthoven 2018). The neuroprotective effect of memantine is due to its role as a NMDA receptor antagonist. In the RTOG 0614 trial, addition of memantine to WBRT (15 × 2.5 Gy) resulted in less decline in delayed recall at 24 weeks (Brown et al. 2013). The difference was not statistically significant, possibly because only 149 patients were evaluable at

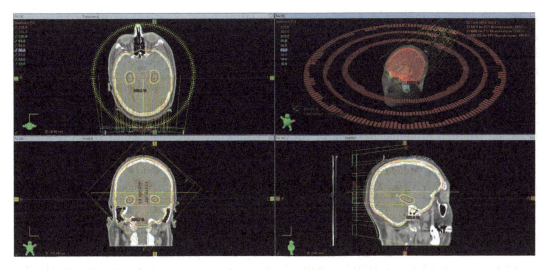

Fig. 1 Example of whole-brain radiotherapy (WBRT) using a hippocampus-sparing technique

24 weeks. However, in the memantine group, time to cognitive decline was significantly longer ($p = 0.01$), and memantine led to significantly better results with respect to specific cognitive functions. Following these promising studies, the authors of RTOG trials 0933 and 0614 performed a randomized phase III trial of 518 patients that compared WBRT plus memantine to hippocampus-sparing WBRT plus memantine (Brown et al. 2020). Hippocampus-sparing led to significantly less neuro-cognitive decline ($p = 0.02$) but no difference in OS or progression-free survival (PFS). The combination of a hippocampus-sparing technique and memantine appears reasonable for patients with good performance and no metastases in the hippocampal areas. Less convincing were the results of a phase III trial of 198 patients investigating donepezil, a reversible acetylcholinesterase inhibitor (Rapp et al. 2015). Patients received partial brain irradiation or WBRT of at least 30 Gy for primary or metastatic brain tumors without intracranial progression during last 3 months. Although Donepezil did not improve overall cognitive composite score (primary outcome), it resulted in modest improvements in specific cognitive functions, particularly in patients with greater impairment prior to treatment.

Although the results of hippocampus-sparing WBRT plus memantine were promising, the best option to avoid neuro-cognitive deficits would be omitting WBRT. Several studies investigated SRS for >4 brain metastases. In 2014, a prospective study (JLGK 0901) of 1194 patients (mainly lung cancer patients) compared SRS with 20–22 Gy for 5–10 lesions ($n = 208$), 2–4 lesions ($n = 531$), and 1 lesion ($n = 455$) (Yamamoto et al. 2014a). Patients had a KPS of ≥ 70, and cerebral lesions had a total volume ≤ 15 mL. Median OS times were 10.8 (5–10 lesions), 10.8 (2–4 lesions), and 13.9 (1 lesion) months. Grade 3–4 adverse events occurred in 3%, 2%, and 2% of patients, respectively. OS was not significantly different between patients with 5–10 lesions and 2–4 lesions ($p = 0.78$). The authors concluded that SRS appeared an alternative to WBRT for up to 10 brain metastases. A retrospective study of 1814 patients (69% lung cancer patients) receiving Gamma Knife radiosurgery compared 2–9 to ≥ 10 lesions (Yamamoto et al. 2014b). After propensity score matching, 360 patients remained in each group for analyses. Median OS times were 6.8 months (2–9 lesions) and 6.0 months (≥ 10 lesions), respectively ($p = 0.10$). No significant differences were observed for cumulative incidence of neurological deterioration ($p = 0.80$) or treatment-related complications ($p = 0.38$). Another retrospective study compared 1515 patients with 5–10 lesions to 804 patients with 11–20 lesions (Yamamoto et al. 2020). Median OS was significantly better in patients with 5–10 lesions (7.7 vs. 6.5 months, $p < 0.001$). SRS may be an option for selected patients with up to 10 brain metastases and possibly even for carefully selected patients with >10 lesions. However, additional randomized trials are required to define the role of SRS alone for >4 lesions.

Another modern approach for multiple brain metastases includes WBRT with a simultaneous integrated boost (SIB) (Fig. 2). In 2020, Zhong et al. presented a prospective series of 13 patients (4 NSCLC patients) receiving 10×2.5 Gy of WBRT + SIB of 10×2.0 Gy (cumulative 45.0 Gy) or 15×2.5 Gy of WBRT + SIB of 15×1.0 Gy (cumulative 52.5 Gy) for 1–10 brain metastases (Zhong et al. 2020). One-year local control and intracranial control rates were 92% (98.6% at lesion level) and 46%, respectively. Several tests did not show significant cognitive decline. In 2021, a retrospective study of 144 lung cancer patients with 1–10 brain metastases was published (Du et al. 2021). Seventy-seven patients received WBRT alone, 39 WBRT + sequential boost, and 28 WBRT + SIB. Median survival times were 7, 11, and 14 months, respectively. WBRT + SIB appeared superior to WBRT alone ($p < 0.001$) and WBRT + sequential boost ($p = 0.037$), which was confirmed in multivariate analyses. Other studies combined WBRT + SIB with a hippocampus-sparing technique. In a single-institution phase II trial of 49 patients (39 lung cancer patients) with 1–8 lesions, hippocampus-sparing WBRT of 10×2 Gy (max. 16 Gy to hippocampi) was combined with a SIB of 10×2 Gy (cumulative dose = 40.0 Gy) (Westover et al. 2020). Median PFS and OS times were 2.9 and 9 months. Cumulative incidences of local and intracranial failure were 8.8% and 21.3%, respectively. Mean cognitive decline at 3 months was only 10.6%. In a retrospective matched-pair study of 124 patients (64 NSCLC patients) with 4–17 lesions, 1-year local control was significantly better with hippocampus-sparing WBRT (12×2.5 Gy) + SIB (12×1.0 or 1.75 Gy) than with WBRT alone (mainly 10×3 Gy or 15×2.5 Gy), i.e., 98% vs. 82%, $p = 0.007$ (Popp et al. 2020). Median intracranial PFS (13.5 vs. 6.4 months, $p = 0.03$) and OS (9.9 vs. 6.2 months, $p = 0.001$) were also better in the SIB-group. Distant brain control at 1 year was better after WBRT alone (82% vs. 69%, $p = 0.016$), probably due to the higher biological effective dose administered to the entire brain. Thus, WBRT + SIB with or without sparing of the hippocampi appears a reasonable option for patients with

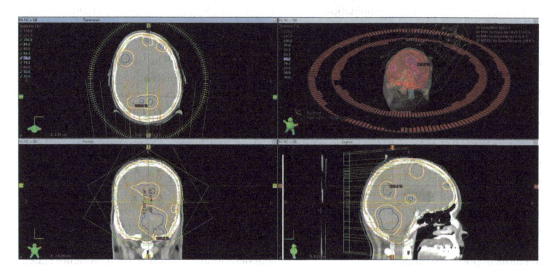

Fig. 2 Example of whole-brain radiotherapy (WBRT) with a simultaneous integrated boost (SIB) for a total of nine brain metastases

multiple brain metastases not amenable or suitable for SRS and FSRT.

3 Radiation Therapy for Single Brain Metastasis

For patients with a single lesion, three small randomized trials compared WBRT alone to WBRT + surgery (Patchell et al. 1990; Vecht et al. 1993; Mintz et al. 1996). In the trial of Patchell et al. ($n = 48$), the combined treatment resulted in longer median OS (9.2 vs. 3.5 months, $p < 0.01$) and fewer local recurrences (20% vs. 52%, $p < 0.02$) (Patchell et al. 1990). Median OS in the study of Vecht et al. ($n = 63$) was 10 months after WBRT + surgery and 6 months after WBRT alone ($p = 0.04$) (Vecht et al. 1993). Mintz et al. ($N = 84$) did not find a significant difference in median OS (5.6 vs. 6.3 months, $p = 0.24$) (Mintz et al. 1996). In a retrospective study of 195 patients, surgery + WBRT resulted in better 1-year OS (48% vs. 26%, $p < 0.001$) and 1-year intracranial control (57% vs. 24%, $p < 0.001$) than WBRT alone (Rades et al. 2008). Moreover, in a randomized trial of 95 patients that compared surgery alone to surgery followed by WBRT, the addition of WBRT resulted in fewer intracranial recurrences (18% vs. 70%, $p < 0.001$) (Patchell et al. 1998). This advantage accounted for the original lesion (10% vs. 46%, $p < 0001$) and new lesions (14% vs. 37%, $p < 0.01$). Deaths due to neurologic causes were fewer after resection + WBRT (14% vs. 44%, $p = 0.003$), whereas median survival was not significantly different (Patchell et al. 1998). According to a retrospective study of 195 patients, the results of surgery + WBRT can be improved with a boost to the metastatic site (Rades et al. 2012b). One-year local control rates were 67% with and 38% without a boost ($p = 0.006$ in the multivariate analysis). One-year OS rates were 60% and 52%, respectively ($p = 0.11$).

Since radiosurgery is less invasive than neurosurgery, it has been questioned whether it can be an alternative to resection for single brain metastases (Fig. 3). In 2008, Muacevic et al. compared resection + WBRT to Gamma Knife radiosurgery alone for single lesions <3 cm (Muacevic et al. 2008). The rate of new brain metastases was lower ($p = 0.04$) in the resection + WBRT group. However, this was more likely due to the WBRT. Moreover, the trial was prematurely closed after 64 patients. In 2012, a retrospective study compared resection + WBRT ($n = 111$) to WBRT + SRS ($n = 41$) for single brain metastasis (Rades et al. 2012c). One-year local control rates were better after WBRT + SRS (87% vs. 56%,

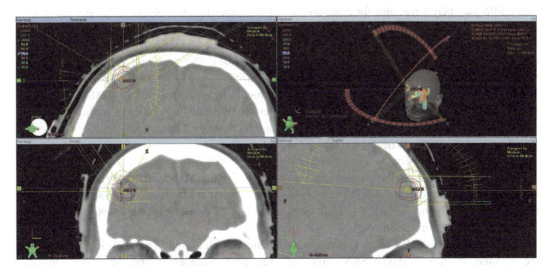

Fig. 3 Example of linear accelerator based stereotactic radiosurgery of a single brain metastasis

$p = 0.005$ in the multivariate analysis). One-year OS rates were 61% and 53%, respectively ($p = 0.16$). Better local control after WBRT + SRS may be explained by potential distribution of tumor cells during neurosurgery. Moreover, the retrospective study design may have introduced a hidden selection bias. Since results of resection + WBRT can be improved with a boost to the metastatic site, another retrospective study compared this approach to WBRT + SRS (Rades et al. 2012d). Forty-six patients receiving resection + WBRT + boost for a single lesion were matched 1:1 for eight characteristics to 46 patients receiving WBRT + SRS. One-year local control rates were 85% after WBRT + SRS compared to 78% after resection + WBRT + boost ($p = 0.35$). One-year intracranial control rates were 74% and 68% ($p = 0.35$), 1-year OS rates 64% and 58% ($p = 0.70$). SRS may be a less invasive alternative to resection for single lesions. When using SRS, addition of WBRT improved local control and freedom from new lesions but not survival (Rades et al. 2012e).

However, these studies did not focus on single brain metastasis from lung cancer. In 2015, Qin et al. presented a systematic review of 18 studies with 713 patients with a single lesion from NSCLC (Qin et al. 2015). Median OS times were 12.7 months after resection and 14.85 months after SRS. OS rates at 1, 2, and 5 years were 59%, 33%, and 19% vs. 62%, 33%, and 14%, respectively. SRS may play a role also for brain metastases from SCLC, particularly if the patients already received prophylactic cranial irradiation (PCI) or experience intracranial failure after WBRT (Cifarelli et al. 2020; Cordeiro et al. 2019). The FIRE-SCLC cohort study compared SRS alone to WBRT alone for single and multiple lesions (propensity-score matching) (Rusthoven et al. 2020). WBRT was associated with significantly longer time to intracranial progression ($p < 0.001$) but similar median intracranial PFS (3.8 vs.4.0 months, $p = 0.79$) and worse OS (5.2 vs. 6.5 months, $p = 0.003$). Thus, SRS alone may be an option for primary treatment of brain metastases from SCLC. Randomized trials are required to properly define SRS's role for these patients.

In addition, several studies investigated a combination of resection and SRS. In 2014, a literature review of 15 publications on postoperative SRS of the resection cavity was presented (Zhang and Chang 2014). More than 50% of the patients had a single lesion, and NSCLC was the most common primary tumor. One-year local control rates ranged from 74% to 91.5%; new lesions occurred in 53.8% (median) after median follow-up of 7.8 months. Symptomatic radionecrosis was found in <10% of patients. In 2017, a single-center phase III trial compared complete resection alone and complete resection + SRS to the resection cavity (maximum diameter ≤ 4 cm) in 132 patients with 1–3 brain metastases from different primary tumors (Mahajan et al. 2017). One-year local control rates were 43% and 72%, respectively ($p = 0.015$). Since 55% of patients in the resection + SRS group developed distant brain metastases, it was questioned whether postoperative WBRT instead of SRS/FSRT would be preferable. In a retrospective study of 132 patients with 141 brain metastases, 36 patients received postoperative WBRT and 96 patients postoperative SRS to the resection cavity (Patel et al. 2014). WBRT resulted in non-significantly better 1-year local control (83% vs. 74%, $p = 0.31$). One-year distant brain control (70% vs. 48%, $p = 0.03$) and 18-months freedom from leptomeningeal disease (87% vs. 69%, $p = 0.045$) rates were significantly higher in the WBRT-group. However, 1-year OS rates were similar (56% vs. 55%, $p = 0.64$), and radiographic leukoencephalopathy was more common after resection + WBRT (47% vs. 7%, $p = 0.001$). The pros and cons of WBRT and SRS/FSRT need to be carefully balanced for each patient (please refer to Sect. 4). Moreover, studies on resection plus adjuvant radiotherapy did not focus on lung cancer patients.

4 Radiation Therapy for a Limited Number of Brain Metastases

Patients with a limited number of brain metastases, most commonly defined as ≤ 3 or ≤ 4 lesions, generally have better survival prognoses than patients with more lesions (Tsao et al. 2012). These patients can benefit from local therapies including SRS, FSRT, and resection. However, neurosurgical resection is generally limited to patients with a single lesion (see Sect. 3).

A retrospective study of 186 patients (69 with lung cancer) with 1–3 lesions found that SRS alone resulted in better 1-year local control of the treated lesions (64% vs. 26%, $p < 0.001$) and 1-year OS (52% vs. 33%, $p = 0.045$) than WBRT alone (Rades et al. 2007b). In a matched-pair study of 304 patients (164 with lung cancer), 152 patients receiving SRS or FSRT alone were matched 1:1 for eight characteristics to 152 patients receiving WBRT alone (Rades et al. 2017a). One-year intracranial control rates were 45% vs. 40% ($p = 0.05$), and 1-year OS rates 45% vs. 40% ($p = 0.65$). Since results of WBRT alone and SRS/FSRT alone were each considered unsatisfactory, several studies investigated the combination of both treatments. The RTOG 9508 phase III trial compared WBRT + SRS-boost to WBRT alone in 331 patients (211 lung cancer patients) with 1–3 brain metastases (Andrews et al. 2004). Higher 1-year local control rates were found after WBRT + SRS (82% vs. 71%, $p = 0.01$). Moreover, in patients with a single lesion, WBRT + SRS was associated with longer median OS (6.5 vs. 4.9 months, $p = 0.039$) than WBRT. In a retrospective matched-pair study of 252 patients (156 lung cancer patients), in which 84 patients receiving WBRT + SRS for 1–3 brain metastases were matched 1:2 for nine characteristics to 168 patients receiving WBRT alone, 1-year intracranial control rates were 71% after WBRT + SRS vs. 48% after WBRT alone ($p = 0.005$) and 1-years OS rates were 53% vs. 45% ($p = 0.10$) (Rades et al. 2017b).

In addition, several studies compared WBRT + SRS to SRS alone. In a randomized controlled trial of 132 patients (88 lung cancer patients) with 1–4 brain metastases, 1-year OS rates were 38.5% after WBRT + SRS vs. 28.4% after SRS alone ($p = 0.42$), and 1-year recurrence rates were 46.8% vs. 76.4% ($p < 0.001$) (Aoyama et al. 2006). In 2011, the results of the EORTC 22,952–26,001 trial were published (Kocher et al. 2011).

A total of 359 patients (190 NSCLC patients) with 1–3 brain metastases (199 receiving SRS and 160 resection) were randomized to local therapy alone or local therapy + WBRT. At 2 years, WBRT led to reduction of local recurrences from 31% to 19% ($p = 0.040$) after SRS and from 59% to 27% ($p < 0.001$) after resection ($p < 0.001$), and to reduction of new brain metastases from 48% to 33% ($p = 0.023$) after SRS and from 42% to 23% ($p = 0.008$) after resection. However, this did not translate into improved median survival (10.9 vs. 10.7 months, $p = 0.89$). Similar results were described in a Cochrane database analysis (Tsao et al. 2018). In that analysis, the addition of WBRT to SRS resulted in significantly improved intracranial control (HR 0.39, 95%-CI 0.25–0.60, $p < 0.0001$), local control (HR 2.73, 95%-CI 1.87–3.99, $p < 0.00001$), and distant brain control (HR 2.34, 95%-CI 1.73–3.18, $p < 0.00001$) but not OS (HR 1.00, 95%-CI 0.80–1.25, $p = 0.99$).

Since the addition of WBRT does not improve survival but can be associated with significant cognitive deficits, physicians have become more reserved regarding its use. Addition of WBRT was recommended for several years, also because Aoyama et al. showed in a subgroup analysis of their trial that cognitive function at 1 and 2 years was better in patients receiving WBRT in addition to SRS, likely due to fewer intracranial recurrences that also cause cognitive deficits (Aoyama et al. 2007). In 2009, Chang et al. presented a phase III trial comparing WBRT + SRS to SRS alone in patients with 1–3 brain metastases (Chang et al. 2009). The trial was prematurely stopped after 58 patients (32 with NSCLC) by the data monitoring board on the basis that there was a probability of 96% that patients after WBRT + SRS significantly more often experienced decline in cognitive function (mean posterior probability of 52%) than after SRS alone (mean posterior probability of 24%) at 4 months. Intracranial control rates at 1 year were 73% after WBRT + SRS and 27% after SRS alone ($p = 0.0003$). However, cognitive function was not investigated at 1 year to evaluate whether the higher rate of intracranial recurrences was associated with more cognitive deficits.

In 2016, an ALLIANCE trial was published that compared WBRT (12 × 2.5 Gy) + SRS (18–22 Gy) to SRS alone (20–24 Gy) in 213 patients (146 with lung cancer) with 1–3 brain metastases (Brown et al. 2016). At 3 months, deterioration of cognitive function was found in 63.5% of patients after SRS alone and in 91.7% of patients after WBRT + SRS ($p < 0.001$). Overall quality of life at 3 months was significantly higher in the SRS alone group ($p = 0.002$). Median survival times were 10.4 months after SRS alone and 7.4 months after WBRT + SRS ($p = 0.92$). Local control rates at 3 months were significantly higher (93.7 vs. 75.3%, $p < 0.001$) and time to intracranial failure was significantly longer after WBRT + SRS. In a subgroup analysis of 28 long-term survivors, cognitive decline was less common after SRS alone at 12 months (60% vs. 94.4%, $p = 0.04$). When interpreting this trial, one should consider that it took 11 years to include 213 patients from 34 institutions. Therefore, patients of this trial likely were highly selected. Moreover, the trials of Chang et al. and Brown et al. (Chang et al. 2009; Brown et al. 2016) did not use a hippocampus-sparing technique or memantine in the WBRT-group that can significantly reduce the risk of cognitive decline (Gondi et al. 2014; Brown et al. 2013, 2020).

As mentioned above, the best option to avoid cognitive deficits is omitting WBRT. To identify patients, who may not require WBRT, a prognostic tool was created in 214 patients (72 patients with NSCLC) to estimate the probability of new brain metastases after SRS alone for 1–3 lesions (Huttenlocher et al. 2014) Based on number/size of lesions, type of primary tumor and extracranial metastases, three groups were created. Six-month rates of freedom from new brain metastases were 36% (16–17 points), 65% (18–20 points), and 60% (21–22 points) ($p < 0.001$). Twelve-month rates were 27%, 44%, and 71%, respectively. Patients of the 16–17 points group could benefit from addition of WBRT.

Few studies exist comparing WBRT + SRS to SRS alone for 1–3 or 1–4 brain metastases that particularly focused on lung cancer. In a retrospective study of 148 lung cancer patients with 1–3 lesions, addition of WBRT significantly improved 1-year distant brain control (83% vs. 48%, $p < 0.001$) but not 1-year local control of the treated lesions (86% vs. 80%, $p = 0.61$) and 1-year OS (59% vs. 49%, $p = 0.32$) (Rades et al. 2014). In 2015, Aoyama et al. presented a secondary analysis of their trial (1–4 lesions) in 88 patients with NSCLC (Aoyama et al. 2007, 2015). They found an improvement in OS with addition of WBRT to SRS in patients with favorable survival prognoses (DS-GPA 2.5–4.0); median OS times were 16.7 months after WBRT + SRS and 10.6 months after SRS alone ($p = 0.04$). For patients with worse survival prognoses (DS-GPA 0–2.0), a survival benefit was not observed ($p = 0.86$). In a secondary analysis of 126 NSCLC patients of the ALLIANCE trial (1–3 lesions), median OS was almost twice as long after WBRT + SRS compared to SRS alone (17.9 vs. 11.6 months, $p = 0.63$) in patients with DS-GPA ≥2.0 although statistical significance was not reached (Brown et al. 2016; Churilla et al. 2017). Summarizing the data of this chapter, addition of WBRT to SRS may be considered for patients with 1–4 brain metastases from NSCLC with favorable survival prognoses and a high risk of developing distant brain metastases after SRS alone.

5 Systemic Treatment in Addition to Radiation Therapy

5.1 Radiosensitizers

Of radiosensitizers evaluated in randomized trials, no agent improved OS when compared to radiotherapy alone (Tsao et al. 2012). In a phase III trial of 554 patients with brain metastases from NSCLC, addition of motexafin gadolinium (MGd) to WBRT led to a non-significantly longer interval to neurologic progression (15 vs. 10 months, $p = 0.12$), and significantly fewer patients in the MGd-group required salvage SRS or resection ($p < 0.001$) (Mehta et al. 2009). The United States Food and Drug Administration (FDA) did not approve MGd for brain metastases from NSCLC (Tsao et al. 2012). Another phase

III trial investigated the efaproxiral (RSR-13) in 515 patients with brain metastases from solid tumors (Suh et al. 2006). Response rates were improved by 7% in the entire cohort and 13% in patients with breast cancer or NSCLC. The FDA oncologic drugs advisory committee did not recommend approval of RSR-13 in addition to WBRT (Tsao et al. 2012).

5.2 "Classic" Chemotherapy

In several phase III trials of patients with brain metastases from lung cancer, addition of chemotherapy to WBRT did not improve OS but significantly increased toxicity. In 2008, the RTOG 0118 trial compared 15 × 2.5 Gy of WBRT plus/minus thalidomide during and following WBRT (Knisely et al. 2008). Accrual was stopped after 183 (of planned 332) patients. Of these, 109 (62%) were lung cancer patients. Median OS time was 3.9 months in both groups ($p = 0.88$). Three-month rates of intracranial progression were 18.7% after WBRT alone and 13.1% after WBRT + thalidomide. Time-to-progression (TTP) curves were not significantly different ($p = 0.097$). However, 48% of patients receiving thalidomide discontinued this treatment due to adverse events. Thus, addition of thalidomide to WBRT was not recommended. Another phase III trial compared 20 × 2 Gy of WBRT plus/minus topotecan in 96 (of planned 320) patients with brain metastases from SCLC or NSCLC (Neuhaus et al. 2009). No significant differences were observed for local response, PFS and OS. However, significantly more grade 3/4 hematological toxicities were observed in patients receiving topotecan (51% vs. 2%). In 2013, the RTOG 0320 trial compared WBRT (15 × 2.5 Gy) + SRS to WBRT + SRS + temozolomide (75 mg/m^2/day × 21 days) or erlotinib (150 mg/day) (Sperduto et al. 2013). Following WBRT + SRS, temozolomide (150–200 mg/m^2/day × 5 days/month) and erlotinib (150 mg/day) could be continued for up to 6 months. This trial was closed early after 126 of 381 patients. Median OS times were 13.4 months after WBRT + SRS alone, 6.3 months after WBRT + SRS + temozolomide and 6.1 months after WBRT + SRS + erlotinib. Six-months rates of intracranial progression were 16%, 29%, and 20%, and median PFS times were 8.1, 4.6, and 4.8 months, respectively. Grade 3–5 toxicity rates were 11%, 41%, and 49% ($p < 0.001$), and deterioration rates of the performance status at 6 months were 53%, 86%, and 86%, respectively.

Summarizing the data from these phase III trials, the addition of "classic" chemotherapy to WBRT cannot be recommended for patients with brain metastases from lung cancer. However, several studies suggested that primary chemotherapy may be an option for patients with asymptomatic brain metastases. In 2001, a phase III trial from France (GFPC 95-1) of 171 patients with brain metastases from NSCLC compared 2–6 cycles of chemotherapy alone with cisplatin (100 mg/m^2 on day 1) and vinorelbine (30 mg/m^2 on days 1, 8, 15, and 22) every 4 weeks to the same chemotherapy plus early WBRT (10 × 3 Gy over 2 weeks, concurrently during the first cycle of chemotherapy) (Robinet et al. 2001). In the chemotherapy alone group, response was evaluated after 2, 4, and 6 cycles. Delayed WBRT was administered in case of intracranial progression, intracranial stable disease after 2 or 4 cycles and after 6 cycles (like for other patients). Intracranial response rates were 27% after 2 cycles of chemotherapy alone and 33% after chemotherapy plus early WBRT ($p = 0.12$). Six-months OS rates (46% vs. 40%) and median OS times (24 vs. 21 weeks) were not significantly different ($p = 0.83$). No significant differences were found regarding hematological and neurological toxicities. Thus, timing of WBRT (early vs. delayed) appeared to have no significant impact on treatment outcomes. Similar results were observed in a randomized pilot study of 48 chemotherapy-naïve patients with NSCLC and synchronous brain metastases, in whom neurologic symptoms were absent or controlled by supportive care. When comparing WBRT followed by chemotherapy to chemotherapy followed by WBRT, intracranial response rates, median PFS, and median OS were not significantly different (Lee et al. 2008). However, grade 3/4 neutropenia was more frequent in the WBRT-first group during subsequent chemotherapy (79% vs. 40%). The authors concluded that primary chemotherapy can be an option for synchronous brain metastases from NSCLC when neurologic symptoms are absent or controlled. In 2015, a phase III trial of 105 (of 176 planned) patients with 1–4 asymptomatic brain metastases from NSCLC compared SRS followed by chemotherapy to upfront chemotherapy (Lim et al. 2015). Median OS times were 14.6 and 15.3 months, respectively ($p = 0.418$). Intracranial response rates were 57% in the SRS-group and 37% in the upfront chemotherapy group ($p = 0.011$). Median time to intracranial progression was non-significantly longer in the SRS-group (9.4 vs. 6.6 months, $p = 0.248$), which was considered a favorable trend by the authors. Median local PFS was significantly longer after SRS plus chemotherapy (not reached vs. 10.2 months, $p < 0.001$), and a trend was found for freedom from new brain lesions (11.9 vs. 8.7 months, $p = 0.247$). Salvage treatment for intracranial disease was required more often in the upfront chemotherapy group ($p = 0.157$). When comparing both groups, one must consider that the proportion of patients with a single brain metastasis was higher in the upfront chemotherapy group (57% vs. 37%). This likely led to a bias favoring the outcomes after upfront chemotherapy. Thus, one may speculate whether significance would have been reached also for superiority of SRS plus chemotherapy for intracranial TTP and freedom from new lesions, if the numbers of lesions were equally distributed in both groups. Based on this trial (Lim et al. 2015) and the study of Robinet et al. (2001), the clinical practice guideline for metastatic NSCLC of the European Society for Medical Oncology (ESMO) stated that for patients with asymptomatic brain metastases who had not yet received systemic treatment, upfront chemotherapy and deferral of WBRT should be considered (Planchard et al. 2018). However, this guideline did not consider the above-mentioned bias in the phase III trial of Lim et al. (2015). Thus, upfront radiotherapy (including WBRT) remains the standard for the majority of patients with multiple (>3–4) brain metastases from NSCLC. Depending on number and size of the lesions, selected patients may receive SRS alone. Highly selected chemotherapy- and immunotherapy-naïve patients with asymptomatic lesions may be considered for upfront chemotherapy.

5.3 Targeted Therapies/Immunotherapy

5.3.1 Tyrosine Kinase Inhibitors

Mutations in the EGFR gene have been reported for approximately 10% of patients with NSCLC (mainly adenocarcinoma) in the Western world and for up to 40% of NSCLC patients in East Asia (Minchom et al. 2014). EGFR-mutated NSCLC shows a high response to EGFR-targeting tyrosine kinase inhibitors (TKIs). First-generation EGFR-TKIs include erlotinib and gefitinib. Several studies investigated the combination of radiotherapy plus TKIs for brain metastases from lung cancer. A phase II trial of 54 patients with multiple brain metastases from adenocarcinoma of the lung compared 10×3 Gy of WBRT alone to WBRT + erlotinib (150 mg/day during and up to 1 month following WBRT) (Zhuang et al. 2013). Median local PFS (10.6 vs. 6.8 months, $p = 0.003$), median PFS (6.8 vs. 5.2 months, $p = 0.009$), and median OS (10.7 vs. 8.9 months) were significantly better after the combined treatment. Outcomes were not different for patients with EGFR mutation and EGFR wild-type. In contrast, a randomized trial of 80 patients with multiple brain metastases from NSCLC did not find a benefit for addition of erlotinib to 5×4 Gy of WBRT (during and after WBRT until disease progression) (Lee et al. 2014). Median neurological PFS was 1.6 months in both arms ($p = 0.84$), and median OS was 3.4 months with and 2.9 months without erlotinib ($p = 0.83$). However, EGFR mutation status was available for only 35 patients, and only one patient (2.9%) had a mutation. In the trial of Sperduto et al. of 1–3 brain metastases from NSCLC, median OS times were longer in the 44 patients receiving WBRT + SRS (13.4 months) than in the 41 patients receiving WBRT + SRS + erlotinib (6.1 months) (Sperduto et al. 2013). According to a meta-analysis of 622 patients with NSCLC from seven studies, addition of gefitinib or erlotinib to WBRT resulted in significantly better response [odds ratio (OR) 3.34, $p = 0.001$], disease-control (OR 3.34, $p = 0.001$), and OS (HR 0.72, $p = 0.002$) (Zheng et al. 2016). These findings were different from a randomized phase III trial presented in 2021 (Yang et al. 2021). A total of 224 patients with ≥2 brain metastases from NSCLC were randomly assigned to 20 × 2 Gy of WBRT or WBRT plus concurrent erlotinib (150 mg/day, starting 6 days before WBRT). Median intracranial PFS was 11.2 vs. 9.2 months ($p = 0.601$), median PFS 5.3 vs. 4.0 months ($p = 0.825$), and median OS 12.9 vs. 10.0 months ($p = 0.545$). Outcomes in EGFR-mutant patients were more favorable than in wild-type patients but also not significantly improved with erlotinib. The authors concluded that addition of EGFR-TKIs to WBRT is not justified for brain metastases from NSCLC, irrespectively of the EGFR mutation status.

These data were supported by a meta-analysis of 2649 patients from 30 studies (Singh et al. 2020). In addition to activating mutations of the EGFR kinase domain, this meta-analysis also considered rearrangements of ALK (oncogenic fusion of two genes, namely ALK and echinoderm microtubule associated protein-like 4). In this meta-analysis, patients with EGFR and ALK mutations had significantly longer median OS (20.9 and 48.5 months) than wild-type patients (9.9 months). WBRT or SRS + TKI did not lead to better OS than radiotherapy alone (28.3 vs.32.2 months, $p = 0.22$) or TKI alone (28.3 vs. 23.9 months, $p = 0.2$). Radiotherapy + TKI resulted in non-significantly longer median PFS than TKI alone (18.6 vs. 13.6 months, $p = 0.06$) but not than radiotherapy alone (18.6 vs. 16.9 months, $p = 0.72$). Subgroup analyses of radiotherapy types did not reveal a benefit for addition of TKIs. Median PFS was 23.2 months after WBRT + TKI vs. 24 months after WBRT alone ($p = 0.72$), and 16.7 months after SRS + TKI vs. 13.6 months after SRS alone ($p = 0.56$). The authors concluded that addition of TKIs to radiotherapy did not provide a benefit regarding PFS and OS. Moreover, TKIs increase the risk of radio-necrosis. In a study from Cleveland (1650 patients with 2843 brain metastases), concurrent targeted therapies significantly increased the 12-month incidence of radio-necrosis after WBRT or SRS (8.8% vs. 5.3%, $p < 0.01$) (Kim et al. 2017). Significant increase was observed for VEGFR-TKIs (14.3% vs. 6.6%, $p = 0.04$) and EGFR-TKIs (15.6% vs. 6.0%, $p = 0.04$).

In addition to studies comparing WBRT + TKI to radiotherapy alone, several retrospective studies investigated whether radiotherapy (WBRT) may be deferred until intracranial progression. A retrospective study of 110 evaluable patients with EGFR-mutant adenocarcinoma compared WBRT with or without sequential erlotinib (n = 32), SRS/FSRT alone ($n = 15$), and erlotinib alone ($n = 63$) (Gerber et al. 2014). Median intracranial TTP was longer in the WBRT group than with erlotinib alone (24 vs. 16 months, $p = 0.04$), and median OS was non-significantly longer (35 vs. 26 months, $p = 0.62$). Magnusson et al. presented two studies including radiotherapy plus sequential TKIs (Magnuson et al. 2016, 2017). In 2016, 50 patients with EGFR-mutant adenocarcinoma were analyzed receiving upfront radiotherapy (17 WBRT, 16 SRS) plus erlotinib (started within 1–2 weeks after radiotherapy) or upfront erlotinib ($n = 17$) plus salvage radiotherapy at progression (Magnuson et al. 2016). Median intracranial PFS (37.9 vs. 10.6 months, $p < 0.001$) and median OS (34.1 vs. 19.4 months, $p = 0.01$) were significantly longer with upfront radiotherapy. In subgroup analyses, the OS benefit was more predominant after SRS (58.4 vs. 19.5 months, $p = 0.01$) than after WBRT (29.9 vs. 19.4 months, $p = 0.09$). In 2017, data of 351 TKI-naïve patients with EGFR-mutant adenocarcinoma from six institutions were reported, who were treated with WBRT followed by TKI ($n = 120$), SRS followed by TKI ($n = 100$), or upfront TKI and salvage radiotherapy at progression ($n = 131$) (Magnuson et al. 2017). Median intracranial TTPs were 24 (WBRT), 23 (SRS), and 17 (TKI) months ($p = 0.025$). The favorable outcome in the WBRT-group was remarkable, since these patients had worse prognostic factors (DS-GPA) than in the other groups. Median OS times were 30, 46, and 25 months, respectively

($p < 0.001$). The authors concluded that deferral of radiotherapy may result in worse OS.

Two other retrospective studies did not find a benefit for addition of radiotherapy to TKIs. In a study of 121 patients with brain metastases at initial diagnosis of EGFR-mutant NSCLC, intracranial response (at least stable disease) rates were 80% after TKI (predominantly gefitinib) + WBRT or SRS and 60% after TKI alone ($p = 0.019$) (Byeon et al. 2016). However, median intracranial PFS (16.6 vs. 21.0 months, $p = 0.492$) and 3-year OS (71.9% vs. 68.2%, $p = 0.675$) were not significantly different. In 2017, Jiang et al. presented of 167 patients with EGFR-mutant NSCLC treated with TKI + WBRT ($n = 51$) or TKI alone ($n = 116$) (Jiang et al. 2016). TKIs included gefitinib, erlotinib, and icotinib. The addition of WBRT did not improve intracranial PFS (6.9 vs. 7.4 months, $p = 0.232$) or OS (21.6 vs. 26.4 months, $p = 0.049$).

In contrast, three recent studies supported the results of Gerber et al. and Magnusson et al. (Gerber et al. 2014; Magnuson et al. 2016, 2017). In 2017, Doherty et al. presented retrospective study of 184 patients with EGFR/ALK-driven NSCLC (Doherty et al. 2017). Treatment regimens including WBRT + TKI were associated with intracranial TTP of 50.5 months, which was significantly longer than after SRS + TKI (12 months) and TKI alone (15 months) ($p = 0.0038$). Median OS times were 21.6, 23.9, and 22.6 months, respectively ($p = 0.67$). Similar findings were reported from the study of Ke et al. including 139 patients with EGFR-mutated adenocarcinoma (Ke et al. 2018). The addition of WBRT to EGFR-TKI (erlotinib) led to longer median intracranial TTP (30.0 vs. 18.2 months, $p = 0.001$) but not OS (48.0 vs. 41.1 months, $p = 0.912$). In the study of Chen et al. from 2019 of 141 patients with brain metastases from EGFR-mutated adenocarcinoma, addition of WBRT to TKI (afatinib, erlotinib, gefitinib, or osimertinib) resulted in significantly better 1-year OS (81.9% vs. 59.6%, $p = 0.002$) (Chen et al. 2019). These results were supported by two meta-analyses (Soon et al. 2015; Du et al. 2018). In the meta-analysis of Soon et al. (363 patients with EGFR-mutated NSCLC from 12 non-comparative observational studies), 4-months intracranial PFS ($p = 0.03$), and 2-year OS ($p = 0.05$) were better with upfront radiotherapy (WBRT plus concurrent TKI, WBRT or SRS alone, WBRT or SRS followed by systemic treatment) than with TKIs alone (Soon et al. 2015). Adverse events were more common in patients receiving upfront radiotherapy. A larger meta-analysis of 1456 patients with EGFR-mutated NSCLC from 13 comparative studies was presented in 2018 (Du et al. 2018). Addition of upfront radiotherapy (WBRT or SRS) alone resulted in significantly better OS (HR 0.78, $p = 0.005$) than TKI alone. Upfront radiotherapy plus TKI showed better OS (HR 0.71, $p = 0.0005$) and intracranial PFS (HR 0.69, $p = 0.04$) than TKI alone. According to subgroup analyses of radiotherapy types, WBRT + TKI resulted in better intracranial PFS (HR 0.64, $p = 0002$) andOS (HR 0.75, $p = 0.05$) than TKI alone, and SRS was associated with better OS (HR 0.37, $p < 0.00001$). The authors concluded that upfront radiotherapy seems critical. However, in addition to first-generation TKIs (including gefitinib, erlotinib, and crizotinib) and second generation TKIs (including alectinib, brigatinib, and ceritinib), third-generation TKIs like the EGFR-TKI osimertinib and the ALK/ROS1-TKI lorlatinib are now available and have shown promising anti-tumor activity in the brain (Wang et al. 2020; Erickson et al. 2020; Bauer et al. 2020). Randomized trials are warranted comparing these new drugs with or without upfront radiotherapy in patients with brain metastases from mutated NSCLC to help clarify optimal therapy.

5.3.2 Immune Checkpoint Inhibitors

Another group of systemic agents increasingly used for metastatic NSCLC is the class of immune checkpoint inhibitors (ICIs). Malignant tumors can develop mechanisms that promote immune tolerance (Protopapa et al. 2019). For example, the immune response is negatively regulated by PD-1 (programmed cell death 1) when it is activated by its ligand PD-L1. Four anti-PD-1/anti-PD-L1 agents were approved for NSCLC, namely anti-PD-1-agents nivolumab and pembrolizumab and anti-PD-L1-agents atezolizumab and durvalumab. To improve the outcomes of patients with brain metastases from NSCLC, several studies investigated combinations of radiotherapy and ICIs.

In 2017, a small retrospective study of 17 patients with brain metastases from NSCLC suggested SRS or FSRT in combination with nivolumab or durvalumab to be feasible (Ahmed et al. 2017). In a larger retrospective study of 163 NSCLC patients, the addition of ICIs to SRS, partial brain irradiation or WBRT, did not significantly increase the rates of any adverse events and grade ≥3 events (Hubbeling et al. 2018). In another retrospective study of 37 NSCLC patients (85 brain metastases), concurrent SRS + ICI (84% nivolumab, 11% atezolizumab, 5% pembrolizumab) was compared to SRS before and SRS after treatment with ICIs. One-year OS rates were 87.3%, 70.0%, and 0% ($p = 0.008$), and 1-year distant brain failure rates were 38.5% vs. 65.8% and 100% ($p = 0.042$) (Schapira et al. 2018). One-year local control was better with SRS administered concurrently or after ICIs than with SRS administered before ICI (100% vs. 72.3%, $p = 0.016$). Grade ≥ 4 adverse events were not observed.

In 2019, Singh et al. performed a retrospective study of 85 patients with brain metastases from NSCLC treated with SRS (Singh et al. 2019). Thirty-nine patients had PD-L1-positive tumors and received anti-P1 treatment; the other 46 patients received chemotherapy. Median OS times were 10 and 11.6 months, respectively ($p = 0.23$). Maximum regression (in %) of brain metastases and time to maximum regression were also not significantly different. In lesions >500 ccm, regression was observed in 90% of lesions after SRS + ICI vs. 47.8% after SRS + chemotherapy ($p = 0.001$), and times to initial response and maximum regression were significantly shorter after SRS + ICI in this subgroup. In 2019, Shepard et al. presented a retrospective matched cohort study of 51 patients with a total of 137 brain metastases from NSCLC treated with SRS plus ICI within 3 months before or after SRS ($n = 17$) or SRS alone ($n = 34$) (Shepard et al. 2019). Patients receiving the combined treatment had a significantly higher rate of complete response (50.0% vs. 15.6%, $p = 0.012$) and shorter time to regression of brain metastases (2.5 vs. 3.1 months, $p < 0.0001$). However, 1-year local control (84.9% vs. 76.3%, $p = 0.94$), cumulative intracranial PFS (HR 2.18, $p = 0.11$) and cumulative OS (HR 0.99, $p = 0.99$) were not significantly different. In 2020, Kim et al. presented a meta-analysis of 12 studies and evaluated the rates of objective (radiologic) response, disease-control and adverse events in patients with brain metastases from NSCLC receiving ICI alone or ICI plus SRS/FSRT (Kim et al. 2020). ICI + SRS/FSRT was associated with significantly higher rates of objective response (95% vs. 24%, $p < 0.01$) and disease-control (97% vs. 44%, $p < 0.01$) than ICI alone. Grade 3/4 adverse events in the central nervous system were not significantly different (5% vs. 4%, $p = 0.93$). Thus, ICI + SRS appeared superior to ICI alone. When using ICIs, the risk of immune-related adverse events (IRAEs) needs to be considered that can be quite severe or even fatal (Leitinger et al. 2018; Zhang et al. 2021). In a retrospective study of 63 patients with brain metastases from NSCLC receiving pembrolizumab, 24 patients (38%) developed IRAEs (Leitinger et al. 2018). Fifty-four patients (86%) received radiotherapy for initial brain metastases. Patients experiencing IRAEs had longer median OS (21 vs. 10 months, $p = 0.004$), intracranial TTP (14 vs. 5 months, $p = 0.001$), and time to extracranial progression (15 vs. 4 months, $p < 0.001$). Randomized trials are required to better define the optimal sequencing and role of ICIs in the treatment of brain metastases from NSCLC.

6 Prophylactic Cranial Irradiation

6.1 Prophylactic Cranial Irradiation for SCLC

Rates of brain metastases of 28% at 1 year and 58% at 2 years were reported after chemotherapy for SCLC (Komaki et al. 1981). According to early randomized trials, PCI significantly improves freedom from brain metastases but not

OS, which led to two meta-analyses (Aupérin et al. 1999; Meert et al. 2001). Aupérin et al. included 987 patients in complete remission after initial treatment from seven trials comparing PCI vs. no PCI for limited-stage (LS-SCLC) or extensive-stage (ES-SCLC) SCLC (Aupérin et al. 1999). Three-year OS rates were 20.7% in the PCI-group and 15.3% without PCI ($p = 0.01$), and 3-year rates of brain metastases were 33.3% and 58.6%, respectively ($p < 0.001$). The other meta-analysis included 1547 patients from 12 randomized trials also comparing PCI vs. no PCI in patients with LS-SCLC and ES-SCLC (Meert et al. 2001). PCI led to decrease in brain metastasis [HR 0.48; 95% confidence interval (CI) 0.39–0.60] and improvement in OS (HR 0.82; 0.71–0.96) in patients with a complete response prior to PCI. Thus, PCI significantly reduces the risk of brain metastases and can improve OS after complete response. However, it can lead to leukoencephalopathy and cognitive decline (Walker et al. 2014; Gondi et al. 2013). PCI is recommended for most patients with LS-SCLC who respond to initial radio-chemotherapy and remain without evidence of brain metastasis on MRI-restaging after completion of radio-chemotherapy (Simone 2nd et al. 2020). Subgroups of patients with LS-SCLC have been identified who are less likely to benefit from PCI including patients with stage I disease (low risk of brain metastases, lack of OS benefit) and patients >70 years (lack of OS benefit, increased risk of late neuro-toxicity) (Simone 2nd et al. 2020). The ASTRO clinical practice guideline recommends that shared decision-making regarding PCI and MRI-based surveillance should be facilitated in case of age > 70 years, limited performance status, significant co-morbidity, or preexisting neurocognitive deficits (Simone 2nd et al. 2020).

The use of PCI for ES-SCLC is still under debate. In 2007, Slotman et al. presented a randomized trial of PCI (5×4 Gy to 12×2.5 Gy) vs. no PCI in patients with ES-SCLC responding to chemotherapy (Slotman et al. 2007). One-year rates of brain metastases were 14.6% and 40.4% ($p < 0.001$), and 1-year OS rates were 27.1% and 13.3%, respectively ($p = 0.003$). Hair loss and fatigue were more common in the PCI-group ($p < 0.001$). Cognitive ($p = 0.07$) and emotional functions ($p = 0.18$) were not significantly different. Another randomized trial investigated PCI (10×2.5 Gy) in patients with ES-SCLC who responded to platinum-based doublet therapy and had no brain metastases on magnetic resonance imaging (MRI) (Takahashi et al. 2017). The trial was closed after an interim analysis of 163 patients because of futility. Median OS was 11.6 months with and 13.7 months without PCI ($p = 0.094$). Cumulative incidences of brain metastases at 18 months were 40% and 64%, respectively ($p < 0.001$). In the no PCI-group, 58% of patients received radiotherapy for brain metastases. The authors concluded that PCI did not improve OS and was not essential for patients with ES-SCLC with negative baseline and periodic brain MRIs.

In addition, three meta-analyses from China were published in 2014 (five studies), 2019 (seven studies), and 2020 (eight studies), respectively (Zhang et al. 2014; Yin et al. 2019; Wen et al. 2020). All these meta-analyses confirmed that PCI significantly reduced the rate of brain metastases in SCLC patients. Conclusions regarding the benefit of PCI with respect to OS are conflicting. Zhang et al. stated that PCI improved OS and should be part of standard treatment for all patients with SCLC (Zhang et al. 2014), whereas Yin et al. concluded that there was little benefit in improving OS when modern imaging showed no brain metastases after initial chemoradiation (Yin et al. 2019). In the most recent meta-analysis that particularly focused on ES-SCLC, PCI significantly improved 1-year OS (HR 1.50; 95% CI 1.23–1.82; $p < 0.0001$) (Wen et al. 2020).

Moreover, large retrospective studies were performed to define the role of PCI for ES-SCLC patients. In 2012, Schild et al. presented a pooled analysis of four phase I and II trials of the North Central Cancer Treatment Group (NCCTG) including 318 with LS-SCLC and 421 with ES-SCLC who achieved at least stable disease with their initial treatment (Schild et al. 2012). Of the entire cohort of 739 patients, 459 received PCI that was associated with significantly longer OS (56% vs. 32% at 1 year and 8% vs. 5% at

3 years, $p < 0.001$). A benefit regarding median OS was found for LS-SCLC (17 vs. 14 months, $p = 0.0045$) and ES-SCLC (10 vs. 8 months, $p = 0.0282$). PCI maintained an OS benefit after adjustment for stage, response, age, performance status, gender, and number of metastatic sites. PCI resulted in more grade ≥ 3 toxicities including alopecia and lethargy (64% vs. 50%, $p = 0.001$). In 2018, Sharma et al. investigated PCI in 4257 patients with ES-SCLC using data from the national cancer database (Sharma et al. 2018). To reduce the risk of bias regarding administration of PCI, patients surviving less than 6 months were excluded and propensity core matching was performed. Median OS was 13.9 months with and 11.1 months without PCI ($p < 0.001$); 1-year OS rates were 61% and 44%, respectively ($p < 0.001$).

In 2009, a randomized trial of 720 patients with LS-SCLC and complete response after chemotherapy and thoracic irradiation was performed to identify the optimal dose-fractionation of PCI (Le Péchoux et al. 2009). This trial compared 25 Gy (10 × 2.5 Gy), which was considered the standard regimen in several countries at that time, to 36 Gy (18 × 2.0 Gy or 24 × 1.5 Gy with two fractions per day). Two-year rates of brain metastases were 29% after 25 Gy and 23% after 36 Gy ($p = 0.18$), and 2-year OS rates were 42% and 37%, respectively ($p = 0.05$). The most common acute toxicities were not significantly different with both regimens. Since 10 × 2.5 Gy was not inferior to 36 Gy, the shorter regimen was considered preferable. However, since the risk of cognitive decline was reported to increase with the dose per fraction, several institutions prefer 15 × 2.0 Gy instead of 10 × 2.5 Gy (De Angelis et al. 1989). In addition, hippocampus-sparing techniques and memantine may be options to reduce cognitive deficits (Gondi et al. 2014; Brown et al. 2013, 2020). In a prospective study of 20 patients with LS-SCLC receiving hippocampus-sparing PCI (mean hippocampal dose <8 Gy), no significant decline in cognitive functions was observed after 6 and 12 months (Redmond et al. 2017). Two patients developed a brain metastasis in the area of the reduced dose without involvement of the dentate gyrus; one lesion was found in the avoidance region. However, both patients had concurrent lesions in areas receiving the full dose. In studies investigating the sites of brain metastases in patients with SCLC, cumulative rates of hippocampal plus peri-hippocampal lesions ranged between 0.8 and 2.7% when considering the number of metastases and 5.1–27.3% (5.1–12.2% without a study of only 11 patients) when considering the number of patients (Guo et al. 2017; Kundapur et al. 2015; Harth et al. 2013; Wan et al. 2013; Gondi et al. 2010). These figures need to be considered when aiming to use hippocampus-sparing PCI. Additional prospective trials are required to properly define the risks and benefits of hippocampus-sparing PCI.

Moreover, after introduction of immune checkpoint inhibitors for ES-SCLC and increasing availability of routine MRI-surveillance, the role of PCI for these patients needs to be re-defined in future trials. Until such trials are available, the use of PCI for ES-SCLC should be considered for each patient on an individual basis considering risks and benefits (Taylor et al. 2020). SWOG is performing a large phase III trial to further address the value of PCI. For brain metastases following PCI, SRS and FSRT can be used as salvage treatment (Cifarelli et al. 2020; Cordeiro et al. 2019; Fairchild et al. 2020).

6.2 Prophylactic Cranial Irradiation for NSCLC

Limited data exist regarding the role of PCI for patients with NSCLC. In a phase III trial of 356 (of targeted 1058) patients with stage III NSCLC, PCI significantly decreased the risk of brain metastases (7.7% vs. 18.0% at 1 year, $p = 0.004$) without improvement in 1-year OS (75.6% vs, 76.9%, $p = 0.86$) and 1-year disease-free survival (56.4% vs. 51.2%, $p = 0.11$) (Gore et al. 2011). Moreover, no significant differences at 1 year were found in any component of quality of life questionnaires despite a significantly greater decline in some specific cognitive functions with PCI (Sun et al. 2011). In addition, two meta-analyses contributed to this topic (Witlox et al. 2018; Al Feghali et al. 2018). One of these meta-analyses included 1462 patients with NSCLC from seven randomized trials, of whom 717 patients received PCI (Witlox et al. 2018). PCI led to a significant reduction in development of brain metastases by 13% [risk ratio (RR) 0.33, 95% CI 0.22–0.45]. Data regarding toxicity and quality of life were limited, and results regarding OS were inconclusive. The other meta-analysis included eight papers and one abstract reporting on six trials (Al Feghali et al. 2018). PCI improved freedom from brain metastases (RR 0.33, 95% CI 0.22–0.45) but not OS (HR 1.08, 95% CI 0.90–1.31). When considering only the two most recent trials of patients with stage III disease, PCI was associated with better disease-free survival (HR 0.67, 95% CI 0.46–0.98) without significant impairment of neuro-cognitive function. PCI may be considered for carefully selected patients with NSCLC, particularly if risk factors for brain metastases exist. Risk factors include non-squamous cell carcinoma (particularly adenocarcinoma), lymph node metastases, and elevated serum levels of carcinogenic embryonic antigen (CEA) or neuron-specific enolase (NSE), lymph node metastases (particularly multiple mediastinal lymph nodes), and age <60 years (An et al. 2018). Additional randomized trials are required that also consider the value of immune checkpoint inhibitors to prevent brain metastasis.

References

Ahmed KA, Kim S, Arrington J et al (2017) Outcomes targeting the PD-1/PD-L1 axis in conjunction with stereotactic radiation for patients with non-small cell lung cancer brain metastases. J Neuro-Oncol 133:331–338

Al Feghali KA, Ballout RA, Khamis AM et al (2018) Prophylactic cranial irradiation in patients with non-small-cell lung cancer: a systematic review and meta-analysis of randomized controlled trials. Front Oncol 8:115

An N, Jing W, Wang H et al (2018) Risk factors for brain metastases in patients with non-small-cell lung cancer. Cancer Med 7:6357–6364

Andrews DW, Scott CB, Sperduto PW et al (2004) Whole brain radiation therapy with or without stereotactic radiosurgery boost for patients with one to three brain metastases: phase III results of the RTOG 9508 randomised trial. Lancet 363:1665–1672

Aoyama H, Shirato H, Tago M et al (2006) Stereotactic radiosurgery plus whole-brain radiation therapy vs stereotactic radiosurgery alone for treatment of brain metastases. A randomized controlled trial. JAMA 295:2483–2491

Aoyama H, Tago M, Kato N et al (2007) Neurocognitive function of patients with brain metastasis who received either whole brain radiotherapy plus stereotactic radiosurgery or radiosurgery alone. Int J Radiat Oncol Biol Phys 68:1388–1395

Aoyama H, Tago M, Shirato H et al (2015) Stereotactic radiosurgery with or without whole-brain radiotherapy for brain metastases: secondary analysis of the JROSG 99-1 randomized clinical trial. JAMA Oncol 1:457–464

Aupérin A, Arriagada R, Pignon JP et al (1999) Prophylactic cranial irradiation for patients with small-cell lung cancer in complete remission. N Engl J Med 341:476–484

Bauer TM, Shaw AT, Johnson ML et al (2020) Brain penetration of lorlatinib: cumulative incidences of CNS and non-CNS progression with lorlatinib in patients with previously treated ALK-positive non-small-cell lung cancer. Target Oncol 15:55–65

Bohlen G, Meyners T, Kieckebusch S et al (2010) Short-course whole-brain radiotherapy (WBRT) for brain metastases due to small-cell lung cancer (SCLC). Clin Neurol Neurosurg 112: 183–187

Borgelt B, Gelber R, Kramer S et al (1980) The palliation of brain metastases: final results of the first two studies by the Radiation Therapy Oncology Group. Int J Radiat Oncol Biol Phys 6:1–9

Brown PD, Pugh S, Laack NN et al (2013) Radiation Therapy Oncology Group (RTOG). Memantine for the prevention of cognitive dysfunction in patients receiving whole-brain radiotherapy: a randomized, double-blind, placebo-controlled trial. Neuro-Oncology 15:1429–1437

Brown PD, Jaeckle K, Ballman KV et al (2016) Effect of radiosurgery alone vs radiosurgery with whole brain radiation therapy on cognitive function in patients with 1 to 3 brain metastases: a randomized clinical trial. JAMA 316:401–409

Brown PD, Gondi V, Pugh S et al (2020) for NRG Oncology: Hippocampal avoidance during whole-brain radiotherapy plus memantine for patients with brain metastases: Phase III trial NRG Oncology CC001. J Clin Oncol 38:1019–1029

Byeon S, Ham JS, Sun JM et al (2016) Analysis of the benefit of sequential cranial radiotherapy in patients with EGFR mutant non-small cell lung cancer and brain metastasis. Med Oncol 33:97

Chang EL, Wefel JS, Hess KR et al (2009) Neurocognition in patients with brain metastases treated with radiosurgery or radiosurgery plus whole-brain irradiation: a randomised controlled trial. Lancet Oncol 10:1037–1044

Chatani M, Matayoshi Y, Masaki N et al (1994) Radiation therapy for brain metastases from lung carcinoma. Prospective randomized trial according to the level of lactate dehydrogenase. Strahlenther Onkol 170:155–161

Chen CH, Lee HH, Chuang HY et al (2019) Combination of whole-brain radiotherapy with epidermal growth factor receptor tyrosine kinase inhibitors improves overall survival in EGFR-mutated non-small cell lung cancer patients with brain metastases. Cancers (Basel) 11:1092

Churilla TM, Ballman KV, Brown PD et al (2017) Stereotactic radiosurgery with or without whole-brain radiation therapy for limited brain metastases: a secondary analysis of the North Central Cancer Treatment Group N0574 (Alliance) randomized controlled trial. Int J Radiat Oncol Biol Phys 99:1173–1178

Cifarelli CP, Vargo JA, Fang W et al (2020) Role of Gamma Knife radiosurgery in small cell lung cancer: a multi-institutional retrospective study of the International Radiosurgery Research Foundation (IRRF). Neurosurgery 87:664–671

Cordeiro D, Xu Z, Shepard M et al (2019) Gamma Knife radiosurgery for brain metastases from small-cell lung cancer: institutional experience over more than a decade and review of the literature. J Radiosurg SBRT 6:35–43

De Angelis LM, Mandell LR, Thaler HAT et al (1989) The role of postoperative radiotherapy after resection of single brain metastasis. Neurosurgery 24:798–805

Doherty MK, Korpanty GJ, Tomasini P et al (2017) Treatment options for patients with brain metastases from EGFR/ALK-driven lung cancer. Radiother Oncol 123:195–202

Du XJ, Pan SM, Lai SZ et al (2018) Upfront cranial radiotherapy vs. EGFR tyrosine kinase inhibitors alone for the treatment of brain metastases from non-small-cell lung cancer: a meta-analysis of 1465 patients. Front Oncol 8:603

Du TQ, Li X, Zhong WS et al (2021) Brain metastases of lung cancer: comparison of survival outcomes among whole brain radiotherapy, whole brain radiotherapy with consecutive boost, and simultaneous integrated boost. J Cancer Res Clin Oncol 147:569–577

Erickson AW, Brastianos PK, Das S (2020) Assessment of effectiveness and safety of osimertinib for patients with intracranial metastatic disease: a systematic review and meta-analysis. JAMA Netw Open 3:e201617

Fairchild A, Guest N, Letcher A et al (2020) Should stereotactic radiosurgery be considered for salvage of intracranial recurrence after prophylactic cranial irradiation or whole brain radiotherapy in small cell lung cancer? A population-based analysis and literature review. J Med Imaging Radiat Sci 51:75–87. e2

Gerber NK, Yamada Y, Rimner A et al (2014) Erlotinib versus radiation therapy for brain metastases in patients with EGFR-mutant lung adenocarcinoma. Int J Radiat Oncol Biol Phys 89:322–329

Gondi V, Tome WA, Marsh J et al (2010) Estimated risk of perihippocampal disease progression after hippocampal avoidance during whole-brain radiotherapy: safety profile for RTOG 0933. Radiother Oncol 95:327–331

Gondi V, Paulus R, Bruner DW et al (2013) Decline in tested and self-reported cognitive functioning after prophylactic cranial irradiation for lung cancer: pooled secondary analysis of Radiation Therapy Oncology Group randomized trials 0212 and 0214. Int J Radiat Oncol Biol Phys 86:656–664

Gondi V, Pugh SL, Tome WA et al (2014) Preservation of memory with conformal avoidance of the hippocampal neural stem-cell compartment during whole-brain radiotherapy for brain metastases (RTOG 0933): a phase II multi-institutional trial. J Clin Oncol 32:3810–3816

Gore EM, Bae K, Wong SJ et al (2011) Phase III comparison of prophylactic cranial irradiation versus observation in patients with locally advanced non-small-cell lung cancer: Primary analysis of Radiation Therapy Oncology Group study RTOG 0214. J Clin Oncol 29:272–278

Guo WL, He ZY, Chen Y et al (2017) Clinical features of brain metastases in small cell lung cancer: an implication for hippocampal sparing whole brain radiation therapy. Transl Oncol 10:54–58

Harth S, Abo-Madyan Y, Zheng L et al (2013) Estimation of intracranial failure risk following hippocampal-sparing whole brain radiotherapy. Radiother Oncol 109:152–158

Harwood AR, Simson WJ (1977) Radiation therapy of cerebral metastases: a randomized prospective clinical trial. Int J Radiat Oncol Biol Phys 2:1091–1094

Hubbeling HG, Schapira EF, Horick NK et al (2018) Safety of combined PD-1 pathway inhibition and intracranial radiation therapy in non-small cell lung cancer. J Thorac Oncol 13:550–558

Huttenlocher S, Dziggel L, Hornung D et al (2014) A new prognostic instrument to predict the probability of developing new cerebral metastases after radiosurgery alone. Radiat Oncol 9:215

Jiang T, Su C, Li X et al (2016) EGFR TKIs plus WBRT demonstrated no survival benefit other than that of TKIs alone in patients with NSCLC and EGFR mutation and brain metastases. J Thorac Oncol 11:1718–1728

Ke SB, Qiu H, Chen JM et al (2018) Therapeutic effect of first-line epidermal growth factor receptor tyrosine kinase inhibitor (EGFR-TKI) combined with whole brain radiotherapy on patients with EGFR mutation-positive lung adenocarcinoma and brain metastases. Curr Med Sci 38:1062–1068

Khuntia D, Brown P, Li J et al (2006) Whole-brain radiotherapy in the management of brain metastasis. J Clin Oncol 24:1295–1304

Kim JM, Miller JA, Kotecha R et al (2017) The risk of radiation necrosis following stereotactic radiosurgery with concurrent systemic therapies. J Neuro-Oncol 133:357–368

Kim DY, Kim PH, Suh CH et al (2020) Immune checkpoint inhibitors with or without radiotherapy in non-small cell lung cancer patients with brain metastases:

a systematic review and meta-analysis. Diagnostics (Basel) 10:1098

Knisely JP, Berkey B, Chakravarti A et al (2008) A phase III study of conventional radiation therapy plus thalidomide versus conventional radiation therapy for multiple brain metastases (RTOG 0118). Int J Radiat Oncol Biol Phys 71:79–86

Kocher M, Sofietti R, Abacioglu U et al (2011) Adjuvant whole-brain radiotherapy versus observation after radiosurgery or surgical resection of one to three cerebral metastases: results of the EORTC 22952-26001 study. J Clin Oncol 29:134–141

Komaki R, Cox JD, Whitson W et al (1981) Risk of brain metastasis from small cell carcinoma of the lung related to length of survival and prophylactic irradiation. Cancer Treat Rep 65:811–814

Kundapur V, Ellchuk T, Ahmed S et al (2015) Risk of hippocampal metastases in small cell lung cancer patients at presentation and after cranial irradiation: a safety profile study for hippocampal sparing during prophylactic or therapeutic cranial irradiation. Int J Radiat Oncol Biol Phys 91:781–786

Le Péchoux C, Dunant A, Senan S et al (2009) Standard-dose versus higher-dose prophylactic cranial irradiation (PCI) in patients with limited-stage small-cell lung cancer in complete remission after chemotherapy and thoracic radiotherapy (PCI 99-01, EORTC 22003-08004, RTOG 0212, and IFCT 99-01): a randomised clinical trial. Lancet Oncol 10:467–474

Lee DH, Han JY, Kim HT et al (2008) Primary chemotherapy for newly diagnosed non-small cell lung cancer patients with synchronous brain metastases compared with whole-brain radiotherapy administered first result of a randomized pilot study. Cancer 113:143–149

Lee SM, Lewanski CR, Counsell N et al (2014) Randomized trial of erlotinib plus whole-brain radiotherapy for NSCLC patients with multiple brain metastases. J Natl Cancer Inst 106:dju151

Leitinger M, Varosanec MV, Pikija S et al (2018) Fatal necrotizing encephalopathy after treatment with nivolumab for squamous non-small cell lung cancer: case report and review of the literature. Front Immunol 9:108

Lim SH, Lee JY, Lee MY et al (2015) A randomized phase III trial of stereotactic radiosurgery (SRS) versus observation for patients with asymptomatic cerebral oligo-metastases in non-small-cell lung cancer. Ann Oncol 26:762–768

Ly S, Lehman M, Liu H et al (2020) Incidence of hippocampal metastases in non-small-cell lung cancer. J Med Imaging Radiat Oncol 64:586–590

Magnuson WJ, Yeung JT, Guillod PD et al (2016) Impact of deferring radiation therapy in patients with epidermal growth factor receptor-mutant non-small cell lung cancer who develop brain metastases. Int J Radiat Oncol Biol Phys 95:673–679

Magnuson WJ, Lester-Coll NH, Wu AJ et al (2017) Management of brain metastases in tyrosine kinase inhibitor-naïve epidermal growth factor receptor-mutant non-small-cell lung cancer: A retrospective multi-institutional analysis. J Clin Oncol 35:1070–1077

Mahajan A, Ahmed S, McAleer MF et al (2017) Postoperative stereotactic radiosurgery versus observation for completely resected brain metastases: a single-centre, randomised, controlled, phase 3 trial. Lancet Oncol 18:1040–1048

Meert AP, Paesmans M, Berghmans T et al (2001) Prophylactic cranial irradiation in small cell lung cancer: a systematic review of the literature with meta-analysis. BMC Cancer 1:5

Mehta MP, Shapiro WR, Phan SC et al (2009) Motexafin gadolinium combined with prompt whole brain radiotherapy prolongs time to neurologic progression in non-small-cell lung cancer patients with brain metastases: results of a phase III trial. Int J Radiat Oncol Biol Phys 73:1069–1076

Minchom A, Yu KC, Bhosle J et al (2014) The diagnosis and treatment of brain metastases in EGFR mutant lung cancer. CNS Oncol 3:209–217

Mintz AH, Kestle J, Rathbone MP et al (1996) A randomized trial to assess the efficacy of surgery in addition to radiotherapy in patients with a single cerebral metastasis. Cancer 78:1470–1476

Muacevic A, Wowra B, Siefert A et al (2008) Microsurgery plus whole brain irradiation versus Gamma Knife surgery alone for treatment of single metastases to the brain: a randomized controlled multicentre phase III trial. J Neuro-Oncol 87:299–307

Mulvenna P, Nankivell M, Barton R et al (2016) Dexamethasone and supportive care with or without whole brain radiotherapy in treating patients with non-small cell lung cancer with brain metastases unsuitable for resection or stereotactic radiotherapy (QUARTZ): results from a phase 3, non-inferiority, randomised trial. Lancet 388:2004–2014

Neuhaus T, Ko Y, Muller RP et al (2009) A phase III trial of topotecan and whole brain radiation therapy for patients with CNS-metastases due to lung cancer. Br J Cancer 100:291–297

Nieder C, Hintz M, Oehlke O et al (2017) Validation of the graded prognostic assessment for lung cancer with brain metastases using molecular markers (lung-molGPA). Radiat Oncol 12:107

Patchell RA, Tibbs PA, Walsh JW et al (1990) A randomized trial of surgery in the treatment of single metastases of the brain. N Engl J Med 322:494–500

Patchell RA, Tibbs PA, Regine WF et al (1998) Postoperative radiotherapy in the treatment of single metastases to the brain. A randomised trial. JAMA 280:1485–1489

Patel KR, Prabhu RS, Kandula S et al (2014) Intracranial control and radiographic changes with adjuvant radiation therapy for resected brain metastases: whole brain radiotherapy versus stereotactic radiosurgery alone. J Neuro-Oncol 120:657–663

Planchard D, Popat S, Kerr K, ESMO Guidelines Committee et al (2018) Metastatic non-small cell lung cancer: ESMO Clinical Practice Guidelines

for diagnosis, treatment and follow-up. Ann Oncol 29(Suppl. 4):iv192–iv237
Popp I, Rau S, Hintz M et al (2020) Hippocampus-avoidance whole-brain radiation therapy with a simultaneous integrated boost for multiple brain metastases. Cancer 126:2694–2703
Priestman TJ, Dunn J, Brada M et al (1996) Final results of the Royal College of Radiologists trial comparing two different radiotherapy schedules in the treatment of cerebral metastases. Clin Oncol 8:308–315
Protopapa M, Kouloulias V, Nikoloudi S et al (2019) From whole-brain radiotherapy to immunotherapy: a multidisciplinary approach for patients with brain metastases from NSCLC. J Oncol 2019:3267409
Qin H, Wang C, Jiang Y et al (2015) Patients with single brain metastasis from non-small cell lung cancer equally benefit from stereotactic radiosurgery and surgery: a systematic review. Med Sci Monit 21:144–152
Rades D, Schild SE, Lohynska R et al (2007a) Two radiation regimens and prognostic factors for brain metastases in nonsmall cell lung cancer patients. Cancer 110:1077–1082
Rades D, Pluemer A, Veninga T et al (2007b) Whole-brain radiotherapy versus stereotactic radiosurgery for patients in recursive partitioning analysis classes 1 and 2 with 1 to 3 brain metastases. Cancer 110:2285–2292
Rades D, Kieckebusch S, Haatanen T et al (2008) Surgical resection followed by whole brain radiotherapy versus whole brain radiotherapy alone for single brain metastasis. Int J Radiat Oncol Biol Phys 70:1319–1324
Rades D, Panzner A, Dziggel L et al (2012a) Dose-escalation of whole-brain radiotherapy for brain metastasis in patients with a favorable survival prognosis. Cancer 118:3853–3859
Rades D, Kueter JD, Gliemroth J et al (2012b) Resection plus whole-brain irradiation versus resection plus whole-brain irradiation plus boost for the treatment of single brain metastasis. Strahlenther Onkol 188:143–147
Rades D, Veninga T, Hornung D et al (2012c) Single brain metastasis: whole-brain irradiation plus either radiosurgery or neurosurgical resection. Cancer 118:1138–1144
Rades D, Kueter JD, Meyners T et al (2012d) Single brain metastasis: resection followed by whole-brain irradiation and a boost to the metastatic site compared to whole-brain irradiation plus radiosurgery. Clin Neurol Neurosurg 114:326–330
Rades D, Hornung D, Veninga T et al (2012e) Single brain metastasis: radiosurgery alone compared with radiosurgery plus up-front whole-brain radiotherapy. Cancer 118:2980–2985
Rades D, Dziggel L, Segedin B et al (2013a) A new survival score for patients with brain metastases from non-small cell lung cancer. Strahlenther Onkol 189:777–781
Rades D, Dziggel L, Segedin B et al (2013b) The first survival score for patients with brain metastases from small cell lung cancer (SCLC). Clin Neurol Neurosurg 115:2029–2032
Rades D, Huttenlocher S, Hornung D et al (2014) Radiosurgery alone versus radiosurgery plus whole-brain irradiation for very few cerebral metastases from lung cancer. BMC Cancer 14:931
Rades D, Janssen S, Dziggel L et al (2017a) A matched-pair study comparing whole-brain irradiation alone to radiosurgery or fractionated stereotactic radiotherapy alone in patients irradiated for up to three brain metastases. BMC Cancer 17:30
Rades D, Janssen S, Bajrovic A et al (2017b) A matched-pair analysis comparing whole-brain radiotherapy with and without a stereotactic boost for intracerebral control and overall survival in patients with one to three cerebral metastases. Radiat Oncol 12:69
Rades D, Hansen HC, Schild SE, Janssen S (2019a) A new diagnosis-specific survival score for patients to be irradiated for brain metastases from non-small cell lung cancer. Lung 197:321–326
Rades D, Hansen HC, Janssen S et al (2019b) Comparison of diagnosis-specific survival scores for patients with small-cell lung cancer irradiated for brain metastases. Cancers (Basel) 11:233
Rapp SR, Case LD, Peiffer A et al (2015) Donepezil for irradiated brain tumor survivors: a phase III randomized placebo-controlled clinical trial. J Clin Oncol 33:1653–1659
Redmond KJ, Hales RK, Anderson-Keightly H et al (2017) Prospective study of hippocampal-sparing prophylactic cranial irradiation in limited-stage small cell lung cancer. Int J Radiat Oncol Biol Phys 98:603–611
Robin TP, Rusthoven CG (2018) Strategies to preserve cognition in patients with brain metastases: a review. Front Oncol 8:415
Robinet G, Thomas P, Breton JL et al (2001) Results of a phase III study of early versus delayed whole brain radiotherapy with concurrent cisplatin and vinorelbine combination in inoperable brain metastasis of non-small-cell lung cancer: Groupe Français de Pneumo-Cancérologie (GFPC) Protocol 95-1. Ann Oncol 12:59–67
Rusthoven CG, Yamamoto M, Bernhardt D et al (2020) Evaluation of first-line radiosurgery vs whole-brain radiotherapy for small cell lung cancer brain metastases: The FIRE-SCLC cohort study. JAMA Oncol 6:1028–1037
Schapira E, Hubbeling H, Yeap BY et al (2018) Improved overall survival and locoregional disease control with concurrent PD-1 pathway inhibitors and stereotactic radiosurgery for lung cancer patients with brain metastases. Int J Radiat Oncol Biol Phys 101:624–629
Schild SE, Foster NR, Meyers JP et al (2012) Prophylactic cranial irradiation in small-cell lung cancer: findings from a North Central Cancer Treatment Group pooled analysis. Ann Oncol 23:2919–2924
Sharma S, McMillan MT, Doucette A et al (2018) Effect of prophylactic cranial irradiation on overall survival in metastatic small-cell lung cancer: a propensity score-matched analysis. Clin Lung Cancer 19:260–269. e3
Shaw MG, Ball DL (2013) Treatment of brain metastases in lung cancer: strategies to avoid/reduce late

complications of whole brain radiation therapy. Curr Treat Opt Oncol 14:553–567

Shepard MJ, Xu Z, Donahue J et al (2019) Stereotactic radiosurgery with and without checkpoint inhibition for patients with metastatic non-small cell lung cancer to the brain: a matched cohort study. J Neurosurg 1–8. online ahead of print

Simone CB 2nd, Bogart JA, Cabrera AR et al (2020) Radiation therapy for small cell lung cancer: an ASTRO clinical practice guideline. Pract Radiat Oncol 10:158–173

Singh C, Qian JM, Yu JB et al (2019) Local tumor response and survival outcomes after combined stereotactic radiosurgery and immunotherapy in non-small cell lung cancer with brain metastases. J Neurosurg 132:512–517

Singh R, Lehrer EJ, Ko S et al (2020) Brain metastases from non-small cell lung cancer with EGFR or ALK mutations: a systematic review and meta-analysis of multidisciplinary approaches. Radiother Oncol 144:165–179

Slotman B, Faivre-Finn C, Kramer G et al (2007) Prophylactic cranial irradiation in extensive small-cell lung cancer. N Engl J Med 357:664–672

Soon YY, Leong CN, Koh WY et al (2015) EGFR tyrosine kinase inhibitors versus cranial radiation therapy for EGFR mutant non-small cell lung cancer with brain metastases: a systematic review and meta-analysis. Radiother Oncol 114:167–172

Sperduto PW, Chao ST, Sneed PK et al (2010) Diagnosis-specific prognostic factors, indexes, and treatment outcomes for patients with newly diagnosed brain metastases: a multi-institutional analysis of 4259 patients. Int J Radiat Oncol Biol Phys 77:655–661

Sperduto PW, Kased N, Roberge D et al (2012) Summary report on the graded prognostic assessment: an accurate and facile diagnosis-specific tool to estimate survival for patients with brain metastases. J Clin Oncol 30:419–425

Sperduto PW, Wang M, Robins HI et al (2013) A phase 3 trial of whole brain radiation therapy and stereotactic radiosurgery alone versus WBRT and SRS with temozolomide or erlotinib for non-small cell lung cancer and 1 to 3 brain metastases: Radiation Therapy Oncology Group 0320. Int J Radiat Oncol Biol Phys 85:1312–1318

Sperduto PW, Yang TJ, Beal K et al (2017) Estimating survival in patients with lung cancer and brain metastases: an update of the Graded Prognostic Assessment for lung cancer using molecular markers (lung-molGPA). JAMA Oncol 3:827–831

Suh JH, Stea B, Nabid A et al (2006) Phase III study of efaproxiral as an adjunct to whole-brain radiation therapy for brain metastases. J Clin Oncol 24:106–114

Sun A, Bae K, Gore EM et al (2011) Phase III trial of prophylactic cranial irradiation compared with observation in patients with locally advanced non–small-cell lung cancer: Neurocognitive and quality-of-life analysis. J Clin Oncol 29:279–286

Sundstrom JT, Minn H, Lertola KK et al (1998) Prognosis of patients treated for intracranial metastases with whole-brain irradiation. Ann Med 30:296–299

Takahashi T, Yamanaka T, Seto T et al (2017) Prophylactic cranial irradiation versus observation in patients with extensive-disease small-cell lung cancer: a multicentre, randomised, open-label, phase 3 trial. Lancet Oncol 18:663–671

Taylor JM, Rusthoven CG, Moghanaki D (2020) Prophylactic cranial irradiation or MRI surveillance for extensive stage small cell lung cancer. J Thorac Dis 12:6225–6233

Tsao MN, Rades D, Wirth A et al (2012) Radiotherapeutic and surgical management for newly diagnosed brain metastasis(es): an American Society for Radiation Oncology evidence-based guideline. Pract Radiat Oncol 2:210–225

Tsao MN, Xu W, Wong RK et al (2018) Whole brain radiotherapy for the treatment of newly diagnosed multiple brain metastases. Cochrane Database Syst Rev 1:CD003869

Vecht CJ, Haaxma-Reiche H, Noordijk EM et al (1993) Treatment of single brain metastasis: radiotherapy alone or combined with neurosurgery? Ann Neurol 33:583–590

Walker AJ, Ruzevick J, Malayeri AA et al (2014) Postradiation imaging changes in the CNS: how can we differentiate between treatment effect and disease progression? Future Oncol 10:1277–1297

Wan JF, Zhang SJ, Wang L et al (2013) Implications for preserving neural stem cells in whole brain radiotherapy and prophylactic cranial irradiation: a review of 2270 metastases in 488 patients. J Radiat Res 54:285–291

Wang N, Zhang Y, Mi Y et al (2020) Osimertinib for EGFR-mutant lung cancer with central nervous system metastases: a meta-analysis and systematic review. Ann Palliat Med 9:3038–3047

Wen P, Wang TF, Li M et al (2020) Meta-analysis of prophylactic cranial irradiation or not in treatment of extensive-stage small-cell lung cancer: the dilemma remains. Cancer Radiother 24:44–52

Westover KD, Mendel JT, Dan T et al (2020) Phase II trial of hippocampal-sparing whole brain irradiation with simultaneous integrated boost for metastatic cancer. Neuro-Oncology 22:1831–1839

Witlox WJA, Ramaekers BLT, Zindler JD et al (2018) The prevention of brain metastases in non-small cell lung cancer by prophylactic cranial irradiation. Front Oncol 8:241

Yamamoto M, Serizawa T, Shuto T et al (2014a) Stereotactic radiosurgery for patients with multiple brain metastases (JLGK0901): a multi-institutional prospective observational study. Lancet Oncol 15:387–395

Yamamoto M, Kawabe T, Sato Y et al (2014b) Stereotactic radiosurgery for patients with multiple brain metastases: a case-matched study comparing treatment results for patients with 2-9 versus 10 or more tumors. J Neurosurg 121 Suppl:16–25

Yamamoto M, Serizawa T, Sato Y et al (2020) Stereotactic radiosurgery results for patients with 5–10 versus 11–20 brain metastases: a retrospective cohort study combining 2 databases totaling 2319 patients. World Neurosurg. S1878-8750(20)32326-3

Yang Z, Zhang Y, Li R, Yisikandaer A et al (2021) Whole brain radiotherapy with and without concurrent erlotinib in NSCLC with brain metastases: a multicentre, open-label, randomized, controlled phase 3 trial. Neuro-Oncol 23:967–978

Yin X, Yan D, Qiu M et al (2019) Prophylactic cranial irradiation in small cell lung cancer: a systematic review and meta-analysis. BMC Cancer 19:95

Zhang Y, Chang EL (2014) Resection cavity radiosurgery for intracranial metastases: a review of the literature. J Radiosurg SBRT 3:91–102

Zhang W, Jiang W, Luan L et al (2014) Prophylactic cranial irradiation for patients with small-cell lung cancer: a systematic review of the literature with meta-analysis. BMC Cancer 14:793

Zhang M, Rodrigues AJ, Pollom EL et al (2021) Improved survival and disease control following pembrolizumab-induced immune-related adverse events in high PD-L1 expressing non-small cell lung cancer with brain metastases. J Neuro-Oncol 152:125–134

Zheng MH, Sun HT, Xu JG et al (2016) Combining whole-brain radiotherapy with gefitinib/erlotinib for brain metastases from non-small-cell lung cancer: a meta-analysis. Biomed Res Int 2016:5807346

Zhong J, Waldman AD, Kandula S et al (2020) Outcomes of whole-brain radiation with simultaneous in-field boost (SIB) for the treatment of brain metastases. J Neuro-Oncol 147:117–123

Zhuang H, Yuan Z, Wang J et al (2013) Phase II study of whole brain radiotherapy with or without erlotinib in patients with multiple brain metastases from lung adenocarcinoma. Drug Des Devel Ther 7:1179–1186

Zimm S, Wampler GL, Stablein D et al (1981) Intracerebral metastases in solid tumor patients: natural history and results of treatment. Cancer 48:384–394

Radiation Therapy for Metastatic Lung Cancer: Bone Metastasis and Metastatic Spinal Cord Compression

Begoña Taboada-Valladares, Patricia Calvo-Crespo, and Antonio Gómez-Caamaño

Contents

1 **Bone Metastases** 780
1.1 Introduction 780
1.2 Conventional Palliative Radiotherapy 780
1.3 Postoperative Palliative Radiotherapy 782
1.4 SBRT 783

2 **Spinal Metastases and Spinal Cord Compression** 784
2.1 Introduction 784
2.2 Conventional Palliative Radiotherapy 786
2.3 SBRT 786

3 **Conclusions** 790

References 790

B. Taboada-Valladares (✉) · P. Calvo-Crespo
A. Gómez-Caamaño
Department of Radiation Oncology,
Santiago de Compostela University Hospital,
Santiago de Compostela, Spain
e-mail: Maria.Begona.Taboada.Valladares@sergas.es;
Patricia.Calvo.Crespo@sergas.es;
Antonio.Gomez.Caamano@sergas.es

Abstract

Non-small cell lung cancer (NSCLC) patients may develop bone metastases (BM) frequently. Depending on the metastases' location, it may affect to a greater or lesser extent the patient's quality of life, with spinal involvement being especially serious if it causes spinal compression. Rapid local treatment is of paramount importance for optimal symptom management.

Radiotherapy (RT) plays a fundamental role in this scenario. A careful screening of patients is essential on the basis of both their general condition and the prognosis of the disease, as assessed by different prognostic scores, published research, and consensus guidelines. At present we have different techniques for the administration of RT: whereas in patients with a poorer prognosis, conventional single-fraction RT is preferred, in patients with a more favorable prognosis technique such as stereotactic body radiation therapy (SBRT), increasing local control (LC) with acceptable toxicity should be considered.

1 Bone Metastases

1.1 Introduction

Between 30% and 40% of patients with NSCLC eventually develop BM during the disease. These may cause skeletal events such as pathological fractures, spinal cord compression (SCC), nerve root compression, or malignant hypercalcemia, all of which have a negative effect on both the patient's quality of life and their functionality (Arnold et al. 2006; Bae et al. 2012).

Among treatment goals for BM we might include pain relief, preservation of mobility, prevention of future complications, minimizing hospitalizations, and optimizing the quality of life (Fairchild 2014).

A number of factors have been associated with the development of BM in patients with NSCLC. Da Silva et al. (2019) analyzed the risk factors associated with developing bone metastases in 1112 NSCLC patients, diagnosed between 2006 and 2014. Median age was 63.4 years with a good Karnofsky index (KPS), 62% were males, 86.6% were with prior smoking history, 51% were with adenocarcinomas, 27.2% were treated with radiochemotherapy (RCT), and 3.3% were with inhibitor tyrosine kinase. BM was detected in 13.2% of the cases during the follow-up. The median time between the diagnosis and the development of metastases was 8.1 months, presenting statistically significant differences across stages (9.6m SI, 8.4m SII, 6.8m SIII, 5.7m SIV, $p < 0.001$). Out of these, 27.2% were vertebral metastases, followed by pelvis and rib metastases. The multivariate analysis found that young age, adenocarcinoma histology, and prior treatment with RT, chemotherapy (CT), or RCT were related to a higher probability of developing BM.

RT is a well-established treatment in this clinical situation and thus considered a gold standard. It is estimated that approximately 40% of patients with BM are treated with RT (Bezjak 2003).

1.2 Conventional Palliative Radiotherapy

Whereas the conventional palliative treatment for bone metastases has a high antalgic response rate (Huisman et al. 2012), LC remains poor, something which is a problem for patients with a favorable prognosis.

Four meta-analyses of more than 20 studies have shown that, when it comes to uncomplicated BM, there exists no benefit in terms of pain, use of analgesia, time to pain improvement, time to pain progression, duration of response, percentage of SCC, acute toxicity, quality of life, and overall survival (OS) between single-fraction RT and fractionated treatments (Sze et al. 2003; Wu et al. 2003; Chow et al. 2007, 2012a).

One of these meta-analyses (Sze et al. 2003), published in 2003, comprised 20 studies with 3621 patients randomized to single- vs. multiple-fraction RT. No differences were found in terms of antalgic response, nor in complete response to pain (34% vs. 32%), but it did find them in terms of retreatment and pathological fractures in the arm of the single fraction.

Another of the abovementioned meta-analyses (Wu et al. 2003) comparing single vs. multiple fraction also differentiated between the administered doses (1 single fraction of 8 Gy vs. 5 fractions of 400 cGy vs. 10 fractions of 300 cGy). No significant differences were found in response to pain, neither a relationship between the response to treatment and the administered dose.

In their 2006 meta-analysis, Chow et al. (2007) included 16 studies, totaling 2513 patients with a single-fraction dose and 2487 with a multiple-fraction one. Although no difference in pain response rates was found, there were more pathological fractures in the arm of the single fraction without them being significant ($p = 0.75$) and more retreatments in the arm of the single fraction ($p < 0.0001$).

In 2012, another meta-analysis (Chow et al. 2012a) compared 2818 patients with single fraction to 2799 ones with fractionated treatment.

The overall response percentage to the single fraction was 60% and complete response was 23%, with no significant differences between the 61% response to fractionated treatment and the 24% of complete responses. Median time to pain response was between 1 and 4 weeks, and the median duration of response was between 12 and 24 months. Regarding toxicity, 3.3% of the single-fraction patients had pathological fracture vs. 3% of the fractionated ones ($p = 0.72$), and 28% suffered SCC in the single-fraction arm vs. 1.9% in the fractionated one ($p = 0.13$). Statistically significant differences in retreatment were found, with 20% for single-fraction patients and 8% for fractionated ones ($p < 0.00001$).

One of the most representative studies is the Dutch trial (Steenland et al. 1999), in which 1157 patients (without SCC, without prior RT, not requiring surgery, and without cervical metastases) between 1996 and 1998 were randomized to a single fraction of 8 Gy vs. 24 Gy in 6 fractions. Out of these, 287 patients were of primary pulmonary origin. 60.2% were responders to treatment and 58% to single fraction. Mean response time was 3 weeks and the duration of the response was 11 weeks. No correlation between histology and initial response ($p = 0.69$) was found. 29.2% featured progression to pain.

A comprehensive review was published in 2018 (Rich et al. 2018) comparing single vs. multiple fraction, with no differences as regards pain response, complete antalgic response, pathological fractures, spinal compression, or acute toxicity. Only statistically significant differences in terms of retreatments (20% in single fraction vs. 8% in multiple one, $p < 0.01$) were found.

A more recent meta-analysis (Chow et al. 2019) has studied the efficacy of the single vs. multiple fraction, being consistent with previous studies: the response rate to treatment is similar in the single-fraction group and the multiple-fraction one, with a higher rate of retreatments in the single-fraction segment.

One of the main problems when it comes to comparing different studies is the criterion with which to define the analgesic response. With the aim of solving this, the International Bone Metastases Consensus Working Party on Palliative RT (Chow et al. 2002) defines a series of categories of response to radiotherapy treatment:

1. Complete response: a pain score of 0 after treatment, without increased analgesia
2. Partial response: reduction in the pain score of 2 or more points on a scale of 0–10, with no increase in analgesia, or with a 25% decrease
3. Pain progression: pain increase of 2 or more points with the same analgesia, or with an increase of 25%
4. Indeterminate response: any response that is not captured by the previous definitions

The ASTRO (Lutz et al. 2017) guidelines on BM were updated in 2017 on the basis of scientific evidence and expert opinion. A series of recommendations were offered:

- For BM, fractionation schemes are equivalent in terms of pain control, with a higher rate of retreatments in single fractions.
- A single fraction of 8 Gy is suitable for the treatment of spinal metastases, especially in those patients with a worse prognosis.
- Those patients with recurrent pain after one month of RT should be considered for retreatment.
- SBRT as the first option for spinal metastases or SCC should be considered within a clinical trial.
- Retreatment with SBRT for spinal metastases can be effective and safe, but it is recommended to do it within a trial.
- The use of surgery, radionuclides, bisphosphonates, or vertebroplasty does not replace treatment with RT in painful BM.

Ganesh et al. (2017) published a review of standard clinical practice patterns in the treatment of uncomplicated BM, describing an increase in the use of the single fraction since 2010, which is less marked in the USA. They concluded that there has been an increase in single-fraction treatment in BM in routine clinical practice, although there are still some clinical guidelines that deem multiple fractionation reasonable depending on the age, performance status (PS), prognosis, and location to be treated.

Optimal fractionation is unresolved. In clinical practice, the choice of fractionation scheme is influenced by the patient's traits (PS, compliance with treatment, life expectancy), tumor-related factors (histology of the primary location, time between diagnosis and BM, time of development of pain or neurological deficit prior to RT), and logistical issues (Wu et al. 2004).

The single fraction is recommended as standard treatment for uncomplicated symptomatic BM, as it has multiple advantages, such as fewer acute adverse effects, fewer hospital trips, less discomfort in position, being more cost effective, and decreased waiting times (Fairchild 2014).

Literature on reradiation is scarce. Retreatment after palliative radiotherapy can be considered as a nonresponse in a previously treated area, as a partial response with the hope of greater benefit when repeating the treatment, or as a pain peak after an initially satisfactory response. Re-irradiation of painful BM (Huisman et al. 2012) in nonresponders or patients with recurrent pain after response occurs in 42% of treated patients. A meta-analysis included 2694 patients, of whom 20% were retreated ones. Twenty-three percent were patients with primary pulmonary tumors. The most frequent sites of re-irradiation were spinal metastases (36%), pelvis metastases (38%), long bone ones (12%), and other sites (14%). The pain response rate was 58%. The complete response to reradiation reached 16–28%. The response time after retreatment was 3–5 weeks and the duration of the response lasted between 15 days and 22 weeks. There is no evidence that the time to progression was shorter in patients previously treated with single fractions.

1.3 Postoperative Palliative Radiotherapy

In long-bone BMs, stabilization is necessary to treat pain and maintain limb functionality (Willeumier et al. 2016) in injuries with risk of fracture. The surgical options depend on the location, size, type of injury, mechanical stability, and morbidity of the procedure in relation to the patient's life expectancy. Prophylactic fixation may be recommended to prevent either pathologic fractures or surgical stabilization of an unstable spine prior to RT. The Mirels scoring system helps predict fracture risk in the setting of metastatic disease in long bones (Mirels 1989).

Multiple reviews on post-surgery radiotherapy in 5–10 fractions suggest that RT prevents bone progression, minimizes the risk of implant failure, and reduces the likelihood of a second procedure (Jacofsky and Haidukewych 2004; Bickels et al. 2009; Biermann et al. 2009; Ruggieri et al. 2010; Malviya and Gerrand 2012; Quinn et al. 2014).

There is a comprehensive review (Willeumier et al. 2016) including two retrospective studies that include lesions treated with surgery, with or without adjuvant radiotherapy, with the primary endpoint being the functional status of the limb (divided into (1) normal function, no pain; (2) normal function, with pain; (3) significantly limited function; (4) no functionality). In the RT group, the percentage of patients with limb functionality was 53% vs. 11.5%. Only postoperative RT proved to be significant in achieving functional status 1 and 2, $p = 0.026$. Better median survival was observed in the RT arm (12.4 months vs. 5.3 months, $p = 0.025$), with no differences in second orthopedic procedures. These results should be taken with caution due to the reduced amount of evidence (adjuvant RT was at the discretion of the surgeon, using nonvalidated score in a heterogeneous population).

Postoperative RT increases the frequency of normal limb use while decreasing pain and the likelihood of implant failure. It also minimizes the risk of disease progression, and reduces the risk of refracture (Chow et al. 2007).

Wolanczyk et al. (2016) examined postoperative outcomes in prophylactically stabilized or pathologic fracture patients who subsequently received RT, bisphosphonates, or both. With a 1-year follow-up, patients treated with radiotherapy or RT and bisphosphonates had less SRE than those treated with bisphosphonates alone (respectively, 9% and 7% vs. 44%).

Doses of 20 Gy/5 fractions or 30 Gy/10 fractions are usually employed, and postoperative treatment is usually started within 2–4 weeks after surgery, once the wound has adequately healed, including the entire surgical field. Complications from the wound are rare.

The ASCO/ASTRO guidelines (Lutz et al. 2011) recommend a 30–20 Gy fractionation scheme in 10–5 fractions, instead of a single fraction given the lack of experience in the postoperative period.

1.4 SBRT

In 1995, Hellman and Weichselbaum proposed the term "oligometastasis" to refer to patients with limited metastatic disease (Hellman and Weichselbaum 1995), in number and location (in one or a limited number of organs), who may have a more indolent biology and a better prognosis than patients with multiple metastases. The incidence of oligometastatic NSCLC is estimated to be around 20–50% of patients with NSCLC depending on the definition used regarding the number of metastases (3 vs. 5) and the time of presentation of the disease (synchronous vs. metachronous) (Bergsma et al. 2017).

Different studies proved a possible benefit in the overall survival in sarcomas with the resection of lung metastases (Pastorino et al. 1997) or liver resections in colorectal carcinoma (Nordlinger et al. 1996). As a result, local ablative treatment with radiotherapy started to be studied.

Over the last decade, advances in RT thanks to guided imagery, planning, and dose escalation have made it possible to achieve ablative doses in SBRT. When comparing SBRT to surgery, it features the advantage of shorter recovery time, fewer side effects, and safety of being able to treat various metastatic lesions. What is more, SBRT could have an abscopal effect on tumors associated with a strong immune response (Zeng et al. 2019).

For oligometastatic patients, SBRT can improve disease-free survival (DFS) and potentially delay systemic treatment (Ost et al. 2016). Screening patients carefully is important, so each case should be discussed in a multidisciplinary committee. Age, PS, comorbidities, and functional capacity are aspects to take into account in decision-making.

Palma et al. (2018) published a phase II treatment with SBRT in oligometastatic patients. Between 2012 and 2016, 99 patients (18 with breast cancer, 18 with lung cancer, 18 with colorectal cancer, and 16 with prostate one) were recruited, being stratified into standard treatment arm vs. standard treatment and SBRT on metastases. A total of 191 metastases were treated, out of which 65 were bone metastases. With a median follow-up of 27 months, better OS was observed in favor of the SBRT arm (28m vs. 41m, $p = 0.09$) and better DFS (6m vs. 12m, $p = 0.001$) at the expense of greater Gr2 toxicity (9% vs. 30%), especially asthenia, dyspnea, and bone pain. No differences were found in the quality of life in both arms.

A follow-up phase III study, SABR-COMET-3, will test the approach in patients with up to three metastatic lesions, and the phase III SABR-COMET-10 will test this approach with lower SBRT doses in patients with up to 10 lesions.

Bedard et al. (2016) conducted a review that included 14 studies on nonspinal bone metastases treated with SBRT. It included primary tumors from various locations, including NSCLC. Patients with less than 5 metastases and a life expectancy greater than 3 months were screened. Due to the different endpoints of the studies it is difficult to analyze the results, but SBRT appears as a safe and feasible treatment option in nonspinal BM, yielding similar results in terms of LC both with a single fraction of SBRT and with multiple fractions, despite obtaining greater toxicity in the arm of the SBRT single fraction. A randomized study comparing single vs. multiple fraction in SBRT would be necessary.

In 2019, a phase II study (Nguyen et al. 2019) comparing SBRT vs. conventional treatment for pain control in nonspinal BM was published. It included 160 patients with painful BM, out of which 81 received SBRT in single fraction (12 Gy if size is >4 cm and 16 Gy if size is <4 cm) and 79 received RT (10 fractions of 3 Gy). The primary endpoint was the response to pain (a progression was considered when they had a 2-point increase in pain score, an increase in the morphine dose >50%, and re-irradiation or pathological fracture). Response to pain was greater in the SBRT arm at 2 weeks (62% vs. 36%, $p = 0.01$), at 3 months (72% vs. 49%, $p = 0.03$), and at 9 months (77% vs. 46%, $p = 0.03$), respectively. Higher rates of LC in the SBRT arm at 1 and 2 years were also found. However, no differences in quality of life, toxicity, or OS were observed. They concluded that SBRT should be considered for painful BM in patients with longer life expectancy.

Ongoing:

- NCT03143322 (Thureau et al. 2021): Extracranial Stereotactic Body Radiation Therapy (SBRT) Added to Standard Treatment Versus Standard Treatment Alone in Solid Tumors Patients with Between 1 and 3 Bone-only Metastases (STEREO-OS). A French study featuring patients with breast prostate and lung carcinoma, with 1–3 bone metastases. The standard treatment + SBRT vs. standard treatment in bone lesions are contrasted in terms of DFS.
- NCT02364115 (ClinicalTrials.gov 2019): Randomized Trial Comparing Conventional Radiotherapy with Stereotactic Radiotherapy in Patients with Bone Metastases, VERTICAL Study (VERTICAL). A Dutch study comparing SBRT in 18 Gy single fraction vs. conventional RT 8 Gy, having as primary endpoint a partial or complete response to pain at 3 months. As secondary endpoints DFS, OS, quality of life, vertebral fracture, and myelopathy, as well as pain response time.

2 Spinal Metastases and Spinal Cord Compression

2.1 Introduction

The spine is a common place for bone metastases, which can lead to major morbidity and mortality. Classic treatment for BM was palliative RT, but improvements in systemic treatments and technological advances of RT make it possible to administer high doses of RT, hence increasing LC and improving the response to pain (Shagal et al. 2008).

The decision to treat in this clinical situation requires a rigorous assessment of life expectancy and the presence of mechanical stability. Jensen et al. define the prognosis of patients with spinal metastases by means of the PRISM (Prognostic Index for Spine Metastases) (Jensen et al. 2017), which divides patients into four groups, from best to worst prognosis, with different medians of OS (Table 1).

Existence of spinal mechanical instability must be evaluated with the SINS (Spinal Instability Neoplastic Score) scale (Fisher et al. 2014) (Table 2). This score considers location, pain, type of bone lesion, spinal alignment, collapse of the vertebral body, and posterolateral involvement. A score between 0 and 18 is generated, being considered as stable if between 0 and 6, potentially unstable when between 7 and 12, and unstable when between 13 and 18. Those potentially unstable or unstable require surgical evaluation.

In cases where spinal metastases involve a soft tissue mass, cord compression may appear. Spinal cord compression is an oncological emergency, whose early diagnosis and treatment are key factors in avoiding severe and irreversible neurological damage (Lawton et al. 2019). Loss of strength and sensitivity and impaired sphincter control are not only an important morbidity, but also related to worse survival. Invasion of the vertebral body caused by hematogenous dissemination is the most frequent cause of spinal cord compression. Sometimes it even creates vertebral mechanical instability, which represents an orthopedic emergency. Pain is the earliest and most frequent symptom. Signs and symptoms appear as the compression progresses, starting from motor weakness and alteration in sensitivity until reaching paralysis to sphincter incontinence as a consequence of complete neurological damage. Medical history and physical examination should hint at the level where spinal compression

Table 1 PRISM score

Variables	Score
Female	+2
Karnofsky	+1 for every 10 patients over 60 on KPS scale
Previous surgery at SSRS site	+2
Previous radiation at SSRS site	−2
Other organ systems involved in metastasis (other than bone)	−1 per system
SSRS for solitary metastasis	+3
Time between diagnosis and metastasis >5 years	+3

Survival groups	Score range
Group 4 (poor prognosis)	<1
Group 3	1–3
Group 2	4–7
Group 1 (excellent prognosis)	>7

Table 2 SINS score

	SINS	Score
Location	Junctional (occipital-C2, C7–T2, T11–L1, L5–S1)	3
	Mobile spine (C3–6, L2–4)	2
	Semirigid (T3–10)	1
	Rigid (S2–5)	0
Pain	Yes	3
	Occasional pain but not mechanical	2
	Pain-free lesion	0
Bone lesion	Lytic	2
	Mixed (lytic/blastic)	1
	Blastic	0
Spinal alignment	Subluxation/translation present	4
	De novo deformity (kyphosis/scoliosis)	2
	Normal alignment	0
Vertebral body collapse	>50% collapse	3
	<50% collapse	2
	Non-collapse with >50% body involved	1
	None of the above	0
Posterolateral involvement of the spinal elements	Bilateral	3
	Unilateral	1
	None of the above	0

Score 0–6: stable spine
Score 7–12: potentially unstable spine
Score 13–18: unstable spine
Recommendation: score > 7 consider surgical intervention

may be developing, with the most important complementary examination being an MRI of the entire spine, which should be requested immediately to decide and start treatment. In general, corticosteroids together with oncological radiotherapy treatment and/or surgery are the most widely used therapeutic weapons.

In the case of epidural disease, the degree and severity of SCC, as well as potential consequences, should be evaluated using the Bilsky score (Bilsky et al. 2010).

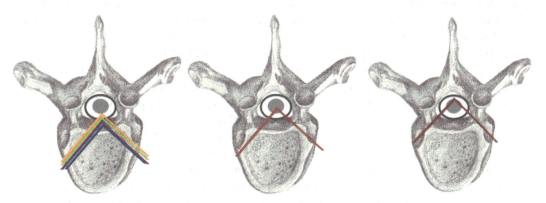

Grade 0: bone-only disease.
Grade 1a: epidural impigement, without deformation of the tecal sac.
Grade 1b: deformation of the tecal sac, without spinal cord abutment.
Grade 1c: deformation of the tecal sac, with spinal cord abutment, but without cord compression.

Grade 2: spinal cord compression, but with CSF visible around the cord.

Grade 3: spinal cord compression, no CSF visible around the cord.

2.2 Conventional Palliative Radiotherapy

Studies have shown that doses of 5 × 400 cGy and 10 × 300 cGy yielded similar results in terms of improved motor function (Rades et al. 2005). However, a prospective nonrandomized study has shown that a long fractionation (10 × 300 cGy) is superior in local PFS versus a short one (5 × 400 cGy) at 6 months (86% vs. 67%, $p = 0.0034$) (Rades et al. 2009). Maranzano et al. (2005) compared different fractionation doses in SCC patients with a life expectancy <6 months, randomizing to a single 8 Gy fraction vs. multiple fractionation. Both fractionations proved effective without significant differences in pain control (56% vs. 59%), motor function (68% vs. 71%), and bladder function (90% vs. 89%). The authors suggest that the single fraction is recommended for SCC and low life expectancy (Maranzano et al. 2009).

In 2005, Patchell et al. published the phase III study (Patchell et al. 2005), comparing decompressive surgery followed by RT versus conventional RT. Both groups received the same doses of corticosteroids and the same doses of RT (30 Gy in 10 fractions of 3 Gy). Decompressive surgery was performed 24 h after randomization and postoperative RT began no later than 2 weeks after surgery. The study included 101 patients (50 in the combined group and 51 in the radiotherapy-only group), out of which 26 patients had a lung cancer diagnosis. The study was stopped after the first interim analysis. The primary objective was to assess the ability to walk. Secondary endpoints included urinary continence, muscle strength, functional status, need for corticosteroids and opiates, as well as survival. Results demonstrated that, although there are no statistically significant differences in terms of survival, a higher percentage of patients treated with decompressive surgery and postoperative radiotherapy maintain the ability to walk, and for longer periods, than patients treated with radiotherapy alone.

The PREMODE study (Rades et al. 2021) screened 44 patients with SCC in terms of local DFS after receiving 5 × 5 Gy at 1, 3, and 6 months. Treatment with VMAT was performed, including the affected vertebra and half of the upper and lower vertebra in the CTV and expanding PTV to 8 mm of margin. Results were compared to a historical group of 213 patients treated with 10 × 300 cGy conventional RT. Local DFS at 6 months was 94% (5 × 5 Gy) vs. 87%, $p = 0.36$, and the OS at 6 months was 43% vs. 38%, $p = 0.74$, with similar response rates, but greater improvement in motor function in the 5 × 5 Gy arm (59% vs. 34%, $p = 0.028$). It was concluded that fractionation of 5 × 5 Gy over 1 week has similar efficacy to 10 × 300 cGy over 2 weeks, although these results should be confirmed in randomized studies.

2.3 SBRT

In SCC patients with mechanical instability, surgical intervention is required. In this scenario, the high local recurrence rates (69.3% at 1 year) (Klekamp and Samii 1998) would justify adjuvant treatments. A traditional approach was to perform conventional RT, although present-day approaches are exploring the field of SBRT, since it is a well-tolerated technique (no toxicities Gr3–4, 9% pain flare), with excellent LC (Tseng et al. 2017). De novo treatment with spinal SBRT achieves LC rates between 80% and 95% in a heterogeneous patient group with varied fractionations, from a single 15 Gy fraction to 30 Gy in three fractions (Wang et al. 2012; Chang et al. 2012). Hall et al. have reported a LC of 90% at 15 months (Hall et al. 2011).

Table 3 shows multiple studies of SBRT in de novo spinal metastases (Jensen et al. 2017) where high rates of LC can be perceived.

Guckenberger et al. (2014) have analyzed the efficacy and safety of SBRT as a treatment for spinal metastases in five centers in the USA, two in Canada, and one in Germany, screening 301 patients with a total of 387 metastases between 2004 and 2013. With a median follow-up of 11.8 months, OS was 19.5 months. OS at 1 and 2 years was 64.9% and 43.7%, respectively. The factors associated with poorer survival were being male, KPS <90%, presence of visceral metastases, uncontrolled systemic disease, and

Table 3 SBRT studies overview

References	Patients/ spinal segments	Histology	Dose fractionation (Gy/fr)	Follow-up duration (median, months)	Local control	Pain response
Tseng et al.	145/279	Mixed	24/2	15	90.3% 1 year 82.4% 2 years	NR
Azad et al.	25/25	Mixed	15–25.5/1–5	18	84%	2/3 had pain relief
Anad et al.	52/76	Mixed	24–27/1–3	8.5	94% 1 year 83% 2 years	90–94% complete pain relief
Bishop et al.	285/332	Mixed	Median tumor dose 43 Gy	19	88% 1 year 82% 3 years	NR
Bate et al.	24/24	Mixed	16–30/1–5	9.8	96% 1 year	NR
Guckenberg et al.	301/387	Mixed	10–60/1–20	11.8	90% 1 year 84% 2 years	44% with severe pretreatment pain, pain free, 56% with mild/moderate pretreatment pain, pain free
Garg et al.	47/47	Mixed	16–24/1	17.8	88% 18 months	18 patients pain free
Chang et al.	93/131	Mixed	NR	23.7	89% 1 year	NR
Gill et al.	14/14	Mixed	30–35/5	34	80% 1 year 73% 2 years	NR
Wang et al.	149/166	Mixed	27–30/3	15.9	81% 1 year 72% 2 year	54% pain free at 6 months, compared to 26% at baseline
Sahgal et al.	14/18	Mixed	24/3	9	72%	NR
Yamada et al.	93/103	Mixed	18–24/1	15	93% 2 years	NR
Chang et al.	17/22	Mixed	27–30/3–5	NR	68%	Narcotic usage fell from 60% at baseline to 36% at 6 months
Ryu et al.	49–61	Mixed	10–16/1	NR	96% 9 months	Overall response 85%

more than one vertebra treated with SBRT. LC at 1 and 2 years was 89.9% and 83.9%, respectively. Only two cases of acute Gr3 toxicity were observed, and no myelopathies.

The longest monoinstitutional experience using 24 Gy in two fractions included 279 spinal SBRTs with 145 patients (Tseng et al. 2018). LC at 1 year was 90.3% and at 2 years was 82.4%, with excellent tolerance.

Sprave et al. (2018a) conducted a phase II study with the primary endpoint of controlling pain. Fifty-five patients were treated with SBRT (24 Gy in a single fraction) vs. conventional 30 Gy RT in ten fractions, using the parameters established by the International Bone Consensus Working Party (Chow et al. 2012b). A higher rate of complete responses was obtained at 3 months (43% vs. 17%, $p = 0.0568$) and at 6 months (53% vs. 10%, $p = 0.0034$) in the SBRT arm. The risk of vertebral fracture was 8.7% at 3 months and 27.8% at 6 months. There was no toxicity greater than G3. Quality of life was not worse for SBRT when compared to conventional treatment (Sprave et al. 2018b).

Reported toxicity with SBRT includes:

1. Pain flare: increased pain during or after completing RT. Whereas with conventional treatment it happens to a third of patients, with SBRT it varies between 14% and 68%. Dexamethasone prevents pain flare and reduces it by 68–19% (Chiang et al. 2013).
2. Vertebral fracture: the high doses administered generate acute inflammation, which can weaken the bone matrix and the risk of fracture. The risk of fracture ranges from 11% to 39% (Faruqi et al. 2018).
3. Myelopathy: it is a late complication from SBRT. A review of 1400 patients reveals myelopathy rates of 0.4% (Hall et al. 2011).

Excellent LC has been achieved in postoperative SBRT, similar to that achieved in de novo metastases. After a vertebrectomy or laminectomy, LC at 1 year is >80%. What is more, in those patients where surgical downgrading of epidural disease is possible, LC is better (Tao et al. 2016).

The RTOG 0631 study (Ryu et al. 2014) is a multicenter phase III study that screened 339 patients featuring between 1 and 3 spinal metastases and who were randomly assigned to receive either SBRT ($n = 209$) at 16 or 18 Gy in one fraction or RT ($n = 130$) in a single 8 Gy fraction in a 2:1 ratio. Minimal epidural lesions at least 3 mm away from the spinal cord were included, and each location could affect up to two contiguous segments of the spine. The primary endpoint was pain control, defined as a 33-point improvement on the Numerical Rating Pain Scale (NRPS), at the treated spine segment at 3 months posttreatment. The study had 80% power to show a 40% improvement in pain response with 2:1 randomization in favor of SRS/SBRT. In a preliminary analysis presented at ASTRO 2019 (Ryu et al. 2019), the results showed that SBRT was not significantly better when compared to RT for symptom control, finding no noteworthy differences in pain response between SBRT and RT at three months (40.3% vs. 57.9%, respectively, $p = 0.99$).

The Canadian Cancer Trials Group/Trans-Tasman Radiation Oncology Group (2021) phase II/III study presented at the ASTRO Annual Meeting in 2020 randomized 229 patients with painful spinal metastases into SBRT (24 Gy in two fractions) or RT (20 Gy in five fractions), concluding that SBRT is superior to conventional RT by significantly improving the complete pain response rate at three (36% vs. 14%) and at six months (33% vs. 16%).

Vertebral re-irradiation is safe, with a 12% of vertebral fracture and a 1.2% of myelopathy. Hashmi et al. (2016) published the results of SBRT retreatment in seven institutions. The median dose treated with conventional RT was 30 Gy in ten fractions and 60% were treated with SBRT. LC was of 83% and there were no cases of myelopathy. With spinal SBRT, the complete antalgic response rate ranges between 46% and 92%, compared to the 24% of complete response obtained with conventional RT.

When planning spinal SBRT, a planning CT with fixation should be performed, fusing it with MRI on T1 and T2 to delineate critical structures. The International Spine Radiosurgery Consortium has published volume definition guidelines for SBRT based on expert opinion with ten representative cases (Cox et al. 2012). GTV should be contoured including the extent of the epidural and paraspinal disease. CTV should include the areas of microscopic extension. If the GTV is present in the vertebral body, pedicle, transverse process, lamina, or spinous process, the entire region must be included. What is more, the adjacent bone region must also be included. PTV should be given a 3 mm margin.

Redmond et al. produced a set of consensus contouring guidelines for postoperative spinal SBRT (Faruqi et al. 2018). Recommendations comprise including preoperative bone extension, epidural disease, and adjacent bone structure as part of the CTV. In the event of specific epidural disease, the CTV should take the shape of a donut. Surgical instrumentation should be excluded from the CTV.

The ideal fractionation for spinal SBRT is unknown. The common patterns of treatment comprise doses of a single fraction of 16–24 Gy, two fractions of 12 Gy, 24–30 Gy in three fractions, 30 Gy in four fractions, and 30–40 Gy in five fractions. When choosing the fractionation, the risk of vertebral fracture (39% in single fraction) (Redmond et al. 2015) and the treatment volume (4–5 fractions are better for larger volumes) must be taken into account. The single fraction is associated to higher risk of pain flare and myelopathy (Ryu et al. 2019).

Due to the difficulty of assessing the response after spinal SBRT, a group of experts developed guidelines for the response to treatment assessment (SPINO) (Thibault et al. 2015). An MRI should be performed every

2–3 months during 2 years and then every 3–6 months, assessed by an expert radiologist. Progression is defined as increased tumor volume, new tumor in the epidural space, and neurological deterioration due to a previously known epidural disease.

Due to the complexity in the therapeutic decision-making for patients with spinal BM, some treatment algorithms have been published (Spratt et al. 2017). These consider which variables should be taken into account for the adequate management of spinal metastatic disease.

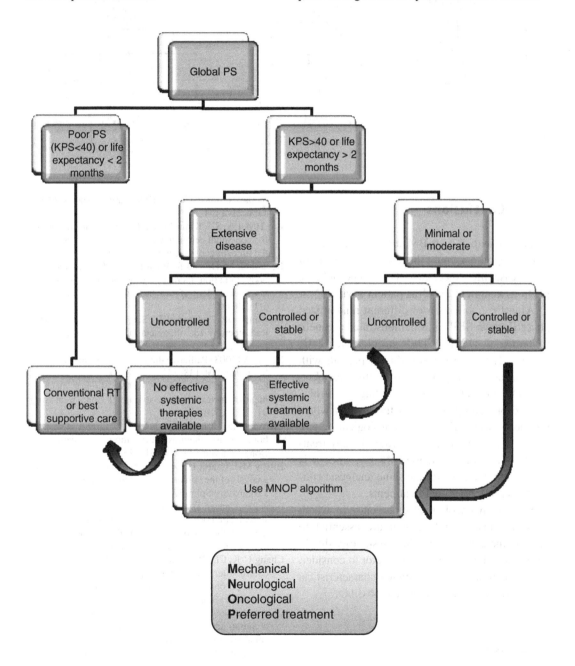

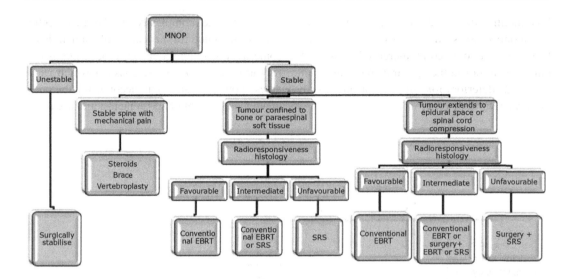

3 Conclusions

Treatment with RT on BM must be individualized taking into account the symptoms, extent of the disease, life expectancy, KPS, comorbidities, previous treatments, and the patient's wishes.

After the publication of different randomized phase II trials, SBRT has demonstrated a benefit in terms of OS and DFS in oligometastatic patients. Therefore, certain NSCLC patients with bone metastases may benefit from this treatment, with a high LC and acceptable antalgic control.

A second group of patients, those with a worse prognosis, worse KPS, and neurological deficit, would benefit from palliative radiotherapy treatment with a single fraction of 8 Gy, since it is more cost effective with the same analgesic control than more fractional treatments.

SCC is an oncological emergency in which early diagnosis and treatment are essential to improve the quality of life. Spinal stability should be assessed, being the primary factor to consider, in conjunction with the patient's characteristics, when offering the best treatment possible.

References

Arnold BN, Thomas DC, Rosen JE et al (2006) Lung cancer in the very young: treatment and survival in the National Cancer Data Base. J Thorac Oncol 11:1121–1131

Bae HM, Lee SH, Kim TM et al (2012) Prognostic factors for non-small cell lung cancer with bone metastasis at the time diagnosis. Lung Cancer 77:572–577

Bedard G, McDonald R, Poon I et al (2016) Stereotactic body radiation therapy for non-spine bone metastases—a review of the literature. Ann Palliat Med 5(1):58–66

Bergsma DP, Salama JK, Singh DP et al (2017) Radiotherapy for oligometastatic lung cancer. Front Oncol 7:210

Bezjak A (2003) Palliative therapy for lung cancer. Semin Surg Oncol 21:138–147

Bickels J, Dadia S, Lidar Z (2009) Surgical management of metastatic bone disease. J Bone Joint Surg 91:1503–1516

Biermann JS, Holt GE, Lewis VO et al (2009) Metastatic bone disease: diagnosis, evaluation, and treatment. J Bone Joint Surg Am 91:1518–1530

Bilsky MH, Laufer I, Fourney DR et al (2010) Reliability analysis of the epidural spinal cord compression scale. J Neurosurg Spine 13:324–328

Canadian Cancer Trials Group (2021) Study comparing stereotactic body radiotherapy vs conventional palliative radiotherapy (CRT) for spinal metastases. https://clinicaltrials.gov/ct2/show/NCT02512965

Chang U-K, Cho W-I, Kim M-S et al (2012) Local tumor control after retreatment of spinal metastasis using stereotactic body radiotherapy; comparison with initial treatment group. Acta Oncol 51:589–595

Chiang A, Zeng L, Zhang L et al (2013) Pain flare is a common adverse event in steroid-naïve patients after spine stereotactic body radiation therapy: a prospective clinical trial. Int J Radiat Oncol Biol Phys 86:638–642

Chow E, Wu J, Hoskin P et al (2002) International consensus on palliative radiotherapy endpoints for future clinical trials in bone metastases. Radiother Oncol 64:275–280

Chow E, Harris K, Fan G et al (2007) Palliative radiotherapy trials for bone metastases: a systematic review. J Clin Oncol 25:1423–1436

Chow E, Zeng L, Salvo N et al (2012a) Update on the systematic review of palliative radiotherapy trials for bone metastases. Clin Oncol (R Coll Radiol) 24:112–124

Chow E, Hoskin P, Mitera G et al (2012b) Update of the international consensus on palliative radiotherapy endpoints for future clinical trials in bone metastases. Int J Radiat Oncol Biol Phys 82(5):1730–1737

Chow R, Hoskin P, Schild S et al (2019) Single vs. multiple fraction palliative radiation therapy for bone metastases: cumulative meta-analysis. Radiother Oncol 141:56–61

ClinicalTrials.gov (2019) Randomized trial comparing conventional radiotherapy with stereotactic radiotherapy in patients with bone metastases, VERTICAL study (VERTICAL)

Cox BW, Spratt DE, Lovelock M et al (2012) International Spine Radiosurgery Consortium consensus guidelines for target volume definition in spinal stereotactic radiosurgery. Int J Radiat Oncol Biol Phys 83:e597–e605

Da Silva G, Bergmann A, Santos Thuler LC (2019) Incidence and risk factors for bone metastasis in non-small cell lung cancer. Asian Pac J Cancer Prev 20(1):45–51

Fairchild A (2014) Palliative radiotherapy for bone metastases from lung cancer: evidence-based medicine? World J Clin Oncol 5(5):845–857

Faruqi S, Tseng C-L, Whyne C et al (2018) Vertebral compression fracture after spine stereotactic body radiation therapy: a review of the pathophysiology and risk factors. Neurosurgery 83:314–322

Fisher CG, Schouten R, Versteeg AL et al (2014) Reliability of the Spinal Instability Neoplastic Score (SINS) among radiation oncologists: an assessment of instability secondary to spinal metastases. Radiat Oncol 9:69

Ganesh V, Chan S, Raman S et al (2017) A review of patterns of practice and clinical guidelines in the palliative radiation treatment of uncomplicated bone metastases Vithusha Ganesh. Radiother Oncol 124:38–44

Guckenberger A, Mantel F, Gerszten P et al (2014) Safety and efficacy of stereotactic body radiotherapy as primary treatment for vertebral metastases: a multi-institutional analysis. Radiat Oncol 9:226

Hall WA, Stapleford LJ, Hadjipanayis CG et al (2011) Stereotactic body radiosurgery for spinal metastatic disease: an evidence-based review. Int J Surg Oncol 2011:979214

Hashmi A, Guckenberger M, Kersh R et al (2016) Re-irradiation stereotactic body radiotherapy for spinal metastases: a multi-institutional outcome analysis. J Neurosurg Spine 25:646–653

Hellman S, Weichselbaum RR (1995) Oligometastases. J Clin Oncol 13:8–10

Huisman M, van den Bosch M, Wijlemans JW et al (2012) Effectiveness of reirradiation for painful bone metastases: a systematic review and meta-analysis. Int J Radiat Oncol Biol Phys 84:8–14

Jacofsky DJ, Haidukewych GJ (2004) Management of pathologic fractures of the proximal femur: state of the art. J Orthop Trauma 18:459–469

Jensen G, Tang C, Hess KR et al (2017) Internal validation of the prognostic index for spine metastasis (PRISM) for stratifying survival in patients treated with spinal stereotactic radiosurgery. J Radiosurg SBRT 5:25–34

Klekamp J, Samii H (1998) Surgical results for spinal metastases. Acta Neurochir 140:957–967

Lawton A, Lee K, Cheville A et al (2019) Assessment and management of patients with metastatic spinal cord compression: a multidisciplinary review. J Clin Oncol 37(1):61–71

Lutz S, Berk L, Chang E et al (2011) Palliative radiotherapy for bone metastases: an ASTRO evidence-based guideline. Int J Radiat Oncol Biol Phys 79:965–976

Lutz S, Balboni T, Jones J et al (2017) Palliative radiation therapy for bone metastases: update of an ASTRO evidence-based guideline. Pract Radiat Oncol 7:4–12

Malviya A, Gerrand C (2012) Evidence for orthopaedic surgery in the treatment of metastatic bone disease of the extremities: a review article. Palliat Med 26:788–796

Maranzano E, Bellavita R, Rossi R et al (2005) Short-course versus split-course radiotherapy in metastatic spinal cord compression: results of a phase III, randomized, multicenter trial. J Clin Oncol 23:3358–3365

Maranzano E, Trippa F, Casale M et al (2009) 8Gy single dose radiotherapy is effective in metastatic spinal cord compression: results of a phase III randomized multicentre Italian trial. Radiother Oncol 93:174–179

Mirels H (1989) Metastatic disease in long bones. A proposed scoring system for diagnosing impending pathologic fractures. Clin Orthop Relat Res 249:256–264

Nguyen Q, Chun S, Chow E et al (2019) Single-fraction stereotactic vs conventional multifraction radiotherapy for pain relief in patients with predominantly nonspine bone metastases. A randomized phase 2 trial. JAMA Oncol 5(6):872–878

Nordlinger B, Guiguet M, Vaillant JC et al (1996) Surgical resection of colorectal carcinoma metastases to the liver. A prognostic scoring system to improve case selection, based on 1568 patients. Association Française de Chirurgie. Cancer 77:1254–1262

Ost P, Jereczek-Fossa BA, As NV et al (2016) Progression-free survival following stereotactic body radiotherapy for oligometastatic prostate cancer treatment-naive recurrence: a multi-institutional analysis. Eur Urol 69:9–12

Palma DA, Olson RA, Harrow S et al (2018) Stereotactic ablative radiation therapy for the comprehensive treatment of oligometastatic tumors (SABR-COMET): results of a randomized trial. Int J Radiat Oncol 102:S3–S4

Pastorino U, Buyse M, Friedel G et al (1997) Long-term results of lung metastasectomy: prognostic analyses based on 5206 cases. J Thorac Cardiovasc Surg 113:37–49

Patchell R, Tibbs P, Regine WF et al (2005) A randomized trial of direct decompressive surgical resection in the treatment of spinal cord compression caused by metastatic cancer. Lancet 366:643–648

Quinn RH, Randall RL, Benevenia J et al (2014) Contemporary management of metastatic bone disease: tips and tools of the trade for general practitioners. Instr Course Lect 63:431

Rades D, Stalpers LJ, Veninga T et al (2005) Evaluation of five radiation schedules and prognosis factors for metastatic spinal cord compression. J Clin Oncol 23:3366–3375

Rades D, Lange M, Veninga T et al (2009) Preliminary results of the SCORE (spinal cord compression recurrence evaluation) study comparing short-course versus long-course radiotherapy for local control of malignant epidural spinal cord compression. Int J Radiat Oncol Biol Phys 73:228–234

Rades D, Cacicedo J, Conde-Moreno A et al (2021) Comparison of 5x 5 Gy and 10x 3 Gy for metastatic spinal cord compression using data from three prospective trials. Radiat Oncol 16:7

Redmond KJ, Sahgal A, Foote M et al (2015) Single versus multiple session stereotactic body radiotherapy for spinal metastasis: the risk-benefit ratio. Future Oncol 11:2405–2415

Rich S, Chow R, Raman S et al (2018) Update of the systematic review of palliative radiation therapy fractionation for bone metastases. Radiother Oncol 126:547–557

Ruggieri P, Mavrogenis AF, Casadei R et al (2010) Protocol of surgical treatment of long bone pathological fractures. Injury 41:1161–1167

Ryu S, Pugh SL, Gerszten PC et al (2014) RTOG 0631 phase 2/3 study of image guided stereotactic radiosurgery for localized (1-3) spine metastases: phase 2 results. Pract Radiat Oncol 4:76–81

Ryu S, Deshmukh S, Timmerman RD et al (2019) Radiosurgery compared to external beam radiotherapy for localized spine metastasis: phase III results of NRG oncology/RTOG 0631. Int J Radiat Oncol Biol Phys 105S:S2

Shagal A, Larson DA, Chang EL (2008) Stereotactic body radiosurgery for spinal metastases: a critical review. Int J Radiat Oncol Biol Phys 71:652–665

Spratt D, Beeler W, Moraes F et al (2017) An integrated multidisciplinary algorithm for the management of spinal metastases: an International Spine Oncology Consortium report. Lancet Oncol 18:e720–e730

Sprave T, Verma V, Förster R et al (2018a) Randomized phase II trial evaluating pain response in patients with spinal metastases following stereotactic body radiotherapy versus three-dimensional conformal radiotherapy. Radiother Oncol 128:274–282

Sprave T, Verma V, Förster R et al (2018b) Quality of life following stereotactic body radiotherapy versus three-dimensional conformal radiotherapy for vertebral metastases: secondary analysis of an exploratory phase II randomized trial. Anticancer Res 38:4961–4968

Steenland E, Leer JW, van Houwelingen H et al (1999) The effect of a single fraction compared to multiple fractions on painful bone metastases: a global analysis of the Dutch Bone Metastasis Study. Radiother Oncol 52:101–109

Sze WM, Shelley MD, Held I et al (2003) Palliation of metastatic bone pain: single fraction versus multifraction radiotherapy - a systematic review of randomised trials. Clin Oncol (R Coll Radiol) 15:345–352

Tao R, Bishop AJ, Brownlee Z et al (2016) Stereotactic body radiation therapy for spinal metastases in the postoperative setting: a secondary analysis of mature phase 1-2 trials. Int J Radiat Oncol Biol Phys 95:1405–1413

Thibault I, Chang EL, Sheehan et al (2015) Response assessment after stereotactic body radiotherapy for spinal metastasis: a report from the SPIne response assessment in Neuro-Oncology (SPINO) group. Lancet Oncol 16:e595–e603

Thureau S, Marchesi V, Vieillard et al (2021) Efficacy of extracranial stereotactic body radiation therapy (SBRT) added to standard treatment in patients with solid tumors (breast, prostate and non-small cell lung cancer) with up to 3 bone-only metastases: study protocol for a randomised phase III trial (STEREO-OS). BMC cancer 21(1):117

Tseng C-L, Eppinga W, Charest-Morin R et al (2017) Spine stereotactic body radiotherapy: indications, outcomes, and points of caution. Glob Spine J 7:179–197

Tseng C-L, Soliman H, Myrehaug S et al (2018) Imaging-based outcomes for 24 Gy in 2 daily fractions for patients with de novo spinal metastases treated with spine stereotactic body radiation therapy (SBRT). Int J Radiat Oncol Biol Phys 102:499–507

Wang XS, Rhines LD, Shiu AS et al (2012) Stereotactic body radiation therapy for management of spinal metastases in patients without spinal cord compression: a phase 1-2 trial. Lancet Oncol 13:395–402

Willeumier J, van der Linden Y, Sander Dijkstra P et al (2016) Lack of clinical evidence for postoperative radiotherapy after surgical fixation of impending or actual pathologic fractures in the long bones in patients with cancer; a systematic review. Radiother Oncol 121:138–142

Wolanczyk MJ, Fakhrian K, Adamietz IA (2016) Radiotherapy, bisphosphonates and surgical stabilization of complete or impending pathologic fractures in patients with metastatic bone disease. J Cancer 7:121–124

Wu JS, Wong R, Johnston M, Bezjak A et al (2003) Meta-analysis of dose-fractionation radiotherapy trials for the palliation of painful bone metastases. Int J Radiat Oncol Biol Phys 55:594–605

Wu JS, Wong RK, Lloyd NS et al (2004) Supportive Care Guidelines Group of Cancer Care Ontario. Radiotherapy fractionation for the palliation of uncomplicated painful bone metastases - an evidence-based practice guideline. BMC Cancer 4:71

Zeng K, Tseng C, Soliman H et al (2019) Stereotactic body radiotherapy (SBRT) for oligometastatic spine metastases: an overview. Front Oncol 9:337

Radiation Therapy for Metastatic Lung Cancer: Liver Metastasis

Fiori Alite and Anand Mahadevan

Contents

1. Introduction 795
2. Incidence 796
3. Non-small Cell Lung Cancer (NSCLC) 797
4. Small Cell Lung Cancer (SCLC) 797
5. Diagnosis 798
6. Management 798
7. Local Therapy in Oligometastatic Lung Cancer 800
8. Liver-Directed Therapies 800
9. Radiation Therapy for Liver Metastasis ... 801

References 805

Abstract

Metastatic cancer is most common cause of mortality in Lung cancer. Hematogenous metastasis of lung cancer is wide spread often involving multiple sites including the brain, bone and adrenals. While colorectal cancer is the most common origin of liver metastasis, liver metastasis from lung cancer is not uncommon. Most patients with liver metastasis are not suitable for liver directed therapy in the definitive or palliative setting. When not suitable for surgical resection, Radiation therapy can offer palliation and ablative radiation can achieve good local control and even be curative in the setting of oligometastasis.

1 Introduction

Metastatic spread of cancer to distant organs is the reason for most cancer deaths (Chen et al. 2009). Mechanistic insights from the classical seed and soil and anatomical/mechanical hypotheses with current knowledge of tumor-stromal interactions (Langley and Fidler 2011) to sequencing of tumor genomes from single cells have enabled the understanding of clonal evolution of cells in the primary tumor and their fate in multiple metastases (Kakiuchi et al. 2003). The

F. Alite · A. Mahadevan (✉)
Radiation Oncology, Geisinger Cancer Institute—Geisinger Health, Geisinger Commonwealth School of Medicine, Danville, PA, USA
e-mail: falite@geisinger.edu; amahadevan@geisinger.edu

epidemiology of cancer metastasis is not clear. Authoritative World Health Organization handbooks on pathology and genetics of tumors and registries using the clinical-anatomical TNM classification report the presence of metastasis at diagnosis without data on location, or on the development of metastasis through the course of the disease and at death. Probably, the largest clinical study originating from MD Anderson Cancer Center, covering 4399 patients from the mid-1990s, somewhat addresses this issue. Other sources of data have been autopsy series, but the validity of this is unclear; autopsies have become very infrequent, and a large recent study reported data from autopsies performed between 1914 and 1943 (Disibio and French 2008). Most patients who die of lung cancer do so from distant metastasis. Lung cancer frequently metastasizes to bone, brain, lung, and liver, causing a shorter survival (Hess et al. 2006).

Metastatic lesions to the liver from other primary sites are not uncommon and can be a significant burden for patients, caregivers, and health-care providers. Liver metastases can cause significant morbidity with pain and anorexia, adversely affecting health-related quality of life. In addition, more extensive liver disease can cause hepatic dysfunction and worsening performance status limiting systemic therapy and increasing mortality (Costi et al. 2014). The most common metastatic lesion in the liver is from colorectal adenocarcinoma where management with surgical hepatic metastasectomy has a long track record with 5-year survival rates of 50–60% and up to 20% achieving long-term disease-free survival in carefully selected patients (Smith and D'Angelica 2015). However, only 10–20% of liver metastases in general are amenable to resection, even less so in metastasis from lung cancer, leaving systemic therapy as the traditional recourse for the majority of patients. For unresectable tumors, despite advances in combination chemotherapy and targeted agents resulting in a doubling of median survival from approximately 10 to 20 months, it is not without significant toxicity (Bekaii-Saab and Wu 2014). Chemotherapy has also been used to downstage lesions, potentially allowing patients to become eligible for liver-directed therapies (Adam et al. 2004). Since most patients with liver metastases remain ineligible for surgery, alternative liver-directed therapies, such as stereotactic body radiotherapy (SBRT), radiofrequency ablation, microwave ablation, radiolabeled microspheres, transarterial chemoembolization, cryoablation, and alcohol injection, have shown some benefit.

2 Incidence

In the Swedish Family-Cancer Database including >14.7 million individuals, a total of 21,169 patients with lung cancer who were diagnosed between 2002 and 2010 were identified, after exclusion of 2874 cases with carcinoids or unspecified histology (Riihimäki et al. 2014). Most patients had adenocarcinoma (43%). About 53% of patients were male, and 80% were diagnosed at age 60 or older (median 70 years for men, 67 years for women). The proportion of patients with metastases also varied between histological subtypes: 62% in adenocarcinoma, 41% in SCC, 61% in SCLC, 56% in LCLC, and 59% in other histology. The most frequently mentioned metastatic sites were nervous system (39% of 9830 patients), bone (34%), liver (20%), respiratory system (18%), and adrenal gland (8%). Patients with adenocarcinoma often had bone (39%) or respiratory system metastases (22%), whereas patients with SCLC had more nervous system (47%) and liver metastases (35%). Overall, 20% of lung cancer patients presented with liver metastasis (equally in men and women of all age groups). However, there was a significantly higher incidence of liver metastasis in patients with SCLC vs. NSCLC (35% vs. 17%; $p < 0.001$). Similarly, another large Japanese study found liver metastasis form

SCLC at twice the rate for NSCLC. They also reported a statistically significant conditional probability of other visceral, bone, and brain metastasis in the presence of liver metastasis (Oikawa et al. 2012).

3 Non-small Cell Lung Cancer (NSCLC)

Approximately 30–40% of NSCLC patients present with metastatic disease at the time of diagnosis. NSCLC recurrence, even after complete resection, is still frequently observed in clinical settings. Many studies have identified some clinicopathological factors, like size and vascular involvement, that could predict the postoperative prognosis of patients with NSCLC (Shimizu et al. 2020).

Liver metastasis is an unfavorable prognostic factor in patients with NSCLC (Tamura et al. 2015). Liver metastatic lesions are rarely associated with severe symptoms, although the majority of NSCLC patients had multiple nodules morphologically. The majority of NSCLC patients with liver metastasis do not respond well or tolerate chemotherapy. NSCLC may cause biliary tract obstruction by metastasizing to the lymph nodes in the porta hepatis or the hepatic parenchyma. The administration of chemotherapy may be complicated by liver metastasis related to the activation or metabolism of several cytotoxic agents commonly used in the treatment of NSCLC. There have been several patients with liver metastases who were unable to continue chemotherapy due to liver dysfunction and associated poor performance status.

4 Small Cell Lung Cancer (SCLC)

Distant metastases upon presentation of small cell lung cancer (SCLC) are a more frequent clinical problem. The four most common sites of metastasis in SCLC at the time of diagnosis appear to be the liver, bone, brain, and lung, with involvement of these sites identified in SCLC patients with newly diagnosed metastatic disease.

In a large series from Japan, while 20% of patients with SCLC presented with liver metastasis, only a third of them had isolated liver metastasis (Tamura et al. 2015). A statistically significant difference was observed in the 1-year survival between the patients with sole liver metastasis and those without metastasis ($p = 0.0009$). According to logistic regression analysis, liver metastasis, brain metastasis, and pleural and/or pericardial fluid are correlated with a poor PS of 2–3. The logistic regression analysis also demonstrated that liver and brain metastases are risk factors of unfavorable response to chemotherapy (reported as stable disease and progressive disease). In a multivariate analysis using Cox proportional hazards model, presence of liver metastasis ($p = 0.0001$), bone metastasis ($p = 0.0401$), brain metastasis ($p = 0.0177$), and pleural and/or pericardial fluids ($p = 0.0020$) were unfavorable prognostic factors.

Investigating the metastatic site-specific time sequence, a Hungarian study of 1009 SCLC patients found that the onset of bone ($p < 0.001$), brain ($p < 0.001$), and pericardial ($p = 0.02$) metastases tended to be late, whereas the development of adrenal gland ($p = 0.005$) and liver ($p < 0.001$) metastases was usually an early event during tumor progression (Megyesfalvi et al. 2021). To investigate whether there are metastasis pairs where one of the metastases usually tends to appear sooner than the other one given that they both appear together in a single patient, they evaluated the order preference of metastatic sites. They found that liver metastases usually precede bone (78% of the cases) and brain (82% of the cases) metastases. Because of its anatomical localization and vascular features, the liver is the most common site of distant metastasis in solid tumors (Gomez et al. 2019). It is not surprising, therefore, that the occurrence of liver metastases tended to be an early event during SCLC progression.

Clinically, treatment for extensive disease (ED)-SCLC consists of systemic chemotherapy and radiotherapy for symptomatic metastatic sites. It is generally accepted that the life expectancy of SCLC patients depends on the extent of disease and the response to chemotherapy. Performance status (PS), gender, disease extent, number of metastatic sites, and response to chemotherapy are poor prognostic factors in ED-SCLC patients, regardless of the location of the metastatic site (Ren et al. 2016).

5 Diagnosis

Several imaging modalities can be used to detect liver metastases from lung cancer. On ultrasound, metastases appear as round or oval hypoechoic lesions; central areas of necrosis may appear hypo- or anechoic. Metastases from mucinous adenocarcinomas and calcifying metastases appear hyperechoic. Unenhanced CT is rarely necessary for the evaluation of liver metastases except for hemorrhagic or calcifying metastases. Metastases from neuroendocrine tumors appear hyperdense on unenhanced CT. On arterial phase helical CT, metastases appear as well-defined or ill-defined hypodense lesions and may show minimal peripheral rim enhancement. Portal venous-phase CT is important in screening for metastases. On portal venous-phase images, metastases appear hypodense to adjacent enhancing liver. Some lesions may show the peripheral washout sign. This refers to peripheral enhancement during the arterial and portal venous phases, which disappears in the delayed phase. On CT arterioportography, metastases appear hypodense. Multidetector CT is superior to conventional CT, and its sensitivity reaches that of CT arterioportography in evaluating liver metastases. On MRI, metastases appear hypointense on T1-weighted images and hyperintense on T2-weighted images, with enhancement patterns similar to those observed with CT. MRI with liver-specific contrast agents was found to be more sensitive than CT in detecting liver metastases (Sahani and Kalva 2004). In a meta-analysis comparing US, CT, MRI, and PET for the detection of liver metastases, Kinkel et al. found that, in studies with a specificity higher than 85%, the mean weighted sensitivity was 55% (95% confidence interval [CI], 41–68) for US, 72% (95% CI, 63–80) for CT, 76% (95% CI, 57–91) for MRI, and 90% (95% CI, 80–97) for FDG PET (Kinkel et al. 2002, Fig. 1).

6 Management

In the past few decades, systemic treatment for advanced lung cancer has remained cytotoxic agents with platinum-based regimens. Activities of daily living (ADL) may be low in a number of patients with liver metastases and may also deteriorate in patients with liver metastases due to pain and liver dysfunction, and the discontinuation of chemotherapy due to the deterioration of ADL in these patients has a clear correlation with poor survival. The administration of chemotherapy may be complicated by metastasis of the liver in the activation or metabolism of several cytotoxic drugs commonly used in the treatment of lung cancer. Many SCLC patients present with multiple nodules, which may cause biliary tract obstruction by metastasizing to lymph nodes in the porta hepatis or hepatic parenchyma.

ECOG1594 was the first trial comparing four different chemotherapy regimens for advanced non-small cell lung cancer (NSCLC) head-to-head (Schiller et al. 2002). All chemotherapy regimens showed almost the same efficacy with objective response rate (ORR) of 19% and 7.9-month median overall survival (OS). The platinum-based doublet chemotherapy approach seemed to reach the plateau in clinical outcomes since then. In 2005, the first-ever trial combining the small molecular targeted agent known as bevacizumab, an anti-vascular endothelial growth factor (VEGF) monoclonal antibody, with doublet chemotherapy, demonstrated superiority of overall survival with this treatment modality in advanced nonsquamous non-small cell lung can-

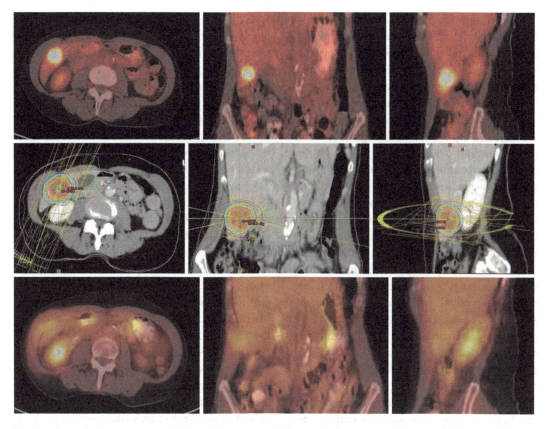

Fig. 1 Metastatic lung cancer with solitary liver metastasis. Top panel: Pretreatment PET scan. Middle panel: SBRT treatment plan 4500 cGy in 3 fractions. Bottom panel: Complete metabolic response 4 months posttreatment

cer patients without brain metastasis (Sandler et al. 2006).

Epidermal growth factor receptor, a well-known biomarker for targeted therapy at present, was first brought up with potential clinical responsiveness to tyrosine kinase inhibitor gefitinib in 2004 (Lee et al. 2013). Since then, the era of targeted therapy was uncovered, and multiple trials demonstrated the efficacy of tyrosine kinase inhibitor (TKI) in oncogene-driven non-small cell lung cancer patients, including tumors with *ALK* rearrangement (Gainor et al. 2013). Up to 69% of patients with advanced NSCLC could harbor actionable driver mutations. In these trials, significantly improved progression-free survival (PFS) was observed compared to traditional chemotherapy; however, no overall survival benefit was identified which may be partly due to high crossover rate after disease progression. Moreover, resistance to tyrosine kinase inhibitors seems inevitable and sequential treatments are warranted (Yu et al. 2013). Since 2013, the advent of immunotherapy has made significant scientific breakthroughs. Efficacy of immunotherapy for those without targetable oncogene mutation was proven in second-line treatment and has evolved to integration in first-line treatment (Carbone et al. 2017). Through long-term follow-up, immunotherapy had also shown itself the greatest potential of long-term clinical benefit. Indeed, similar to targeted therapy, patients may eventually develop resistance to immunotherapy (Carbone et al. 2017), and some may even suffer hyperprogression after immunotherapy (Champiat et al. 2017). The desire of novel agents that showed better efficacy, prolonged survival benefit, and overcame resistance promoted the development of new potential targets and corresponding drugs with numerous emerging agents and their superior clinical responsiveness.

Standard-of-care first-line treatment for extensive-stage small cell lung cancer remains platinum chemotherapy (carboplatin or cisplatin) with etoposide (Sun et al. 2019). Despite response rates of 60–65%, limited progress has been made in more than two decades; outcomes remain poor, with a median overall survival of approximately 10 months. Despite small cell lung cancer having a high mutation rate, which suggests that these tumors may be immunogenic and could respond to immune checkpoint inhibitors, clinical outcomes with immunotherapy have not been as robust as NSCLC. Adding immunotherapy to chemotherapy may enhance antitumor immunity and improve outcomes beyond those achieved with our current therapeutic armamentarium. Clinical activity of immunotherapies has been observed in patients with refractory or metastatic small cell lung cancer; however, a phase II single-group study of maintenance pembrolizumab and a phase III study of ipilimumab plus chemotherapy showed no improved efficacy in the first-line treatment of extensive-stage small cell lung cancer. The addition of atezolizumab to chemotherapy in the first-line treatment of extensive-stage small cell lung cancer resulted in significantly longer overall survival and progression-free survival than chemotherapy alone (Horn et al. 2018).

7 Local Therapy in Oligometastatic Lung Cancer

In a systematic review of the literature, data were obtained on 757 NSCLC patients with 1–5 synchronous or metachronous metastases treated with surgical metastasectomy, stereotactic radiotherapy/radiosurgery, or radical external beam radiotherapy, and curative treatment of the primary lung cancer, from hospitals worldwide (Ashworth et al. 2014). Factors predictive of overall survival (OS) and progression-free survival were evaluated using Cox regression. Risk groups were defined using recursive partitioning analysis (RPA). Analyses were conducted on training and validating sets (two-thirds and one-third of patients, respectively). Median OS was 26 months, 1-year OS 70.2%, and 5-year OS 29.4%. Surgery was the most commonly used treatment for the primary tumor (635 patients [83.9%]) and metastases (339 patients [62.3%]). Factors predictive of OS were synchronous versus metachronous metastases ($p < 0.001$), N-stage ($p < 0.002$), and adenocarcinoma histology ($p < 0.036$); the model remained predictive in the validation set (c-statistic 0.682). In RPA, three risk groups were identified: low-risk, metachronous metastases (5-year OS, 47.8%); intermediate-risk, synchronous metastases and N0 disease (5-year OS, 36.2%); and high-risk, synchronous metastases and N1/N2 disease (5-year OS, 13.8%).

In a multicenter, randomized, phase II trial that enrolled patients with stage IV NSCLC, three or fewer metastases, and no progression at 3 or more months after frontline systemic therapy (Gomez et al. 2019), patients were randomly assigned (1:1) to maintenance therapy or observation (MT/O) or to LCT to all active disease sites. The primary end point was PFS; secondary endpoints were OS, toxicity, and appearance of new lesions. All analyses were two sided, and p values less than 0.10 were deemed significant. With a median follow-up time of 38.8 months (range 28.3–61.4 months), the PFS benefit was durable (median 14.2 months [95% CI, 7.4–23.1 months] with LCT vs. 4.4 months [95% CI, 2.2–8.3 months] with MT/O; $p = 0.022$). The study also found an OS benefit in the LCT arm (median 41.2 months [95% CI, 18.9 months to not reached] with LCT vs. 17.0 months [95% CI, 10.1–39.8 months] with MT/O; $p = 0.017$). No additional grade 3 or greater toxicities were observed. Survival after progression was longer in the LCT group (37.6 months with LCT vs. 9.4 months with MT/O; $p = 0.034$). Of the 20 patients who experienced progression in the MT/O arm, 9 received LCT to all lesions after progression, and the median OS was 17 months (95% CI, 7.8 months to not reached).

8 Liver-Directed Therapies

In patients with limited metastatic disease and good performance status and who are responding or not tolerating systemic therapy, liver-directed therapies may be appropriate.

Since most patients with liver metastases remain ineligible for surgery, alternative liver-directed therapies, such as stereotactic body radiotherapy (SBRT), radiofrequency ablation, microwave ablation, radiolabeled microspheres, transarterial chemoembolization, cryoablation, and alcohol injection, have shown some benefit.

9 Radiation Therapy for Liver Metastasis

Radiation therapy is an established palliative modality, and for patients experiencing painful liver metastasis, even a single fraction of external beam radiotherapy directed to the whole liver can achieve meaningful symptomatic relief and improved quality of life in a majority of patients (Soliman et al. 2013). However, for eradicating metastatic disease, conventional radiation therapy techniques treating large areas of the liver parenchyma are largely ineffective owing to the low tolerance of the liver to high-dose irradiation due to the risk of radiation-induced liver disease (RILD) (Dawson et al. 2002). With the emergence of more sophisticated treatment planning software and methods of image guidance in the past two decades, more tightly focused treatment fields are now possible, allowing for delivery of higher more compact doses in fewer fractions to discrete individual liver lesions, while sparing the uninvolved liver. With this combination of spatial precision and the administration of tumoricidal radiation doses with SBRT, it is feasible to achieve high rates of tumor control while minimizing the irradiation of surrounding healthy tissue, thereby reducing the risk of RILD (Dawson and Balter 2004). Multiple retrospective and prospective series have explored the feasibility, efficacy, and safety of SBRT for liver metastasis. The first clinical series of SBRT in extracranial tumors was published over 20 years ago by the investigators from Karolinska Institute in Sweden, who reported on the first 42 lesions of the lung, liver, and retroperitoneal space in 31 patients treated with "stereotactic high-dose fraction radiation therapy" (Blomgren et al. 1995). With a wide range of doses and fractionations, ranging from 1 to 4 fractions, the local control rate was 80%, and 50% of the tumors either decreased in size or disappeared. These data fueled further interest in this SBRT approach, and multiple trials have subsequently evaluated the use of SBRT for liver tumors.

Early studies of liver SBRT investigated single-fraction regimens, extrapolating from the single-fraction approach used in radiosurgery for the brain. Investigators from the University of Heidelberg were the first to report prospective outcomes of single-fraction SBRT for liver metastases (Herfarth et al. 2001). A total of 37 patients, with 55 liver metastases, were treated with single-fraction SBRT on a dose escalation scheme starting at 14 Gy and increasing to 26 Gy. The 18-month local control rate was 67% for all patients, but it was significantly higher for patients treated at 22–26 Gy vs. those treated at 14–20 Gy (81% vs. 0%). The investigators did present the caveat that this result may have been due to a learning phase, as investigators had noted that local control also improved in patients who were enrolled later in the study, as more appropriate margin expansions were applied. No significant toxicity was reported. Stanford University Medical Center performed a phase I single-fraction dose escalation study for primary and metastatic liver tumors, which included 19 of 26 patients with hepatic metastases (Goodman et al. 2010). The single-fraction radiation dose was escalated from 18 to 30 Gy in 4 Gy increments. At a median follow-up of 17 months, there were no dose-limiting toxicities. There was one acute grade 2 (duodenal ulcer 1 month after treatment) and two late grade 2 gastrointestinal toxicities, and both duodenal ulcers manifested by gastrointestinal bleeding, at 8 and 25 months posttreatment. Of note, 20 months after treatment, the second patient received an additional 56 Gy using intensity-modulated radiotherapy with conventional fractionation to the porta hepatitis region for a recurrence in the treated (18 Gy) lesion and developed an ulcer, 3 months after completion of the additional radiotherapy. All three of the duodenal ulcers were among patients treated to sites in the porta hepatis. The 1-year cumulative incidence of local control for all patients was 77%. For patients with liver metastases, the 1-year and 2-year overall survival rates were 62% and 49%, respectively. Although the results of single-fraction liver SBRT appeared promising, the potential toxicity of ultrahigh-dose radiotherapy in the abdomen led many groups to investigate hypofractionated regimens. Hoyer et al. reported outcomes of 44 hepatic metastases treated with SBRT 45 Gy in 3 fractions, with a 2-year actuarial local control rate of 79%. One- and 2-year overall survival rates were 67% and 38%, respectively (Hoyer et al. 2006). Treatment-related toxicity included one patient who died of hepatic failure, one patient with colonic perforation requiring surgical management, and two patients with duodenal ulceration treated conservatively. Of note, margins to planning target volumes (PTV) were used for respiratory motion, and tracking or gating to manage respiratory motion was not used in this study which could account for the high peri-hepatic gastrointestinal toxicity. A phase I/II study of 3-fraction SBRT in patients with primary and metastatic liver lesions was conducted in the Netherlands. A total of 34 liver metastases were treated to 37.5 Gy in 3 fractions with a 2-year local control rate of 86%. One- and 2-year overall survival rates were 85% and 62%, respectively.

One of the largest series of patients treated in the real world is from the RSSearch Registry (Mahadevan et al. 2018). The study included 427 patients with 568 liver metastases from 25 academic and community-based centers. Median age was 67 years (31–91 years). Colorectal adenocarcinoma (CRC) was the most common primary cancer. Seventy-three percent of patients received prior chemotherapy. Median tumor volume was 40 cc (1.6–877 cc), and median SBRT dose was 45 Gy (12–60 Gy) delivered in a median of 3 fractions (Chen et al. 2009; Langley and Fidler 2011; Kakiuchi et al. 2003; Disibio and French 2008; Hess et al. 2006). At a median follow-up of 14 months (1–91 months) the median overall survival (OS) was 22 months. Median OS was greater for patients with CRC (27 months), breast (21 months), and gynecological (25 months) metastases compared to lung (10 months), other gastrointestinal (GI) (18 months), and pancreatic (6 months) primaries ($p < 0.0001$). Smaller tumor volumes (<40 cc) correlated with improved OS (25 vs. 15 months, $p = 0.0014$). BED10 $\geq$100 Gy was also associated with improved OS (27 vs. 15 months, $p < 0.0001$). Local control (LC) was evaluable in 430 liver metastases from 324 patients. Two-year LC rates were better for BED10 $\geq$100 Gy (77.2% vs. 59.6%), and the median LC was better for tumors <40 cc (52 vs. 39 months). There was no difference in LC based on the histology of the primary tumor.

A summary of select prospective trials using SBRT for liver metastases is presented in Table 1 and is described in more detail. To date, there are no published phase III data. The studies, as in the RSSearch Registry real-world database study, vary in dose heterogeneity, primary histology, tumor volumes, total radiation dose, and dose per fraction.

Investigators at the University of Colorado performed a prospective phase I/II trial of 3-fraction SBRT for patients with three or fewer liver metastases, measuring less than 6 cm. In the phase I portion of the trial, which included 18 patients, the dose of SBRT was escalated from 36 to 60 Gy in 3 fractions, and no dose-limiting toxicity was observed. In the subsequent report of the combined phase I/II multi-institutional results, 47 patients were treated to 63 liver metastases at 7 participating institutions (Rusthoven et al. 2009). Thirty-eight patients received the phase II dose of 60 Gy in 3 fractions. With a median follow-up of 16 months, the 1- and 2-year actuarial in-field local control rates were 95% and 92%, respectively. Among lesions <3 cm, the 2-year actuarial local control rate was 100%. The 2-year overall survival rate was 30%, and only one patient experienced grade 3 or higher toxicity (2%). A phase I study of 6-fraction SBRT for liver metastases was performed at Princess Margaret Hospital (Lee et al. 2009). The tumor dose was determined by the effective liver volume (V_{eff}) irradiated concept and the risk of RILD. V_{eff} is defined as the normal liver volume minus all gross tumor volumes, which if irradiated uniformly to the treated dose would be associated with the same risk of toxicity as the nonuniform

Table 1 Outcomes in published literature for SBRT for liver metastasis

Study	Number of lesions	Number of patients	Primary	Dose/fractionation	Toxicity	Median follow-up (months)	Local control	Survival
Blomgren et al. (1995)	Variable	31	Mixed	8–66 Gy/1–4	2 hemorrhagic gastritis	1.5–3.8	80%	NR
Herfarth et al. (2001)	1–3	37	NR	14–26 Gy/1	NR	Mean 14.9	18 months: 67%	1 year: 76% 2 years: 55%
Hoyer et al. (2006)	1–6 (<6 cm)	44	Mixed majority CRC	45 Gy/3	1 liver failure 2 severe late GI	52	2 years: 86%	1 year: 67% 2 years: 38%
Méndez Romero et al. (2006)	1–3 (<7 cm)	25	Mixed majority CRC	37.5 Gy/3	4 acute grade ≥3 1 late grade 3	12.9	2 years: 86%	1 year: 85% 2 years: 62%
Rusthoven et al. (2009)	1–3 (<6 cm)	47	Mixed majority CRC	60 Gy/3	<2% late grade ≥3	16	2 years: 92% <3 cm: 100%	Median 17.6
Lee et al. (2009)	Variable	68	Mixed majority CRC	28–60 Gy/3	8 acute grade 3 1 grade 4	10.8	1 year: 71%	18 months: 47%
Ambrosino et al. (2009)	1–3 (<6 cm)	27	Mixed majority CRC	25–60 Gy/3	NR	13	74%	NR
Goodman et al. (2010)	1–5 (<5 cm)	26	Mixed majority CRC	18–30 Gy/1	4 late grade 2	17.3	1 year: 77%	1 year: 62% 2 years: 49%
Rule et al. (2011)	1–5	27	Mixed majority CRC	30 Gy/3 50–60 Gy/5	No ≥grade 2	20	30 Gy: 56% 50 Gy: 89% 60 Gy: 100%	30 Gy: 56% 2 years 50 Gy: 67% 2 years 60 Gy: 50% 2 years
Scorsetti et al. (2013)	1–3 (<6 cm)	61	Mixed majority CRC	52.5–75/3	No ≥grade 3	24	91%	1 year: 80% 2 years: 70%
Mahadevan et al. (2018)	Variable	427	Mixed majority CRC	45 (12–60)/3 (1–5)	NR	14 (1–91)	Median: 52 months 1 year: 84% 2 years: 72%	Median: 22 months 1 year: 74% 2 years: 49%

dose distribution delivered. Individualized radiation doses were based on normal tissue complication probability (NTCP)-calculated risk of RILD at three risk levels (5%, 10%, and 20%). The median SBRT dose was 41.8 Gy in 6 fractions over 2 weeks. Among 68 patients, there were only two grade 3 liver enzyme changes, but no RILD or other grade 3 or higher toxicity. With a median follow-up of 10.8 months, the 1-year local control rate was 71%, and the 18-month overall survival rate was 47% (Lee et al. 2009). The authors commented in their discussion that the use of V_{eff} might have led to an overestimation of toxicity risk and thus led to overly conservative prescription doses, and they cautioned against an overreliance on models that convert dose constraints applicable to conventionally fractionated radiotherapy to the SBRT setting. A prospective study from Italy evaluated 27 patients with liver metastases treated with 25–60 Gy (median 36 Gy) delivered in 3 fractions (Ambrosino et al. 2009). Mean tumor volume was 35.9 mL. At a median follow-up of 13 months, crude local control rate was 74%. Mild-to-moderate transient hepatic dysfunction was observed in nine patients, pleural effusions in two, and partial portal vein thrombosis, pulmonary embolism, and upper gastrointestinal tract bleeding in one patient each. The University of Texas Southwestern reported results from their phase I SBRT dose escalation trial, with three dose groups, 30 Gy/3 fractions, 50 Gy/5 fractions, and 60 Gy/5 fractions (Rule et al. 2011). At 2 years, local control rates were 56%, 89%, and 100%. Two-year overall survival rates were 56%, 67%, and 50%, accordingly. Further, there appeared to be a significant dose-response relationship between 30 and 60 Gy arms ($p = 0.009$). There was no grade 4–5 toxicity, and one grade 3 asymptomatic transaminitis occurred in the 50 Gy cohort.

More recently, the group from Milan reported findings from a phase II trial including 61 patients with 76 liver metastases treated to 25 Gy in 3 fractions (Scorsetti et al. 2013). At a median follow-up of 12 months, the overall local control rate was 95%. One- and 2-year overall survival rates were 80% and 70%, respectively. There was no reported RILD; one patient experienced late grade 3 chest wall pain.

The Radiation Therapy Oncology Group (RTOG) has conducted a phase I trial of hypofractionated RT for hepatic metastases (RTOG 0438) (Dawson et al. 2019). A total of 26 patients were enrolled, and 4 dose levels were achieved: 35–50 Gy in 5 Gy increments delivered in 10 fractions. There were no dose-limiting toxicities reported. Four patients (two patients at 45 Gy and two patients at 50 Gy) developed grade 3 toxicity. No other late toxicities were observed with a potential median follow-up of 66.1 months.

Several studies have evaluated potential prognostic factors for local control with SBRT for liver metastases. Smaller tumors and those receiving a higher dose have been associated with better local control (Rusthoven et al. 2009). A pooled analysis of prognostic factors following SBRT for liver metastases from colorectal cancer demonstrated that total dose of radiation, dose per fraction, and biologically effective dose were significantly associated with local control (Chang et al. 2011). Local control rate exceeding 90% was achieved when doses of 46–52 Gy in 3 fractions were delivered, and the authors concluded that doses of 48 Gy or higher in 3 fractions should be offered if feasible. Interestingly, there have been several studies indicating that histology may affect outcomes with colorectal metastases having worse local control than metastatic lesions from other primary sites; thus, the higher dose of 48 Gy may be necessary in these tumors, while lower doses may be sufficient for non-colorectal histologies (Klement et al. 2017).

One unique feature of treating liver tumors with radiation is the need to account for the respiratory motion of the liver and the tumor within it. A potential advantage of the capability to track tumor motion leads to a reduced margin (typically 3–5 mm) in comparison with systems that use abdominal compression, breath-hold techniques, or respiratory gating, where the tumor position is generated from different phases of respiration and typically includes a 5–10 mm margin to compensate for tumor motion with an addition small margin for setup uncertainty. This reduction in margin may spare adjacent normal liver from receiving high doses of radiation, potentially resulting in lower toxicities. The decreased volume of liver receiving 15 Gy (V_{15}) and reduced mean liver doses can be achieved with type real-time respiratory motion management, thereby decreasing the likelihood of RILD and allowing higher dose to be delivered for larger tumors. In principle, SBRT treatments are designed to deliver maximum prescribed dose to the tumor with a rapid falloff of dose to the surrounding normal tissue. There is scarcity of literature on the comparative clinical outcomes and toxicity of various SBRT techniques (Colvill et al. 2016). Furthermore, future studies need to be done to assess the effects of SBRT on long-term outcomes on tumors located near the porta hepatis.

The overall data suggest that patient selection is critical in identifying the subset of metastatic NSCLC patients who are most likely to benefit from ablative treatments and experience long-term survival. However, in the absence of appropriately matched and randomized controls, one cannot discern whether the prolonged survivals in this highly selected population are simply a reflection of the natural history of young, fit patients with minimal, indolent metastatic disease, or rather a result of the complete eradication and "cure" of truly oligometastatic cancer. Ultimately, randomized controlled trials are required to assess whether an oligometastatic state exists in NSCLC. Results from several ongoing phase III trials assessing the efficacy of local consolidative therapy for oligometastatic disease and particularly in NSCLC patients after induction chemotherapy, in NRG LU002 (clinicaltrials.gov-NCT 03137771), are awaited and expected to help answer these important clinical questions.

References

Adam R, Delvart V, Pascal G et al (2004) Rescue surgery for unresectable colorectal liver metastases downstaged by chemotherapy: a model to predict long-term survival. Ann Surg 240(4):644–657; discussion 657–658

Ambrosino G, Polistina F, Costantin G et al (2009) Image-guided robotic stereotactic radiosurgery for unresectable liver metastases: preliminary results. Anticancer Res 29(8):3381–3384

Ashworth AB, Senan S, Palma DA et al (2014) An individual patient data meta-analysis of outcomes and prognostic factors after treatment of oligometastatic non-small-cell lung cancer. Clin Lung Cancer 15(5):346–355. https://doi.org/10.1016/j.cllc.2014.04.003

Bekaii-Saab T, Wu C (2014) Seeing the forest through the trees: a systematic review of the safety and efficacy of combination chemotherapies used in the treatment of metastatic colorectal cancer. Crit Rev Oncol Hematol 91(1):9–34. https://doi.org/10.1016/j.critrevonc.2014.01.001

Blomgren H, Lax I, Näslund I, Svanström R (1995) Stereotactic high dose fraction radiation therapy of extracranial tumors using an accelerator. Clinical experience of the first thirty-one patients. Acta Oncol (Stockholm, Sweden) 34(6):861–870

Carbone DP, Reck M, Paz-Ares L et al (2017) First-line nivolumab in stage IV or recurrent non-small-cell lung cancer. N Engl J Med 376(25):2415–2426. https://doi.org/10.1056/NEJMoa1613493

Champiat S, Dercle L, Ammari S et al (2017) Hyperprogressive disease is a new pattern of progression in cancer patients treated by anti-PD-1/PD-L1. Clin Cancer Res 23(8):1920–1928. https://doi.org/10.1158/1078-0432.CCR-16-1741

Chang DT, Swaminath A, Kozak M et al (2011) Stereotactic body radiotherapy for colorectal liver metastases: a pooled analysis. Cancer 117(17):4060–4069. https://doi.org/10.1002/cncr.25997

Chen LL, Blumm N, Christakis NA, Barabási AL, Deisboeck TS (2009) Cancer metastasis networks and the prediction of progression patterns. Br J Cancer 101(5):749–758. https://doi.org/10.1038/sj.bjc.6605214

Colvill E, Booth J, Nill S et al (2016) A dosimetric comparison of real-time adaptive and non-adaptive radiotherapy: a multi-institutional study encompassing robotic, gimbaled, multileaf collimator and couch tracking. Radiother Oncol 119(1):159–165. https://doi.org/10.1016/j.radonc.2016.03.006

Costi R, Leonardi F, Zanoni D, Violi V, Roncoroni L (2014) Palliative care and end-stage colorectal cancer management: the surgeon meets the oncologist. World J Gastroenterol 20(24):7602–7621. https://doi.org/10.3748/wjg.v20.i24.7602

Dawson LA, Balter JM (2004) Interventions to reduce organ motion effects in radiation delivery. Semin Radiat Oncol 14(1):76–80. https://doi.org/10.1053/j.semradonc.2003.10.010

Dawson LA, Normolle D, Balter JM, McGinn CJ, Lawrence TS, Ten Haken RK (2002) Analysis of radiation-induced liver disease using the Lyman NTCP model. Int J Radiat Oncol Biol Phys 53(4):810–821

Dawson LA, Winter KA, Katz AW et al (2019) NRG oncology/RTOG 0438: a phase 1 trial of highly conformal radiation therapy for liver metastases. Pract Radiat

Oncol 9(4):e386–e393. https://doi.org/10.1016/j.prro.2019.02.013

Disibio G, French SW (2008) Metastatic patterns of cancers: results from a large autopsy study. Arch Pathol Lab Med 132(6):931–939. https://doi.org/10.1043/1543-2165(2008)132[931:MPOCRF]2.0.CO;2

Gainor JF, Varghese AM, Ou SH et al (2013) ALK rearrangements are mutually exclusive with mutations in EGFR or KRAS: an analysis of 1,683 patients with non-small cell lung cancer. Clin Cancer Res 19(15):4273–4281. https://doi.org/10.1158/1078-0432.CCR-13-0318

Gomez DR, Tang C, Zhang J et al (2019) Local consolidative therapy vs. maintenance therapy or observation for patients with oligometastatic non-small-cell lung cancer: long-term results of a multi-institutional, phase II, randomized study. J Clin Oncol 37(18):1558–1565. https://doi.org/10.1200/JCO.19.00201

Goodman KA, Wiegner EA, Maturen KE et al (2010) Dose-escalation study of single-fraction stereotactic body radiotherapy for liver malignancies. Int J Radiat Oncol Biol Phys 78(2):486–493. https://doi.org/10.1016/j.ijrobp.2009.08.020

Herfarth KK, Debus J, Lohr F et al (2001) Stereotactic single-dose radiation therapy of liver tumors: results of a phase I/II trial. J Clin Oncol 19(1):164–170. https://doi.org/10.1200/JCO.2001.19.1.164

Hess KR, Varadhachary GR, Taylor SH et al (2006) Metastatic patterns in adenocarcinoma. Cancer 106(7):1624–1633. https://doi.org/10.1002/cncr.21778

Horn L, Mansfield AS, Szczęsna A et al (2018) First-line atezolizumab plus chemotherapy in extensive-stage small-cell lung cancer. N Engl J Med 379(23):2220–2229. https://doi.org/10.1056/NEJMoa1809064

Hoyer M, Roed H, Traberg Hansen A et al (2006) Phase II study on stereotactic body radiotherapy of colorectal metastases. Acta Oncol (Stockholm, Sweden) 45(7):823–830. https://doi.org/10.1080/02841860600904854

Kakiuchi S, Daigo Y, Tsunoda T, Yano S, Sone S, Nakamura Y (2003) Genome-wide analysis of organ-preferential metastasis of human small cell lung cancer in mice. Mol Cancer Res 1(7):485–499

Kinkel K, Lu Y, Both M, Warren RS, Thoeni RF (2002) Detection of hepatic metastases from cancers of the gastrointestinal tract by using noninvasive imaging methods (US, CT, MR imaging, PET): a meta-analysis. Radiology 224(3):748–756. https://doi.org/10.1148/radiol.2243011362

Klement RJ, Guckenberger M, Alheid H et al (2017) Stereotactic body radiotherapy for oligo-metastatic liver disease—influence of pre-treatment chemotherapy and histology on local tumor control. Radiother Oncol 123(2):227–233. https://doi.org/10.1016/j.radonc.2017.01.013

Langley RR, Fidler IJ (2011) The seed and soil hypothesis revisited—the role of tumor-stroma interactions in metastasis to different organs. Int J Cancer 128(11):2527–2535. https://doi.org/10.1002/ijc.26031

Lee MT, Kim JJ, Dinniwell R et al (2009) Phase I study of individualized stereotactic body radiotherapy of liver metastases. J Clin Oncol 27(10):1585–1591. https://doi.org/10.1200/JCO.2008.20.0600

Lee CK, Brown C, Gralla RJ et al (2013) Impact of EGFR inhibitor in non-small cell lung cancer on progression-free and overall survival: a meta-analysis. J Natl Cancer Inst 105(9):595–605. https://doi.org/10.1093/jnci/djt072

Mahadevan A, Blanck O, Lanciano R et al (2018) Stereotactic body radiotherapy (SBRT) for liver metastasis—clinical outcomes from the international multi-institutional RSSearch® Patient Registry. Radiat Oncol 13(1):26. https://doi.org/10.1186/s13014-018-0969-2

Megyesfalvi Z, Tallosy B, Pipek O et al (2021) The landscape of small cell lung cancer metastases: organ specificity and timing. Thorac Cancer 12(6):914–923. https://doi.org/10.1111/1759-7714.13854

Méndez Romero A, Wunderink W, Hussain SM et al (2006) Stereotactic body radiation therapy for primary and metastatic liver tumors: a single institution phase I–II study. Acta Oncol (Stockholm, Sweden). 45(7):831–837. https://doi.org/10.1080/02841860600897934

Oikawa A, Takahashi H, Ishikawa H, Kurishima K, Kagohashi K, Satoh H (2012) Application of conditional probability analysis to distant metastases from lung cancer. Oncol Lett 3(3):629–634. https://doi.org/10.3892/ol.2011.535

Ren Y, Dai C, Zheng H et al (2016) Prognostic effect of liver metastasis in lung cancer patients with distant metastasis. Oncotarget 7(33):53245–53253. https://doi.org/10.18632/oncotarget.10644

Riihimäki M, Hemminki A, Fallah M et al (2014) Metastatic sites and survival in lung cancer. Lung Cancer 86(1):78–84. https://doi.org/10.1016/j.lungcan.2014.07.020

Rule W, Timmerman R, Tong L et al (2011) Phase I dose-escalation study of stereotactic body radiotherapy in patients with hepatic metastases. Ann Surg Oncol 18(4):1081–1087. https://doi.org/10.1245/s10434-010-1405-5

Rusthoven KE, Kavanagh BD, Cardenes H et al (2009) Multi-institutional phase I/II trial of stereotactic body radiation therapy for liver metastases. J Clin Oncol 27(10):1572–1578. https://doi.org/10.1200/JCO.2008.19.6329

Sahani DV, Kalva SP (2004) Imaging the liver. Oncologist 9(4):385–397. https://doi.org/10.1634/theoncologist.9-4-385

Sandler A, Gray R, Perry MC et al (2006) Paclitaxel-carboplatin alone or with bevacizumab for non-small-cell lung cancer. N Engl J Med 355(24):2542–2550. https://doi.org/10.1056/NEJMoa061884, pii: 355/24/2542

Schiller JH, Harrington D, Belani CP et al (2002) Comparison of four chemotherapy regimens for advanced non-small-cell lung cancer. N Engl J Med 346(2):92–98. https://doi.org/10.1056/NEJMoa011954, pii: 346/2/92

Scorsetti M, Arcangeli S, Tozzi A et al (2013) Is stereotactic body radiation therapy an attractive option for unresectable liver metastases? A preliminary report from a phase 2 trial. Int J Radiat Oncol Biol Phys 86(2):336–342. https://doi.org/10.1016/j.ijrobp.2012.12.021

Shimizu R, Kinoshita T, Sasaki N et al (2020) Clinicopathological factors related to recurrence patterns of resected non-small cell lung cancer. J Clin Med 9(8). https://doi.org/10.3390/jcm9082473

Smith JJ, D'Angelica MI (2015) Surgical management of hepatic metastases of colorectal cancer. Hematol Oncol Clin North Am 29(1):61–84. https://doi.org/10.1016/j.hoc.2014.09.003

Soliman H, Ringash J, Jiang H et al (2013) Phase II trial of palliative radiotherapy for hepatocellular carcinoma and liver metastases. J Clin Oncol 31(31):3980–3986. https://doi.org/10.1200/JCO.2013.49.9202

Sun A, Durocher-Allen LD, Ellis PM et al (2019) Initial management of small-cell lung cancer (limited- and extensive-stage) and the role of thoracic radiotherapy and first-line chemotherapy: a systematic review. Curr Oncol 26(3):e372–e384. https://doi.org/10.3747/co.26.4481

Tamura T, Kurishima K, Nakazawa K et al (2015) Specific organ metastases and survival in metastatic non-small-cell lung cancer. Mol Clin Oncol 3(1):217–221. https://doi.org/10.3892/mco.2014.410

Yu HA, Arcila ME, Rekhtman N et al (2013) Analysis of tumor specimens at the time of acquired resistance to EGFR-TKI therapy in 155 patients with EGFR-mutant lung cancers. Clin Cancer Res 19(8):2240–2247. https://doi.org/10.1158/1078-0432.CCR-12-2246

Advances in Supportive and Palliative Care for Lung Cancer Patients

Michael J. Simoff, Javier Diaz-Mendoza, A. Rolando Peralta, Labib G. Debiane, and Avi Cohen

Contents

1	Introduction	809
2	**Dyspnea**	810
2.1	Hypoxia	810
2.2	Chronic Obstructive Pulmonary Disease	810
3	**Dyspnea in Malignant Airway Obstruction**	811
3.1	Bronchoscopy	812
3.2	Thermal Techniques	812
3.3	Nonthermal Techniques	815
3.4	Airway Stents	817
4	**Pleural Disease**	818
5	**Tracheoesophageal Fistula**	821
6	Cough	823
7	Hemoptysis	823
8	Conclusion	825
References		825

M. J. Simoff (✉)
Interventional Pulmonology and Lung Cancer Screening, Henry Ford Hospital/Wayne State University School of Medicine, Detroit, MI, USA
e-mail: msimoff1@hfhs.org

J. Diaz-Mendoza
Interventional Pulmonology Fellowship and Education, Pulmonary and Critical Care Medicine, Henry Ford Hospital/Wayne State University School of Medicine, Detroit, MI, USA

A. R. Peralta
Pulmonary, University of California, San Diego, CA, USA

L. G. Debiane
Interventional Pulmonology, Pulmonary and Critical Care Medicine, Henry Ford Hospital/Wayne State University School of Medicine, Detroit, MI, USA

A. Cohen
Interventional Pulmonology, Henry Ford Hospital/Wayne State University School of Medicine, Detroit, MI, USA

1 Introduction

The majority of patients with lung cancer will experience some symptoms (dyspnea, cough, and/or hemoptysis) during the course of their disease. These symptoms not only can greatly affect the quality of life of these patients, but may also influence the therapeutic modalities that their physician may want to employ to deliver further therapy.

Most physicians would define palliation as the relief or soothing of symptoms of a disease, but not affecting cure. The term palliation has often been associated with end-of-life care of patients with cancer. In this chapter, a broader view of palliation is used. As an example of this, relief of an airway obstruction in a patient with end-stage lung cancer may allow them to not suffocate as their cause of death, versus a patient diagnosed with an airway obstruction, subsequently proven to be cancer. This patient's airway obstruction is relieved, and the patient can breathe better and thereby undergo more aggressive therapy as well as have a diminished risk of a post-obstructive pneumonia. Although "cure" may not be affected by the direct intervention, many palliative techniques can increase survival of patients in addition to improving their quality of life. In the study by Brutinel et al., in a patient population affected by airway obstruction, 84–92% of their patients had symptomatic palliation of symptoms solely with laser resection of the endobronchial tumor. Survival at 7 months was better in the laser bronchoscopy group (60%, $n = 71$) than in the control group (0%, $n = 25$) (Brutinel et al. 1987). This idea is an expansion on the traditional view of palliation; with more modern tools and techniques, this broader view should be a part of all treating physicians' thinking.

Symptoms patients with lung cancer may experience include dyspnea, cough, and hemoptysis. Many different manifestations of lung cancer (local invasion, metastasis, or paraneoplastic syndromes) may be responsible for any or all of these. The goal of this chapter is to expand the treating physician's awareness of a variety of these etiologies and a variety of possible therapeutic interventions.

2 Dyspnea

Dyspnea will affect 65% of all patients with lung cancer during some time in their disease course (Jacox et al. 1994; World Health Organization 1990). The etiologies of dyspnea can vary including hypoxia, progression of underlying diseases (i.e., chronic obstructive pulmonary disease [COPD], asthma, congestive heart failure [CHF]), airway obstruction, pleural disease, and deconditioning from inactivity brought on from therapy or from extended stays in the hospital; depression and malnutrition can also be causes as these also occur in many patients (Hoegler 1997).

Dyspnea is a very complex problem as the myriad of etiologies or combinations of conditions can lead to a difficult time for patients and physicians. If the etiology for dyspnea can be identified correctly, it can be managed successfully. With some type of palliative treatment, the patient may have a much greater tolerance for further interventions (whether it be radiation therapy, chemotherapy, or surgery), which might have been impossible except for the intervention.

2.1 Hypoxia

When a patient is short of breath, it is often an automatic response by patients, nurses, and physicians that the patient needs oxygen. Hypoxia is a common complication in patients with lung cancer. Hypoxia is defined as an oxygen saturation of $\leq 88\%$. Some patients will have hypoxia at rest. Other patients will maintain adequate oxygenation while resting but quickly desaturate with activity developing dyspnea. Supplemental oxygen is a very common intervention to help relieve dyspnea due to desaturations in patients with hypoxia both at rest and with exertion (Escalante et al. 1996). When patients are hypoxic with rest or with activity, the use of oxygen with sleep can often help improve rest. The prescription of oxygen particularly with activity should be titrated to ensure that patients are receiving the appropriate doses.

Hypoxia is an objective diagnosis, dyspnea is not. The simple technique of directing a handheld fan toward your face can help diminish the sense of shortness of breath. Galbraith et al. (2010) have demonstrated this in their study published in 2010, which supports the hypothesis that a handheld fan directed to the face reduces the sensation of breathlessness. It must be remembered by practitioners that oxygen should be prescribed for patients with hypoxia, but if a patient is not hypoxic other etiologies of dyspnea should be looked for.

2.2 Chronic Obstructive Pulmonary Disease

It is not uncommon for patients with lung cancer to have other underlying diseases of their lungs, particularly chronic obstructive pulmonary disease (COPD). During therapy for lung cancer, the treatments themselves and/or infections brought on by immunosuppression of the treatments can lead to exacerbations of a patient's chronic underlying disorder. Beta-2 agonists, antibiotics, and sometimes steroid use can often improve the tracheobronchitis and/or bronchospasm associated with the flare-ups. The use of aggressive treatment regimens can assist in controlling some of the underlying lung disease, which can manifest as worsening shortness of breath. Checking airway mechanics with objective testing such as spirometry can assist in the assessment of patients with increasing shortness of breath and underlying disease. Telltale reductions in dynamic airway volumes (FEV_1 and FVC) can help guide therapeutic approaches and measure response of those therapies with return to baseline values.

3 Dyspnea in Malignant Airway Obstruction

Between 2009 and 2015, over 61% of newly diagnosed lung cancer in the United States was detected at an advanced stage (Siegel et al. 2020). More than half of these patients will have central airway involvement with airway compromise caused by intraluminal tumor growth, extraluminal tumor compression, or a combination of both (Fig. 1). Humans have a great capacity of reserve in our ability to breath. When the central airway diameter is obstructed by >50%, patients will encounter significant dyspnea that affects the quality of life (Beamis et al. 2002). Not all endobronchial disease causes complete obstruction of the airways. Patients who have partial airway obstruction (<50%) will often develop worsening shortness of breath as their therapy progresses, particularly during radiation treatments. When radiation treatments involve the areas of obstruction, mucosal inflammation and edema rapidly progress to further airway obstruction. When this becomes greater than 50%, symptoms will begin. Therefore, endobronchial techniques should be considered not only as the end stage of lung cancer management but also at the beginning and throughout the ongoing oncological care (Cortese and Edell 1993).

Most patients with airway obstruction-related dyspnea are at home with limited performance status. A smaller population are hospitalized due to the severity of dyspnea symptoms, while some are critically ill and rely on invasive and noninvasive mechanical ventilatory support. The majority of procedures performed in the United States for airway obstructions are therefore performed on an outpatient basis. Those patients hospitalized due to dyspnea, post-obstructive pneumonia, or respiratory failure, due to an airway obstruction, commonly improve rapidly after intervention. These patients are often extubated soon postoperatively. This rapid symptomatic improvement allows patients to remain ambulatory with an improved quality of life and with greater potential for therapy. It may also allow them to continue with or begin additional oncological treatment that would otherwise be held due to infections or inpatient status. Although interventional procedures are not definitive therapies, they often provide partial to total relief of the severe dyspnea produced by nearly complete airway occlusion.

It should be noted that the severity of illness does not preclude patients from undergoing endobronchial therapies. In fact, the acuity of illness does not directly correlate with achieving palliative outcomes. The technical success rates for airway recanalization are overall high. Endobronchial therapy should not be withheld from patients solely based on the perioperative and preoperative risk. Patients who had endobronchial obstruction, complete lobar obstruction, or significant pre-procedural dyspnea were more likely to demonstrate clinically significant improvement in their quality of life and dyspnea after bronchoscopic intervention (Ost et al. 2015).

Interventional pulmonary programs that include endobronchial therapeutic procedures should include an armamentarium of modalities rather than a single invasive approach to manage patients with complicated lung cancer. As each patient's anatomy differs, the manner in which the patient's cancer leads to symptoms varies. Several procedures used in conjunction (i.e., laser and stenting) may be necessary to provide the most effective treatment. The necessity of multiple modalities can also be affected by the patient's medical condition. For instance, patients with high oxygen requirements cannot be treated with traditional thermal energy modalities. Regarding endobronchial prosthesis, the use of both metallic and silastic stents is very important

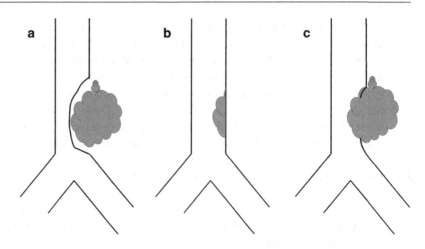

Fig. 1 Types of malignant central airway obstruction. A diagram of the trachea with the three main types of malignant central airway obstruction. (**a**) Extraluminal; (**b**) intraluminal; and (**c**) mixed obstruction

as each stent type has great advantages over the other. A program offering a wide variety of modalities allows the best selection of approaches for any given patient (Beamis et al. 2002).

The following sections discuss a variety of techniques and tools available to the interventionalist. In many cases, no one technique is better than the other, and some combination of these techniques often offers the greatest benefit to the patient.

3.1 Bronchoscopy

Since the inception of flexible fiber-optic bronchoscopy (Fig. 2) in the late 1960s in Japan and in 1970 in the United States, it has become the most widespread tool for evaluating and diagnosing diseases of the airways and lungs (Ikeda 1970). The rigid bronchoscope, the predecessor to the flexible bronchoscope, was in many regards forgotten as a tool until the practice of interventional pulmonology evolved in the 1980s. Interventional pulmonology is offered by pulmonologists who have undergone additional training in the field (Beaudoin et al. 2015; Mullon et al. 2017). A frequent tool used for therapeutic and palliative purposes by interventional pulmonologist is the rigid bronchoscope.

The rigid bronchoscope is a large straight stainless steel tube with a beveled distal end (Fig. 3). While the patient is under general anesthesia, the trachea can be directly intubated. The proximal end of the rigid bronchoscope has a central opening and several side ports that can be used for ventilation, light and imaging, and instrumentation. The varying tube diameters (3–18 mm) allow for a gamut of sophisticated instruments and techniques that would otherwise not be possible with flexible bronchoscopy. Overall, both the flexible bronchoscope and the rigid bronchoscope are necessary for the practice of interventional pulmonology. When compared to a flexible bronchoscope, the rigid bronchoscope allows for higher suction capability, simultaneous use of multiple instruments at a time, and placement of silicone stents. These unique capacities of the rigid bronchoscope lend it to be most commonly used for palliative and therapeutic management of central airway obstruction (Diaz-Mendoza et al. 2018).

3.2 Thermal Techniques

There are numerous tools available for the management of airway tumors and obstructions. Mechanical debulking is often complicated by significant hemorrhage. Thermal ablative techniques such as laser, electrocautery, and argon plasma coagulation allow for rapid debulking while providing coagulation effects through devascularization. The availability of such techniques propelled the field of palliative and rapid bronchoscopic approach to symptom relief.

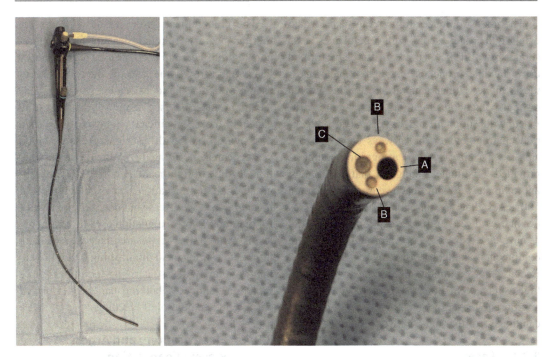

Fig. 2 Flexible bronchoscope. The flexible bronchoscope pictured on the left is available in different tip and channel diameters depending on the procedure at hand. On the right, the tip of the bronchoscope is shown with the (A) working channel, (B) light sources, and (C) camera

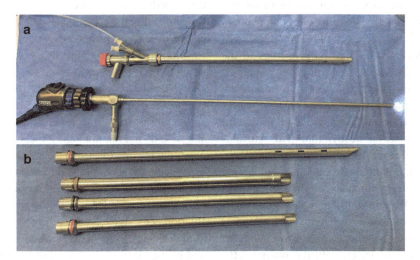

Fig. 3 Rigid bronchoscope. (**a**) The camera head and a light source attached to the telescope are inserted into a rigid bronchoscope as pictured through the red sealing cap. The rigid bronchoscope provides two channels for additional tool insertion including a large-caliber suction catheter. The ventilator circuit is connected to a ventilation port. (**b**) There are different diameter sizes available for use. A bronchial scope is longer in length with side ventilation ports that remain in the trachea while the tip of the bronchial scope is in a mainstem bronchus

Thermal techniques are preferably performed using rigid bronchoscopy with general anesthesia (Prakash et al. 1991). They can also be performed using flexible bronchoscopy with topical anesthesia alone. Under general anesthesia or even during spontaneous breathing, the patient is provided with supplemental oxygen. The oxygen-rich environment in the airways can lead to a catastrophic airway fire if an ignition source is provided. Estimates suggest that there are approximately 700 fires each year with more than 500 cases that are unreported on near misses (Akhtar et al. 2016). It is exceptionally essential to have an experienced operator and appropriate equipment available for these modalities. Because of such limitations, patients who require high supplementation of oxygen to maintain appropriate tissue oxygenation may not be ideal candidates for thermal ablative techniques.

3.2.1 Laser

Laser technology utilizes radiant energy and light amplification to deliver a narrowband of a specific wavelength. By delivering this energy via a quartz monofilament fiber to a surface, one can achieve variable responses ranging from superficial penetration in the millimeter range up to complete tissue destruction. The degree of response depends on both the properties of the laser (i.e., wavelength, frequency, power output) and the tissue characteristics (i.e., absorption rate and water content).

Several types of lasers are currently used within the airways: neodymium (Nd) yttrium-aluminum-garnet (YAG), potassium titanyl phosphate (KTP), holmium (Ho), and carbon dioxide (CO_2). Each laser produces a light at a different wavelength. Water has different absorption coefficients at different wavelengths (Fig. 4). For example, Nd:YAG emits at a wavelength of 1064 nm. At this wavelength, the water coefficient of absorption is fairly low making Nd:YAG laser better suited for coagulation effect while the cutting effect remains low. Alternatively, CO_2 laser emits at a higher wavelength of 10,600 nm. This in turn results in high tissue absorption making this laser effective at cutting rather than coagulation.

The predominant tissue effects of lasers are thermal necrosis (photodesiccation) and photocoagulation. Thermal necrosis uses higher energy levels to destroy tissue, causing the formation of eschar or actual photodesiccation of tissue. This technique must be used cautiously as most lung cancers have significant vascularity. When destroying tissue with laser energy, large blood vessels can be perforated with the tissue destruction, leading to significant hemorrhage. The technique of photodesiccation is an excellent tool for managing airway disease but does require a skillful operator. Photocoagulation uses lower energy levels with longer exposure intervals, causing tumors to "shrink" and diminishing blood flow to that region. By devascularizing the tumor, more rapid mechanical debulking can be performed with improved control of bleeding.

3.2.2 Electrocautery and Argon Plasma Coagulation

Electrocautery is the use of an electrical current to heat tissue. By creating a voltage differential between a source probe and the target tissue, electrons flow toward and through a higher resistance medium (i.e., tissue), thus generating heat. By controlling the current density, electrocautery can be used to perform coagulation, cutting, fulguration, and vaporization. Argon plasma coagulation (APC) uses ionized argon gas jet flow (also known as plasma) to conduct electrons in a non-contact technique.

In contrast to laser technology, electrocautery and APC do not require highly specialized equipment that is often exclusive to large hospital centers. Electrical generators are found in almost all hospitals that offer any surgical services. Another stark difference between the two methods of ablation is the associated depth of tissue penetration. With laser, light photons significantly scatter within the deep tissue creating a considerable heat sink effect. Electrons on the other hand do not scatter in the deep layers but rather focus their energy at the point of contact (Bolliger 2006).

Electrocautery is different from APC in the sense that it requires direct contact with the tissue to transmit the electrons. The contact probes for electrocautery come in multiple sizes and shapes

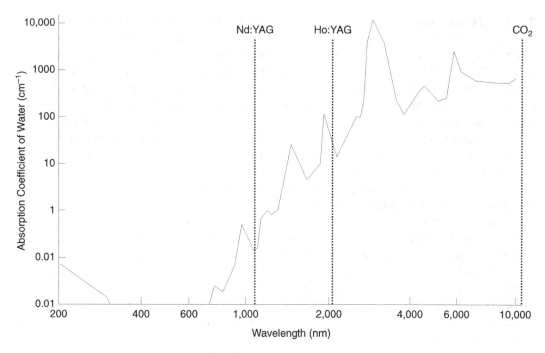

Fig. 4 Absorption of the main chromophores. The degree of absorption of each laser's wavelength determines that laser's ability to cut and coagulate tissue. Increased absorption allows for cutting and ablation. Decreased absorption causes coagulation. Continuous-line H_2O; broken-line HbO_2. Vertical lines represent wavelengths of three medical lasers (Nd:YAG, Ho:YAG, CO_2). HbO_2 does not absorb wavelengths above 1000 nm. (Adapted from Squiers et al. 2014)

such as forceps, knife, and snare. Some tumor configurations within the airways may not be amenable to direct contact for which the APC may be a more suitable tool. As the generated plasma will fire toward the path of least resistance, APC allows for a noncontact focus of energy that can go around corners in a skilled operator's hands.

As with laser, APC and electrocautery can be sources of ignition for an airway fire. It is very important to maintain the fraction of inhaled oxygen below 40% during the use of these modalities. Albeit highly unlikely, there have been reported cases of life-threatening gas embolisms occurring with both laser and APC (Reddy et al. 2008). Unlike laser, APC and electrocautery should be cautiously used in patients with an automatic implantable cardioverter defibrillator (AICD) or pacemaker if the electrical current changes can trigger a false discharge. These patients should undergo preoperative device interrogation and setting changes to accommodate for the use of electrocautery and APC.

3.3 Nonthermal Techniques

Other techniques used to relieve airway obstruction and improve respiratory symptoms are not based on the use of heat energy. These modalities have a delayed effect in comparison with the immediate effects of thermal energy. Cryotherapy, photodynamic therapy, and brachytherapy are examples of these modalities. Endobronchial intratumoral injection of chemotherapy (paclitaxel) under rigid bronchoscopy guidance is under study and could help in the relief of airway obstruction (Yarmus et al. 2019). Brachytherapy will be discussed in another section of this book.

3.3.1 Cryotherapy

Lowering the temperature to −40 °C at a rate of −100 °C per minute is needed to achieve adequate cell death (90%) within an area being treated; cryotherapy uses extreme cold to destroy tissue obstructing the airways. Cryoprobes use a compressed gas such as liquid nitrogen (−196 °C), nitrous oxide (−80 °C), and carbon dioxide, which is allowed to rapidly expand in an enclosed volume. By the Joule-Thomson effect, the temperature of the compressed gas drops significantly and freezes the adjacent tissue. The tissue is frozen and then thawed, typically in 30-s cycles. The flash freezing of tissue leads to formation of crystals in the intra- and extracellular space, causing damage of organelles and fluid shifting. Local vasoconstriction and thrombosis further lead to ischemia and delayed cell death (Gage and Baust 1998).

Since tissue necrosis is delayed, formation of debris within the airways can be seen at 48–72 h, making the need for a repeat bronchoscopy for removal of this tissue very likely, and in some cases, repeating treatments are needed. Due to this delayed effect, this mode should not be used in critical endobronchial obstruction caused by tumors. Cryotherapy has shown to be safe and effective for palliation of inoperable lung cancer, as well as in metastatic lung tumors (de Baere et al. 2015). The largest series of endobronchial cryotherapy (476 patients) has been reported by Maiwand et al. (2004). His team showed a 69% improvement of cough, 59% improvement of dyspnea, and 76% improvement of hemoptysis after using endobronchial cryotherapy. Complications reported have remained less than 1% and include respiratory distress, bleeding, and pneumothorax (Maiwand et al. 2004). Cryotherapy has also been used in combination with other ablative modalities, airway stenting, as well as chemotherapy (Xu et al. 2020a).

The advantage of this mode, and all other delayed modes of tissue destruction, is that it can be used at any level of oxygen (FiO_2) a patient may require to correct hypoxia. This is a big difference with all the other heat modalities like laser that require an FiO_2 below 40% in order to avoid ignition and fire.

3.3.2 Photodynamic Therapy

Photodynamic therapy (PDT) is a procedure that incorporates the use of a photosensitizing agent in combination with a specific light to stimulate a photooxidative reaction, producing singlet oxygen that leads to cell death through apoptosis, necrosis, and autophagocytosis of cancer. The photosensitizer (porfimer sodium is the most commonly used in the United States) is administered intravenously and penetrates all cells systematically, with significant clearance by most cells, concentrating in cancer cells. An argon dye or diode laser is used via bronchoscopy to provide 632 nm wavelength light energy, which is then used to activate the photosensitizer and start the photooxidative process. Again, as all the other delayed-effect modalities, formation of bronchial debris from tumor necrosis will require a bronchoscopic intervention 36 h later to clean the airways.

PDT can effectively reduce airway obstruction and improve respiratory function and quality of life in advanced inoperable non-small cell lung cancer (NSCLC) (Moghissi et al. 1999; Minnich et al. 2010). PDT can help control vessel bleeding and improve hemoptysis (Jones et al. 2001). Traditionally, due to its delayed effects, PDT is not used for airway obstructions, but to manage other manifestations of malignant airway disease.

PDT has been combined effectively with external beam radiation therapy and brachytherapy. A series of 32 patients with bulky endobronchial NSCLC treated with PDT followed by brachytherapy reported 81% local control, 94% distant metastasis-free survival, and 100% overall survival after 24 months (Freitag et al. 2004).

The effect of PDT as neoadjuvant therapy for NSCLC has also been demonstrated leading to conversion of inoperable patients into resectable or diminishing the degree of surgery required, i.e., initially planned pneumonectomies converted into lobectomies (Okunaka et al. 1999; Ross et al. 2006).

PDT is an excellent therapeutic modality for early-stage NSCLC and has shown a significant response (Furuse et al. 1993) in patients with roentgenographically occult bronchogenic carcinomas, with high overall survival rates (Endo et al. 2009).

3.4 Airway Stents

Airway stents have been a cornerstone in the management of malignant airway obstruction of different types (extrinsic compression or mixed) since Dumon described the creation of the first dedicated airway stent (made of silicone) and its use in 1990 (Dumon 1990). Since that time, multiple airway stents have been developed based on various structural materials, deploying systems, etc. Overall, we can divide stents into three groups: silicone based, metal based, and others (Fig. 5, Table 1).

Some of the advantages of silicone stents include that they are easily removed and replaced, customization is straightforward, and they are of much lower cost. Disadvantages of silastic stents include that they require rigid bronchoscopy to be placed, a higher risk of migration, and difficulty when airways have different diameters due to anatomy and/or tissue/tumor changes (Ost et al. 2012).

Self-expanding metal stents are easier to insert (can be placed without rigid bronchoscopy), conform better to the airways, and have a good wall/internal diameter relationship. Their main disadvantages include having an increased risk of infection (Ost et al. 2012), tumor or granulation tissue ingrowth leading to obstruction, and difficulty of stent repositioning or removal (in the case of partially or fully uncovered stents) once it has been seated completely in the airway. These characteristics, both good and bad, are becoming more similar to silastic stents with the use of newer fully covered metallic stents. Their engineering has begun to eliminate some of the advantages that initially made them very popular.

All stents have different degrees of secretion adherence depending on the material of the stent, its covering, and shape characteristics. This needs to be taken into consideration whenever a patient is being managed with an airway stent. Many of the stents placed prior to the principal therapy for malignancy should be thought of as temporary, and patients evaluated for removal after treatment.

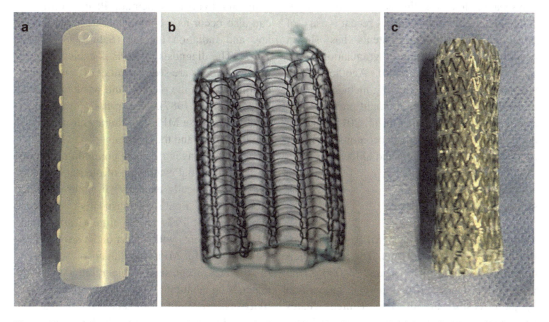

Fig. 5 The two most common types of airway stents include silicone and metal stents. Figure shows tubular silicone stent (**a**), metal stent uncovered (Ultraflex™) (**b**), and metal stent covered (Merit Endotek™) (**c**)

Table 1 Types of airway stents (based on their main structural material)

Silicone stents[a]	Metal stents	Others
Montgomery T-tube Tubular silicone (with its variations) Silicone Y-stent	Ultraflex™ (nitinol with or without silicone cover) Merit Endotek™ (nitinol with polyurethane cover) Bonastent[R] (nitinol with silicone cover) iCast™ (stainless steel with polytetrafluoroethylene covers)	Dynamic stent (silicone with C-shaped stainless steel support) Polyflex stent (polyester mesh combined with silicone)

[a]Silicone stents are made 100% of silicone

Airway stenting has been shown to improve dyspnea in patients with airway obstruction caused by NSCLC and other types of malignancies. Its prolonged effect over dyspnea when used with mechanical debulking of the tumor has been found in a randomized study (Dutau et al. 2020). While most studies have shown the positive effect of airway stenting on the relief of dyspnea (Ost et al. 2015), its effect on quality of life and survival is still being debated (Ost et al. 2015; Marchese et al. 2020). Most airway stents are placed in central airways (trachea, mainstem bronchi), although airway stenting of lobar airways can also be performed. However, its long-term effectiveness still needs to be studied (Marchese et al. 2020).

The formation of granulation tissue in the airways leading to obstruction is a potential complication caused by stents; recent use of paclitaxel-eluting silicone stents has shown promise to the prevention of granulation tissue formation (Xu et al. 2020b). Another recent advancement in airway stenting includes the use of bioabsorbable stents that could prevent long-term complications (Dutau et al. 2015) and the use of 3D printed stents that accommodate better to the airway shape (Young and Gildea 2017).

4 Pleural Disease

Malignant pleural effusions (MPE) occur commonly among cancer patients. The annual incidence is estimated to be around 50,000 cases/year in the United Kingdom and more than 150,000 cases/year in the United States (American Thoracic Society 2000; Rahman et al. 2010), greater than half of whom develop dyspnea (Chernow and Sahn 1977). The mechanism of dyspnea with pleural effusions is unclear. It is believed to be due to mechanical factors influencing the chest wall, mediastinum, pleural space, lung, and probably most significantly diaphragm. Any of these changes individually or more commonly in combination contribute to the sensation of dyspnea in the patient with a pleural effusion.

Pleural effusions in the setting of lung cancer may be malignant or para-malignant (Sahn 1985, 1987, 1997). With para-malignant pleural effusions, there is not a direct involvement of the pleura with tumor. They can result from local tumor effects (such as lymphatic obstruction and superior vena cava syndrome) or from systemic effects of the tumor (such as pulmonary embolism and hypoalbuminemia). Pleural effusions can also occur as a complication of chemotherapy and radiation therapy (Sahn 1985, 1987, 1997). The diagnosis of MPE is achieved when malignant cells are seen on either cytopathologic examination of the pleural fluid or pleural tissue biopsy (Sahn 1987). The primary techniques used to diagnose MPEs are thoracentesis, closed needle biopsy, and thoracoscopy.

Thoracentesis is the most common technique used in the initial evaluation of pleural effusion. MPEs are typically exudative in nature but can meet the light's transudative criteria approximately 19% of the time (Light et al. 1972). In patients with cancer and a strong clinical suspicion for MPE, the diagnostic sensitivity of initial thoracentesis with pleural fluid cytology depends on the tumor type, with the lowest sensitivity observed with mesothelioma, sarcoma, and head and neck cancer and the highest sensitivity seen with breast and pancreatic cancer (Grosu et al. 2018). For lung cancer, the pleural fluid obtained by thoracentesis yields positive cytology for malignant cells in 62–90% of true MPE (Grosu et al. 2018; Hsu 1987; Loddenkemper et al. 1983; Starr and Sherman 1991; van de Molengraft and Vooijs 1988), the highest sensitivity (90%) seen with lung adenocarcinoma (Grosu et al. 2018).

Closed needle pleural biopsy can also be performed for the evaluation of an MPE. However, its diagnostic yield for the most part has been historically considered to be lower than that of thoracentesis, ranging between 40% and 65% (Loddenkemper et al. 1983; Poe et al. 1984; Prakash and Reiman 1985; Loddenkemper 1998; Chakrabarti et al. 2006). There is a 7–12% additive yield from closed needle biopsy over cytology alone (Prakash and Reiman 1985; Loddenkemper 1998; Escudero Bueno et al. 1990). The practice of closed needle pleural biopsies has diminished over time perhaps because of its small added benefit and the general push by clinicians for a higher yield tissue diagnosis via thoracoscopy.

Medical thoracoscopy, or pleuroscopy, is a procedure more commonly being used by nonsurgeons for the diagnosis and treatment of pleural effusions. This technique has excellent results in the diagnosis and treatment of MPEs in appropriate populations. In a study of patients being evaluated for MPE, all enrolled patients had cytologic assessment by thoracentesis and closed needle pleural biopsies, followed by thoracoscopy. This representative study demonstrated diagnostic yields of 62% for thoracentesis and 44% for closed needle pleural biopsy, with a combined sensitivity of 74%, and a diagnostic yield of 95% for medical thoracoscopy (Loddenkemper 1998). Other studies have demonstrated similar result (Boutin et al. 1981; Cantó et al. 1977; Menzies and Charbonneau 1991; Oldenburg and Newhouse 1979). After medical thoracoscopy had been performed, less than 10% of effusions remain undiagnosed (Loddenkemper 1981, 1998; Boutin et al. 1981; Cantó et al. 1977; Mårtensson et al. 1985).

In institutions where medical thoracoscopy is not performed, most thoracic surgeons can perform video-assisted thoracoscopic surgery (VATS). VATS differs from medical thoracoscopy in that patients undergoing VATS will have general rather than moderate anesthesia; they will be intubated, usually with double-lumen endotracheal tube, rather than be spontaneously breathing; and three incisions will be made rather than the typical one (two for certain procedures). VATS is an excellent procedure but is considered a fairly invasive diagnostic procedure for an otherwise uncomplicated pleural effusion. In addition, it is not uncommon that patients with lung cancer suffer from advanced chronic obstructive pulmonary disease with diminished physiologic reserves making them poor surgical candidates for a VATS procedure.

The major indication for treating a pleural effusion is to achieve symptomatic relief from dyspnea. Once the diagnosis of MPE has been made, a therapeutic plan warrants to be established with the patients and their families and an in-depth discussion of expectations and goals of care should take place, remembering that the etiology of dyspnea is more complex than the amount of fluid identified in the pleural space (Agustí et al. 1997; Brown et al. 1978; Estenne et al. 1983; Karetzky et al. 1978; Krell and Rodarte 1985; Light et al. 1986) and may be related to problems with the lung itself (lymphangitic spread of tumor, atelectasis, or direct tumor invasion). The limitation of diaphragmatic movement caused by fluid accumulation is believed to be a major mechanism of dyspnea in patients with untreated pleural effusions. Trapped lung due to parenchymal or pleural disease will minimize the magnitude of the symptomatic relief typically observed with pleural fluid drainage. Therefore, initially, a large-volume thoracentesis should be performed to assess the effects upon breathlessness by fluid removal and the ability of the lung to re-expand, as well as the rate and degree of re-accumulation. A chest X-ray is recommended before and after large-volume thoracentesis to evaluate for the degree of lung re-expansion as this may help guide management (Feller-Kopman et al. 2018). If the trapped lung is believed to be due to endobronchial obstruction, therapeutic bronchoscopy should be considered to attempt to recanalize the airway and as such optimize lung expansion.

Chest radiographs and thoracic ultrasonography should be used to assess whether the pleural fluid is free flowing or loculated and to evaluate for the presence of any mediastinal shifts with respect to the pleural effusion. In general, a contralateral shift of the mediastinum with large effusions suggests that evacuation of the pleural fluid should provide relief of dyspnea to the patient. Ipsilateral mediastinal shift on the other hand suggests the presence of a trapped lung or an endobronchial obstruction, potentially limiting the relief of dyspnea a patient may experience with evacuation of pleural fluid. Expert opinion suggests stopping the pleural fluid drainage as soon as the patient experiences dyspnea, chest pain, hemodynamic changes, intractable cough, or any new emerging symptoms. The chest pain or discomfort is believed to be the result of the precipitous buildup of negative intrathoracic pressure in the context of a trapped lung physiology. Limited removal of fluid ($\leq$300 mL) by thoracentesis is suggested in this subpopulation to minimize reducing the pleural pressure rapidly (American Thoracic Society 2000).

Pleural pressure monitoring can be performed before, during, and after thoracentesis; has been hypothesized for long to help guide the amount of fluid drainage; and can help assess for the presence of a trapped lung at the time of thoracentesis in patients with MPE (Lan et al. 1997). However, a multicenter single-blind randomized controlled trial in 2019 (Lentz et al. 2019) compared large-volume thoracentesis guided by symptoms plus pleural manometry to drainage guided by symptoms alone (control) and found that measurement of pleural pressure by manometry did not alter procedure-related chest discomfort. There was also no difference in breathlessness between both groups. About 10% of the control group developed asymptomatic pneumothorax ex vacuo compared to none in the pleural manometry group (Lentz et al. 2019). Overall, while pleural pressure monitoring may convey a more objective assessment for the presence of trapped lung compared to chest radiograph, it is considered to be complex and without enough evidence to support its regular use.

Therapeutic modalities for managing MPEs include repeated thoracentesis, chemical pleurodesis via a chest tube or thoracoscopy, pleuroperitoneal shunting, pleural drainage catheters, and systemic therapy. Repeated large-volume thoracentesis is a viable option for those patients with poor performance status, slow fluid re-accumulation, advanced disease, and limited life expectancy (Roberts et al. 2010). There are no studies upon which to base repeated thoracentesis. A large multicenter cohort study found a 30% cumulative incidence of recurrence of effusion by day 15 (Grosu et al. 2019). If the MPE continues to accumulate, a more definitive procedure can be considered.

A variety of sclerosant agents have been used for pleurodesis including talc, tetracycline, doxycycline, bleomycin, *C. parvum*, iodine, and interferon, among others (Clive et al. 2016), with a Cochrane database from 2004 reporting an overall successful chemical pleurodesis rate of about 84% and talc being the sclerosant agent of choice (Shaw and Agarwal 2004). Talc can be used either via chest tube placement with pleural evacuation and talc slurry instillation or during medical thoracoscopy or video-assisted thoracoscopic surgery, with talc poudrage. Poudrage and slurry pleurodesis methods demonstrated a clinical success rate of 91% with no significant difference in recurrence rates of effusions (Fentiman et al. 1983, 1986; Hamed et al. 1989; Hartman et al. 1993; Kennedy et al. 1994; Todd et al. 1980; Yim et al. 1996). A more recent multicenter randomized controlled trial in the United Kingdom compared thoracoscopic talc poudrage (4 g) to talc slurry (4 g) via a chest tube and found comparable pleurodesis failure rates at 90 days (22% vs. 24%, respectively) (Bhatnagar et al. 2019). The greatest concern with the use of talc is 1% risk of developing fatal acute respiratory distress syndrome (ARDS) and 4% risk of nonfatal ARDS reported in the literature. Most of the ARDS complications have been reported in the United States. It has been suggested that this may be due to the size of talc particles used in the United States versus those used in Europe (Milanez

Campos et al. 1997; Rehse et al. 1999). Recently, a large-particle-size talc (Steritalc®, Novatech, France) was approved by the Food and Drug Administration (FDA) to be used in the United States.

Other pleurodesis agents used include doxycycline, which when compared to historical controls had a similar success rate as previous studies with tetracycline, 80–85% (Heffner et al. 1994; Patz et al. 1998; Pulsiripunya et al. 1996). Bleomycin has been used and compared in randomized testing to tetracycline and found to have similar complete response rates (Hartman et al. 1993; Martínez-Moragón et al. 1997; Moffett and Ruckdeschel 1992). Doxycycline when compared directly with bleomycin had a 79% complete response to bleomycin's 72% (Hayata et al. 1993). When bleomycin was compared to talc, talc demonstrated superior complete response rate of 81% versus 65% (Xia et al. 2014). Antineoplastic agents had a reported complete response at initial pleurodesis of 44% (Walker-Renard et al. 1994).

For MPEs due to small-cell lung cancer, the lung cancer therapy of choice is systemic chemotherapy. Often, these patients will respond with resolution of pleural effusions and dyspnea (Livingston et al. 1982).

The use of pleuroperitoneal shunting has been reported for the management of malignant and other intractable pleural effusions. All of these studies are case series rather than randomized in any fashion. Initial data looks promising, but it has not been evaluated in head-to-head studies with more conventional treatment methods (i.e., chest tube drainage with chemical pleurodesis) (Petrou et al. 1995; Ponn et al. 1991; Pope and Joseph 1989; Reich et al. 1993; Schulze et al. 2001).

Lately, tunneled indwelling pleural catheters (TIPCs) have gained popularity in the management of MPEs. TIPCs are less invasive, allow for an entirely outpatient approach for the management of recurrent symptomatic MPEs, and provide significant relief of dyspnea. The greatest improvements in dyspnea are seen in patients with more severe dyspnea at baseline and those who have subsequently received chemotherapy and/or radiation therapy (Ost et al. 2014; Tremblay and Michaud 2006; Warren et al. 2008). TIPCs are also favored in patients with a trapped lung (Pien et al. 2001). Spontaneous pleurodesis (or auto-pleurodesis) can occur with TIPC, and the rate of pleurodesis has been reported in a systematic review in 2011 to be around 45% (Van Meter et al. 2011). The optimal frequency drainage of TIPC has been evaluated in multiple trials; daily drainage resulted in a significantly higher incidence proportion of pleurodesis compared to every-other-day drainage (Wahidi et al. 2017) and to symptom-guided drainage; however, the mean daily breathlessness did not differ (Muruganandan et al. 2018). Dyspnea relief from TIPC was further evaluated by comparing it to chemical pleurodesis by talc slurry; there was no significant difference in dyspnea relief over the first 42 days but TIPC performed better at 6 months (Davies et al. 2012). With respect to hospital length of stay, patients with TIPC have a statistically significant lower hospital length of stay than those who undergo talc slurry (Thomas et al. 2017). With outpatient administration of talc through a TIPC, a higher successful rate of pleurodesis was achieved compared to treatment with TIPC alone (Bhatnagar et al. 2018).

In the latest published guidelines by the American Thoracic Society in 2018, either TIPC or chemical pleurodesis is recommended as the first-line therapy for patients with MPE with an expandable lung following large-volume thoracentesis. For patients with a nonexpandable lung, prior failed pleurodesis, or a loculated effusion, TIPC is favored over chemical pleurodesis (Feller-Kopman et al. 2018). Future clinical trials are needed to further evaluate the optimal approach to the management of MPEs.

5 Tracheoesophageal Fistula

The term tracheoesophageal fistula (TEF) is used to describe an abnormal communication between the respiratory and digestive tract, which leads to spillage of gastric and oral contents into the respiratory tract. Although a fistula can occur between the esophagus and trachea or main bronchi (TEF and BEF, respectively), we will use the term TEF interchangeably for the purpose of this review.

The proximal esophagus is at the level of the larynx and extends around 19–25 cm to the gastroesophageal sphincter. It lies immediately posterior to the trachea and left mainstem bronchus. The membranous trachea and esophagus each have a 4 mm wall thickness and are separated by only a thin layer of connective areolar tissue. It is these anatomical characteristics that render the trachea and esophagus susceptible to fistula formation when their integrity is disrupted.

TEF is broadly classified as congenital and acquired. Congenital TEF is identified in childhood and occurs due to abnormalities in the development of the anterior foregut as it gives rise to the dorsal esophagus and ventral trachea; these are usually related to esophageal atresia. An H-type TEF has been identified in adults as a rare cause of chronic cough and dysphagia (Bank et al. 2020). Acquired TEF is more frequently seen in adults and is classified as benign and malignant, with each category accounting for around half of the acquired cases (Reed and Mathisen 2003).

Benign TEF can occur due to prolonged mechanical ventilation, excessive cuff pressure of an endotracheal or tracheostomy tube, traumatic endotracheal intubation or tracheostomy placement, penetrating or blunt trauma, complications of laryngeal or esophageal surgery, granulomatous mediastinal infection (i.e., tuberculosis, actinomycosis), ingestion of corrosive products, foreign body aspiration or ingestion, stent-related injuries, and inflammatory disorders (rheumatoid arthritis) (Muniappan et al. 2013; Shen et al. 2010). With the increased use of mechanical ventilation, TEF fistula related to endotracheal and tracheostomy tubes has surpassed infections as the most common etiology of benign TEF (Diddee and Shaw 2006).

The majority of cases of malignant TEF are related to esophageal and lung cancer (77% and 16%, respectively) (Burt et al. 1991). The overall incidence of TEF in esophageal cancer is 4–12% and 0.3% for lung cancer (Burt et al. 1991; Balazs et al. 2008). Additionally, therapeutic interventions can themselves lead to or hasten the development of TEF. Esophageal stenting, a technique frequently used in the treatment of esophageal cancer, can lead to stent-associated esophagorespiratory fistula (SERF) in 4% of the cases at a median of 5 months (0.4–53 months). The risk is higher when the location of the stent is in the proximal or mid esophagus, compared to the distal esophagus (6% vs. 14% vs. 0%) (Bick et al. 2013). Radiation therapy leads to esophageal perforation in 5% of the patients up to 40 weeks after completion (Chen et al. 2014).

Patients with TEF may present with cough, aspiration, fever, dysphagia, recurrent respiratory tract infections, hemoptysis, and chest pain. The impaired oral route and recurrent infections frequently lead to worsening nutritional status and dehydration. Patients with benign TEF due to endotracheal or tracheostomy tubes may present with abdominal bloating, inadequate ventilation and/or oxygenation, and difficulty weaning from mechanical ventilation (Kim et al. 2020).

TEF is diagnosed with a combination of radiologic and endoscopic findings. Barium esophagography can show the spillage of contrast material into the respiratory tract. Upper endoscopy and flexible bronchoscopy are important in determining the location and size of the fistula and offer guidance on therapeutic interventions.

The treatment of malignant TEF is mainly palliative. Surgical correction in such instances should be discouraged given the generally poor functional status and limited life expectancy. The overall goal is to protect the airways from further spillage of gastric contents, maintain an adequate nutritional status, and improve the quality of life (Simoff et al. 2013).

Survival with supportive measures alone is short at 1–6 weeks (Reed and Mathisen 2003). General measures include placing the patient in the semi-recumbent position, acid-suppressive therapy with PPI or H2 receptor antagonist, removal of nasogastric and orogastric tubes, and complete avoidance of the oral route. Nutrition can be maintained via a gastrostomy or jejunostomy tube, and in certain instances parenteral nutrition may be necessary.

Double stenting (esophagus and airway) or esophageal stenting alone using self-expanding metallic stents is recommended to manage malignant TEF (Simoff et al. 2013). Double stenting appears to have higher success rates compared to single stenting (Ke et al. 2015; Freitag et al. 1996); however, they both lead to similar improvements in QoL measures (Herth et al. 2010). If double stenting is chosen, placing the airway stent first is recommended to decrease the risk of airway compromise (Simoff et al. 2013).

Patients with benign TEF should be managed surgically if they are considered good surgical candidates. Those patients who are not stable for surgery should be stabilized and bridged to surgery if possible. If surgical correction is not feasible, double or single stenting may be used (Kim et al. 2020).

6 Cough

Cough is a common symptom in patients with lung cancer, seen in 25–84% of patients at the time of diagnosis. Despite its prevalence in this patient population, it is often underrecognized and undertreated, thus significantly affecting the QoL (Harle et al. 2012).

Cough can be caused by cancer-specific mechanisms like endobronchial disease, airway obstruction, pleural disease, or tracheoesophageal fistula or cancer therapies like radiation-induced pneumonitis, chemotherapy, or postsurgical changes. Additionally, patients may have underlying comorbidities which manifest with cough such as gastrointestinal reflux disease, COPD, bronchiectasis, or interstitial lung disease (Simoff et al. 2013). There is a paucity of literature regarding the management of cough in patients with lung cancer, and the overall recommendations rely heavily on expertise. More research in this area is needed (Molassiotis et al. 2010, 2015).

A comprehensive evaluation for all the potential causes of cough is recommended. In those cases, in which a specific cause is identified, this should be managed per available guidelines (i.e., management of COPD or TEF). Cough secondary to chemotherapy or radiation-induced pneumonitis can be treated with corticosteroids (Simoff et al. 2013).

Symptomatic management is strongly recommended for those patients without an identifiable cause or with refractory cough. Nonopioid cough suppressants can be tried initially, followed by centrally acting opioids (codeine) if the former fail. Morphine and methadone could be considered before introducing peripherally acting opioids such as Levodropropizine, Moguisteine, or Levocloperastine. Constipation should be anticipated and prophylactically managed when opioids are prescribed (Molassiotis et al. 2010).

7 Hemoptysis

Hemoptysis is defined as the expectoration of blood originating from the lower respiratory tract. The correct identification of the source of bleeding is important as blood from the upper respiratory or upper gastrointestinal tract (also known as pseudohemoptysis) can also be expectorated and is frequently confused for hemoptysis.

Hemoptysis is classified into mild, moderate, and massive based upon the amount and rate of bleeding. The severity of bleeding is paramount because the airways have a dead space of around 150 mL and even a small amount of blood can rapidly lead to clot formation and asphyxiation (Jean-Baptiste 2000). Historically, the term "massive hemoptysis" was used to identify patients who need emergent interventions. However, the cutoff value in the literature is quite variable (100–1000 mL in 24 h) and therefore clinical parameters, such as hemodynamic or respiratory instability, and baseline patient characteristics, should also be taken into consideration (Yendamuri 2015; Ibrahim 2008). The terms "non-life-threatening" and "life-threatening hemoptysis" may provide a more clinically valuable classification. It is the authors' opinion that any airway bleeding that is life-threatening should be considered massive and therefore warrants prompt attention and interventions.

Hemoptysis is common in lung cancer, being the presenting symptom in 7% of cases and occurring in around 20% of patients at some point during the course of their disease (Simoff et al. 2013; Kvale et al. 2007). There are many other etiologies for hemoptysis including but not limited to airway diseases (bronchitis, bronchiectasis), pulmonary infections, rheumatic and autoimmune disorders, pulmonary parenchymal and vascular disorders, traumatic, iatrogenic, coagulopathies, and idiopathic (Yendamuri 2015). Although any condition that leads to non-life-threatening hemoptysis can also lead to life-threatening hemoptysis, bronchiectasis, tuberculosis, fungal infections, and primary or metastatic lung lesions account for most of those cases (Xi et al. 2018).

The diagnostic workup of hemoptysis includes a medical history, physical examination, laboratory testing, chest imaging including chest X-ray and computed tomography, and bronchoscopy. This workup, however, can only be entertained when the patient is in a stable condition, and therefore lifesaving interventions should not be delayed.

The initial priorities in cases of life-threatening hemoptysis are protecting the airway to ensure adequate oxygenation and ventilation, assuring hemodynamic stability, and correcting coagulopathies. If the site of bleeding is known, rotating the patient with the bleeding side down should be done immediately as it will decrease the spillage of blood to the unaffected lung. Endotracheal intubation using a large-size single-lumen endotracheal tube is recommended over double-lumen tubes as this provides superior access to the airway for diagnostic and therapeutic interventions. Selective right or left mainstem bronchus intubation can be performed to protect the nonbleeding lung (Kathuria et al. 2020; Davidson and Shojaee 2020).

Computed tomography is successful in detecting the site of bleeding in most patients. Additionally, it offers information on extrapulmonary causes of hemoptysis and can help delineate the bronchial arterial system in cases where embolization is required (Sakr and Dutau 2010). The value of CT may be limited in cases of known lung cancer where the source of bleeding is already known.

Bronchoscopy is recommended to lateralize and—if possible—identify a specific segment or lesion as the source of bleeding (Simoff et al. 2013). Non-life-threatening hemoptysis may be managed with flexible bronchoscopy. Rigid bronchoscopy is preferred in cases of life-threatening hemoptysis if the expertise is readily available and only after a careful clinical evaluation is performed. Rigid bronchoscopy has the advantage of securing the airway while simultaneously allowing the use of large suction catheters and therapeutic tools.

Multiple endobronchial strategies have been tried in cases where the area of bleeding is known but no specific lesion is identified. These include iced saline lavage, balloon tamponade techniques, vasoactive drugs, local delivery of silicone spigots, instillation of tranexamic acid, instillation of gelatin-thrombin, and others (Kathuria et al. 2020; Davidson and Shojaee 2020; Dutau et al. 2006; Peralta et al. 2018; Tsai et al. 2020). When an endobronchial source of bleeding is identified, more direct therapies such as electrocautery and laser photocoagulation using laser or argon plasma coagulation can be used with good results (Jalilie et al. 2016; Han et al. 2007; Morice et al. 2001).

Following stabilization and localization of the bleeding, prompt angioembolization is recommended. This should also be pursued in cases where endobronchial therapies are not readily available or when the severity of bleeding precludes their consideration. Pre-procedural computed tomography and bronchoscopy can help delineate target areas and decrease the time and contrast load required during embolization. The bronchial arteries are the most common culprit vessels; the intercostal, internal mammary, and subclavian artery and its branches are less commonly affected. Bronchial artery embolization for hemoptysis has a clinical success of 70–99%; however, this should be tempered with the high recurrence rate of 10–57% (Panda et al. 2017).

Radiation therapy has an important role after initial stabilization and localization of the source of bleeding. It has a palliation rate of 76–95% for primary lung lesions and 86% for metastatic lung lesions (Fleming et al. 2017). Surgery for the management of life-threatening hemoptysis in patients with lung cancer is generally not indicated due to the generally advanced stage of disease. Additionally, emergent surgery for life-threatening hemoptysis carries a high mortality of around 34% (Andréjak et al. 2009).

8 Conclusion

There are many symptoms associated with lung cancer that can be palliated to allow patients the opportunity to maximize other more definitive treatments of their lung cancer. With newer tools and techniques, we can provide much more advanced care to patients today than ever before. Understanding what can be done is the responsibility of treating physicians. Consultation with a team of experts in the assessment of pulmonary, airways, or pleural disease at your facility or a regional referral center will allow the quickest assessment of a patient's complaints and the most rapid institution of therapeutic measures.

References

Agustí AG, Cardús J, Roca J, Grau JM, Xaubet A, Rodriguez-Roisin R (1997) Ventilation-perfusion mismatch in patients with pleural effusion: effects of thoracentesis. Am J Respir Crit Care Med 156(4 Pt 1):1205–1209

Akhtar N, Ansar F, Baig MS, Abbas A (2016) Airway fires during surgery: management and prevention. J Anaesthesiol Clin Pharmacol 32(1):109–111

American Thoracic Society (2000) Management of malignant pleural effusions. Am J Respir Crit Care Med 162(5):1987–2001

Andréjak C et al (2009) Surgical lung resection for severe hemoptysis. Ann Thorac Surg 88(5):1556–1565

Balazs A, Kupcsulik PK, Galambos Z (2008) Esophagorespiratory fistulas of tumorous origin. Non-operative management of 264 cases in a 20-year period. Eur J Cardiothorac Surg 34(5):1103–1107

Bank J, Voaklander R, Sossenheimer M (2020) H-type tracheoesophageal fistula: a rare cause of cough and dysphagia in adults. ACG Case Rep J 7(12):e00492

Beamis JF, Becker HD, Cavaliere S, Colt H, Diaz-Jimenez JP, Dumon JF, Edell E, Kovitz KL, Macha HN, Mehta AC, Marel M, Noppen M, Strausz J, Sutedja TG (2002) ERS/ATS statement on interventional pulmonology: chairmen: C.T. Bolliger, P.N. Mathur. Eur Respir J 19(2):356–373

Beaudoin EL, Chee A, Stather DR (2015) Interventional pulmonology: an update for internal medicine physicians. Minerva Med 105(3):197–209

Bhatnagar R, Keenan EK, Morley AJ et al (2018) Outpatient talc administration by indwelling pleural catheter for malignant effusion. N Engl J Med 378(14):1313–1322

Bhatnagar R, Piotrowska HEG, Laskawiec-Szkonter M et al (2019) Effect of thoracoscopic talc poudrage vs talc slurry via chest tube on pleurodesis failure rate among patients with malignant pleural effusions: a randomized clinical trial. JAMA 323(1):60–69

Bick BL et al (2013) Stent-associated esophagorespiratory fistulas: incidence and risk factors. Gastrointest Endosc 77(2):181–189

Bolliger CT (2006) Therapeutic bronchoscopy with immediate effect: laser, electrocautery, argon plasma coagulation and stents. Eur Respir J 27(6):1258–1271

Boutin C, Viallat JR, Cargnino P, Farisse P (1981) Thoracoscopy in malignant pleural effusions. Am Rev Respir Dis 124(5):588–592

Brown NE, Zamel N, Aberman A (1978) Changes in pulmonary mechanics and gas exchange following thoracocentesis. Chest 74(5):540–542

Brutinel WM, Cortese DA, McDougall JC et al (1987) A two-year experience with the neodymium-YAG laser in endobronchial obstruction. Chest 91:159–165

Burt M et al (1991) Malignant esophagorespiratory fistula: management options and survival. Ann Thorac Surg 52(6):1222–1228; discussion 1228–1229

Cantó A, Blasco E, Casillas M et al (1977) Thoracoscopy in the diagnosis of pleural effusion. Thorax 32(5):550–554

Chakrabarti B, Ryland I, Sheard J, Warburton CJ, Earis JE (2006) The role of Abrams percutaneous pleural biopsy in the investigation of exudative pleural effusions. Chest 129(6):1549–1555

Chen HY et al (2014) Esophageal perforation during or after conformal radiotherapy for esophageal carcinoma. J Radiat Res 55(5):940–947

Chernow B, Sahn SA (1977) Carcinomatous involvement of the pleura: an analysis of 96 patients. Am J Med 63(5):695–702

Clive AO, Jones HE, Bhatnagar R, Preston NJ, Maskell N (2016) Interventions for the management of malignant pleural effusions: a network meta-analysis. Cochrane Database Syst Rev (5):CD010529

Cortese DA, Edell ES (1993) Role of phototherapy, laser therapy, brachytherapy, and prosthetic stents in the management of lung cancer. Clin Chest Med 14(1):149–159

Davidson K, Shojaee S (2020) Managing massive hemoptysis. Chest 157(1):77–88

Davies HE, Mishra EK, Kahan BC et al (2012) Effect of an indwelling pleural catheter vs chest tube and talc pleurodesis for relieving dyspnea in patients with malignant pleural effusion: the TIME2 randomized controlled trial. JAMA 307(22):2383–2389

de Baere T et al (2015) Evaluating cryoablation of metastatic lung tumors in patients—safety and efficacy: the ECLIPSE trial—interim analysis at 1 year. J Thorac Oncol 10(10):1468–1474

Diaz-Mendoza J, Peralta AR, Debiane L, Simoff MJ (2018) Rigid bronchoscopy. Semin Respir Crit Care Med 39(6):674–684

Diddee R, Shaw IH (2006) Acquired tracheo-oesophageal fistula in adults. Continuing education in anaesthesia. Crit Care Pain 6(3):105–108

Dumon JF (1990) A dedicated tracheobronchial stent. Chest 97(2):328–332

Dutau H et al (2006) Endobronchial embolization with a silicone spigot as a temporary treatment for massive hemoptysis: a new bronchoscopic approach of the disease. Respiration 73(6):830–832

Dutau H et al (2015) Biodegradable airway stents—bench to bedside: a comprehensive review. Respiration 90(6):512–521

Dutau H et al (2020) Impact of silicone stent placement in symptomatic airway obstruction due to non-small cell lung cancer—a French multicenter randomized controlled study: the SPOC trial. Respiration 99(4):344–352

Endo C et al (2009) Results of long-term follow-up of photodynamic therapy for roentgenographically occult bronchogenic squamous cell carcinoma. Chest 136(2):369–375

Escalante CP, Martin CG, Elting LS et al (1996) Dyspnea in cancer patients. Etiology, resource utilization, and survival implications in a managed care world. Cancer 78:1314–1319

Escudero Bueno C, García Clemente M, Cuesta Castro B et al (1990) Cytologic and bacteriologic analysis of fluid and pleural biopsy specimens with Cope's needle. Study of 414 patients. Arch Intern Med 150(6):1190–1194

Estenne M, Yernault JC, De Troyer A (1983) Mechanism of relief of dyspnea after thoracocentesis in patients with large pleural effusions. Am J Med 74(5):813–819

Feller-Kopman DJ, Reddy CB, DeCamp MM et al (2018) Management of malignant pleural effusions. An official ATS/STS/STR clinical practice guideline. Am J Respir Crit Care Med 198(7):839–849

Fentiman IS, Rubens RD, Hayward JL (1983) Control of pleural effusions in patients with breast cancer. A randomized trial. Cancer 52(4):737–739

Fentiman IS, Rubens RD, Hayward JL (1986) A comparison of intracavitary talc and tetracycline for the control of pleural effusions secondary to breast cancer. Eur J Cancer Clin Oncol 22(9):1079–1081

Fleming C et al (2017) Palliative efficacy and local control of conventional radiotherapy for lung metastases. Ann Palliat Med 6(Suppl 1):S21–S27

Freitag L et al (1996) Management of malignant esophagotracheal fistulas with airway stenting and double stenting. Chest 110(5):1155–1160

Freitag L et al (2004) Sequential photodynamic therapy (PDT) and high dose brachytherapy for endobronchial tumour control in patients with limited bronchogenic carcinoma. Thorax 59(9):790–793

Furuse K et al (1993) [Photodynamic therapy (PDT) in roentgenographically occult lung cancer by photofrin II and excimer dye laser]. Gan To Kagaku Ryoho 20(10):1369–1374

Gage AA, Baust J (1998) Mechanisms of tissue injury in cryosurgery. Cryobiology 37(3):171–186

Galbraith S, Fagan P, Perkins P, Lynch A, Booth S (2010) Does the use of a handheld fan improve chronic dyspnea? A randomized, controlled crossover trial. J Pain Symptom Manage 29:831–838

Grosu HB, Kazzaz F, Vakil E, Molina S, Ost D (2018) Sensitivity of initial thoracentesis for malignant pleural effusion stratified by tumor type in patients with strong evidence of metastatic disease. Respiration 96(4):363–369

Grosu HB, Molina S, Casal R et al (2019) Risk factors for pleural effusion recurrence in patients with malignancy. Respirology (Carlton, Vic) 24(1):76–82

Hamed H, Fentiman IS, Chaudary MA, Rubens RD (1989) Comparison of intracavitary bleomycin and talc for control of pleural effusions secondary to carcinoma of the breast. Br J Surg 76(12):1266–1267

Han CC, Prasetyo D, Wright GM (2007) Endobronchial palliation using Nd:YAG laser is associated with improved survival when combined with multimodal adjuvant treatments. J Thorac Oncol 2(1):59–64

Harle AS et al (2012) Understanding cough and its management in lung cancer. Curr Opin Support Palliat Care 6(2):153–162

Hartman DL, Gaither JM, Kesler KA, Mylet DM, Brown JW, Mathur PN (1993) Comparison of insufflated talc under thoracoscopic guidance with standard tetracycline and bleomycin pleurodesis for control of malignant pleural effusions. J Thorac Cardiovasc Surg 105(4):743–747; discussion 747–748

Hayata Y, Kato H, Konaka C, Okunaka T (1993) Photodynamic therapy (PDT) in early-stage lung cancer. J Thorac Oncol 9(1–6):287–293

Heffner JE, Standerfer RJ, Torstveit J, Unruh L (1994) Clinical efficacy of doxycycline for pleurodesis. Chest 105(6):1743–1747

Herth FJ et al (2010) Combined airway and oesophageal stenting in malignant airway-oesophageal fistulas: a prospective study. Eur Respir J 36(6):1370–1374

Hoegler D (1997) Radiotherapy for palliation of symptoms in incurable cancer. Curr Probl Cancer 21:129–183

Hsu C (1987) Cytologic detection of malignancy in pleural effusion: a review of 5,255 samples from 3,811 patients. Diagn Cytopathol 3(1):8–12

Ibrahim WH (2008) Massive haemoptysis: the definition should be revised. Eur Respir J 32(4):1131–1132

Ikeda S (1970) Flexible bronchofiberscope. Ann Otol Rhinol Laryngol 79(5):916–923

Jacox A, Carr DB, Payne R et al (1994) Management of cancer pain: clinical practice guidelines No. 9. AHCPR Publication No. 94-0592, Mar 1994. Agency for Health Care Policy and Research, U.S. Department of Health and Human Services, Public Health Service, Rockville, MD

Jalilie A et al (2016) [Electrocautery and bronchoscopy as a first step for the management of central airway obstruction and associated hemoptysis]. Rev Med Chil 144(11):1417–1423

Jean-Baptiste E (2000) Clinical assessment and management of massive hemoptysis. Crit Care Med 28(5):1642–1647

Jones BU et al (2001) Photodynamic therapy for patients with advanced non-small-cell carcinoma of the lung. Clin Lung Cancer 3(1):37–41; discussion 42

Karetzky MS, Kothari GA, Fourre JA, Khan AU (1978) Effect of thoracentesis on arterial oxygen tension. Respiration 36(2):96–103

Kathuria H et al (2020) Management of life-threatening hemoptysis. J Intensive Care 8:23

Ke M, Wu X, Zeng J (2015) The treatment strategy for tracheoesophageal fistula. J Thorac Dis 7(Suppl 4):S389–S397

Kennedy L, Rusch VW, Strange C, Ginsberg RJ, Sahn SA (1994) Pleurodesis using talc slurry. Chest 106(2):342–346

Kim HS et al (2020) Management of tracheo-oesophageal fistula in adults. Eur Respir Rev 29(158):200094

Krell WS, Rodarte JR (1985) Effects of acute pleural effusion on respiratory system mechanics in dogs. J Appl Physiol (Bethesda, Md: 1985) 59(5):1458–1463. https://doi.org/10.1152/jappl.1985.59.5.1458

Kvale PA, Selecky PA, Prakash UB (2007) Palliative care in lung cancer: ACCP evidence-based clinical practice guidelines (2nd edition). Chest 132(3 Suppl):368s–403s

Lan RS, Lo SK, Chuang ML, Yang CT, Tsao TC, Lee CH (1997) Elastance of the pleural space: a predictor for the outcome of pleurodesis in patients with malignant pleural effusion. Ann Intern Med 126(10):768–774

Lentz RJ, Lerner AD, Pannu JK et al (2019) Routine monitoring with pleural manometry during therapeutic large-volume thoracentesis to prevent pleural-pressure-related complications: a multicentre, single-blind randomized controlled trial. Lancet Respir Med 7(5):447–455

Light RW, Macgregor MI, Luchsinger PC, Ball WC Jr (1972) Pleural effusions: the diagnostic separation of transudates and exudates. Ann Intern Med 77(4):507–513

Light RW, Stansbury DW, Brown SE (1986) The relationship between pleural pressures and changes in pulmonary function after therapeutic thoracentesis. Am Rev Respir Dis 133(4):658–661

Livingston RB, McCracken JD, Trauth CJ, Chen T (1982) Isolated pleural effusion in small cell lung carcinoma: favorable prognosis. A review of the Southwest Oncology Group experience. Chest 81(2):208–211

Loddenkemper R (1981) Thoracoscopy: results in non-cancerous and idiopathic pleural effusions. Poumon Coeur 37(4):261–264

Loddenkemper R (1998) Thoracoscopy—state of the art. Eur Respir J 11(1):213–221

Loddenkemper R, Grosser H, Gabler A, Mai J, Preussler H, Brandt H (1983) Prospective evaluation of biopsy methods in the diagnosis of malignant pleural effusions-intrapatient comparison between pleural fluid cytology, blind needle-biopsy and thoracoscopy. Am Rev Respir Dis 127:114

Maiwand MO et al (2004) The application of cryosurgery in the treatment of lung cancer. Cryobiology 48(1):55–61

Marchese R et al (2020) Secondary carina and lobar bronchi stenting in patients with advanced lung cancer: is it worth the effort? A clinical experience. Ann Thorac Cardiovasc Surg 26(6):320–326

Mårtensson G, Pettersson K, Thiringer G (1985) Differentiation between malignant and non-malignant pleural effusion. Eur J Respir Dis 67(5):326–334

Martínez-Moragón E, Aparicio J, Rogado MC, Sanchis J, Sanchis F, Gil-Suay V (1997) Pleurodesis in malignant pleural effusions: a randomized study of tetracycline versus bleomycin. Eur Respir J 10(10):2380–2383

Menzies R, Charbonneau M (1991) Thoracoscopy for the diagnosis of pleural disease. Ann Intern Med 114(4):271–276. https://doi.org/10.7326/0003-4819-114-4-271

Milanez Campos J, Werebe C, Vargas F, Jatene F, Light RJL (1997) Respiratory failure due to insufflated talc. Lancet 349(9047):251–252

Minnich DJ et al (2010) Photodynamic laser therapy for lesions in the airway. Ann Thorac Surg 89(6):1744–1748; discussion 1748–1749

Moffett MJ, Ruckdeschel JC (1992) Bleomycin and tetracycline in malignant pleural effusions: a review. Semin Oncol 19(2 Suppl 5):59–62; discussion 62–63

Moghissi K et al (1999) The place of bronchoscopic photodynamic therapy in advanced unresectable lung cancer: experience of 100 cases. Eur J Cardiothorac Surg 15(1):1–6

Molassiotis A et al (2010) Clinical expert guidelines for the management of cough in lung cancer: report of a UK task group on cough. Cough 6:9

Molassiotis A et al (2015) Interventions for cough in cancer. Cochrane Database Syst Rev 5(5):CD007881

Morice RC et al (2001) Endobronchial argon plasma coagulation for treatment of hemoptysis and neoplastic airway obstruction. Chest 119(3):781–787

Mullon JJ, Burkart KM, Silvestri G, Hogarth DK, Almeida F, Berkowitz D, Eapen GA, Feller-Kopman D, Fessler HE, Folch E, Gillespie C, Haas A, Islam SU, Lamb C, Levine SM, Majid A, Maldonado F, Musani AI, Piquette C et al (2017) Interventional pulmonology fellowship accreditation standards: executive summary of the Multisociety Interventional Pulmonology Fellowship Accreditation Committee. Chest 151(5):1114–1121

Muniappan A et al (2013) Surgical treatment of nonmalignant tracheoesophageal fistula: a thirty-five-year experience. Ann Thorac Surg 95(4):1141–1146

Muruganandan S, Azzopardi M, Fitzgerald DB et al (2018) Aggressive versus symptom-guided drainage of malignant pleural effusion via indwelling pleural catheters (AMPLE-2): an open-label randomized trial. Lancet Respir Med 6(9):671–680

Okunaka T et al (1999) Lung cancers treated with photodynamic therapy and surgery. Diagn Ther Endosc 5(3):155–160

Oldenburg FA Jr, Newhouse MT (1979) Thoracoscopy. A safe, accurate diagnostic procedure using the rigid thoracoscope and local anesthesia. Chest 75(1):45–50

Ost DE et al (2012) Respiratory infections increase the risk of granulation tissue formation following airway stenting in patients with malignant airway obstruction. Chest 141(6):1473–1481

Ost DE, Jimenez CA, Lei X et al (2014) Quality-adjusted survival following treatment of malignant pleural effusions with indwelling pleural catheters. Chest 145(6):1347–1356

Ost DE, Ernst A, Grosu HB, Lei X, Diaz-Mendoza J, Slade M, Gildea TR, Machuzak MS, Jimenez CA, Toth J, Kovitz KL, Ray C, Greenhill S, Casal RF, Almeida FA, Wahidi MM, Eapen GA, Feller-Kopman D, Morice RC et al (2015) Therapeutic bronchoscopy for malignant central airway obstruction: success rates and impact on dyspnea and quality of life. Chest 147(5):1282–1298

Panda A, Bhalla AS, Goyal A (2017) Bronchial artery embolization in hemoptysis: a systematic review. Diagn Interv Radiol 23(4):307–317

Patz EF Jr, McAdams HP, Erasmus JJ et al (1998) Sclerotherapy for malignant pleural effusions: a prospective randomized trial of bleomycin vs. doxycycline with small-bore catheter drainage. Chest 113(5):1305–1311

Peralta AR, Chawla M, Lee RP (2018) Novel bronchoscopic management of airway bleeding with absorbable gelatin and thrombin slurry. J Bronchology Interv Pulmonol 25(3):204–211

Petrou M, Kaplan D, Goldstraw P (1995) Management of recurrent malignant pleural effusions. The complementary role talc pleurodesis and pleuroperitoneal shunting. Cancer 75(3):801–805

Pien GW, Gant MJ, Washam CL, Sterman DH (2001) Use of an implantable pleural catheter for trapped lung syndrome in patients with malignant pleural effusion. Chest 119(6):1641–1646

Poe RH, Israel RH, Utell MJ, Hall WJ, Greenblatt DW, Kallay MC (1984) Sensitivity, specificity, and predictive values of closed pleural biopsy. Arch Intern Med 144(2):325–328

Ponn RB, Blancaflor J, D'Agostino RS, Kiernan ME, Toole AL, Stern H (1991) Pleuroperitoneal shunting for intractable pleural effusions. Ann Thorac Surg 51(4):605–609

Pope AR, Joseph JH (1989) Pleuroperitoneal shunt for pneumonectomy cavity malignant effusion. Chest 96(3):686–688

Prakash UB, Reiman HM (1985) Comparison of needle biopsy with cytologic analysis for the evaluation of pleural effusion: analysis of 414 cases. Mayo Clin Proc 60(3):158–164. https://doi.org/10.1016/s0025-6196(12)60212-2

Prakash UB, Offord KP, Stubbs SE (1991) Bronchoscopy in North America: the ACCP survey. Chest 100(6):1668–1675

Pulsiripunya C, Youngchaiyud P, Pushpakom R, Maranetra N, Nana A, Charoenratanakul S (1996) The efficacy of doxycycline as a pleural sclerosing agent in malignant pleural effusion: a prospective study. Respirology (Carlton, Vic) 1(1):69–72

Rahman NM, Ali NJ, Brown G et al (2010) Local anaesthetic thoracoscopy: British Thoracic Society pleural disease guideline 2010. Thorax 65(Suppl):2

Reddy C, Majid A, Michaud G, Feller-Kopman D, Eberhardt R, Herth F, Ernst A (2008) Gas embolism following bronchoscopic argon plasma coagulation: a case series. Chest 134(5):1066–1069

Reed MF, Mathisen DJ (2003) Tracheoesophageal fistula. Chest Surg Clin N Am 13(2):271–289

Rehse DH, Aye RW, Florence MG (1999) Respiratory failure following talc pleurodesis. Am J Surg 177(5):437–440

Reich H, Beattie EJ, Harvey JC (1993) Pleuroperitoneal shunt for malignant pleural effusions: a one-year experience. Semin Surg Oncol 9(2):160–162

Roberts ME, Neville E, Berrisford RG, Antunes G, Ali NJ (2010) Management of a malignant pleural effusion: British Thoracic Society pleural disease guideline 2010. Thorax 65(Suppl 2):ii32–ii40

Ross P Jr et al (2006) Incorporation of photodynamic therapy as an induction modality in non-small cell lung cancer. Lasers Surg Med 38(10):881–889

Sahn SA (1985) Malignant pleural effusions. Clin Chest Med 6(1):113–125

Sahn SA (1987) Malignant pleural effusions. Semin Respir Med 9:43–53

Sahn SA (1997) Pleural diseases related to metastatic malignancies. Eur Respir J 10(8):1907–1913

Sakr L, Dutau H (2010) Massive hemoptysis: an update on the role of bronchoscopy in diagnosis and management. Respiration 80(1):38–58

Schulze M, Boehle AS, Kurdow R, Dohrmann P, Henne-Bruns D (2001) Effective treatment of malignant pleural effusion by minimal invasive thoracic surgery: thoracoscopic talc pleurodesis and pleuroperitoneal shunts in 101 patients. Ann Thorac Surg 71(6):1809–1812

Shaw P, Agarwal R (2004) Pleurodesis for malignant pleural effusions. Cochrane Database Syst Rev (1):CD002916

Shen KR et al (2010) Surgical management of acquired nonmalignant tracheoesophageal and bronchoesophageal fistulae. Ann Thorac Surg 90(3):914–918; discussion 919

Siegel RL, Miller KD, Jemal A (2020) Cancer statistics, 2020. CA Cancer J Clin 70(1):7–30

Simoff MJ et al (2013) Symptom management in patients with lung cancer: diagnosis and management of lung cancer, 3rd ed: American College of Chest Physicians evidence-based clinical practice guidelines. Chest 143(5 Suppl):e455S–e497S

Squiers J, Teeter W, Hoopman J, Piepenbrok K, Wagner R, Ferguson R, Nagji A, Peltz M, Wait M, DiMaio JM (2014) Holmium: YAG laser bronchoscopy ablation of benign and malignant airway obstructions: an 8-year experience. Lasers Med Sci. 29:1437–1443

Starr RL, Sherman ME (1991) The value of multiple preparations in the diagnosis of malignant pleural effusions. A cost-benefit analysis. Acta Cytol 35(5):533–537

Thomas R, Fysh ETH, Smith NA et al (2017) Effect of an indwelling pleural catheter vs talc pleurodesis on hospitalization days in patients with malignant pleural effusion: the AMPLE randomized clinical trial. JAMA 318(19):1903–1912

Todd TR, Delarue NC, Ilves R, et al (1980) Talc poudrage for malignant pleural effusion. Chest. 78:542

Tremblay A, Michaud G (2006) Single-center experience with 250 tunneled pleural catheter insertions for malignant pleural effusion. Chest 129(2):362–368

Tsai YS et al (2020) Effects of tranexamic acid on hemoptysis: a systematic review and meta-analysis of randomized controlled trials. Clin Drug Investig 40(9):789–797

van de Molengraft FJ, Vooijs GP (1988) The interval between the diagnosis of malignancy and the development of effusions, with reference to the role of cytologic diagnosis. Acta Cytol 32(2):183–187

Van Meter ME, McKee KY, Kohlwes RJ (2011) Efficacy and safety of tunneled pleural catheters in adults with malignant pleural effusions: a systematic review. J Gen Intern Med 26(1):70–76

Wahidi MM, Reddy C, Yarmus L et al (2017) Randomized trial of pleural fluid drainage frequency in patients with malignant pleural effusions. The ASAP trial. Am J Respir Crit Care Med 195(8):1050–1057

Walker-Renard PB, Vaughan LM, Sahn SA (1994) Chemical pleurodesis for malignant pleural effusions. Ann Intern Med 120(1):56–64

Warren WH, Kalimi R, Khodadadian LM, Kim AW (2008) Management of malignant pleural effusions using the Pleur(x) catheter. Ann Thorac Surg 85(3):1049–1055

World Health Organization (1990) Cancer pain relief and palliative care: report of a WHO Expert Committee. World Health Organization technical report series, 804. World Health Organization, Geneva, pp 1–75

Xi Y et al (2018) [Cause of massive hemoptysis in critical patients and the effect of bronchial artery embolization]. Zhonghua Wei Zhong Bing Ji Jiu Yi Xue 30(7):671–676

Xia H, Wang XJ, Zhou Q, Shi HZ, Tong ZH (2014) Efficacy and safety of talc pleurodesis for malignant pleural effusion: a meta-analysis. PLoS One 9(1):e87060

Xu F et al (2020a) Clinical study of systemic chemotherapy combined with bronchoscopic interventional cryotherapy in the treatment of lung cancer. BMC Cancer 20(1):1089

Xu J et al (2020b) Paclitaxel-eluting silicone airway stent for preventing granulation tissue growth and lung cancer relapse in central airway pathologies. Expert Opin Drug Deliv 17(11):1631–1645

Yarmus L et al (2019) Prospective multicentered safety and feasibility pilot for endobronchial intratumoral chemotherapy. Chest 156(3):562–570

Yendamuri S (2015) Massive airway hemorrhage. Thorac Surg Clin 25(3):255–260

Yim AP, Chan AT, Lee TW, Wan IY, Ho JK (1996) Thoracoscopic talc insufflation versus talc slurry for symptomatic malignant pleural effusion. Ann Thorac Surg 62(6):1655–1658

Young BP, Gildea TR (2017) Initial clinical experience using 3D printing and patient-specific airway stents: compassionate use of 3D printed patient-specific airway stents. Am J Respir Crit Care Med 195: A1711

Part VIII

Other Intrathoracic Malignancies

Thymic Cancer

Gokhan Ozyigit and Pervin Hurmuz

Contents

1   Introduction.. 833
2   Histopathology... 834
3   Prognosis.. 834
4   Workup... 835
5   Staging... 835
6   Treatment... 837
6.1 Surgery... 837
6.2 Radiotherapy.. 838
6.3 Chemotherapy.. 839
6.4 Radiotherapy Technique.............................. 839
6.5 Treatment Volumes....................................... 840
6.6 Treatment Planning....................................... 840
6.7 Recommended Treatment Algorithm...... 845
7   Follow-Up... 846
References.. 846

G. Ozyigit (✉) · P. Hurmuz
Department of Radiation Oncology, Faculty of Medicine, Hacettepe University, Ankara, Turkey
e-mail: gozyigit@hacettepe.edu.tr

1 Introduction

The thymus gland is a capsulated lymphoepithelial organ located in the anterior mediastinum. It is composed of an outer cortex consisting of epithelial cells, and medulla composed of degenerated keratinized epithelial cells (Hassall's corpuscles), myoid cells, thymic lymphocytes, and B lymphocytes. The gland weighs approximately 15 g at birth and 40 g at puberty; however, it slowly involutes in adulthood (Pearse 2006). In early life, the thymus functions in T-lymphocyte differentiation and maturation and releases T lymphocytes into the circulation.

Thymic neoplasms are rare tumors arising from the epithelial cells of thymus and they account for roughly 50% of anterior mediastinal masses. Thymoma and thymic carcinoma are the most frequent anterior mediastinal neoplasms in adults. Thymomas appear benign histologically; however, they may exhibit invasive clinical behavior. Thymic carcinomas (type C thymomas) are highly invasive with higher metastatic potential. Neuroendocrine tumors of the thymus are rare accounting for less than 5% of all neoplasms of the anterior mediastinum and behave aggressively with high local invasion and regional lymph node metastases (Kondo and Monden 2003).

No environmental or infectious factors have been demonstrated to play a role in the pathogenesis of thymic epithelial tumors. Reports on the development of thymoma after radiation, solid-organ transplantation, and immunosuppression, including the context of human immunodeficiency virus infection, are rare. Genetic risk factors, such as multiple endocrine neoplasia 1, may influence the development of thymomas and thymic carcinoids (Girard et al. 2015; Kojima et al. 2006).

Thymoma is mainly seen between ages 40 and 60 with equal gender distribution. It can be associated with myasthenia gravis and a variety of systemic and autoimmune disorders, such as pure red cell aplasia, pancytopenia, hypogammaglobulinemia, and collagen vascular disease (Tomaszek et al. 2009).

Thymic carcinomas are distinct from invasive thymomas both pathologically and clinically with higher capsule invasion and metastasis rates (Eng et al. 2004). Patients with thymic carcinoma are typically middle aged or elderly, and there is a slight male predominance.

2 Histopathology

The WHO classification, developed in 1999 and last revised in 2015, is the most widely accepted system used for the evaluation of thymic epithelial tumors (Marx et al. 2015). This includes several subtypes of thymic tumor based on the relative proportion of epithelial and lymphocytic cells as shown in Table 1.

3 Prognosis

The two most important prognostic factors for thymoma and thymic carcinoma are invasiveness (stage) and completeness of surgical resection. The 5-year and 10-year survival rates for well-encapsulated thymomas without invasion are more than 90%, and for

Table 1 WHO classification of tumors of the thymus

WHO type	Morphologic characteristics
Thymomas	
A	• Bland oval/spindle epithelial cells, rare or no lymphocytes
Atypical A	• Type A thymoma and • ≥4 mitoses/10 HPF and/or • Coagulative tumor necrosis and/or • Hypercellularity
AB	• Types A + B1 or A + B2 • Comprised of at least 10% of each subtype • Subtypes can be intermingled or separated
B	• B1 to B3 • Increase in tumor cells (in relation to thymocytes) • Emergence of cytologic atypia of tumor cells • Presence (B1 > B2) or absence (B3 > B2) of medullary islands
B1	• Medullary elements (paler areas [medullary islands]) with or without Hassall's corpuscle-like elements) • Scattered epithelial cells (<3 contiguous epithelial cells)
B2	• Mixture of epithelial cells and lymphocytes • Medullary elements on occasion
B3	• Polygonal epithelial cells, rare lymphocytes
Uncommon types of thymoma	
Metaplastic thymoma	• Biphasic morphology • Component A: Strands/nests of bland, darker, oval to spindle tumor cells, reminiscent of type A thymoma • Component B: Paler, more elongated spindle cells reminiscent of fibroblasts • Paucity of lymphocytes
Micronodular thymoma with lymphoid stroma	• Nests/nodules of bland oval to spindle tumor cells, reminiscent of type A thymoma (nodular appearance of the tumor on low magnification) • Interspersed reactive lymphoid cells; predominantly of B-cell phenotype-forming follicles with germinal centers; only scattered TdT-positive thymocytes along the interface to the tumor cell nests

Table 1 (continued)

WHO type	Morphologic characteristics
Microscopic thymoma	• Incidental finding within an otherwise benign-appearing thymic gland • Unencapsulated nodule • <1 mm in greatest dimensions • Bland oval to spindle tumor cells, reminiscent of type A thymoma
Sclerosing and/or ossifying thymoma	• Extensive sclerosing fibrosis and/or ossification • Usually at least a few cellular foci comprised of a mixture of lymphocytes and epithelioid cells (Girard et al. 2015; Kojima et al. 2006)
Thymic carcinomas	• Distorted architecture; possibly single-tumor cells • Desmoplasia • Usually more cytologic atypia of tumor cells
Thymic neuroendocrine tumors	
Typical carcinoid tumor	• <2 mitoses/2 mm^2 • No necrosis
Atypical carcinoid tumor	• ≥2 to 10 mitoses/2 mm^2 and/or • Necrosis
Large cell neuroendocrine carcinoma	• >10 mitoses/2 mm^2
Small cell carcinoma	• >10 mitoses/2 mm^2

Abbreviations: *WHO* World Health Organization; *HPF* high-power fields; *TdT* terminal deoxynucleotidyl transferase

invasive thymomas, the rates range from 30% to 70%. In case of thymic carcinoma extensive lymph node dissection (>10 nodes) is needed and disease-free survival (DFS) can be as high as 90% in patients with N0 disease compared to 33% in patients with lymph node-positive disease.

4 Workup

Most thymic tumors are discovered during myasthenia gravis workup or incidentally on chest imaging. Some patients might have cough, chest pain, dyspnea, hoarseness, or superior vena cava syndrome due to local extent of the disease and up to 70% of thymomas may be associated with paraneoplastic syndromes. Initial workup should include physical examination, complete blood count, comprehensive blood chemistry (including serum beta-human chorionic gonadotropin and alpha-fetoprotein to rule out germ cell tumors), and chest computerized tomography (CT) with IV contrast. Chest magnetic resonance imaging (MRI) can be used in case of suspicious thymic cyst and pericardial or great vessel invasion. The role of positron-emission tomography (PET) has not been well established due to variations in fluorodeoxyglucose (FDG) uptake in thymomas. However, PET/CT can help to distinguish thymomas from thymic carcinomas but not for predicting the histologic grade of thymoma (Nakagawa et al. 2017; Benveniste et al. 2013).

The definitive diagnosis of a thymoma or thymic carcinoma requires a tissue diagnosis. For patients thought to have a thymoma that is amenable to complete resection, the initial step is surgical resection. In case of suspicion in imaging and patients with a tumor that is not considered amenable to complete resection or in whom surgery is contraindicated because of age or comorbidity, a tissue diagnosis with a core needle biopsy or an open biopsy is required prior to therapy (Drevet et al. 2019; Gomez et al. 2014). All patients should be managed by a multidisciplinary team experienced in the management of thymoma and thymic cancers.

5 Staging

Masaoka system with the modification proposed by Koga et al. has long been used for staging of thymic epithelial tumors (Koga et al. 1994; Masaoka et al. 1981). This system is based on pathological findings after surgery (Table 2). The first tumor, node, metastasis (TNM) staging system by the American Joint Committee on Cancer (AJCC) for thymic cancers was published in the eighth edition (Table 3).

Table 2 Masaoka-Koga staging system of thymic epithelial tumors

Stage	Definition
I	Grossly and microscopically completely encapsulated
II	(a) Microscopic transcapsular invasion
	(b) Macroscopic invasion into surrounding fatty tissue or grossly adherent to but not through mediastinal pleura or pericardium
III	Macroscopic invasion of neighboring organ (e.g., pericardium, great vessels, or lung)
IV	(a) Pleural or pericardial dissemination
	(b) Lymphogenous or hematogenous metastasis

Table 3 Tumors of the thymus TNM staging AJCC UICC eighth edition

Primary tumor (T)[a,b]

T category	T description
TX	Primary tumor cannot be assessed
T0	No evidence of primary tumor
T1	Tumor encapsulated or extending into the mediastinal fat; may involve the mediastinal pleura
T1a	Tumor with no mediastinal pleura involvement
T1b	Tumor with direct invasion of mediastinal pleura
T2	Tumor with direct invasion of the pericardium (either partial or full thickness)
T3	Tumor with direct invasion into any of the following: lung, brachiocephalic vein, superior vena cava, phrenic nerve, chest wall, or extrapericardial pulmonary artery or veins
T4	Tumor with invasion into any of the following: aorta (ascending, arch, or descending), arch vessels, intrapericardial pulmonary artery, myocardium, trachea, esophagus

Regional lymph nodes (N)[c]

N category	N description
NX	Regional lymph nodes cannot be assessed
N0	No regional lymph node metastasis
N1	Metastasis in anterior (perithymic) lymph nodes
N2	Metastasis in deep intrathoracic or cervical lymph nodes

Distant metastasis (M)

M category	M description
M0	No pleural, pericardial, or distant metastasis
M1	Pleural, pericardial, or distant metastasis
M1a	Separate pleural or pericardial nodule(s)
M1b	Pulmonary intraparenchymal nodule or distant organ metastasis

Prognostic stage groups

The T, N, and M categories are organized into stage groups, as shown in the table. This schema was developed based primarily on outcomes; in the lower stages, recurrence rates in patients with complete resections were judged most relevant, whereas in higher stages, survival in all patients, regardless of the resection status, was weighed more heavily. Practical applicability and clinical implications were also considered. Differences among the stage groups were subjected to statistical analysis and generally were found to have a stepwise progression toward worse survival in multiple patient cohorts (e.g., R0, R-any[d])

When T is …	And N is …	And M is …	Then the stage group is …
T1a,b	N0	M0	I
T2	N0	M0	II
T3	N0	M0	IIIA

Table 3 (continued)

T4	N0	M0	IIIB
Any T	N1	M0	IVA
Any T	N0, N1	M1a	IVA
Any T	N2	M0, M1a	IVB
Any T	Any N	M1b	IVB

Abbreviations: *TNM* tumor, node, metastasis; *AJCC* American Joint Committee on Cancer; *UICC* Union for International Cancer Control

[a] Involvement must be microscopically confirmed in pathological staging, if possible

[b] T categories are defined by "levels" of invasion; they reflect the highest degree of invasion regardless of how many other (lower level) structures are invaded. T1, level 1 structures: Thymus, anterior mediastinal fat, mediastinal pleura; T2, level 2 structures: pericardium; T3, level 3 structures: lung, brachiocephalic vein, superior vena cava, phrenic nerve, chest wall, hilar pulmonary vessels; T4, level 4 structures: aorta (ascending, arch, or descending), arch vessels, intrapericardial pulmonary artery, myocardium, trachea, esophagus

[c] Involvement must be microscopically confirmed in pathological staging, if possible

[d] R0: no residual tumor; R-any: any type of resection (no residual tumor, microscopic residual tumor, or macroscopic residual tumor at the primary cancer site or regional nodal sites)

6 Treatment

6.1 Surgery

Surgery is the primary treatment for thymic tumors. Complete resection that includes total removal of thymus (thymectomy) with surrounding mediastinal fat is an important prognostic factor for survival (Davenport and Malthaner 2008; Strobel et al. 2004; Safieddine et al. 2014). Sometimes resection of the pericardium or lung parenchyma might be required to achieve complete resection with histologically negative margins. Patients with signs or symptoms of myasthenia gravis should be carefully evaluated and treated medically preoperatively due to increased surgical risks. Bilateral phrenic nerve dissection should be avoided to prevent respiratory failure. Pleural spaces should be evaluated for possible tumor implants.

Lymph node dissection has not been routinely performed; however, a standardized lymph node mapping system was proposed by the ITMIG/International Association for the Study of Lung Cancer (IASLC) Thymic Epithelial Tumors Staging Project for reporting and staging (Bhora et al. 2014). In this system, N1 nodes were classified as anterior region nodes, and N2 nodes were classified as deep region nodes. N1 nodes include anterior mediastinal nodes (perithymic, prevascular, para-aortic, and supradiaphragmatic nodes) and anterior cervical nodes. N2 nodes include tracheobronchial and aortopulmonary window nodes, internal mammary nodes, deep cervical nodes, and supraclavicular nodes. For patients with early-stage resectable thymoma total thymectomy is the standard of care while it is recommended to add lymph node dissection in invasive thymomas. For those with thymic carcinoma systematic dissection of minimum ten lymph nodes from N1 to N2 is recommended (Park et al. 2013). If complete resection is not possible due to invasion of tumor to the phrenic nerve, innominate vein, or heart/great vessels neoadjuvant treatment (chemotherapy ± radiotherapy) might be used for making tumor amenable to surgery (Falkson et al. 2009).

Open thymectomy with sternotomy has been the standard surgical approach; however, there is an increasing interest in minimally invasive thymectomy (MIT) approaches like video-assisted thoracic surgery and robotic-assisted thoracic surgery. MIT is associated with less perioperative morbidity and shorter lengths of hospital stay; currently these are not considered as the standard of care due to lack of long-term data. Complete resection remains as one of the most important prognostic factors in thymic neoplasms and is associated with improved survival rates (Corona-Cruz et al. 2018). MIT can achieve similar R0 resection rates to open thymectomy for thymoma; however, long-term follow-up is necessary to evaluate the local recurrence rates (Burt et al. 2017).

6.2 Radiotherapy

6.2.1 Thymoma

6.2.1.1 Masaoka-Koga Stage 1

Complete surgical resection of the entire thymus gland, including all mediastinal tissues anterior to the pericardium, aorta, and superior vena cava from phrenic nerve to phrenic nerve laterally and from the diaphragm inferiorly to the level of the thyroid gland superiorly, including the upper poles of the thymus, is recommended as the standard of care (Falkson et al. 2009). Neither adjuvant nor neoadjuvant chemotherapy or radiotherapy is recommended for R0 resection due to low recurrence rates of 0–2%. Chemoradiation or radiation alone should be considered for patients who are medically unfit for surgery.

6.2.1.2 Masaoka-Koga Stage 2

Complete surgical resection is the standard of care. The role of PORT in stage II disease is controversial. Several retrospective studies suggested that patients with completely resected stage II disease did not have any advantage after PORT, whereas there are other studies including two meta-analyses that suggest that RT might improve local control and survival (Jackson et al. 2017; Song et al. 2020; Liu et al. 2016; Forquer et al. 2010; Utsumi et al. 2009; Singhal et al. 2003; Korst et al. 2009; Zhou et al. 2016). Routine adjuvant radiation is not recommended for stage IIA disease. However, patients with stage IIB disease and stage IIA with high-risk features (larger tumor size, aggressive histology (type B2–B3), or microscopic or grossly positive surgical margins), and postoperative radiotherapy (PORT) appear to reduce the risk of recurrence to that of patients with R0 resections and lower risk features (Drevet et al. 2019).

Neither adjuvant nor neoadjuvant systemic therapy is recommended for stage II disease. Chemoradiation or radiation alone should be considered for patients who are medically unfit for surgery.

6.2.1.3 Masaoka-Koga Stage 3

Surgery should be considered either initially or after neoadjuvant therapy, with the aim being complete removal of the tumor with wide surgical margins. An analysis of the International Thymic Malignancies Interest Group Retrospective Database in 1263 patients with completely resected (R0) stage II or III thymoma evaluated the role of PORT. The 5- and 10-year OS rates for patients having surgery plus PORT were 95% and 86%, respectively, compared with 90% and 79% for patients receiving surgery alone ($p = 0.002$). This OS benefit was valid for stage II ($p = 0.02$) and stage III thymoma ($p = 0.0005$) (Rimner et al. 2016). On multivariate analysis, earlier stage, younger age, absence of paraneoplastic syndrome, and PORT were significantly associated with improved OS.

Another national database analysis for the role of PORT in 4056 patients with Masaoka stage I–IV thymoma and thymic carcinoma was reported. On multivariate analysis of OS in the thymoma cohort adjusted for age, WHO histologic subtype, Masaoka-Koga stage group, surgical margins, and chemotherapy administration, PORT was associated with superior OS ($p = 0.001$). Propensity score-matched analyses confirmed the survival advantage associated with PORT. The study concluded that PORT was associated with longer OS, with the greatest relative benefits observed for stage IIB to III disease and positive margins (Jackson et al. 2017).

Lim et al. evaluated the Surveillance, Epidemiology, and End Results (SEER) database for 529 patients with thymoma for PORT (Lim et al. 2015). Before and after propensity score matching, overall survival ($p = 0.018$ and 0.008, respectively) and disease-specific survival ($p = 0.007$ and 0.008, respectively) were better in the PORT group. In the subgroup analyses, PORT was associated with favorable OS in stages III and IV ($p = 0.049$ and 0.012, respectively) and DSS in stage III disease ($p = 0.005$).

In patients with stage III–IVA disease that is not amenable to initial surgery initial biopsy should be performed followed by induction chemotherapy followed by subsequent surgery or radiotherapy (Girard et al. 2015).

6.2.1.4 Masaoka-Koga Stage IVB
RT should be individualized to the needs of the patient. RT can be used for palliation and possibly as curative therapy in oligometastatic disease.

6.2.2 Thymic Carcinoma
Thymic carcinoma is often associated with severe outcomes and systemic involvement whereas thymomas mostly present with local and regional progression. Complete surgical resection is the mainstay of treatment and an independent prognostic factor of favorable outcome (Safieddine et al. 2014).

Patients with thymic carcinoma have higher local recurrence risks of 20–30% in stage I up to 80% in advanced disease (Drevet et al. 2019; Fu et al. 2016; Detterbeck et al. 2014). Although data is limited it has been shown that patients with R0 resection and who received PORT have improved OS and RFS (Jackson et al. 2017; Fu et al. 2016; Omasa et al. 2015; Ruffini et al. 2014). According to current evidence PORT might be optional in stage I disease and should be considered in stage II disease with R0 resection but is highly recommended after R1 and R2 resection and in stage III–IVA thymic carcinoma (Girard et al. 2015; Drevet et al. 2019; Komaki and Gomez 2014). For patients with R1 resection PORT may be accompanied with systemic chemotherapy, while those with R2 resection, chemoradiotherapy should be utilized especially in thymic carcinoma (Gomez et al. 2014; Komaki and Gomez 2014).

6.2.3 Definitive Radiotherapy
Definitive radiation therapy is generally used for patients with thymic tumors who are not candidates for surgery due to the extent of disease or medical conditions at diagnosis. Addition of chemotherapy to radiotherapy increases the efficiency of radiotherapy. Preoperative chemoradiotherapy appears to increase the rate of complete resection of stage III and IVA thymomas and unresectable thymic carcinomas (Girard et al. 2015; Detterbeck and Parsons 2004).

6.3 Chemotherapy

Chemotherapy is used as the initial therapy in potentially resectable, unresectable, metastatic, or recurrent disease. Induction chemotherapy is standard in nonresectable advanced thymic epithelial tumors. Cisplatin-based combination regimens including combinations of cisplatin, doxorubicin, and cyclophosphamide, and cisplatin and etoposide, should be administered.

6.4 Radiotherapy Technique

6.4.1 Target Volume Determination and Delineation Guidelines
The ITMIG initiative established definitions and reporting guidelines for radiation therapy for thymic malignancies (Gomez et al. 2011). Radiotherapy is predominantly used after surgery, to reduce the risk of mediastinal relapse. However, it can be used as part of definitive treatment for patients that are not medically operable, as a part of preoperative treatment for tumors that are not resectable after neoadjuvant chemotherapy, or for recurrent disease.

6.4.2 Patient Positioning and Simulation

The simulation procedure is similar to that in lung cancer. Patients should be strictly immobilized in a supine position with the neck slightly extended and with their arms over their head, if possible, to move arms away from possible beam angles. CT simulation should be performed with slice thickness of ≤3 mm. Intravenous contrast may be considered to better differentiate the target and normal structures. When available, a four-dimensional (4D) CT scan should be performed, to assess for internal motion during treatment planning; other motion-encompassing options could be slow CT scanning covering the whole breathing cycle or obtaining CT both at inspiratory and expiratory phases to define internal motion (Gomez and Komaki 2010; Keall et al. 2006). A fusion of the treatment planning CT scan with diagnostic FDG PET/CT scan can be helpful in target delineation.

6.5 Treatment Volumes

Gross tumor volume (GTV): If present, it involves gross disease and any macroscopic invasion into thymic or surrounding fatty tissue or organs (mediastinal pleura, pericardium, great vessels, lung, etc.) plus any grossly involved lymph nodes (nodes that are >1 cm in diameter or have a necrotic center or are positive on PET) which should be delineated as determined from CT, MRI, or FDG PET/CT scans (Epstein et al. 2016).

Internal Target Volume (ITV) or Internal GTV (iGTV): The GTV contouring is based on 4D CT data (respiratory datasets are "binned" by phase: 0–100% at 10% intervals) and iGTV is contoured by using the maximum-intensity projection (MIP) settings, with modifications based on visual verification of contours in individual respiratory phases.

Clinical target volume (CTV): CTV encompasses any possible microscopic spread and areas at risk for microscopic spread in addition to the iGTV of the primary tumor and involved nodes, plus the preoperative extent and operative bed if surgery has been done. In the postoperative setting, target volumes should be delineated using a combination of the patient's preoperative and postoperative imaging plus intraoperative findings, including the placement of surgical clips to indicate regions at particular risk for persistent disease. Previously the whole mediastinum was included in CTV; however, with the use of CT-based treatment planning the volumes are more limited. The margin over the iGTV is 0.5–1.0 cm.

Planning Target Volume (PTV): Target margins are dependent on the techniques used during simulation (use of 4D CT simulation for internal motion or not) and use of daily image guidance (e.g., kV-cone beam CT). PTV for setup error depends on the institution, but generally is a 0.5–1 cm expansion from the CTV when using daily image guidance.

Acceptable PTV margins are as follows:

- CTV to PTV margin, without 4D CT simulation (or equivalent) and without daily kV imaging: 1.0–1.5 cm
- ITV to PTV margin, with 4D CT simulation (or equivalent) but without daily kV imaging: 0.5–1.0 cm
- ITV to PTV margin, with 4D CT simulation and daily kV imaging: 0.5 cm

Organs at Risk (OAR): Guidelines for delineating organs at risk have been standardized in RTOG atlases (Roach III et al. 2003).

6.6 Treatment Planning

Historically, 2D radiotherapy technique has been used for the treatment of thymic neoplasms exposing large amounts of uninvolved normal tissues to high doses of radiation. 3D conformal radiation and intensity-modulated radiation (IMRT) with motion management should be considered to improve conformity and spare normal tissues. Current evidence for treatment of thymic tumors is summarized in Table 4.

Radiation for R1 or R2 thymic malignancies should be started within 3 months of surgical

Table 4 Selective adjuvant radiotherapy studies

Author, year	Number of patients	Dose	5-year LC	5-year DFS	5-year OS	Comments
Nakahara et al. (1988)	141	PORT 30–50 Gy	–	–	Stage I: 100% Stage II: 91.5% Stage III: 87.8% Stage IV: 46.6% 97.6% (complete resection) 68.2% (subtotal resection) 25% (biopsy)	Complete resection plus radiation therapy resulted in best survival rates
Curran Jr. et al. (1988)	103	PORT 32–60 Gy	100% (R0, stages II–III) 79% (R1–R2, stages II–III)	Stage I: 100% Stage II: 58% Stage III: 53%	Stage I: 67% Stage II: 86% Stage III: 69%	No recurrence occurred for stage I after R0 resection; PORT improved local control stages II–III
Jackson and Ball (1991)	28	PORT 40–50 Gy	61%	–	53%	High rate of radiation toxicity (11%)
Haniuda et al. (1992)	70	PORT 40–50 Gy	Stage I and stage II R0 with or without PORT: 100% Stage II R1 with PORT: 100% Stage II R1 without PORT: 63.6%	–	Stage II: 74%	PORT is effective in patients with pleural adhesion, without microinvasion
Pollack et al. (1992)	36	PORT/preoperative 40–60 Gy (median 50 Gy)	–	74% for patients who had total resection, 60% for subtotal resection, and 20% for biopsy alone	Stage I: 70% Stage II: 75% Stage III: 58% Stage IVA: 57%	Patients with R1–R2 resections did worse; multimodality treatment is recommended
Cowen et al. (1995)	149	22–50 Gy preoperative 30–70 Gy PORT ± chemotherapy (median, 40–55 Gy)	78.5% Stage I: 100% Stage II: 98% Stage III: 69% Stage IVA: 59%	59.5%	–	Stage and extent of resection effects, local control, and survival

(continued)

Table 4 (continued)

Author, year	Number of patients	Dose	5-year LC	5-year DFS	5-year OS	Comments
Mornex et al. (1995)	90	PORT 30–70 Gy	Stage IIIA: 86% Stages IIIB–IVA: 59%	–	51%	PORT improved LC; doses greater than 50 Gy recommended for incompletely resected tumors
Latz et al. (1997)	43	PORT 10–72 Gy	81%	–	Stage II: 90% Stage III: 67% Stage IV: 30%	Role of radiotherapy for completely resected stage II thymomas is uncertain
Kondo and Monden (2003)	1320	PORT 40 Gy	Stage I: 99.1% Stage II: 95.9% Stage III: 71.6% Stage IV: 65.7%	–	Stage I: 100% Stage II: 98% Stage III: 89% Stage IV: 71%	R0 resection is the most important factor in the treatment
Singhal et al. (2003)	70	PORT 45–55 Gy	98.6%	–	91%	R0 resection alone is sufficient treatment for stage I and II thymoma
Zhu et al. (2004)	175	PORT 50–55 Gy (R0) 60–65 Gy (R1–R2)	Stage II: 96% Stage III: 56% Stage IVA: 43% Stage IVB: 22%	–	Stage II: 96% Stage III: 78% Stage IVA: 57% Stage IVB: 36%	No LC or OS benefit for extended-field versus involved-field radiation therapy
Chang et al. (2011)	76	PORT (43.2–66 Gy) (median 50 Gy)	Median time to recurrence 37.4 in surgery and 50.6 months in PORT	Surgery: 80% PORT: 97.8%	95.3%	PORT was beneficial in stage II and III thymoma
Omasa et al. (2015)	155 thymic carcinomas, 1110 thymoma	–	–	PORT for stage II and III TC, hazard ratio, 0.48, $p = 0.03$ PORT for stage II and III thymoma: NS	PORT for stage II and III TC, hazard ratio, 0.94 $p = 0.53$ PORT for stage II and III thymoma: NS	PORT was beneficial in stage II and III TC

Abbreviations: *PORT* postoperative radiotherapy; *RT* radiotherapy, *TC* thymic carcinoma; *LC* local control; *DFS* disease-free survival; *OS* overall survival resection (Komaki and Gomez 2014; Gomez et al. 2011). PORT doses above 45 Gy have been shown to improve DFS and OS in patients with invasive stage II thymoma (Kundel et al. 2007). It was thought that 40–45 Gy is sufficient for the control of R0 or R1 disease but in a retrospective study, Zhu et al. revealed that increasing the dose above 50 Gy is a prognostic factor for 5-year survival in unresectable disease and there are other studies stating that doses above 60 Gy are necessary for incompletely resected or gross disease (Mornex et al. 1995; Zhu et al. 2004; Ogawa et al. 2002; Ciernik et al. 1994; Fuller et al. 2010).

ITMIG guidelines propose that the minimum postoperative adjuvant dose for patients with R0 resection for thymoma should be 40 Gy in 1.8–2 Gy per fractions; doses below 54 Gy are not recommended for gross residual disease; and doses above 64 Gy are not considered appropriate in the postoperative setting (Gomez et al. 2011). Proton radiation therapy can be used to reduce cardiac dose in cases in which the treatment volume is very large due to its dose distribution advantages. Recommended doses are shown in Table 5.

Normal tissue constraints can be based on the quantitative analysis of normal tissue effects in the clinic (QUANTEC) guidelines with normal tissue complication probability models (Table 6) (Gomez et al. 2011; Marks et al. 2010).

Figure 1 shows radiotherapy volumes and treatment planning in a patient receiving adjuvant radiotherapy.

Table 5 Recommended radiotherapy treatment doses

Status	Total dose (1.8–2 Gy/fraction)
Adjuvant radiotherapy	
Clear/close margins	45–50 Gy
R1	54 Gy
R2	60–70 Gy
Unresectable disease	60–70 Gy
	54 Gy with concomitant chemotherapy

Table 6 Dosimetric constraints to be used and reported in the treatment of thymic malignancies

	RT alone	Chemotherapy and RT	Chemotherapy and RT before surgery
Spinal cord	Dmax <45 Gy	Dmax <45 Gy	Dmax <45 Gy
Lung	MLD ≤20 Gy	MLD ≤20 Gy	MLD ≤20 Gy
	V20 ≤40%	V20 ≤35%	V20 ≤30%
		V10 ≤45%	V10 ≤40%
		V5 ≤65%	V5 ≤55%
Heart	V30 ≤45%	V30 ≤45%	V30 ≤45%
	Mean dose	Mean dose	Mean dose
	<26 Gy	<26 Gy	<26 Gy
Esophagus	Dmax ≤80 Gy	Dmax ≤80 Gy	Dmax ≤80 Gy
	V70 <20%	V70 <20%	V70 <20%
	V50 <50%	V50 <40%	V50 <40%
	Mean dose	Mean dose	Mean dose
	<34 Gy	<34 Gy	<34 Gy
Kidney	20 Gy <32% of bilateral kidney	20 Gy <32% of bilateral kidney	20 Gy <32% of bilateral kidney
Liver	V30 ≤40%	V30 ≤40%	V30 ≤40%
	Mean dose	Mean dose	Mean dose
	<30 Gy	<30 Gy	<30 Gy

Abbreviations: *RT* radiotherapy; *MLD* mean lung dose; *Dmax* maximal dose; *PTV* planning target volume; *CTV* clinical target volume; *GTV* gross tumor volume

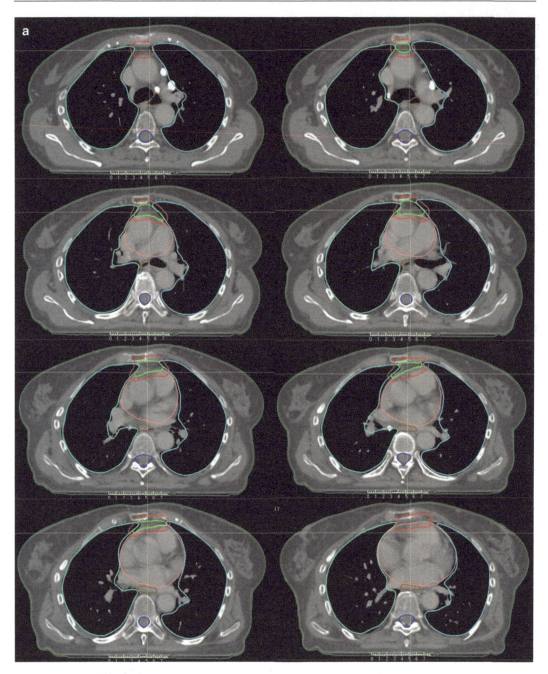

Fig. 1 A 72-year-old female patient with 2.2 × 1.7 cm mass in anterior mediastinum underwent surgery. Pathology report revealed that the mass was thymoma (WHO type B2) invading the mediastinal fatty tissue and it was removed with clear surgical margins (Masaoka-Koga stage IIB, R0 resection). (**a**) The clinical target volume (green) and planning target volume (red) were defined and 50 Gy in 25 fractions was prescribed to cover the preoperative mass and operative area. (**b**) Intensity-modulated radiotherapy treatment plan of the patient

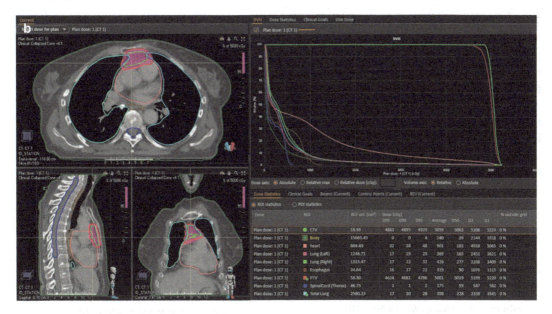

Fig. 1 (continued)

6.7 Recommended Treatment Algorithm

The initial treatment for thymic tumors is surgery if feasible. Adjuvant radiotherapy should be considered for patients with features at high risk for recurrence. Definitive radiation can be considered for a nonresectable or inoperable tumor. The recommended algorithm for the treatment of thymoma and thymic carcinoma is summarized in Table 7.

The following guidelines should be considered:

- Patients with stage I thymoma should not receive adjuvant therapy after a complete thymectomy (R0 resection, negative margins) with close interval surveillance imaging.
- Patients with stage II thymoma with R1 or R2 resection may benefit from adjuvant RT. Doses of 50–60 Gy are generally recommended.
- Patients with stage II thymic carcinoma can be treated with adjuvant radiation after R0 resection to doses of 50–54 Gy.
- Patients with stage III–IVA thymic neoplasms are recommended to receive adjuvant radiotherapy after R0.

Table 7 Recommended treatment algorithm for thymoma and thymic carcinoma according to the Masaoka-Koga staging system

WHO pathology	Stage I		Stage II		Stage III		Stage IVA
	R0	R1–R2	R0	R1–R2	R0	R1–R2	R1–R2
A–B1	–	RT	–	RT	RT	RT	CRT
B2, B3, TCa	–	RT	RT	CRT	RT/CRT	CRT	CRT

Abbreviations: *R0* complete resection; *R1–R2* microscopic/gross residual disease; *RT* postoperative radiotherapy; *CRT* concurrent or sequential chemotherapy and radiotherapy

- Patients with thymic neoplasms and R1–R2 resection benefit from adjuvant radiotherapy. Doses of 50–60 Gy are generally recommended. Radiation doses below 54 Gy are inadequate for gross residual disease.
- Management of unresectable disease is controversial. These can be treated with induction chemotherapy ± neoadjuvant chemoradiation followed by surgery.
- If surgery is not possible definitive radiotherapy can be delivered.

7 Follow-Up

Follow up with chest CT with IV contrast every 6 months for 2 years, then annually for 5 years for thymic carcinoma, and 10 years for thymoma is recommended (Gomez et al. 2014). Complete remission through clinical examination and imaging studies is necessary. MRI and FDG PET/CT might be helpful to distinguish viable residual or slowly regressing tumor or post-therapy changes in case of suspicion.

References

Benveniste MFK, Moran CA, Mawlawi O et al (2013) FDG PET-CT aids in the preoperative assessment of patients with newly diagnosed thymic epithelial malignancies. J Thorac Oncol 8:502–510

Bhora FY, Chen DJ, Detterbeck FC et al (2014) The ITMIG/IASLC thymic epithelial tumors staging project: a proposed lymph node map for thymic epithelial tumors in the forthcoming 8th edition of the TNM classification of malignant tumors. J Thorac Oncol 9:S88–S96

Burt BM, Yao X, Shrager J et al (2017) Determinants of complete resection of thymoma by minimally invasive and open thymectomy: analysis of an international registry. J Thorac Oncol 12:129–136

Chang JH, Kim HJ, Wu H-G, Kim JH, Kim YT (2011) Postoperative radiotherapy for completely resected stage II or III thymoma. J Thorac Oncol 6:1282–1286

Ciernik IF, Meier U, Lütolf UM (1994) Prognostic factors and outcome of incompletely resected invasive thymoma following radiation therapy. J Clin Oncol 12:1484–1490

Corona-Cruz JF, López-Saucedo RA, Ramírez-Tirado LA et al (2018) Extended resections of large thymomas: importance of en bloc thymectomy. J Thorac Dis 10:3473–3481

Cowen D, Richaud P, Mornex F et al (1995) Thymoma: results of a multicentric retrospective series of 149 non-metastatic irradiated patients and review of the literature. FNCLCC trialists. Fédération Nationale des Centres de Lutte Contre le Cancer. Radiother Oncol 34:9–16

Curran WJ Jr, Kornstein MJ, Brooks JJ, Turrisi AT III (1988) Invasive thymoma: the role of mediastinal irradiation following complete or incomplete surgical resection. J Clin Oncol 6:1722–1727

Davenport E, Malthaner RA (2008) The role of surgery in the management of thymoma: a systematic review. Ann Thorac Surg 86:673–684

Detterbeck FC, Parsons AM (2004) Thymic tumors. Ann Thorac Surg 77:1860–1869

Detterbeck FC, Stratton K, Giroux D et al (2014) The IASLC/ITMIG Thymic Epithelial Tumors Staging Project: proposal for an evidence-based stage classification system for the forthcoming (8th) edition of the TNM classification of malignant tumors. J Thorac Oncol 9:S65–S72

Drevet G, Collaud S, Tronc F, Girard N, Maury J-M (2019) Optimal management of thymic malignancies: current perspectives. Cancer Manag Res 11:6803–6814

Eng TY, Fuller CD, Jagirdar J, Bains Y, Thomas CR Jr (2004) Thymic carcinoma: state of the art review. Int J Radiat Oncol Biol Phys 59:654–664

Epstein JI, Egevad L, Amin MB et al (2016) The 2014 International Society of Urological Pathology (ISUP) consensus conference on Gleason grading of prostatic carcinoma definition of grading patterns and proposal for a new grading system. Am J Surg Pathol 40:244–252

Falkson CB, Bezjak A, Darling G et al (2009) The management of thymoma: a systematic review and practice guideline. J Thorac Oncol 4:911–919

Forquer JA, Rong N, Fakiris AJ, Loehrer PJ Sr, Johnstone PA (2010) Postoperative radiotherapy after surgical resection of thymoma: differing roles in localized and regional disease. Int J Radiat Oncol Biol Phys 76:440–445

Fu H, Gu ZT, Fang WT et al (2016) Long-term survival after surgical treatment of thymic carcinoma: a retrospective analysis from the Chinese Alliance for Research of Thymoma Database. Ann Surg Oncol 23:619–625

Fuller CD, Ramahi EH, Aherne N, Eng TY, Thomas CR Jr (2010) Radiotherapy for thymic neoplasms. J Thorac Oncol 5:S327–S335

Girard N, Ruffini E, Marx A, Faivre-Finn C, Peters S (2015) Thymic epithelial tumours: ESMO Clinical Practice Guidelines for diagnosis, treatment and follow-up. Ann Oncol 26(Suppl 5):v40–v55

Gomez D, Komaki R (2010) Technical advances of radiation therapy for thymic malignancies. J Thorac Oncol 5:S336–S343

Gomez D, Komaki R, Yu J, Ikushima H, Bezjak A (2011) Radiation therapy definitions and reporting guidelines for thymic malignancies. J Thorac Oncol 6:S1743–S1748

Gomez D, Komaki R, Yu J, Ikushima H, Bezjak A (2014) [Radiation therapy definitions and reporting guidelines for thymic malignancies]. Zhongguo Fei Ai Za Zhi 17:110–115

Haniuda M, Morimoto M, Nishimura H, Kobayashi O, Yamanda T, Iida F (1992) Adjuvant radiotherapy after complete resection of thymoma. Ann Thorac Surg 54:311–315

Jackson MA, Ball DL (1991) Post-operative radiotherapy in invasive thymoma. Radiother Oncol 21:77–82

Jackson MW, Palma DA, Camidge DR et al (2017) The impact of postoperative radiotherapy for thymoma and thymic carcinoma. J Thorac Oncol 12:734–744

Keall PJ, Mageras GS, Balter JM et al (2006) The management of respiratory motion in radiation oncology report of AAPM Task Group 76. Med Phys 33:3874–3900

Koga K, Matsuno Y, Noguchi M et al (1994) A review of 79 thymomas: modification of staging system and reappraisal of conventional division into invasive and non-invasive thymoma. Pathol Int 44:359–367

Kojima Y, Ito H, Hasegawa S, Sasaki T, Inui K (2006) Resected invasive thymoma with multiple endocrine neoplasia type 1. Jpn J Thorac Cardiovasc Surg 54:171–173

Komaki R, Gomez DR (2014) Radiotherapy for thymic carcinoma: adjuvant, inductive, and definitive. Front Oncol 3:330

Kondo K, Monden Y (2003) Therapy for thymic epithelial tumors: a clinical study of 1,320 patients from Japan. Ann Thorac Surg 76:878–884; discussion 884–885

Korst RJ, Kansler AL, Christos PJ, Mandal S (2009) Adjuvant radiotherapy for thymic epithelial tumors: a systematic review and meta-analysis. Ann Thorac Surg 87:1641–1647

Kundel Y, Yellin A, Popovtzer A et al (2007) Adjuvant radiotherapy for thymic epithelial tumor: treatment results and prognostic factors. Am J Clin Oncol 30:389–394

Latz D, Schraube P, Oppitz U et al (1997) Invasive thymoma: treatment with postoperative radiation therapy. Radiology 204:859–864

Lim YJ, Kim HJ, Wu HG (2015) Role of postoperative radiotherapy in nonlocalized thymoma: propensity-matched analysis of surveillance, epidemiology, and end results database. J Thorac Oncol 10:1357–1363

Liu Q, Gu Z, Yang F et al (2016) The role of postoperative radiotherapy for stage I/II/III thymic tumor-results of the ChART retrospective database. J Thorac Dis 8:687–695

Marks LB, Yorke ED, Jackson A et al (2010) Use of normal tissue complication probability models in the clinic. Int J Radiat Oncol Biol Phys 76:S10–S19

Marx A, Chan JKC, Coindre J-M et al (2015) The 2015 World Health Organization classification of tumors of the thymus: continuity and changes. J Thorac Oncol 10:1383–1395

Masaoka A, Monden Y, Nakahara K, Tanioka T (1981) Follow-up study of thymomas with special reference to their clinical stages. Cancer 48:2485–2492

Mornex F, Resbeut M, Richaud P et al (1995) Radiotherapy and chemotherapy for invasive thymomas: a multicentric retrospective review of 90 cases. The FNCLCC trialists. Fédération Nationale des Centres de Lutte Contre le Cancer. Int J Radiat Oncol Biol Phys 32:651–659

Nakagawa K, Takahashi S, Endo M, Ohde Y, Kurihara H, Terauchi T (2017) Can (18)F-FDG PET predict the grade of malignancy in thymic epithelial tumors? An evaluation of only resected tumors. Cancer Manag Res 9:761–768

Nakahara K, Ohno K, Hashimoto J et al (1988) Thymoma: results with complete resection and adjuvant postoperative irradiation in 141 consecutive patients. J Thorac Cardiovasc Surg 95:1041–1047

Ogawa K, Uno T, Toita T et al (2002) Postoperative radiotherapy for patients with completely resected thymoma: a multi-institutional, retrospective review of 103 patients. Cancer 94:1405–1413

Omasa M, Date H, Sozu T et al (2015) Postoperative radiotherapy is effective for thymic carcinoma but not for thymoma in stage II and III thymic epithelial tumors: the Japanese Association for Research on the Thymus Database Study. Cancer 121:1008–1016

Park IK, Kim YT, Jeon JH et al (2013) Importance of lymph node dissection in thymic carcinoma. Ann Thorac Surg 96:1025–32; discussion 32

Pearse G (2006) Normal structure, function and histology of the thymus. Toxicol Pathol 34:504–514

Pollack A, Komaki R, Cox JD et al (1992) Thymoma: treatment and prognosis. Int J Radiat Oncol Biol Phys 23:1037–1043

Rimner A, Yao X, Huang J et al (2016) Postoperative radiation therapy is associated with longer overall survival in completely resected stage II and III thymoma-an analysis of the International Thymic Malignancies Interest Group Retrospective Database. J Thorac Oncol 11:1785–1792

Roach M III, DeSilvio M, Lawton C et al (2003) Phase III trial comparing whole-pelvic versus prostate-only radiotherapy and neoadjuvant versus adjuvant combined androgen suppression: Radiation Therapy Oncology Group 9413. J Clin Oncol 21:1904–1911

Ruffini E, Detterbeck F, Van Raemdonck D et al (2014) Tumours of the thymus: a cohort study of prognostic factors from the European Society of Thoracic Surgeons database. Eur J Cardiothorac Surg 46:361–368

Safieddine N, Liu G, Cuningham K et al (2014) Prognostic factors for cure, recurrence and long-term survival after surgical resection of thymoma. J Thorac Oncol 9:1018–1022

Singhal S, Shrager JB, Rosenthal DI, LiVolsi VA, Kaiser LR (2003) Comparison of stages I-II thymoma treated by complete resection with or without adjuvant radiation. Ann Thorac Surg 76:1635–1641; discussion 1641–1642

Song SH, Suh JW, Yu WS et al (2020) The role of postoperative radiotherapy in stage II and III thymoma: a Korean multicenter database study. J Thorac Dis 12:6680–6689

Strobel P, Bauer A, Puppe B et al (2004) Tumor recurrence and survival in patients treated for thymomas and thymic squamous cell carcinomas: a retrospective analysis. J Clin Oncol 22:1501–1509

Tomaszek S, Wigle DA, Keshavjee S, Fischer S (2009) Thymomas: review of current clinical practice. Ann Thorac Surg 87:1973–1980

Utsumi T, Shiono H, Kadota Y et al (2009) Postoperative radiation therapy after complete resection of thymoma has little impact on survival. Cancer 115:5413–5420

Zhou D, Deng XF, Liu QX, Zheng H, Min JX, Dai JG (2016) The effectiveness of postoperative radiotherapy in patients with completely resected thymoma: a meta-analysis. Ann Thorac Surg 101:305–310

Zhu G, He S, Fu X, Jiang G, Liu T (2004) Radiotherapy and prognostic factors for thymoma: a retrospective study of 175 patients. Int J Radiat Oncol Biol Phys 60:1113–1119

Advances in Radiation Therapy for Malignant Pleural Mesothelioma

Gwendolyn M. Cramer, Charles B. Simone II, Theresa M. Busch, and Keith A. Cengel

Contents

1	Introduction	850
2	RT for MPM	850
3	Palliative RT for MPM Symptom Management	852
4	Surgical Cytoreduction and RT	852
5	Neoadjuvant Hemithoracic RT Prior to EPP	853
6	Adjuvant Hemithoracic RT Following EPP	853
7	Adjuvant Hemithoracic RT Following eP/D	855
8	SBRT Salvage	856
9	Adjuvant Prophylactic RT to Interventional Sites	856
10	RT and Immunotherapies	857
11	Future Roles for RT in MPM	858
	References	859

Abstract

Malignant pleural mesothelioma (MPM) is a relatively rare, aggressive, and heterogeneous disease in both tumor architecture and treatment response. This intratumoral and intertumoral heterogeneity necessitates a multidisciplinary treatment plan for patients that is modified over the course of their disease. Currently, radiation therapy (RT) is most commonly used in the palliative setting to manage symptoms in patients with advanced disease. Definitive standard treatment options in patients incorporate RT in conjunction with surgical cytoreduction and chemotherapy, although local tumor recurrence is still common. Advances in RT delivery technology to improve tumor selectivity, in combination with immunotherapies and advances in surgical techniques, will increase the potential for RT-assisted durable local control for MPM. Continued innovation in RT, supported by clinical trials to determine optimal multidisciplinary care strategies, has enormous potential to improve morbidity and survival in patients with MPM.

G. M. Cramer · T. M. Busch · K. A. Cengel (✉)
Department of Radiation Oncology, Hospital of the University of Pennsylvania, Perelman School of Medicine, Philadelphia, PA, USA
e-mail: keith.cengel@pennmedicine.upenn.edu

C. B. Simone II
Department of Radiation Oncology, New York Proton Center, New York, NY, USA

1 Introduction

The asbestos-associated malignant pleural mesothelioma (MPM) is a relatively rare and highly aggressive malignancy of the mesothelial lining of the pleura. It is a heterogeneous disease in both tumor architecture and treatment response; the intratumoral and intertumoral heterogeneity necessitates a multidisciplinary treatment plan for patients that is modified over the course of their disease. The various histologic subtypes of MPM include approximately 60% epithelioid and 40% nonepithelioid types (including subtypes of sarcomatoid, spindle, desmoplastic, fibrous, biphasic, and not otherwise specified) (Inai 2008). While epithelioid histology and early-stage disease are associated with better prognoses, median survival for MPM patients generally ranges from only 6 to 18 months. Patients are often diagnosed at an advanced stage and can present with a variety of symptoms, including significant dyspnea due to pleural effusion (in earlier stages) or tumor bulk-induced respiratory restriction (in later stages), chest wall/thoracic pain, and anorexia.

Treatment usually consists of chemotherapy, and in surgical candidates, definitive standard treatment options also incorporate radiation therapy (RT) in conjunction with cytoreduction through extrapleural pneumonectomy (EPP) or extended pleurectomy/decortication (eP/D) with improved survival. Since local tumor recurrence is still common even with these multimodal therapies, additional strategies suggested to improve tumor control include fluorescence-guided resection (Predina et al. 2019), hyperthermic intraoperative chemotherapy (Burt et al. 2018), intraoperative photodynamic therapy (Rice et al. 2019), immunotherapies (Aggarwal et al. 2018), and neoadjuvant hemithoracic RT. Currently, RT is most commonly used in the palliative setting for MPM to manage symptoms in patients with advanced disease. It is also used as part of the trimodal therapy for patients receiving chemotherapy, surgical resection, and postoperative RT, and it has an emerging role as a definitive treatment in patients not eligible for surgery.

2 RT for MPM

While RT can provide durable local control for MPM, the relative radiosensitivity of surrounding organs and the disseminated nature of the disease/pleura limit the ability to safely deliver optimal RT doses for MPM patients. Advances in RT delivery technology are supporting greater roles for RT at various stages of MPM. 2D/3D conformal treatment planning consists of geometric field shapes (portals) defined by multileaf collimator (MLC) blocks, typically delivered from 1 to 4 beam angles. Photon dose distribution complexity can be further refined by modulating the fluence across each portal with multiple MLC configurations per portal (intensity-modulated radiation therapy, IMRT). Alternatively, conformality can be achieved by moving the gantry in a rotational arc with continuous MLC adjustments during beam delivery (volumetric modulated arc therapy, VMAT). The increased dose gradient conformality gained from both of these techniques is achieved at the cost of an increased volume of normal tissues receiving low doses of radiation, described as a "low-dose wash" effect.

While these treatment planning techniques have decreased toxicity compared to older techniques, the trade-off of increased radiation to normal tissues is particularly concerning in MPM due to the low RT tolerance of nearby healthy organs. This normal tissue radiosensitivity hinders the delivery of a curative RT dose to all pleural surfaces using conventional RT (photons/electrons) while preserving normal/sufficient cardiopulmonary function.

Because protons have different physical characteristics in tissues, including the potential for no exit dose, proton RT has the potential to provide a greater degree of spatial control and deliver increased doses to tumor or areas at risk of recurrence while sparing dose to critical normal tissues. Reports of proton RT as a part of a multimodality management schema demonstrate the potential to achieve dramatic and long-lasting clinical benefits for patients with MPM (Li et al. 2015; Pan et al. 2015). Still, proton RT is limited by the risk of RT-induced toxicities to the

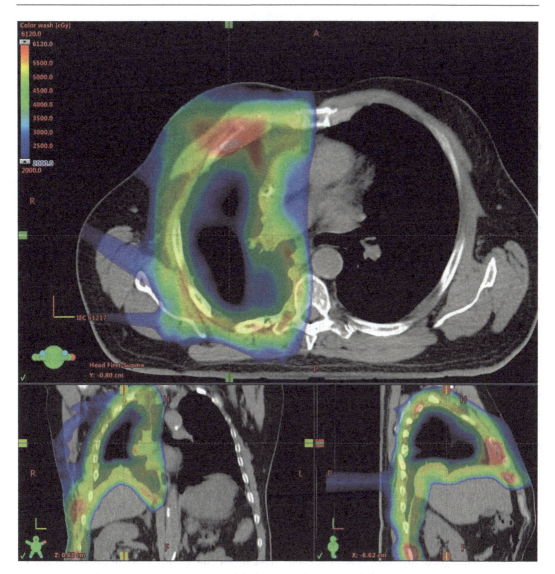

Fig. 1 Hemithoracic IMPT dose distribution for a patient with multifocal recurrent disease approximately 2 years after surgery. Dose prescribed was 50.4 Gy (1.8 Gy/fraction) to entire pleura with a simultaneous in field boost to 61.6 Gy (2.2 Gy/fraction) given in 28 fractions

ipsilateral lung. Attempting to treat the entirety of the pleura, including the major/minor fissures, typically results in very little dose sparing for the ipsilateral lung. Thus, in clinical trials of pleural RT with intact lung, RT has been typically limited to the treatment of peripheral pleural surfaces in the definitive or adjuvant settings or to treating specific, symptomatic regions in the palliative setting. Proton RT to the entire peripheral pleura can also be used to successfully treat multifocal pleural recurrences after lung-sparing surgery (Fig. 1). In select patients with few comorbidities, RT with definitive intent can lead to significantly higher median survivals than has been reported with palliative therapies. For example, in the absence of surgical resection, RT has been used definitively in selected patients to treat bulky areas of disease or even all glycolytically active (FDG-avid) diseases (Feigen et al. 2011).

3 Palliative RT for MPM Symptom Management

Symptoms of dyspnea and pain in MPM patients arise from complex etiological factors. Dyspnea can be caused by compressive atelectasis of the lung by a tumor mass and/or pleural effusion, decreased lung compliance/ventilation with a restrictive pattern due to circumferential involvement of lung by tumor, and alteration in ventilation-perfusion matching. MPM invasion into structures such as the chest wall, spinal nerve roots/intercostal nerves, or diaphragm can be identified as an anatomic correlate of regional/localized pain based on the review of patient pain symptoms and cross-sectional imaging. Pain can also result from diffuse pleural involvement by MPM, contracture of the pleural tumor rind leading to impingement-related pain as the ipsilateral ribs are drawn closer together, or malignant pleural effusion. Palliative therapies for these symptoms include physiologically directed therapies such as drainage of pleural effusions, medically directed therapies such as chemotherapy, and symptom-directed therapies such as narcotic analgesics or nerve blocks. RT is also the standard of care in the palliative setting to relieve symptoms arising from MPM compression or invasion of normal structures and organs. In general, palliative RT aims to identify and alleviate the most proximal or significant cause of distress and can be highly successful, especially for symptoms with good anatomic correlates on cross-sectional imaging caused by a limited extent of the total tumor burden.

Despite the known sensitivity of MPM cells to RT, the ideal RT dose fractionation strategy and response rates in the palliative setting often go unreported. One retrospective study of RT in 54 patients with advanced MPM reported an in-field radiologic response rate of 43% at 2 months, which compares favorably with objective response rates for multiagent chemotherapy (Jenkins et al. 2011). Since MPM tumors can take several months to reach minimal size following RT, this 2-month time point may actually underestimate the true objective response rate for RT. It is also important to note that a decrease in painful symptoms is frequently reported by patients prior to, or in the absence of, objective tumor shrinkage. This can be seen in the comparison of the 43% 2-month response rate noted above with a systematic review of the largely retrospective or descriptive studies present in the literature in which the reported RT response rates for pain range from 50 to 69% (Macleod et al. 2014). To better measure response rates and help define a more standard approach to palliative RT in patients with MPM, Macleod et al. undertook a phase II trial (SYSTEMS) of RT for pain palliation. In this study, 40 patients were recruited from three oncology centers in the United Kingdom, and 35 of these patients (88%) went on to receive palliative RT (MacLeod et al. 2015). Five weeks after receiving 20 Gy in five daily fractions, 47% of the 30 assessable patients experienced an improvement in pain scores and 14/19 patients achieved either a partial response or a stable disease by modified RECIST 1.1 criteria for an overall response rate of 74% at 12 weeks. These encouraging results have led the investigators to initiate the SYSTEMS-2 trial, a randomized trial of 20 Gy in five fractions vs. 36 Gy in six fractions to determine whether dose escalation might further improve pain palliation.

4 Surgical Cytoreduction and RT

Due to both the locally extensive nature of MPM and risk of systemic spread, multiple treatment modalities are typically combined in definitive approaches to managing patients. The combination of aggressive local and systemic treatment strategies to address this is nevertheless limited by the potential morbidities of these treatment regimens. While no single approach is entirely effective in the definitive management of MPM, the strategy in any definitive surgery-based multimodal treatment plan is to employ surgical cytoreduction to a macroscopic complete resection (MCR) and then utilize other therapies such as intraoperative adjuvants to control the inevitably present microscopic residual disease. There are two main surgical strategies for achieving

MCR for MPM. One method involves an extrapleural pneumonectomy (EPP), in which the parietal pleura, diaphragm, pericardium, and lung are all resected en bloc. The other commonly used method is a lung-sparing pleurectomy/decortication (P/D), which is often referred to as an extended P/D (eP/D) or radical pleurectomy when performed to attain MCR. There is no single surgical standard of care to achieve MCR for MPM patients, and both EPP and eP/D are performed at high-volume MPM surgical centers (Rusch et al. 2013; Taioli et al. 2015) depending on the patient presentation and surgeon's discretion. Notably, patients with epithelioid histology appear to benefit most from surgery; sarcomatoid histology is generally associated with the same or worse survival after treatment plans that incorporate surgical cytoreduction compared with systemic therapy alone.

5 Neoadjuvant Hemithoracic RT Prior to EPP

Preoperative RT is performed as the standard treatment for many malignancies, including lung (Chen et al. 2018) and colorectal cancers (van Gijn et al. 2011). A recent phase I–II trial (Surgery for Mesothelioma After Radiation Therapy, SMART) tested the feasibility of this method for MPM. Patients received 25 Gy in five daily fractions to the entire hemithorax with a simultaneous in-field boost to 30 Gy to areas of high-risk disease. Patients then went on to receive an EPP typically within 1 week of radiotherapy completion. Although there was a relatively high morbidity rate, this treatment combination was clinically feasible and led to a median overall survival of 24.4 months. In patients with epithelioid histology, median overall survival was 42.8 months. These results are one of the highest survival rates for MPM treatment involving EPP, but Cho et al. emphasize that this treatment combination should only be performed in experienced surgical institutions due to the risk of morbidities (Cho et al. 2021). They are currently recruiting for the next trial of oligofractionated radiotherapy followed by resection (SMARTER trial, NCT04028570), which allows for either EPP or eP/D.

However, even with proton RT, it is often difficult to deliver high doses to all pleural surfaces without unacceptable toxicities to the intact lung underneath. Thus, RT is more commonly performed in an adjuvant fashion after MCR via either EPP or eP/D to reduce the total dose required to achieve durable local control.

6 Adjuvant Hemithoracic RT Following EPP

There are a number of techniques for adjuvant irradiation of the ipsilateral chest wall following EPP. The entire hemithorax can be treated to a total dose of 30–40 Gy using 3D conformal photon RT techniques with a boost to a total dose of 50–60 Gy for high-risk regions. Data on 3D techniques for RT after EPP demonstrate significant acute and late toxicities. These include pulmonary vascular damage, esophagitis, pericarditis, pneumonitis, pulmonary fibrosis, and pneumothorax. More modern techniques include mixed photon-electron (Yajnik et al. 2003) and hemithoracic IMRT techniques (Forster et al. 2003). A mixed photon-electron technique can limit low-dose irradiation exposure to the contralateral lung but can still result in significant doses to ipsilateral hemithoracic normal tissues (Hill-Kayser et al. 2009). The use of IMRT or VMAT approaches has increased conformality and consistency in delivery but commonly increases dose to the contralateral lung and heart. Despite the potential for simplicity and reproducibility with the inverse treatment planning process needed for IMRT or VMAT, there remains a significant learning curve for treatment planning using these techniques, with experienced centers demonstrating clearly superior plans in terms of dose to target vs. normal tissues (Patel et al. 2012).

Trials of adjuvant RT to the involved hemithorax following EPP have established improved local control when compared to EPP alone, at the cost of serious but potentially tolerable toxicities. The typical multimodal protocol in these studies has consisted of neoadjuvant chemotherapy, EPP,

Table 1 Selected large studies of EPP followed by hemithoracic RT

References	Total no. of patients (%)			Stage I–II vs. III–IV	RT dose	Median OS (months)	
	Initial	EPP	RT			ITT	RT
Weder et al. (2007)	61 (100)	45 (74)	36 (59)	64% vs. 26%	50–60 Gy	19.8	NR
Krug et al. (2009)	77 (100)	57 (74)	40 (59)	52% vs. 48%	54 Gy	16.8	29.1
de Perrot et al. (2009)	60 (100)	45 (75)	30 (50)	58% vs. 42%	50–60 Gy	14	59 (N0), 14 (N+)
Van Schil et al. (2010)	58 (100)	42 (72)	37 (64)	88% vs. 12%	54 Gy	18.4	32.9
Gomez et al. (2013)	NR	136 (100)	86 (64)	50% N0; 50% N+	45–60 Gy	NR	14.7
Federico et al. (2013)	54 (100)	45 (83)	25 (46)	60% vs. 40%	50.4–54 Gy	15.5	NR
Thieke et al. (2015)	NR	NR	62	NR	50–54 Gy	NR	20.4
Hasegawa et al. (2016)	42 (100)	30 (71)	17 (40)	64% vs. 36%	54 Gy	19.9	39
Stahel et al. (2015) and Riesterer et al. (2019)	151 (100)	27 (50)	27 (50)	70% vs. 30%	45–46 Gy	15	19.3

EPP extrapleural pneumonectomy, *ITT* intent to treat, *OS* overall survival, *NR* not reported

and postoperative hemithoracic RT, and results have been replicated across a number of centers in North America, Europe, and Asia (Krug et al. 2009; de Perrot et al. 2009; Hasegawa et al. 2016; Gomez et al. 2013; Federico et al. 2013; Weder et al. 2007; Van Schil et al. 2010; Thieke et al. 2015) (Table 1). In these studies, about two-thirds of patients were at earlier stage (AJCC 7th edition Stage I/II) and generally treated with total doses of 50–60 Gy in 1.8–2 Gy fractions. When analyzed by an intent to treat (ITT) that includes all patients who started neoadjuvant chemotherapy in the survival analysis, this approach yields a median overall survival ranging from 14 to 20 months. When analyzed by methods that exclude patients who did not complete the full course of trimodality treatment, median overall survivals are significantly improved to 15–40 months. However, 20–25% of patients did not undergo surgery primarily due to disease progression on planned neoadjuvant chemotherapy (EPP column in Table 1), and only 40–60% of patients completed the full trimodality course (RT column in Table 1). In one study of EPP with intraoperative cisplatin, adjuvant cisplatin/pemetrexed, and 54 Gy IMRT, 6 of 13 patients (46%) developed fatal radiation pneumonitis. Analysis of these data suggests that low RT doses to the contralateral lung likely contributed to these fatal pulmonary toxicities (Allen et al. 2006). This clearly demonstrates the relatively steep learning curve required to produce RT plans that minimize the dose to normal tissues, but even patients treated at experienced centers have significant risks of radiation pneumonitis that is fatal in 3–10% of cases.

As noted above, these data have been compared in a nonrandomized, retrospective fashion to institutional data to suggest that patients who complete RT have superior progression-free and overall survival when compared to EPP alone. Since patients who undergo EPP without RT are often too moribund to receive RT or have rapidly progressive disease, there is an intrinsic potential for bias in these comparisons. To quantify the potential magnitude of benefit of post-EPP RT, the Swiss Group for Clinical Cancer Research (SAKK) conducted a randomized clinical trial of preoperative chemotherapy followed by EPP with or without RT at 14 centers in Switzerland, Belgium, and Germany (SAKK 17/04), shown in the bottom row of Table 1 (Stahel et al. 2015; Riesterer et al. 2019). In this trial, 151 patients with stage I–III MPM received preoperative chemotherapy consisting of cisplatin/pemetrexed every 21 days for three cycles, with 113 patients (75%) continuing to EPP. Of the patients who underwent EPP, an 85% MCR rate (96/113) was achieved that represented 64% of the original 151 patients who started chemotherapy. Fifty-four of these 96 patients (56%) underwent randomization to observation vs. postoperative IMRT (27 in each group or 18% of the original patients). Final analysis of these data failed to demonstrate a statistically significant improvement in the overall survival. Critiques of this study noted that the radiotherapy cohort consisted of only 27 patients out of the original 151 who were treated at 14 centers with 3 different dose fractionation schemes without central radiotherapy quality assurance and also noted the aforementioned impact of center RT experience on the quality of plans (Rimner et al. 2016a). Moreover, the 15-month overall survival for all 151 patients was on the lower end of the ITT overall survival ranges in Table 1. Nevertheless, these findings, along with the generally superior results of protocols including lung-sparing surgery, raise a cautionary note for the future of EPP/RT in the management of patients with MPM.

7 Adjuvant Hemithoracic RT Following eP/D

More recently, lung-sparing surgery using eP/D is increasingly performed as the preferred approach, when possible, for achieving MCR in MPM patients. However, with the lung intact, it can be more challenging to design an RT treatment plan with an ideal tumor dose and acceptable toxicities to adjacent organs. Development of radiation pneumonitis in the ipsilateral lung is of particular concern. As noted above, postoperative RT cannot easily be delivered to all pleural surfaces, including the major/minor fissures, even with the most advanced RT techniques/technology. However, investigators at Memorial Sloan Kettering Cancer Center have pioneered a technique using IMRT to treat the peripheral pleural space that carries the highest risk of local recurrence, as detailed in the IMPRINT study (Rimner et al. 2016b). In this study, 45 patients with MPM were treated with neoadjuvant chemotherapy, with 21 patients (47%) proceeding to lung-sparing surgery and 16 (36%) proceeding to postoperative RT. An additional 11 patients (24%) went on to RT without surgical resection for a total of 27 patients (60%) who received RT to the external pleural surfaces. Of the patients who received RT, the median dose was 46.8 Gy and the median overall survival was 23.7 months. Comparable results have been reported by other groups, with 20 patients experiencing a 33-month median overall survival in one study and 20 patients experiencing a median overall survival of 28.4 months in another (Chance et al. 2015; Minatel et al. 2014).

Furthermore, Trovo et al. have recently completed a phase III trial that included patients with nonmetastatic MPM receiving lung-sparing surgery and chemotherapy who were randomized to radical hemithoracic radiation therapy (RHR) versus palliative RT (Trovo et al. 2021). The 55 patients randomized to RHR received 50 Gy in 25 fractions to the pleural cavity, with residual disease receiving a simultaneous integrated boost of 60 Gy. For palliative RT (53 patients), doses ranged from 21 Gy in 3 fractions to 20–30 Gy in 5–10 fractions. The 2-year overall survival rate was 58% after RHR versus 28% after PR, and median survivals were 8.5 and 17.6 months, respectively, again suggesting a dose response with radiotherapy treatment. Notably, these patients died mostly from distant progression rather than local relapse.

The toxicity rates for IMRT to the external pleura are generally lower than what has been reported previously with older RT delivery techniques. Shaikh and colleagues have compared outcomes for 78 patients after IMPRINT to 131 patients who previously received lung-sparing surgery and conventional RT delivery (Shaikh et al. 2017). They found that, in the context of modern chemotherapy and lung-sparing surgery, pleural IMRT as a part of modern trimodality treatment in MPM is associated with improved outcomes including higher overall survival and lower rates of severe toxicity. Based on the above prior studies, a phase III trial (NCT04158141) has been recently opened through NRG Oncology (NRG-LU006) that randomizes patients with MPM who receive eP/D and standard chemotherapy to adjuvant pleural IMRT versus observation. Taken together with the median survivals that are comparable or potentially superior to those achieved with EPP and RT, these results suggest that RT to the external pleura has potential clinical application in both operative/adjuvant and nonoperative settings.

8 SBRT Salvage

The prevalence of recurrent disease after multimodal therapies requires standardized treatment recommendations for effective salvage strategies. Stereotactic body radiation therapy (SBRT), that is well established for non-small cell lung cancer and parenchymal lung metastases, has also recently been demonstrated to achieve excellent local control for a range of isolated pleural recurrences following systemic therapy or surgery. SBRT may be an effective option for patients with recurrent MPM because it can deliver a local ablative dose of RT with a tolerable toxicity profile. Of the studies listed in Table 2, only one patient experienced a SBRT-related grade ≥3 toxicity (esophageal toxicity with upper gastrointestinal bleeding (Schröder et al. 2019)). Based upon these results observed by Schröder et al. (2019), Ghirardelli et al. (2021), and Barsky et al. (2021), pleural SBRT for oligoprogressive MPM can achieve durable local control for a range of isolated pleural recurrences following chemotherapy, immunotherapy, and/or surgery and can delay the time until initiating subsequent therapy courses without adding substantial toxicity. Barsky et al. (2021) postulate that Ghirardelli and Schröder reported lower local control rates due to the use of lower BED treatments. We recommend that high BED SBRT, with close respect to organ-at-risk tolerances, is more likely to maximize the therapeutic ratio and benefit of salvage RT for MPM.

9 Adjuvant Prophylactic RT to Interventional Sites

MPM tends to recur in subcutaneous tissues and the chest wall after interventional procedures such as biopsy, thoracoscopy, or thoracotomy. Superficial (orthovoltage X-rays or electrons) RT is often employed in prophylactic irradiation of interventional tracts (PIT) in an attempt to reduce recurrence. In the absence of RT, the rates of intervention-site metastases demonstrate significant variability, with the control (no prophylactic radiation) arm of the three published, randomized clinical trials of PIT showing 10–40% of patients developing intervention-site metastases (Boutin et al. 1995; Bydder et al. 2004; O'Rourke et al. 2007) (Table 3). However, the ability of PIT to reduce the rate of intervention-site recurrence remains an open question, with these randomized trial data demonstrating conflicting results. While some radiation oncologists have continued to recommend PIT, it is not clear which patients might benefit most from this therapy.

A more recent multicenter phase III trial with greater patient numbers specifically compared prophylactic versus delayed RT for large-bore interventions that failed to show any benefits in

Table 2 Retrospective studies of pleural SBRT for oligoprogressive MPM

References	Patients	RT details	Local control			TFST months (95% CI)
			6 months	12 months	24 months	
Schröder et al. (2019)	21	20–50 Gy of 2.5–12.5 Gy/Fx in 3–20 Fxs	NR	73.5%	NR	NR
Ghirardelli et al. (2021)	37	25–56 Gy of SBRT >5 Gy/Fx or hypoRT <5 Gy/Fx	84%	76%	NR	6 (4.9–7.1)
Barsky et al. (2021)	15	30–50 Gy in 4–5 Fxs	100%	100%	100%	10.9 (5.7–27.8)

NR not reported, *TFST* time to further systemic therapy

Table 3 Randomized trials of prophylactic irradiation of surgical tracts (PIT) in patients with MPM

References	Patients	RT details	Tract relapse rate No PIT	PIT	p
Boutin et al. (1995)	40	21 Gy/3 Fx <15 days postprocedure	40%	0%	<0.001
Bydder et al. (2004)	43	10 Gy/1 Fx <15 days postprocedure	10%	7%	n.s.
O'Rourke et al. (2007)	61	21 Gy/3 Fx <21 days postprocedure	13%	10%	n.s.
Clive et al. (2016)	203	21 Gy/3 Fx <42 days postprocedure	16%	9%	n.s.
Bayman et al. (2019)	374	21 Gy/3 Fx <42 days postprocedure	10%	6%	n.s.

terms of tract relapse rates, survival, or quality of life (Clive et al. 2016). Additionally, another multicenter randomized phase III trial of PIT vs. observation (Bayman et al. 2016) set up to improve our understanding of the potential benefits of PIT in patients with MPM has recently been completed. This trial was larger than any of the earlier trials, and it similarly showed no significant benefits (Bayman et al. 2019). A recent retrospective review that limited pooled analyses to these two recent trials found that PIT can modestly but significantly reduce the risk of intervention-site metastases, but it is unlikely to alter the disease course or overall survival (Lee et al. 2021). Nevertheless, based on these newer trials, recent guidelines now advise against the routine use of PIT to prevent surgical tract metastases (NCCN 2021). As long as patients receive careful follow-up after procedures, metastases to these sites can be managed as they arise.

10 RT and Immunotherapies

Early studies of immunotherapy in MPM included cytokine therapies such as interleukin-2 (IL-2) and interferon α-2a/b (IFN-α). Although systemic toxicities have limited the efficacy of these treatments, they showed some promise in both palliation of symptoms and reduction of tumor burden (Castagneto et al. 2001; Alley et al. 2017). More recent immunotherapy strategies have focused on targeting the PD-1/PD-L1 and CTLA-4 immune checkpoint pathways. Thus far, CTLA-4 blockade alone has had only minimal impacts, with the most recent randomized phase III study of tremelimumab vs. placebo in previously treated MPM showing no benefits in the overall survival. PD-1/PD-L1 blockade has shown more promise, although a randomized phase III study investigating the efficacy of pembrolizumab versus single-agent chemotherapy (gemcitabine or vinorelbine) in relapsed MPM patients did not demonstrate survival improvement (Popat et al. 2020). These results highlight the need for identifying patients most likely to respond to checkpoint inhibitors as well as identify combination treatment strategies that augment immunotherapy efficacy. Progress in combination immunotherapy was recently reported in the CheckMate 743 phase III randomized trial that showed that nivolumab plus ipilimumab significantly improved overall survival versus standard-of-care chemotherapy, with this combination now emerging as an FDA-approved first-line option for previously untreated unresectable MPM (Baas et al. 2021).

Another potentially attractive combination is the use of RT with immunotherapy. RT is known to have immunomodulatory effects that can, in some cases, lead to abscopal responses. The potential for localized RT to activate or improve antitumor immunity in conjunction with immunotherapies such as checkpoint inhibitors is beginning to be explored in clinical trials for patients with MPM (Alley et al. 2017). For example, the SMART trial and related preclinical work noted immune system activation after RT and even upregulation of PD-L1 status and thus are amenable to combinations with immunotherapies to potentially improve survival (De La Maza et al. 2017; de Perrot et al. 2020). So far, there have not been sufficient studies on optimizing RT delivery strategies that will best enhance this effect, but ideal techniques may include either SBRT or protons. By delivering ablative doses of irradiation, SBRT can induce a more robust immune response that allows for the upregulation of major histocompatibility complex I, immunomodulatory cytokines, inflammatory mediators, heat-shock proteins, death receptors, etc., which can augment the antitumor immune responses in combination with immunotherapy (Finkelstein et al. 2011). Additionally, due to the immunologic effects of proton therapy and its potential to better spare critical normal tissues in the thorax from excessive irradiation (Simone and Rengan 2014; Chang et al. 2016), this may also be a promising RT modality.

There is almost no clinical data on combinations of RT and immunotherapies at present. One recent case report of an MPM patient who received intrapleural IFN-α gene therapy and later palliative RT resulting in local and abscopal tumor responses shows the potential of these combinations (Barsky et al. 2019). Two trials have recently been initiated to determine the feasibility of RT in combination with PD-1/PD-L1 blockade for MPM. The phase I trial at MD Anderson (NCT02959463) will include 24 patients with intact lungs (i.e., excluding those undergoing EPP) who receive hemithoracic or palliative RT, both followed by pembrolizumab (anti-PD-1) infusions. The phase I–II trial at Memorial Sloan Kettering (NCT03399552) will include 15 patients with MPM who have received at least one prior line of systemic therapy who will receive one dose of avelumab (anti-PD-L1) infusion every other week and a short course of SBRT after the first two doses.

11 Future Roles for RT in MPM

Advances in RT delivery technology will continue to improve spatial selectivity of tumor tissue and reduce normal tissue toxicities, a key concern for thoracic malignancies. Technologies such as image guidance, stereotactic body radiation therapy, intensity-modulated radiation therapy, and proton therapy will only increase the ability to create regions of local control with acceptable normal tissue damage to surrounding structures (Shaikh et al. 2017). Another novel approach utilizes ultrahigh-dose-rate (FLASH) RT of at least 40–60 Gy/s compared to standard dose rates of less than 1 Gy/s. Ongoing research has shown that whole abdomen and thoracic FLASH-RT is clinically tolerable in mice, and these studies support the value of FLASH for minimizing RT-induced toxicities while achieving the same, or potentially even improved, tumor kill as standard-dose-rate RT (Durante et al. 2018; Diffenderfer et al. 2020; Levy et al. 2019). The biological and physical mechanisms that govern FLASH vs. standard-dose-rate sparing of normal tissues have yet to be determined, but a combination of differences in DNA damage-induced apoptosis (Levy et al. 2020), cytokine upregulation (such as TGF-β) (Favaudon et al. 2014; Buonanno et al. 2019), effects on immune and stem cells (Fouillade et al. 2020), and oxygen depletion/response to hypoxia (Adrian et al. 2020) comprises the current hypothesis. Proton FLASH-RT may be particularly beneficial as a surgical adjuvant or in combination with immunotherapies because of its potential lower side effect profile, since this technique combines the increased spatial selectivity of proton RT with the enhanced normal tissue protection provided by the FLASH dose rate.

Advances in surgical techniques along with new immune therapies will continue to extend survival, increasing the potential for RT-assisted durable local control to contribute to the management of these patients. The ability to spatially target high doses of RT using technologies such as SBRT allows treatment to oligoprogressive or oligometastatic sites to provide durable control, although the impact of this therapy on MPM prognosis must still be determined. Thus, continued biological and clinical innovation in RT has a tremendous potential to improve both morbidity and survival of patients with MPM. Further clinical trials are needed to determine the optimal strategies for combining advanced RT delivery techniques in the multidisciplinary care of these patients.

Acknowledgments This work was supported in part by a grant from the National Institutes of Health P01-CA087971.

References

Adrian G, Konradsson E, Lempart M, Bäck S, Ceberg C, Petersson K (2020) The FLASH effect depends on oxygen concentration. Br J Radiol 93:20190702

Aggarwal C, Haas AR, Metzger S et al (2018) Phase I study of intrapleural gene-mediated cytotoxic immunotherapy in patients with malignant pleural effusion. Mol Ther 26:1198–1205

Allen AM, Czerminska M, Janne PA et al (2006) Fatal pneumonitis associated with intensity-modulated radiation therapy for mesothelioma. Int J Radiat Oncol Biol Phys 65:640–645

Alley EW, Katz SI, Cengel KA, Simone CB (2017) Immunotherapy and radiation therapy for malignant pleural mesothelioma. Transl Lung Cancer Res 6:212–219

Baas P, Scherpereel A, Nowak AK et al (2021) First-line nivolumab plus ipilimumab in unresectable malignant pleural mesothelioma (CheckMate 743): a multicentre, randomised, open-label, phase 3 trial. Lancet 397:375–386

Barsky AR, Cengel KA, Katz SI, Sterman DH, Simone CB (2019) First-ever abscopal effect after palliative radiotherapy and immuno-gene therapy for malignant pleural mesothelioma. Cureus 11:e4102

Barsky AR, Yegya-Raman N, Katz SI, Simone CB, Cengel KA (2021) Managing oligoprogressive malignant pleural mesothelioma with stereotactic body radiation therapy. Lung Cancer 157:163–164

Bayman N, Ardron D, Ashcroft L et al (2016) Protocol for PIT: a phase III trial of prophylactic irradiation of tracts in patients with malignant pleural mesothelioma following invasive chest wall intervention. BMJ Open 6:e010589

Bayman N, Appel W, Ashcroft L et al (2019) Prophylactic irradiation of tracts in patients with malignant pleural mesothelioma: an open-label, multicenter, phase III randomized trial. J Clin Oncol 37:1200–1208

Boutin C, Rey F, Viallat JR (1995) Prevention of malignant seeding after invasive diagnostic procedures in patients with pleural mesothelioma. A randomized trial of local radiotherapy. Chest 108:754–758

Buonanno M, Grilj V, Brenner DJ (2019) Biological effects in normal cells exposed to FLASH dose rate protons. Radiother Oncol 139:51–55

Burt BM, Richards WG, Lee HS et al (2018) A phase I trial of surgical resection and intraoperative hyperthermic cisplatin and gemcitabine for pleural mesothelioma. J Thorac Oncol 13:1400–1409

Bydder S, Phillips M, Joseph DJ et al (2004) A randomised trial of single-dose radiotherapy to prevent procedure tract metastasis by malignant mesothelioma. Br J Cancer 91:9–10

Castagneto B, Zai S, Mutti L et al (2001) Palliative and therapeutic activity of IL-2 immunotherapy in unresectable malignant pleural mesothelioma with pleural effusion: results of a phase II study on 31 consecutive patients. Lung Cancer 31:303–310

Chance WW, Rice DC, Allen PK et al (2015) Hemithoracic intensity modulated radiation therapy after pleurectomy/decortication for malignant pleural mesothelioma: toxicity, patterns of failure, and a matched survival analysis. Int J Radiat Oncol Biol Phys 91:149–156

Chang JY, Jabbour SK, De Ruysscher D et al (2016) Consensus statement on proton therapy in early-stage and locally advanced non-small cell lung cancer. Int J Radiat Oncol Biol Phys 95:505–516

Chen D, Wang H, Song X, Yue J, Yu J (2018) Preoperative radiation may improve the outcomes of resectable IIIA/N2 non-small-cell lung cancer patients: a propensity score matching-based analysis from surveillance, epidemiology, and end results database. Cancer Med 7:4354–4360

Cho BCJ, Donahoe L, Bradbury PA et al (2021) Surgery for malignant pleural mesothelioma after radiotherapy (SMART): final results from a single-centre, phase 2 trial. Lancet Oncol 22:190–197

Clive AO, Taylor H, Dobson L et al (2016) Prophylactic radiotherapy for the prevention of procedure-tract metastases after surgical and large-bore pleural procedures in malignant pleural mesothelioma (SMART): a multicentre, open-label, phase 3, randomised controlled trial. Lancet Oncol 17:1094–1104

De La Maza L, Wu M, Wu L et al (2017) In situ vaccination after accelerated hypofractionated radiation and surgery in a mesothelioma mouse model. Clin Cancer Res 23:5502–5513

de Perrot M, Feld R, Cho BC et al (2009) Trimodality therapy with induction chemotherapy followed by extrapleural pneumonectomy and adjuvant high-dose hemithoracic radiation for malignant pleural mesothelioma. J Clin Oncol 27:1413–1418

de Perrot M, Wu L, Cabanero M et al (2020) Prognostic influence of tumor microenvironment after hypofractionated radiation and surgery for mesothelioma. J Thorac Cardiovasc Surg 159:2082–91.e1

Diffenderfer ES, Verginadis II, Kim MM et al (2020) Design, implementation and in vivo validation of a novel proton FLASH radiotherapy system. Int J Radiat Oncol Biol Phys 106(2):440–448

Durante M, Brauer-Krisch E, Hill M (2018) Faster and safer? FLASH ultra-high dose rate in radiotherapy. Br J Radiol 91:20170628

Favaudon V, Caplier L, Monceau V et al (2014) Ultrahigh dose-rate FLASH irradiation increases the differential response between normal and tumor tissue in mice. Sci Transl Med 6:245ra93

Federico R, Adolfo F, Giuseppe M et al (2013) Phase II trial of neoadjuvant pemetrexed plus cisplatin followed by surgery and radiation in the treatment of pleural mesothelioma. BMC Cancer 13:22

Feigen M, Lee ST, Lawford C et al (2011) Establishing locoregional control of malignant pleural mesothelioma using high-dose radiotherapy and (18) F-FDG PET/CT scan correlation. J Med Imaging Radiat Oncol 55:320–332

Finkelstein SE, Timmerman R, McBride WH et al (2011) The confluence of stereotactic ablative radiotherapy and tumor immunology. Clin Dev Immunol 2011:439752

Forster KM, Smythe WR, Starkschall G et al (2003) Intensity-modulated radiotherapy following extrapleural pneumonectomy for the treatment of malignant mesothelioma: clinical implementation. Int J Radiat Oncol Biol Phys 55:606–616

Fouillade C, Curras-Alonso S, Giuranno L et al (2020) FLASH irradiation spares lung progenitor cells and limits the incidence of radio-induced senescence. Clin Cancer Res 26:1497–1506

Ghirardelli P, Franceschini D, D'Aveni A et al (2021) Salvage radiotherapy for oligo-progressive malignant pleural mesothelioma. Lung Cancer 152:1–6

Gomez DR, Hong DS, Allen PK et al (2013) Patterns of failure, toxicity, and survival after extrapleural pneumonectomy and hemithoracic intensity-modulated radiation therapy for malignant pleural mesothelioma. J Thorac Oncol 8:238–245

Hasegawa S, Okada M, Tanaka F et al (2016) Trimodality strategy for treating malignant pleural mesothelioma: results of a feasibility study of induction pemetrexed plus cisplatin followed by extrapleural pneumonectomy and postoperative hemithoracic radiation (Japan Mesothelioma Interest Group 0601 Trial). Int J Clin Oncol 21:523–530

Hill-Kayser CE, Avery S, Mesina CF et al (2009) Hemithoracic radiotherapy after extrapleural pneumonectomy for malignant pleural mesothelioma: a dosimetric comparison of two well-described techniques. J Thorac Oncol 4:1431–1437

Inai K (2008) Pathology of mesothelioma. Environ Health Prev Med 13:60–64

Jenkins P, Milliner R, Salmon C (2011) Re-evaluating the role of palliative radiotherapy in malignant pleural mesothelioma. Eur J Cancer 47:2143–2149

Krug LM, Pass HI, Rusch VW et al (2009) Multicenter phase II trial of neoadjuvant pemetrexed plus cisplatin followed by extrapleural pneumonectomy and radiation for malignant pleural mesothelioma. J Clin Oncol 27:3007–3013

Lee CC, Soon YY, Vellayappan B, Leong CN, Koh WY, Tey JCS (2021) Prophylactic irradiation of tracts in patients with malignant pleural mesothelioma: a systematic review and meta-analysis of randomized trials. Crit Rev Oncol Hematol 160:103278

Levy KN, Suchitra N, Wang J, Chow S et al (2019) FLASH irradiation enhances the therapeutic index of abdominal radiotherapy in mice. Nat Commun. (Under review)

Levy K, Natarajan S, Wang J et al (2020) Abdominal FLASH irradiation reduces radiation-induced gastrointestinal toxicity for the treatment of ovarian cancer in mice. Sci Rep 10:21600

Li Y, Alley E, Friedberg J et al (2015) Prospective assessment of proton therapy for malignant pleural mesothelioma. International Association for the Study of Lung Cancer Annual Meeting, Denver, CO

Macleod N, Price A, O'Rourke N, Fallon M, Laird B (2014) Radiotherapy for the treatment of pain in malignant pleural mesothelioma: a systematic review. Lung Cancer 83:133–138

MacLeod N, Chalmers A, O'Rourke N et al (2015) Is radiotherapy useful for treating pain in mesothelioma?: a phase II trial. J Thorac Oncol 10:944–950

Minatel E, Trovo M, Polesel J et al (2014) Radical pleurectomy/decortication followed by high dose of radiation therapy for malignant pleural mesothelioma. Final results with long-term follow-up. Lung Cancer 83:78–82

NCCN (2021) National Comprehensive Cancer Network guidelines: malignant pleural mesothelioma (Version 2.2021). [cited March 27, 2021]. https://www.nccn.org/professionals/physician_gls/pdf/mpm.pdf

O'Rourke N, Garcia JC, Paul J, Lawless C, McMenemin R, Hill J (2007) A randomised controlled trial of intervention site radiotherapy in malignant pleural mesothelioma. Radiother Oncol 84:18–22

Pan HY, Jiang S, Sutton J et al (2015) Early experience with intensity modulated proton therapy for lung-intact mesothelioma: a case series. Pract Radiat Oncol 5:e345–e353

Patel PR, Yoo S, Broadwater G et al (2012) Effect of increasing experience on dosimetric and clinical outcomes in the management of malignant pleural mesothelioma with intensity-modulated radiation therapy. Int J Radiat Oncol Biol Phys 83:362–368

Popat S, Curioni-Fontecedro A, Dafni U et al (2020) A multicentre randomised phase III trial comparing pembrolizumab versus single-agent chemotherapy for advanced pre-treated malignant pleural mesothelioma: the European Thoracic Oncology Platform (ETOP) 9-15) PROMISE-meso trial. Ann Oncol 31:1734–1745

Predina JD, Newton AD, Corbett C et al (2019) A clinical trial of TumorGlow to identify residual disease during pleurectomy and decortication. Ann Thorac Surg 107:224–232

Rice SR, Li YR, Busch TM et al (2019) A novel prospective study assessing the combination of photodynamic therapy and proton radiation therapy: safety and outcomes when treating malignant pleural mesothelioma. Photochem Photobiol 95:411–418

Riesterer O, Ciernik IF, Stahel RA et al (2019) Pattern of failure after adjuvant radiotherapy following extrapleural pneumonectomy of pleural mesothelioma in the SAKK 17/04 trial. Radiother Oncol 138:121–125

Rimner A, Simone CB 2nd, Zauderer MG, Cengel KA, Rusch VW (2016a) Hemithoracic radiotherapy for mesothelioma: lack of benefit or lack of statistical power? Lancet Oncol 17:e43–ee4

Rimner A, Zauderer MG, Gomez DR et al (2016b) Phase II study of hemithoracic intensity-modulated pleural radiation therapy (IMPRINT) as part of lung-sparing multimodality therapy in patients with malignant pleural mesothelioma. J Clin Oncol 34:2761–2768

Rusch V, Baldini EH, Bueno R et al (2013) The role of surgical cytoreduction in the treatment of malignant pleural mesothelioma: meeting summary of the

International Mesothelioma Interest Group Congress, September 11–14, 2012, Boston, Mass. J Thorac Cardiov Sur 145:909–910

Schröder C, Opitz I, Guckenberger M et al (2019) Stereotactic body radiation therapy (SBRT) as salvage therapy for oligorecurrent pleural mesothelioma after multi-modality therapy. Front Oncol 9:961

Shaikh F, Zauderer MG, von Reibnitz D et al (2017) Improved outcomes with modern lung-sparing trimodality therapy in patients with malignant pleural mesothelioma. J Thorac Oncol 12:993–1000

Simone CB, Rengan R (2014) The use of proton therapy in the treatment of lung cancers. Cancer J 20:427–432

Stahel RA, Riesterer O, Xyrafas A et al (2015) Neoadjuvant chemotherapy and extrapleural pneumonectomy of malignant pleural mesothelioma with or without hemithoracic radiotherapy (SAKK 17/04): a randomised, international, multicentre phase 2 trial. Lancet Oncol 16:1651–1658

Taioli E, Wolf AS, Flores RM (2015) Meta-analysis of survival after pleurectomy decortication versus extrapleural pneumonectomy in mesothelioma. Ann Thorac Surg 99:472–480

Thieke C, Nicolay NH, Sterzing F et al (2015) Long-term results in malignant pleural mesothelioma treated with neoadjuvant chemotherapy, extrapleural pneumonectomy and intensity-modulated radiotherapy. Radiat Oncol 10:267

Trovo M, Relevant A, Polesel J et al (2021) Radical hemithoracic radiotherapy versus palliative radiotherapy in non-metastatic malignant pleural mesothelioma: results from a phase 3 randomized clinical trial. Int J Radiat Oncol Biol Phys 109:1368–1376

van Gijn W, Marijnen CA, Nagtegaal ID et al (2011) Preoperative radiotherapy combined with total mesorectal excision for resectable rectal cancer: 12-year follow-up of the multicentre, randomised controlled TME trial. Lancet Oncol 12:575–582

Van Schil PE, Baas P, Gaafar R et al (2010) Trimodality therapy for malignant pleural mesothelioma: results from an EORTC phase II multicentre trial. Eur Respir J 36:1362–1369

Weder W, Stahel RA, Bernhard J et al (2007) Multicenter trial of neo-adjuvant chemotherapy followed by extrapleural pneumonectomy in malignant pleural mesothelioma. Ann Oncol 18:1196–1202

Yajnik S, Rosenzweig KE, Mychalczak B et al (2003) Hemithoracic radiation after extrapleural pneumonectomy for malignant pleural mesothelioma. Int J Radiat Oncol Biol Phys 56:1319–1326

Primary Tracheal Tumors

Shrinivas Rathod

Contents

1 Epidemiology 864
2 Risk Factors 864
3 Presentation 864
4 **Investigations** 865
4.1 Imaging 865
4.2 Endoscopic Techniques 866
4.3 Pulmonary Function Test 866
5 **Outcomes and Epidemiological Prognostic Factors** 866
6 **Management** 867
6.1 Surgery 867
6.2 Radiation 872
6.3 Systemic Therapy 874
6.4 Endobronchial Treatments 874
7 **Patterns of Failure** 874
8 **Current Challenges and Future Direction** 875
9 **Conclusion** 875
References 875

Abstract

Primary tracheal tumors are sporadic and represent 0.1% of all malignancy. The low index of suspicion and nonspecific symptoms often result in diagnostic delays. Surgery is the primary treatment with the optimal survival rates. Radiation can play a vital role in adjuvant, curative (unresectable), and palliative settings.

Lack of a standard staging system is a significant challenge, and the current state of primary tracheal cancer literature reflects a lack of a high level of evidence interventions. The management relies on available low-quality evidence, with databases lacking complete details and jeopardized by geographical bias. Using a standard staging system, creating a central/national level rare disease database, and rigorous data recording would help overcome some of the current shortcomings. Managing these rare tumors in experienced centers with multidisciplinary expertise is recommended.

S. Rathod (✉)
Department of Radiation Oncology, BC Cancer Agency, Abbotsford, BC, Canada
e-mail: shrinivas.rathod@bccancer.bc.ca

1 Epidemiology

Primary tracheal tumors are sporadic, and primary tracheal carcinoma (PTC) represents less than 0.1% of all and less than 2% of upper airway malignancies (Bhattacharyya 2004). The reported incidence of PTC is 1–2.6 cases per 100,000 population per year (Rostom and Morgan 1978; Manninen et al. 1991; Urdaneta et al. 2011; Licht et al. 2001). There is a paucity of data on the incidence trends of PTC over the last several decades (Urdaneta et al. 2011; Webb et al. 2006). There are significant differences in racial distribution, and over 75% of affected are white, which could reflect bias in geographical representation (Urdaneta et al. 2011; Xie et al. 2012; He et al. 2017).

The WHO classification groups PTC with tumors of the hypopharynx, larynx, and parapharyngeal space (Gale et al. 2017). Histologically, squamous cell carcinoma and adenoid cystic carcinoma are the two most common types and account for over 66–70% of PTC (Honings et al. 2009a). Surveillance epidemiology and end results (SEER) showed that 50% was tracheal squamous cell carcinoma (TSCC) and 16% was tracheal adenoid cystic carcinoma (TACC) (Urdaneta et al. 2011). However, a recent individual patient data (IPD) meta-analysis involving 733 cases found both TSCC and TACC equally prevalent and accounted for 31% and 34% of cases, respectively (He et al. 2017; Mallick et al. 2019). Carcinoid, lymphoma, melanoma, mucoepidermoid carcinoma, and sarcoma are rare to represent a small proportion of PTC (Madariaga and Gaissert 2018).

There are significant epidemiological differences between TSCC and TACC as detailed in Table 1. TSCC is exophytic or ulcerative morphology and exhibits aggressive behavior with regional and metastatic spread (Honings et al. 2009a; Macchiarini 2006). TSCC commonly predominantly affects males (male-to-female ratio 4.4:1) and peaks in the sixth–seventh decades of life (Mallick et al. 2019).

In contrast, TACC manifests as a slow-growing indolent cancer with nodular/stenosing

Table 1 Clinical characteristics of tracheal cancer

	Squamous cell ca	Adenoid cystic ca
Incidence	31–50%	16–34%
Age	6th–7th decades	4th–5th decades
Gender	Predominantly males	Equal to skewed females
Morphology	Exophytic or ulcerative	Nodular
Spread	Nodal and metastatic involvement	Perineural involvement
Clinical course	Aggressive	Indolent

growth with perineural involvement (Maziak et al. 1996). TACC affects the younger population with a peak incidence in the fifth decade of life and equal to marginally higher female involvement (male-to-female ratio 0.85:1) (Webb et al. 2006; Mallick et al. 2019). Nodal (25%) and metastatic (15%) involvement is common in TACC but relatively rare in TACC (Webb et al. 2006; Allen et al. 2007; He et al. 2017; Yang et al. 1997).

2 Risk Factors

The current knowledge of risk factors and the strength of the association is limited. Smoking is a common risk factor and reported in 80–90% of TSCC (Webb et al. 2006; Mallick et al. 2019). The association is relatively less strong in TACC and noted in 33–42% of cases (Webb et al. 2006; Mallick et al. 2019). Few studies report a high proportion of drinking habits (Webb et al. 2006). Studies report PTC association with synchronous or metachronous cancers of oropharynx, larynx, and lung (Napieralska et al. 2016; Grillo 1990).

3 Presentation

The rarity poses unique challenges at presentation and diagnostic delays (Meyers and Mathisen 1997). The nonspecific symptoms could mimic laryngeal or pulmonary etiology. With a low index of suspicion for PTC, these cases are often misdiagnosed as asthma or chronic obstructive pulmonary disease (Parrish et al. 1983). About one-third of cases, unfortunately, face a diagnostic delay of up to 6-month post-initial presentation (Yang et al. 1997). These delays are prevalent in young individuals and TACC histologies (Yang et al. 1997).

Dyspnea and hemoptysis are the most common presenting symptoms (Meyers and Mathisen 1997). Cough, wheeze, pneumonia, hoarseness, and weight loss could also be other common symptoms. In a series of 67 patients of PTC from Veteran General Hospital, cough (70%), dyspnea (65%), hemoptysis (39%), stridor (39%), hoarseness (31%), weight loss (22%), and wheezing (19%) were common presenting symptoms (Yang et al. 1997). MDACC series of 74 patients of PTC reported dyspnea (55%), hemoptysis (48%), cough (42%), and hoarseness (35%) as the most common presenting symptoms (Webb et al. 2006).

These symptoms, in the majority of cases, represent advanced local disease burden. Dyspnea is typically associated with significant luminal compromise (Macchiarini 2006). Dyspnea on exertion and dyspnea at rest suggest 50% and 75% luminal compromise, respectively (Licht et al. 2001; Wood 2002; Weber et al. 1978). A small proportion, 5–10%, of cases are asymptomatic and diagnosed incidentally (Meyers and Mathisen 1997).

4 Investigations

4.1 Imaging

The diagnostic utility of X-ray chest in PTC is minimal, and less than 18–28% of cases are identified on X-ray chest (Manninen et al. 1991; Honings et al. 2009b). However, it could serve to be a useful tool to assess concomitant pulmonary processes.

CT neck and chest are regarded as standard imaging investigations and help identify the lesion, location, size, invasion, involvement of adjacent structures, lymph node or vascular involvement, metastasis, and synchronous lesions (Fig. 1) (Park et al. 2009). Conventional CT techniques might underestimate the depth of invasion and impact resectability in up to 10% of cases (Shadmehr et al. 2011).

Advances in techniques as volumetric and dynamic imaging may help enhance imaging details (Shepard et al. 2018; Barnes et al. 2017; Javidan-Nejad 2010). Virtual endoscopy and optical coherence tomography techniques could further enhance the diagnostic abilities and aid bronchoscopy (McInnis et al. 2018; Han et al. 2005).

TSCC typically presents as a focal polypoid or sessile lesion, or eccentric narrowing or circumferential wall thickening of wall lumen (Park et al. 2009). On the contrary, TACC shows a propensity for the submucosal spread and presents

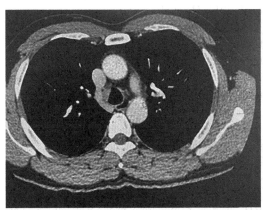
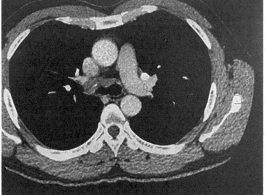

Fig. 1 Distal tracheal lesion with carinal involvement

with smooth circumferential or infiltrative growth (Park et al. 2009).

MRI does not offer a specific advantage over CT, and its role in PTC is minimal (Macchiarini 2006). The utility of PET/CT is variable and unclear in PTC. PET/CT could be useful in TSCC histologies as it tends to have increased FDG avidity (Park et al. 2009; Waki et al. 1998). However, TACC has a varying degree of FDG avidity correlating with the degree of differentiation, and high- and intermediate-grade tumors are FDG avid rather than low-grade tumors (Jeong et al. 2007).

4.2 Endoscopic Techniques

Endoscopic assessment of laryngo-tracheobronchial airway is a standard diagnostic investigation (Jamjoom et al. 2014). It offers the direct visualization and accurate evaluation of the location, extent, surface, shape, endoluminal compromise, resectability, and, importantly, tissue for pathological confirmation (Wood 2001). Procedure-induced risk of edema and bleeding could aggravate the airway obstruction. Rigid bronchoscopy helps to secure the airway and is preferred over flexible bronchoscopy (Diaz-Mendoza et al. 2019).

Endobronchial ultrasound (EBUS) is useful to assess the thickness, extent of tracheal wall invasion, and peritracheal extension. Kurimoto et al. compared EBUS with histological assessment and reported 95% concordance for the depth of invasion (Kurimoto et al. 1999). The role of esophagoscopy is limited and can be helpful to assess the suspected esophageal invasion/fistula (Meyers and Mathisen 1997).

4.3 Pulmonary Function Test

Pulmonary function tests help identify obstructive patterns and assess inspiratory–expiratory loop flattening (Macchiarini 2006).

4.3.1 Staging System
There is no standard or widely accepted staging system available for PTC. Bhattacharyya reported primary tumor and nodal staging for tracheal carcinoma (Bhattacharyya 2004). This contemporary system classifies primary tumor confined to trachea (size <2 cm), confined to trachea (size >2 cm), spread outside the trachea but not to adjacent organs or structures, spread to adjacent organs or structures, or unknown or cannot be assessed as T1, T2, T3, T4, and Tx, respectively. No evidence of regional nodal disease, positive regional nodal disease, and unknown or cannot be assessed were classified as N0, N1, and Nx, respectively. Stages were grouped as stage I (T1N0), stage II (T2N0), stage III (T3N0), and stage IV (T4N0 or any N1 disease).

Previous SEER data series classified PTC as localized (confined to trachea), regional (adjacent tissue involving vessels and bones), and distant disease (Urdaneta et al. 2011). In a separate SEER data-based series, a modified tracheal extension-based grouping was used. Tracheal extension confined to trachea, localized with spread outside the trachea but not to adjacent organs, tumor that involved adjacent organs or other structures (including vessels, nerves, pretracheal fascia, cricoid, esophagus, esophagus, pleura, main bronchi, sternum, thymus, thyroid gland, vertebral column), and tumor that involved further contiguous extension were grouped as E1, E2, E3, and E4, respectively. Mediastinal, paratracheal, pretracheal, and tracheoesophageal lymph nodes were classified as N1 and distant nodes grouped as N2 (He et al. 2017). Several other staging systems exist; however, none of these are validated or widely accepted (Urdaneta et al. 2011; He et al. 2017).

Macchiarini proposed TNM classification for tracheal cancers; however, its effectiveness is unclear and awaits further validation (Macchiarini 2006). Currently, there is no accepted TNM staging system available for PTC.

5 Outcomes and Epidemiological Prognostic Factors

PTC carries a moderate prognosis, and 5-year overall survival is 25–30% (Urdaneta et al. 2011). Age at diagnosis is a prognostic factor, and young age <50 years predicts better survival (Urdaneta et al. 2011; He et al. 2017; Mallick et al. 2019; Yang et al. 1997; Hararah et al. 2020). Poor outcomes with advancing age could be related to associated comorbidity, tolerance to surgery, and TSCC histology (Mallick et al. 2019).

Histology is a significant prognostic factor, and TSCC has significantly worse outcomes than TACC (Urdaneta et al. 2011; Webb et al. 2006). SEER data showed that TSCC carries a dismal prognosis with 5-year overall survival rate of 12%, contrary to 74% observed in TACC (Urdaneta et al. 2011). In subgroup analysis confined to localized disease, the survival difference persisted (5-year overall survival rate of 25% in TSCC vs. 91% in TACC; $p < 0.01$).

The extent of disease also predicts survival outcomes, and localized disease has a better 5-year overall survival of 46% over regional (5-year overall survival rate of 26%) and distant disease (5-year overall survival rate of 4%) (Urdaneta et al. 2011). Similarly, lymph node involvement is prognostic, and node-negative PTC expects a better survival (5-year overall survival rate of 52.7% vs. 10.4%; $p = 0.05$) (Urdaneta et al. 2011).

6 Management

Surgery is the primary treatment in the management of PTC. With limited supportive evidence, radiation plays an important role in adjuvant, radical, and palliative setting. Summary of these treatments in select recent publications is shown in Table 2.

6.1 Surgery

Surgical resection is considered the standard and preferred modality. Young (<50 years), white males, higher education level, academic centers, small tumor size, and TACC are more likely to undergo surgical resection (Agrawal et al. 2017; Benissan-Messan et al. 2020). Involvement of greater than 50% length of trachea, significant mediastinal invasion, multiple positive lymph nodes, and presence of distant metastasis, especially in TSCC, generally indicate unresectability (Meyers and Mathisen 1997). Curative surgical procedure includes laryngectomy with upper tracheal resection, laryngotracheal resection, tracheal resection, or carinal resection ± pulmonary resection (Meyers and Mathisen 1997).

Surgical outcomes improved over the past several decades, and 5-year overall survival rate has exceeded 50% (Agrawal et al. 2017; Benissan-Messan et al. 2020; Honings et al. 2007). A recent survey of practice in the United States treated between 2004 and 2015 suggests 5-year overall survival rate of 71% after resection, 39% after surgical debulking, and 31% without surgery ($p < 0.001$) (Benissan-Messan et al. 2020). This could be related to improvement in diagnostic techniques, anesthesia and surgery over time, and reduced mortality and morbidity and influenced by selection bias. IPD meta-analysis showed that surgically treated PTC survived significantly longer than nonsurgically treated PTC (180 vs. 36 months; $p < 0.001$) (Mallick et al. 2019). Similarly, SEER data analysis showed that PTC undergoing oncological surgery did better than those having no surgery (Urdaneta et al. 2011). Agarwal et al. showed that surgery improved overall survival (HR 2.63, 95% CI: 2.16–3.13, $p < 0.001$) and cancer-specific survival (HR 2.50, 95% CI: 1.96–3.13, $p < 0.001$).

The extent of surgery plays a vital role in the management of PTC. Total/complete resection improved survival outcomes, and positive margins are associated with inferior outcomes (Grillo 1990; Regnard et al. 1996).

In a TSCC-specific series of 532 cases, nearly 20% were treated with limited or curative surgery, and an additional 20% were treated with limited or curative surgery with adjuvant treatment. In a multivariate analysis, curative surgery (HR 0.42, 95% CI: 0.26–0.69), curative surgery with adjuvant therapy (HR 0.44, 95% CI: 0.27–0.72), and limited surgery with adjuvant therapy (HR 0.53, 95% CI: 0.36–0.77) were associated with reduced risk of death. IPD meta-analysis showed that the median OS for surgically treated TACC was numerically better than nonsurgically treated PTC (180 vs. 108 months; $p = 0.25$) (Mallick et al. 2019).

Table 2 Summary of treatments in select recent publications

	Author (reference)	Publication type	Year	Number of patients	Histology	Treatments	Radiation doses	Outcomes		Key findings
1	Mallick et al. (2019)	Individual patient data meta-analysis	2020	733	TACC 33%	Surgery 42%	Radical radiation 70 Gy	Median OS	Whole group—96 months	Surgery improves OS
					TSCC 31%	Radiation 38%	Adjuvant radiation 60 Gy	Median OS	Surgery vs. no surgery—180 vs. 36 months	Surgery better over radiation
								Median OS	Surgery vs. no radiation—180 vs. 48 months	
2	Ran et al. (2021)	Systematic review	2021	1252	TACC 100%	Surgery alone 40%	Radical radiation 60 Gy	5-year OS	Surgery alone: 86%	Surgery alone and surgery with postoperative radiation are commonly used
						Surgery and post-op radiation 37%	Adjuvant radiation	5-year OS	Surgery and radiation: 97%	Surgery alone and surgery with postoperative radiation offer good control rates
						Radiation alone 19%	54 Gy	5 year OS	Radiation alone: 5-year OS 35%	
								5 year OS	Surgery, radiation and chemotherapy: 90%	

#	Study type	Year	N	Histology	Treatment	Radiation dose	Outcome metric	Result	Conclusions
3	Yusuf et al. (2019)	Retrospective cohort	2019	549	TSCC 43%	Surgery 100%	> 30 Gy	Median OS	Whole group—6.88 years	Adjuvant radiation did not improve survival
					TACC 33%	Post-op radiation alone 37%		Median OS	TSCC 2.4 years	Use of adjuvant radiation common with positive margins and TACC
						Post-op concurrent chemoradiation—18%		Median OS	TACC 10.2 years	Adjuvant radiation did not improve survival in positive margins
										Adjuvant radiation improved survival in positive margins in SCC (median OS 2.40 vs. 1.25 years) but not statistically significant ($p = 0.1897$)
4	He et al. (2017)	Retrospective cohort	2017	287	TSCC 35%	Surgery 68%	NR	5-year OS	Whole group 49%	Old age, large tumor size, advanced extension, or no surgery associated with worse prognosis
					Adenocarcinoma 35%	Radiation 39%				
					Epithelial 10%					

(continued)

Table 2 (continued)

	Author (reference)	Publication type	Year	Number of patients	Histology	Treatments	Radiation doses	Outcomes		Key findings
5	Xie et al. (2012)	Retrospective cohort	2011	156	TSCC 42%	Surgery and radiation 62%—in radiation cohort	NR	Median OS	Surgery and radiation 60 months	Better overall survival in the radiation vs. the no-radiation group ($p = 0.015$)
					TACC 15%	RT alone 38%—in radiation cohort			Surgery alone 55 months	SCC, regional disease extension, or those who did not undergo surgery, the use of radiation improved survival
									In patients undergoing surgery, overall survival was better in those undergoing postoperative RT (in no case was RT given preoperatively in the SCC group) vs. no RT (5-year survival 58.2% vs. 6.7%; median survival 91 months vs. 12 months, respectively, $p = 0.0003$)	
									In those without surgery, overall survival was also better in those treated with RT vs. no RT (4-year survival 41.0% vs. 8.8%; median survival 33 months vs. 5 months, respectively, $p = 0.010$)	
6	Yang et al. (1997)	Retrospective cohort	2020	132	TACC 100%	Surgery 100%	Dose 60 Gy or more—47%	5-year OS	Positive margins 82%	TACC is associated with high rates of margin positivity
						Adjuvant radiation 72%			Negative margins 80%	Adjuvant radiation not associated with an overall survival benefit
						Positive margins—60%			Positive margins with radiation 82%	
						% of population with positive margins receiving radiation—79%			Negative margins with radiation 82%	

	Study	Design	Year	N	Histology	Treatment		Outcome measure	Outcome	Conclusion
7	Hararah et al. (2020)	Retrospective cohort	2020	532	TSCC 100%	Any surgery 40%	Dose 60 Gy or more—45%	5 year OS	Whole group 25%	Curative surgery and adjuvant treatment, chemoradiation, and radiation alone were associated with decreased likelihood of death compared to no treatment
						Curative surgery 16%		Median OS	Whole group—20 months	Worse outcomes are associated with elderly patients and those with poor performance status
						Limited surgery and adjuvant treatment 20%			Curative surgery and adjuvant treatment 42 months	
						Curative surgery and adjuvant treatment 20%			Curative surgery 41 months	
						Chemoradiation 26%			Chemoradiation 26 months	
						Radiation alone 17%			Limited surgery and adjuvant treatment 17 months	
									Radiation alone 16 months	
						No treatment 16%			Limited surgery 15 months	
									No treatment 6 months	
8	Urdaneta et al. (2011)	Retrospective cohort	2011	578	TSCC 45%	Surgery (type known/unknown) 65%	NR	5-year OS	Whole group 27%	Surgery improved survival

OS overall survival, *NR* not reported, *TSCC* tracheal squamous cell carcinoma, *TACC* tracheal adenoid cystic carcinoma

Owing to the risk of submucosal spread and perineural invasion, TACC is associated with high margin positivity rates. Yang et al. reported post-resection margin positivity rates as high as 60%. In this series, clinical T4 status was the only factor associated with positive margin in the multivariate model (odds ratio 7.71; 95% CI: 1.94–30.67; $p < 0.01$) (Yang et al. 2020). Positive margins did not impact overall survival at 5 years (positive margin 82.2% vs. negative margin 82.2%, $p = 0.97$) and were insignificant after multivariable adjustment (HR = 1.73; 95% CI: 0.62–4.84; $p = 0.30$).

6.2 Radiation

Radiation is a commonly used treatment modality. A recent meta-analysis suggests that radiation therapy was used in 37% of cases, including 18% who received radical intent radiation (Mallick et al. 2019).

6.2.1 Adjuvant Radiation

Radiation treatment is commonly used as an adjuvant treatment in the presence of positive margins, advanced disease, perineural or lymphovascular invasion, nodal involvement, and/or extracapsular extension (Fiorentino et al. 2021; Yusuf et al. 2019). These indications are primarily based on the extrapolation of practice across other common tumor sites. The direct evidence to support some of these indications is limited and variable across studies.

Xie et al. evaluated the SEER database and conducted a matched-pair analysis to assess the impact of radiation (Xie et al. 2012). In this cohort, radiation therapy was associated with significantly improved overall survival (median survival 41 vs. 14 months, $p = 0.015$) and significantly lower cumulative incidence of death from tracheal cancer ($p = 0.041$). A radiation-associated overall survival benefit was noted with TSCC histology (median survival 73 vs. 7 months, $p < 0.001$), regional disease extension (median survival 24 vs. 6 months, $p = 0.03$), or unresectable tumors (median survival 12 vs. 5 months, $p = 0.04$) (Xie et al. 2012).

In the MDACC series, adjuvant radiation did not significantly affect ($p = 0.159$) overall survival. However, in the subset analysis limited to TSCC (Webb et al. 2006), adjuvant radiation benefited disease-specific survival. Webb et al. recommended the use of adjuvant radiation to most cases of TSCC including negative margins and TACC as they are typically associated with high margin positivity and perineural spread. In a recent analysis of 287 PTC cases, the use of radiation did not have a statistically significant association (HR = 0.755; 95% CI: 0.471–1.212; $p = 0.245$) with survival (He et al. 2017). Similarly, previous SEER database analysis of 578 PTC did not show a survival benefit with radiation treatment (Urdaneta et al. 2011). Possible selection bias and lack of radiation dose/technique details in the SEER database limit any meaningful interpretation of the role of radiation in these studies (Urdaneta et al. 2011).

Honing et al. reported 8% macroscopic and 55% microscopic positivity rates in resected TACC (Honings et al. 2010). Evidence showed that high doses (>60 Gy) of adjuvant radiation to TACC with positive margins improve local control and survival (Ogino et al. 1995; Azar et al. 1998). Yang et al. assessed the role of adjuvant radiation in TACC with positive margins identified through the National Cancer Database (Yang et al. 2020). In this cohort of 132 cases, 79 had positive margins, of which 62 received adjuvant radiation. Adjuvant radiation did not impact the overall survival at 5 years (adjuvant RT—82.0% vs. no adjuvant RT—82.4% $p = 0.80$) and was insignificant after multivariable adjustment (HR = 1.04; 95% CI: 0.21–5.25; $p = 0.96$) (Yang et al. 2020). Recent SEER data and individual patient data meta-analysis showed no overall survival benefit ($p = 0.5$) with adjuvant radiation (Urdaneta et al. 2011; Mallick et al. 2019). Authors suggested that this could reflect selection bias, and no definitive conclusions on the role of radiation could be drawn from this data.

A recent systematic review of tracheal TACC studied 1252 cases, and 36% received adjuvant radiation. Adjuvant radiation improved 5-year OS from 86% to 97% supporting its role in TACC (Ran et al. 2021).

In summary, limited evidence supports the role of adjuvant radiation post-surgery. In the studies not meeting statistical significance, authors correctly suggest that given the lack of complete radiation dose/technique details and selection biases, no definitive conclusions on the role of radiation can be drawn from this data.

6.2.2 Curative Radiation

The role of curative radiation alone is limited primarily to unresectable PTC. Jeremic et al. reported a series of unresectable PTC of TSCC histology treated with radical radiation (60–70 Gy using 1.8–2 Gy per day 5 days a week regimen) (Jeremic et al. 1996). The cohort achieved a good response with a median survival of 24 months and 5-year survival rate of 27%. There was no significant difference between 60 and 70 Gy group in terms of 5-year survival (60 Gy—22% vs. 70 Gy—31%; $p = 0.5$) or delayed toxicity (60 Gy—11% vs. 70 Gy—38%, $p = 0.16$) (Jeremic et al. 1996). High-dose radiation alone is an appropriate option in a suitable scenario, and doses of at least 60 Gy are recommended to achieve long-term control (Chow et al. 1993; Chao et al. 1998; Mornex et al. 1998). Unresectable TACC can also be treated with radical radiation (at least 60 Gy) to achieve long-term survival and good local control of 20–70% (Napieralska et al. 2016; Levy et al. 2018).

Je et al. reported excellent local progression-free survival at 5- and 10-year rates of 67% and 27% in the definitive RT group (Je et al. 2017). A recent systematic review by Ran et al. showed encouraging long-term survival (5 years 35% and 10 years 16%) in TACC undergoing radical RT (Ran et al. 2021).

External beam radiation followed by brachytherapy boost could also serve as an appropriate option. Harms et al. reported in a series of 25 cases of PTC that 10 were treated with EBRT (50 Gy) followed by endotracheal brachytherapy (15 Gy) and achieved excellent 3-year actuarial survival of 32%. Brachytherapy boost did not increase acute toxicity. A total of 5 of 25 experienced late toxicity, of which 4 received brachytherapy boost. Authors suggested that this is primarily related to higher total dose in the brachytherapy group over those who did receive brachytherapy boost (Harms et al. 2000).

In summary, unresectable patients' radical radiation can achieve good long-term survival and serve as an appropriate radical option.

6.2.3 Palliative Radiation

Palliative radiation plays a vital role in achieving symptomatic relief. Palliative radiation can be offered through external beam radiation alone and/or brachytherapy. Excellent symptomatic relief with palliative radiation was noted with obstruction (82%), hemoptysis (72%), dyspnea (56%), and cough (47%) (Makarewicz and Mross 1998). Various EBRT fractionations as 20 Gy in 5 fractions over 1 week, 30 Gy in 10 fractions over 2 weeks, or, in select cases, 8 Gy in 1 fraction can be considered. EBRT and brachytherapy (2–3 Fr of 6–7.5 Gy each) combination could be another alternative (Makarewicz and Mross 1998).

6.2.4 Radiation Technique, Doses, and Volumes

Use of IMRT or VMAT should be preferred for adjuvant and curative cases of PTC (Fig. 2). These techniques could reduce radiation-induced acute and late toxicity.

Commonly, radiation dose ranges of 60–70 Gy (2 Gy per day 5 days a week over 6–7 weeks) are used in radical settings. In the brachytherapy boost setting, most commonly an external beam radiation dose of 50 Gy followed by four sessions of brachytherapy was used. In adjuvant setting, 60–66 Gy is a favored regimen (2 Gy per day 5 days a week over 6–5.5 weeks) (Mallick et al. 2019).

In palliative settings, various EBRT fractionations as 20 Gy in 5 fractions over 1 week, 30 Gy in 10 fractions over 2 weeks, or, in select cases, 8 Gy in 1 fraction can be considered.

For radical intent treatments, delineation of gross primary disease with 2–3 cm margins (especially in TACC) involved nodes, and adjacent draining lymph node region is a reasonable approach (Jeremic et al. 1996; Harms et al. 1999). For palliative intent treatments, target volume should encompass gross disease with adequate margins of 2–3 cm (Makarewicz and Mross 1998).

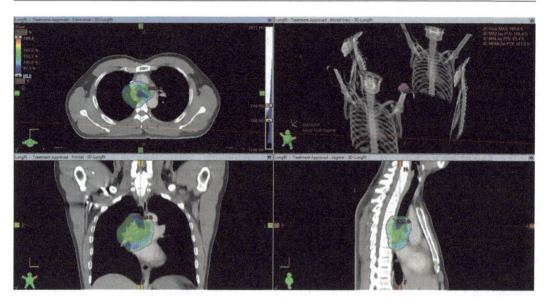

Fig. 2 Radiation planning images of PTC

6.3 Systemic Therapy

The role of systemic therapy in PTC is limited and unclear. Multiple combinations as paclitaxel-carboplatin, cisplatin-etoposide, and cisplatin-vinorelbine are explored (Webb et al. 2006; Allen et al. 2007; Napieralska et al. 2016). However, the indication, optimal combination, and dosing remain a question warranting further investigation.

6.4 Endobronchial Treatments

Endobronchial treatments are primarily used in the palliative scenario for obstructing lesions (Wood 2002). Stenting is commonly used in intrinsic or extrinsic airway obstruction or tracheoesophageal fistula. Silicone or self-expanding metallic/hybrid are commonly used stents and are available in different shapes and sizes. It usually offers immediate symptomatic and quality-of-life improvement (Aboudara et al. 2020; Guibert et al. 2016). Stenting in experienced hand carries high (>90%) success and low (<10%) complication rates (Guibert et al. 2016).

Several other endobronchial treatment techniques as mechanical debulking, laser, electrocoagulation, argon plasma coagulation, photodynamic therapy, and cryotherapy can be used for intrinsic airway narrowing or obstruction (American College of Chest Physicians and Health and Science Policy Committee 2003; Ernst et al. 2003; Bolliger et al. 2002). With life-threatening or significant intrinsic obstruction, modalities with immediate action as mechanical debulking, laser, electrocoagulation, and argon plasma coagulation are commonly explored. On the contrary, photodynamic therapy and cryotherapy with delayed effect are reserved for non-life-threatening or minimally obstructing scenarios (Ernst et al. 2003; Bolliger et al. 2002).

7 Patterns of Failure

There is minimal data available on patterns of failures. Mallick et al. reported 16% recurrences (120 of 733 patients) with a median time to progression of 22.5 months. Limited information on the site was available, and 30 recorded distant metastases involved lung, bone, liver, brain, epidural lesions, ileum, and nose (Mallick et al. 2019). There were no significant differences by histology (48—TACC and 43—TSCC). In another TSCC-specific series, 418 reported regional and distant metastases. Of these, 93 (22%) were nodal, and 104 (25%) were distant metastasis. Lung (46/104, 44.2%) was the most common site of distant metastasis (Ran et al. 2021). Another Canadian series of 38 TACC reported 17 hematogenous metastasis, of which 13 involved lung (Maziak et al. 1996). Distant metastasis is reported as a common site of failure in TACC (Je et al. 2017).

8 Current Challenges and Future Direction

Rarity is the prime issue and poses a significant challenge in the management of PTC. Current management of PTC is based on the available low-quality evidence as case series and retrospective cohorts. Understandably, these often lack complete details, and bias remains a significant concern, further jeopardizing the evidence quality.

Radiation is commonly used in PTC; however, the supportive evidence in adjuvant settings is limited and variable across different studies. Unfortunately, radiation technique and dose details were not recorded in the SEER database and significantly limited the analysis. The characteristics of plausible majority population undergoing radiation were advanced age, stage, poor performance status, positive margin, unresectable, or treated with palliative intent. These would introduce significant selection bias making an assessment of radiation extremely challenging.

The importance of nodal involvement is unclear and requires research. The lack of a uniform staging system is a significant concern affecting reporting, assessing prognostic and therapeutic factors, and comparing the reported literature. Development, validation, and standard staging system adaptation would help standard recording of disease burden and comparison across different groups.

The creation of a central/national level rare disease database and rigorous recording of demographic, treatment, toxicity, and outcome would help overcome some of the current shortcomings with quality of evidence.

Undoubtedly, PTC literature's current state reflects a lack of a high level of evidence interventions and warrants further research (Sharifnia et al. 2017). Till then, these should be managed in multidisciplinary settings, ideally in centers with experience in PTC.

9 Conclusion

PTC is extremely rare, and the current management of PTC is based on the available low-quality evidence. Surgery and radiation continue to play a vital role in the management of PTC. These should be managed in multidisciplinary settings ideally in centers with experience in PTC.

There are several important questions regarding staging, nodal status, and role of radiation that deserve further research and clarification. Creation of central/national level rare disease databases and rigorous recording of demographic, treatment, toxicity, and outcome would help overcome some of the current shortcomings with quality of evidence.

Conflict of Interest Statement I do not have any conflict of interest to disclose.

References

Aboudara M, Rickman O, Maldonado F (2020) Therapeutic bronchoscopic techniques available to the pulmonologist: emerging therapies in the treatment of peripheral lung lesions and endobronchial tumors. Clin Chest Med 41:145–160

Agrawal S, Jackson C, Celie KB et al (2017) Survival trends in patients with tracheal carcinoma from 1973 to 2011. Am J Otolaryngol 38:673–677

Allen AM, Rabin MS, Reilly JJ et al (2007) Unresectable adenoid cystic carcinoma of the trachea treated with chemoradiation. J Clin Oncol 25:5521–5523

American College of Chest Physicians, Health and Science Policy Committee (2003) Diagnosis and management of lung cancer: ACCP evidence-based guidelines. American College of Chest Physicians. Chest 123:D–G, 1S–337S

Azar T, Abdul-Karim FW, Tucker HM (1998) Adenoid cystic carcinoma of the trachea. Laryngoscope 108:1297–1300

Barnes D, Gutierrez Chacoff J, Benegas M et al (2017) Central airway pathology: clinic features, CT findings with pathologic and virtual endoscopy correlation. Insights Imaging 8:255–270

Benissan-Messan DZ, Merritt RE, Bazan JG et al (2020) National utilization of surgery and outcomes for primary tracheal cancer in the United States. Ann Thorac Surg 110:1012–1022

Bhattacharyya N (2004) Contemporary staging and prognosis for primary tracheal malignancies: a population-based analysis. Otolaryngol Head Neck Surg 131:639–642

Bolliger CT, Mathur PN, Beamis JF et al (2002) ERS/ATS statement on interventional pulmonology. European Respiratory Society/American Thoracic Society. Eur Respir J 19:356–373

Chao MW, Smith JG, Laidlaw C et al (1998) Results of treating primary tumors of the trachea with radiotherapy. Int J Radiat Oncol Biol Phys 41:779–785

Chow DC, Komaki R, Libshitz HI et al (1993) Treatment of primary neoplasms of the trachea. The role of radiation therapy. Cancer 71:2946–2952

Diaz-Mendoza J, Debiane L, Peralta AR et al (2019) Tracheal tumors. Curr Opin Pulm Med 25:336–343

Ernst A, Silvestri GA, Johnstone D et al (2003) Interventional pulmonary procedures: guidelines from the American College of Chest Physicians. Chest 123:1693–1717

Fiorentino A, Gregucci F, Desideri I et al (2021) Radiation treatment for adult rare cancers: oldest and newest indication. Crit Rev Oncol Hematol 159:103228

Gale N, Poljak M, Zidar N (2017) Update from the 4th edition of the World Health Organization classification of head and neck tumours: what is new in the 2017 WHO blue book for tumours of the hypopharynx, larynx, trachea and parapharyngeal space. Head Neck Pathol 11:23–32

Grillo HC (1990) Primary tracheal tumors: treatment and results. Ann Thorac Surg 49:69–77

Guibert N, Mhanna L, Droneau S et al (2016) Techniques of endoscopic airway tumor treatment. J Thorac Dis 8:3343–3360

Han S, El-Abbadi NH, Hanna N et al (2005) Evaluation of tracheal imaging by optical coherence tomography. Respiration 72:537–541

Hararah MK, Stokes WA, Oweida A et al (2020) Epidemiology and treatment trends for primary tracheal squamous cell carcinoma. Laryngoscope 130:405–412

Harms W, Latz D, Becker H et al (1999) HDR-brachytherapy boost for residual tumour after external beam radiotherapy in patients with tracheal malignancies. Radiother Oncol 52:251–255

Harms W, Latz D, Becker H et al (2000) Treatment of primary tracheal carcinoma. The role of external and endoluminal radiotherapy. Strahlenther Onkol 176:22–27

He J, Shen J, Huang J et al (2017) Prognosis of primary tracheal tumor: a population-based analysis. J Surg Oncol 115:1004–1010

Honings J, van Dijck JA, Verhagen AF et al (2007) Incidence and treatment of tracheal cancer: a nationwide study in the Netherlands. Ann Surg Oncol 14:968–976

Honings J, Gaissert HA, Ruangchira-Urai R et al (2009a) Pathologic characteristics of resected squamous cell carcinoma of the trachea: prognostic factors based on an analysis of 59 cases. Virchows Arch 455:423–429

Honings J, Gaissert HA, Verhagen AF et al (2009b) Undertreatment of tracheal carcinoma: multidisciplinary audit of epidemiologic data. Ann Surg Oncol 16:246–253

Honings J, Gaissert HA, Weinberg AC et al (2010) Prognostic value of pathologic characteristics and resection margins in tracheal adenoid cystic carcinoma. Eur J Cardiothorac Surg 37:1438–1444

Jamjoom L, Obusez EC, Kirsch J et al (2014) Computed tomography correlation of airway disease with bronchoscopy—part II: tracheal neoplasms. Curr Probl Diagn Radiol 43:278–284

Javidan-Nejad C (2010) MDCT of trachea and main bronchi. Radiol Clin North Am 48:157–176

Je HU, Song SY, Kim DK et al (2017) A 10-year clinical outcome of radiotherapy as an adjuvant or definitive treatment for primary tracheal adenoid cystic carcinoma. Radiat Oncol 12:196

Jeong SY, Lee KS, Han J et al (2007) Integrated PET/CT of salivary gland type carcinoma of the lung in 12 patients. AJR Am J Roentgenol 189:1407–1413

Jeremic B, Shibamoto Y, Acimovic L et al (1996) Radiotherapy for primary squamous cell carcinoma of the trachea. Radiother Oncol 41:135–138

Kurimoto N, Murayama M, Yoshioka S et al (1999) Assessment of usefulness of endobronchial ultrasonography in determination of depth of tracheobronchial tumor invasion. Chest 115:1500–1506

Levy A, Omeiri A, Fadel E et al (2018) Radiotherapy for tracheal-bronchial cystic adenoid carcinomas. Clin Oncol (R Coll Radiol) 30:39–46

Licht PB, Friis S, Pettersson G (2001) Tracheal cancer in Denmark: a nationwide study. Eur J Cardiothorac Surg 19:339–345

Macchiarini P (2006) Primary tracheal tumours. Lancet Oncol 7:83–91

Madariaga MLL, Gaissert HA (2018) Overview of malignant tracheal tumors. Ann Cardiothorac Surg 7:244–254

Makarewicz R, Mross M (1998) Radiation therapy alone in the treatment of tumours of the trachea. Lung Cancer 20:169–174

Mallick S, Benson R, Giridhar P et al (2019) Demography, patterns of care and survival outcomes in patients with malignant tumors of trachea: a systematic review and individual patient data analysis of 733 patients. Lung Cancer 132:87–93

Manninen MP, Antila PJ, Pukander JS et al (1991) Occurrence of tracheal carcinoma in Finland. Acta Otolaryngol 111:1162–1169

Maziak DE, Todd TR, Keshavjee SH et al (1996) Adenoid cystic carcinoma of the airway: thirty-two-year experience. J Thorac Cardiovasc Surg 112:1522–1531; discussion 1531–1532

McInnis MC, Weisbrod G, Schmidt H (2018) Advanced technologies for imaging and visualization of the tracheobronchial tree: from computed tomography and MRI to virtual endoscopy. Thorac Surg Clin 28:127–137

Meyers BF, Mathisen DJ (1997) Management of tracheal neoplasms. Oncologist 2:245–253

Mornex F, Coquard R, Danhier S et al (1998) Role of radiation therapy in the treatment of primary tracheal carcinoma. Int J Radiat Oncol Biol Phys 41:299–305

Napieralska A, Miszczyk L, Blamek S (2016) Tracheal cancer - treatment results, prognostic factors and incidence of other neoplasms. Radiol Oncol 50:409–417

Ogino T, Ono R, Shimizu W et al (1995) Adenoid cystic carcinoma of the tracheobronchial system: the role of postoperative radiotherapy. Radiat Med 13:27–29

Park CM, Goo JM, Lee HJ et al (2009) Tumors in the tracheobronchial tree: CT and FDG PET features. Radiographics 29:55–71

Parrish RW, Banks J, Fennerty AG (1983) Tracheal obstruction presenting as asthma. Postgrad Med J 59(698):775–776

Ran J, Qu G, Chen X et al (2021) Clinical features, treatment and outcomes in patients with tracheal adenoid cystic carcinoma: a systematic literature review. Radiat Oncol 16:38

Regnard JF, Fourquier P, Levasseur P (1996) Results and prognostic factors in resections of primary tracheal tumors: a multicenter retrospective study. The French Society of Cardiovascular Surgery. J Thorac Cardiovasc Surg 111:808–813; discussion 813–814

Rostom AY, Morgan RL (1978) Results of treating primary tumours of the trachea by irradiation. Thorax 33:387–393

Shadmehr MB, Farzanegan R, Graili P et al (2011) Primary major airway tumors; management and results. Eur J Cardiothorac Surg 39:749–754

Sharifnia T, Hong AL, Painter CA et al (2017) Emerging opportunities for target discovery in rare cancers. Cell Chem Biol 24:1075–1091

Shepard JO, Flores EJ, Abbott GF (2018) Imaging of the trachea. Ann Cardiothorac Surg 7:197–209

Urdaneta AI, Yu JB, Wilson LD (2011) Population based cancer registry analysis of primary tracheal carcinoma. Am J Clin Oncol 34:32–37

Waki A, Kato H, Yano R et al (1998) The importance of glucose transport activity as the rate-limiting step of 2-deoxyglucose uptake in tumor cells in vitro. Nucl Med Biol 25:593–597

Webb BD, Walsh GL, Roberts DB et al. (2006) Primary tracheal malignant neoplasms: the University of Texas MD Anderson Cancer Center experience. J Am Coll Surg 202:237–46. https://doi.org/10.1016/j.jamcollsurg.2005.09.016. Epub 2005 Nov 21. PMID: 16427548

Weber AL, Shortsleeve M, Goodman M et al (1978) Cartilaginous tumors of the larynx and trachea. Radiol Clin North Am 16:261–267

Wood DE (2001) Bronchoscopic preparation for airway resection. Chest Surg Clin N Am 11:735–748

Wood DE (2002) Management of malignant tracheobronchial obstruction. Surg Clin North Am 82:621–642

Xie L, Fan M, Sheets NC et al (2012) The use of radiation therapy appears to improve outcome in patients with malignant primary tracheal tumors: a SEER-based analysis. Int J Radiat Oncol Biol Phys 84:464–470

Yang KY, Chen YM, Huang MH et al (1997) Revisit of primary malignant neoplasms of the trachea: clinical characteristics and survival analysis. Jpn J Clin Oncol 27:305–309

Yang CJ, Shah SA, Ramakrishnan D et al (2020) Impact of positive margins and radiation after tracheal adenoid cystic carcinoma resection on survival. Ann Thorac Surg 109:1026–1032

Yusuf M, Gaskins J, Trawick E et al (2019) Effects of adjuvant radiation therapy on survival for patients with resected primary tracheal carcinoma: an analysis of the National Cancer Database. Jpn J Clin Oncol 49:628–638

Pulmonary Carcinoid

Roshal R. Patel, Brian De, and Vivek Verma

Contents

1 Etiology and Epidemiology 880
2 Histopathology and Biology 880
3 Clinical Presentation and Workup 880
4 Staging 882
5 Treatment 882
5.1 Surgical Resection 882
5.2 Symptom Management 888
5.3 Radionuclides 888
5.4 Chemotherapy 889
5.5 Targeted Therapy 889
5.6 Radiation Therapy 890
6 Prognosis 900
References 901

Abstract

Pulmonary carcinoid tumors are uncommon neuroendocrine tumors of the lung that lack invasive characteristics. They are histologically characterized as typical (low grade) or atypical (high grade) carcinoids based on mitotic activity and presence of necrosis. Pulmonary carcinoid tumors most commonly present as asymptomatic, incidental findings on chest radiographs. Diagnosis is confirmed via tissue sampling, although advanced imaging modalities such as somatostatin-based imaging may prove useful. Surgical resection is the primary treatment for these tumors; however, systemic therapies or radiation treatments may be considered in more advanced or medically inoperable setting. Medical therapies may be appropriate for patients with paraneoplastic syndromes, including carcinoid syndrome. Prognosis for patients with typical carcinoids is relatively favorable, although worse in patients with atypical carcinoids.

R. R. Patel (✉)
Albany Medical College, Albany, NY, USA
e-mail: patel.roshal@gmail.com

B. De · V. Verma
The University of Texas MD Anderson Cancer Center, Houston, TX, USA

First described in 1907 by Siegfried Oberndorfer, the term "carcinoid" represents a carcinoma-like lesion that lacks invasive characteristics. Pulmonary carcinoids are neuroendocrine tumors of the lung that are relatively uncommon. They vary in terms of clinical presentation and lack the aggressiveness of other neuroendocrine lung neoplasms such as large cell neuroendocrine carcinoma and small cell carcinoma. Often previously described as bronchial adenomas, pulmonary carcinoids were later found to have malignant potential. Pulmonary carcinoids are often characterized as typical versus atypical based on presentation and histologic characteristics.

1 Etiology and Epidemiology

Pulmonary carcinoid tumors are relatively rare lung tumors that are found in both smokers and nonsmokers; these neoplasms account for less than 2% of pulmonary malignancies. The incidence is fewer than 2 per 100,000; however, rates have been slowly increasing over the last several decades and potentially influenced by diagnostic tools and practices (Hemminki and Li 2001; Modlin et al. 2003; Dasari et al. 2017). Although males are more likely to have noncarcinoid pulmonary tumors, the development of pulmonary carcinoid is nearly twice as likely in females and more common in those of Caucasian descent (Modlin et al. 2003). Typical carcinoid tumors occur in over 80% of cases, with atypical carcinoids representing the remaining 20% (Soga and Yakuwa 1999; Rugge et al. 2008).

Compared to more aggressive neuroendocrine tumors, pulmonary carcinoids tend to present in younger patients and have a better prognosis. The role of smoking in the development of pulmonary carcinoids is disputed, although there is stronger evidence to suggest the implication of smoking in patients with atypical carcinoid tumors (Fink et al. 2001; Hassan et al. 2008). No other risk factors, including environmental exposure, have been shown to confer increased rates of pulmonary carcinoid development (Leoncini et al. 2016).

2 Histopathology and Biology

The 2015 World Health Organization classification of lung tumors describes lung neuroendocrine tumors as a scale across low grade (typical carcinoids), intermediate grade (atypical carcinoids), and high grade (large cell neuroendocrine carcinoma and small cell lung cancer) (Travis et al. 2015). Histologically, this is characterized by typical carcinoids having fewer than two mitoses per 2 mm^2 and no necrosis. Atypical carcinoids have 2–10 mitoses per 2 mm^2 or presence of necrosis.

Typical carcinoids are usually centrally located within the bronchopulmonary tree and are generally smaller. Atypical carcinoids are usually peripherally located and larger. These two major histologic classifications correlate with differences in survival outcomes, as 5-year overall survival for typical carcinoids ranges from 75 to 96%, whereas for atypical carcinoids it is 27–72% (Travis et al. 1998; Skuladottir et al. 2002; García-Yuste et al. 2007).

The cells of origin of pulmonary carcinoids are widely considered to be the enterochromaffin cells from embryonic divisions of the foregut. They are histologically defined by small, uniform polygonal cells comprised of membrane-bound eosinophilic neurosecretory vesicles, "salt-and-pepper" chromatin, and inconspicuous nuclei. Pulmonary carcinoids have a mutational rate of 0.4 mutations per megabase, significantly lower than other pulmonary malignancies. The most commonly mutated genes include *MEN1* and *ARID1A*—genes that play a role in chromatin remodeling (Fernandez-Cuesta et al. 2014; Simbolo et al. 2017).

3 Clinical Presentation and Workup

Pulmonary carcinoids most commonly present as asymptomatic disease noted as an incidental finding on a chest radiograph as a mass in the mediastinum or hilum. While typical carcinoids usually present with localized disease, atypical carcinoids often present as locally advanced or even metastatic in some instances.

When symptomatic, functional pulmonary carcinoids can present with carcinoid syndrome. Observed in 8% of pulmonary carcinoid cases, carcinoid syndrome is less prevalent than in neuroendocrine tumors of other sites such as the pancreas or small bowel (Halperin et al. 2017). The clinical presentation of carcinoid syndrome includes episodic skin flushing, tachycardia, shortness of breath, wheezing, and diarrhea. These symptoms are caused by the systemic release of vasoactive amines and polypeptides such as 5-hydroxyindoleacetic acid (5-HIAA). Such substances can be identified via 24-h urine or plasma 5-HIAA testing. Symptoms can be elicited or worsened by states of stress such as emotional turmoil as well as food and alcohol.

Approximately 1–2% of pulmonary carcinoid tumors present with Cushing's syndrome (Scanagatta et al. 2004; Kulke and Mayer 1999). Ectopic production of adrenocorticotropic hormone by the carcinoid tumor can lead to symptoms of central weight gain (often in the face, neck, and torso), abdominal striae, hyperglycemia, hypertension, hirsutism, and depression, as well as others. Initial screening can be conducted via several tests including a midnight dexamethasone suppression test, midnight salivary cortisol, or 24-h urinary free cortisol followed by adrenocorticotropic hormone tests to determine adrenal versus extra-adrenal causes.

Although extremely rare, cases of other neuroendocrine hormone-releasing tumors have been reported. Such vasoactive substances that can be released include corticotropin, dopamine, histamine, growth hormone, neurotensin, prostaglandins, and substance P (Fazel et al. 2008; Feldman 1985; Gustafsen et al. 1988; Kim et al. 2015; Bhansali et al. 2002; Krug et al. 2016; Feldman et al. 1974).

In a patient with a suspected lung mass, the differential diagnoses include lung carcinomas, metastasis from an extrapulmonary source, pulmonary carcinoids, and benign conditions (e.g., hamartomas, granulomas). Thorough history and physical examination should be conducted to identify clinical concerns and associated symptoms. Workup for patients with symptomatic carcinoid or Cushing's syndromes can include urine and plasma tests as previously mentioned.

Diagnostic imaging should begin with a CT chest with contrast if possible. While extrathoracic disease at diagnosis in patients with pulmonary carcinoids is rare, considerations for abdominal multiphasic CT or MRI as well as brain MRI may be considered based on clinical presentation. Somatostatin receptor-based imaging using ^{68}gallium-DOTATATE with PET/CT or ^{111}indium-octreotide with somatostatin receptor scintigraphy with PET/CT can also be considered (Jiang et al. 2019; Kuyumcu et al. 2012) as roughly 80% of pulmonary carcinoid tumors (whether functional or nonfunctional) express somatostatin receptors on immunohistochemistry (Kayani et al. 2009; Chong et al. 2007). These modalities targeting somatostatin receptors have been shown to be more reliable than PET/CT alone in differentiating between carcinoids and atelectasis (Jiang et al. 2019). Furthermore, somatostatin receptor-based imaging has demonstrated value in identifying recurrences as well (Musi et al. 1998).

As most pulmonary carcinoid tumors are centrally located, bronchoscopy is an important diagnostic tool, during which transbronchial biopsies can be obtained. For more peripheral tumors, CT or ultrasound can be used to guide fine needle aspiration biopsies of the tumor. Hematoxylin and eosin staining may be able to identify atypical versus typical versus other neuroendocrine phenotypes based on the previously described metrics of mitotic activity per 2 mm^2 and the presence of necrosis. Ki-67 immunostaining can be helpful in differentiating carcinoid versus noncarcinoid neuroendocrine tumors but cannot differentiate between typical and atypical carcinoid phenotypes (Pelosi et al. 2014). Furthermore, immunohistochemical staining for neuroendocrine and epithelial differentiation may be useful as well. Such markers include synaptophysin, chromogranin A, CD56 (neural cell adhesion molecule), cytokeratin, and thyroid transcription factor-1. Similar to Ki-67 immunostaining, these immunohistochemical markers are useful in differentiating carcinoid from noncarcinoid pathologies, but cannot differentiate typical versus atypical phenotypes.

4 Staging

At present, pulmonary carcinoid tumors are not staged differently than other lung malignancies such as non-small cell or small cell lung cancers. Staging is conducted using the 8th edition (2017) of the American Joint Committee on Cancer/Union for International Cancer Control TNM system guidelines, wherein T stage is assigned largely based on tumor size and/or degree of radiologically apparent invasion and N staging is based on the particular location of nodal involvement. Typical pulmonary carcinoid tumors present most often as stage I tumors. However, up to nearly half of atypical carcinoids may present as stage II–III due to bronchopulmonary or mediastinal node involvement (García-Yuste et al. 2007; Mezzetti et al. 2003). Retrospective analysis of data from the International Association for the Study of Lung Cancer and the National Cancer Institute's Surveillance Epidemiology and End Results database found that TNM staging (7th edition) correlated with the prognosis for pulmonary carcinoid tumors (Travis et al. 2008).

5 Treatment

5.1 Surgical Resection

Surgery, whenever possible, is widely considered the cornerstone for managing bronchopulmonary carcinoids. However, this has not been proven by randomized data, largely on account of the relative rarity of this disease. Nevertheless, initial evaluation for resection is a preferred approach at most centers, similar to the current standard of care for other earlier stage cancers of the lung. Table 1 summarizes several notable publications of surgery for these neoplasms.

Also similar to that for other lung neoplasms, surgical evaluation should consist of a complete history and physical examination with evidence of pulmonary function adequate enough to tolerate the proposed resection approach. Careful examination of thoracic imaging is essential to determine the type of surgical approach that is most optimal for addressing areas of clinically apparent or subclinical spread while preserving baseline lung function as best as possible. The goal of surgical resection is complete extirpation, without microscopic or macroscopic residual disease.

For localized disease, there is currently no consensus on the use of lobectomy versus sublobar approaches. At many centers, a conservative extent of resection is generally preferred because there is currently no prospective/robust evidence that more limited resection yields a higher rate of positive surgical margins, poorer disease-related outcomes, or both. Hence, approaches such as wedge resection, segmentectomy, and other sublobar techniques are very often utilized for localized tumors, provided that the tumor location and/or size is not prohibitive. Accordingly, the National Comprehensive Cancer Network (NCCN) guidelines at the time of writing state that either lobectomy or sublobar techniques are appropriate (National Comprehensive Cancer Network 2020). Carcinoid tumors situated more centrally may require sleeve approaches (e.g., sleeve lobectomy).

For more advanced disease, lobectomy is the consensus approach. Similar to the case for locally advanced non-small cell lung cancer (NSCLC), there is little role for pneumonectomy; this largely stems from the profound physiological changes caused by removal of an entire lung. As a result, resection could be relatively contraindicated if the disease extent/location would lend itself to a pneumonectomy, and referral for definitive radiation-based therapy in those cases may be the preferred approach. The utility of debulking surgery (without the goal of achieving a microscopic complete resection) remains understudied and currently unknown for pulmonary carcinoids.

The role of mediastinal lymph nodal evaluation is also unresolved to date—also largely on account of a large lack of evidence in this rare disease—in particular, whether lymph nodal dissection is required in all cases or whether more limited nodal sampling is adequate. It is unlikely that the extent of lymph node removal directly impacts survival, but rather may serve as a better

Table 1 Patients treated with primary surgery

First author (reference)	Year	# of patients	Treatments used	Surgery details	Outcomes	Key conclusions
Ferguson (2000)	2000	109 (78%) typical	Surgery alone	90 (65%) lobectomy 22 (16%) wedge or segmental resection 20 (14%) bilobectomy 4 (3%) pneumonectomy 3 (2%) bronchial sleeve	Typical: 5-year OS 90%	Survival favorable regardless of histology Local recurrence more common among atypical subtypes
		26 (19%) atypical			Atypical 5-year OS 70%	
Fink (2001)	2001	128 (90%) typical	Surgery alone	77 (56%) lobectomy 22 (16%) pneumonectomy	Typical: 5-year OS 89% 10-year OS 82%	Excellent long-term prognosis with aggressive surgical therapy
		14 (10%) atypical		18 (13%) wedge resection 9 (7%) bilobectomy 4 (3%) segmentectomy 4 (3%) sleeve resection 1 (1%) endobronchial laser therapy	Atypical: 5-year OS 75% 10-year OS 56%	
Fiala (2003)	2003	77 (80%) typical	Surgery alone	49 (51%) lobectomy 14 (15%) bronchoplastic procedure	Typical: 5-year OS 99% 10-year OS 88%	Very good prognosis even in node-positive patients with surgical management
		19 (20%) atypical		11 (11%) atypical resection and segmentectomy 9 (9%) sleeve lobectomy 7 (7%) pneumonectomy 5 (5%) enucleation	Atypical: 5-year OS 95% 10-year OS 74%	
Mezzetti (2003)	2003	88 (90%) typical	Surgery alone	Typical: 62 (70%) lobectomy 23 (26%) sparing resection 3 (3%) pneumonectomy	Typical: 5-year OS 92% 10-year OS 90%	Favorable prognoses among patients; parenchyma-sparing resections appropriate for typical, avoid limited resections for atypical
		10 (10%) atypical		Atypical: 7 (70%) lobectomy 2 (20%) sparing resection 1 (10%) pneumonectomy	Atypical: 5-year OS 71% 10-year OS 60%	

(continued)

Table 1 (continued)

First author (reference)	Year	# of patients	Treatments used	Surgery details	Outcomes	Key conclusions
Schrevens (2004)	2004	59 (88%) typical	Surgery alone	40 (60%) lobectomy 14 (21%) bilobectomy 9 (13%) pneumonectomy 4 (6%) limited resection	Typical: 5-year OS 92%	Radical excision with detailed lymph node evaluation is important in carcinoid
		8 (12%) atypical			Atypical: 5-year OS 67%	
Cardillo (2004)	2004	121 (74%) typical	Surgery alone	112 (69%) lobectomy 21 (13%) bilobectomy 12 (7%) pneumonectomy 9 (6%) wedge resection 8 (5%) sleeve lobectomy 1 (1%) segmental resection	N0 typical or atypical 5-year OS 100% N1 typical 5-year OS 90%	Nodal status is a stronger predictor of prognosis than histological subtype; N2 carcinoid tumors have a dismal prognosis
		42 (26%) atypical			N1 atypical 5-year OS 79% N2 atypical 5-year OS 22%	
Rea (2007)	2007	174 (69%) typical 78 (31%) atypical	Surgery alone	121 (48%) lobectomy 76 (30%) sleeve or bronchoplastic resection 18 (7%) bilobectomy 14 (6%) segmentectomy 13 (5%) wedge resection 10 (4%) pneumonectomy	5-year OS 90% 10-year OS 83% (typical 93%, atypical 64%) 15-year OS 77%	Typical histology and N0 status are most important prognostic factors
Ferolla (2009)	2009	100 (81%) typical	Surgery alone	92 (75%) lobectomy or bilobectomy 12 (10%) sleeve lobectomy or bronchial sleeve	Typical: 5-year OS 98% 10-year OS 96% 15-year OS 84%	Major surgical procedures with systemic nodal dissection are required for optimal treatment
		23 (19%) atypical		6 (5%) pneumonectomy 4 (3%) segmentectomy 2 (2%) wedge resection 2 (2%) bronchoplasty 2 (2%) enucleation 1 (1%) tracheal resection	Atypical: 5-year OS 72% 10-year OS 57% 15-year OS 24%	

Study	Year	Histology	Treatment	Surgery Type	Survival	Conclusions
Machuca (2010)	2010	110 (87%) typical	Surgery alone	58 (46%) lobectomy 26 (21%) sleeve lobectomy 19 (15%) sublobar resection 9 (7%) bronchoplasty 8 (6%) bilobectomy 6 (5%) pneumonectomy 2 (2%) sleeve segmentectomy	Typical: 5-year OS 91% 10-year OS 89%	Bronchial carcinoid tumors only. Surgery is safe and adequate
		16 (13%) atypical			Atypical: 5-year OS 56% 10-year OS 47%	
Aydin (2011)	2011	84 (81%) typical	Surgery alone	49 (47%) lobectomy 17 (16%) bilobectomy 15 (14%) pneumonectomy 11 (11%) bronchoplasty (w/ or w/o lobectomy) 7 (7%) sleeve lobectomy 4 (4%) wedge resection 1 (1%) segmentectomy	Typical: 5-year OS 92% 10-year OS 83%	Histologic subtype, disease stage, and type of surgery were prognostic
		20 (19%) atypical			Atypical: 5-year OS 73% 10-year OS 46%	
Johnson (2011)	2011	43 (83%) typical	Surgery alone[a]	27 (52%) lobectomy 10 (19%) wedge resection 5 (10%) segmentectomy 5 (10%) bilobectomy 4 (8%) sleeve resection 1 (2%) pneumonectomy	Typical: 5-year OS 97% 10-year OS 72%	Histology may be more prognostic than nodal involvement
		9 (17%) typical			Atypical: 5-year OS 35% 10-year OS 0%	
Zhong (2012)	2012	106 (81%) typical	Surgery alone	34 (26%) sleeve lobectomy 32 (24%) lobectomy 31 (24%) pneumonectomy 26 (20%) bilobectomy 6 (5%) bronchoplastic procedure w/o resection 2 (2%) segmentectomy	Typical: 5-year OS 98% 10-year OS 90% 15-year OS 74%	Histology and nodal status were significant independent prognostic factors for survival
		25 (19%) atypical			Atypical: 5-year OS 86% 10-year OS 74% 15-year OS 24%	

(continued)

Table 1 (continued)

First author (reference)	Year	# of patients	Treatments used	Surgery details	Outcomes	Key conclusions
Stolz (2015)	2015	95 (69%) typical	Surgery alone	110 (80%) lobectomy or bilobectomy 15 (11%) sleeve lobectomy 6 (4%) pneumonectomy 4 (3%) wedge resection 2 (1%) bronchial resection	Typical: 5-year OS 97% 10-year OS 90%	Histology, age, and nodal status were associated with better prognosis. Systematic lymphadenectomy should always be performed
		42 (31%) atypical			Atypical: 5-year OS 71% 10-year OS 62%	
Okereke (2016)	2016	96 (79%) typical	Surgery alone	108 (89%) anatomic resection 13 (11%) minimally invasive, video assisted	Typical: 5-year OS 96% 10-year OS 77%	Nodal metastases and tumor size are not associated with recurrence or survival. Number of mitoses independently associated with survival
		25 (21%) atypical			Atypical: 5-year OS 87% 10-year OS 69%	
Ramirez (2017)	2017	113 (67%) typical	Surgery or observation	121 (72%) underwent resection	Typical: 5-year OS 90% 10-year OS 81%	Ki-67, Nodal status, differentiation status, and carcinoid phenotype were prognostic
		46 (27%) atypical 10 (6%) unknown			Atypical: 5-year OS 84% 10-year OS 59%	
Pikin (2017)	2017	23 (92%) typical 2 (8%) atypical	Surgery alone	25 (100%) endoscopic resection followed by bronchoplasty	5-year OS 100% 10-year OS 92% Local control 100% at last follow-up	Endobronchial carcinoid tumors only
Sadowski (2018)	2018	83 (73%) typical	Surgery alone[a]	52 (46%) lobectomy 17 (15%) wedge resection 11 (10%) undefined surgery 9 (8%) segmentectomy 3 (3%) bilobectomy 2 (2%) pneumonectomy 2 (2%) bronchial resection	Typical: Mean DFS 74 months Mean OS 86 months	SwissNET analysis. Atypical histology confers worse outcomes
		14 (12%) atypical 16 (14%) unknown			Atypical: Mean DFS 48 months Mean OS 48 months	

| Filosso (2019) | 2019 | 876 typical (stage I only, 100%) | Surgery alone | 616 (70%) lobectomy 122 (14%) wedge resection 75 (9%) segmentectomy 63 (7%) sleeve lobectomy | Typical: All patients 5-year OS 94% Lobectomy 5-year OS 96% Segmentectomy 5-year OS 94% HR for death with wedge resection 1.98 ($P =$ ss) 5-year LC 94% | European Society of Thoracic Surgeons retrospective database of the Neuroendocrine Tumors of the Lung Working Group analysis. Anatomic surgical resection is superior for stage I typical carcinoid tumors |

Percentages may add to less than or more than 100% in several cases due to missing information or multiple procedures conducted for patients
[a]Several patients received adjuvant chemotherapy in these studies; however, limited details regarding timing and outcomes are provided

indicator of the necessity for adjuvant therapy, since an increasing number of harvested lymph nodes increases the likelihood that "true" pN0 disease is present and adjuvant therapy can be omitted. Reported rates of nodal involvement in pulmonary carcinoids vary markedly—clinically apparent involvement in roughly 8–10% of typical carcinoids and 25% of atypical cases, and pathologic involvement in 17% for typical carcinoids and 39–46% for atypical histology (Steuer et al. 2015; Kneuertz et al. 2018). These findings, although derived from retrospective data, suggest that mediastinal lymph node dissection should be considered for the vast majority of atypical carcinoids and larger sized typical carcinoids. However, whether nodal sampling alone for smaller sized typical carcinoids is adequate enough remains unclear. Thus, clinicians should weigh the advantages and disadvantages of both approaches in such patients on a case-by-case basis. Ideally, intraoperative pathologic examination of the sampled lymphatics may better inform the necessity for a complete dissection (i.e., if the intraoperative evaluation confirms nodal spread).

Endobronchial modalities (e.g., laser ablation and cryotherapy) to treat pulmonary carcinoid are gaining popularity, largely owing to the reduced invasiveness. Unlike the surgical techniques mentioned above, the goal of endobronchial approaches is not to achieve a complete resection, but rather to debulk only. The rationale is that debulking alone may be required for low-grade typical carcinoids (ideally smaller sized), because they display relatively low-grade growth and the patient may not require full-scale surgery. Hence, the primary advantage of this approach is to spare the lung parenchyma, whereas a key disadvantage is the inability to examine the lymphatics. The outcomes of endobronchial therapies for pulmonary carcinoids have been limited to very few studies, largely retrospective and mostly in typical cases (Reuling et al. 2019). The results reveal recurrence rates and outcomes comparable to surgery and a low complication rate; however, a critical caveat is that they largely comprise a highly enriched population of well-selected patients. Thus, it is unlikely that the data apply equally well to the general population of pulmonary carcinoids. As a result, on account of a large lack of data, these modalities are recommended only if surgery and radiation therapy are both contraindicated (National Comprehensive Cancer Network 2020). If these modalities are considered, however, careful patient selection by a multidisciplinary panel is highly recommended.

5.2 Symptom Management

Somatostatin analogs such as octreotide or lanreotide are considered first-line therapy in patients presenting with symptoms of carcinoid syndrome or in the large proportion of patients that may have positive somatostatin receptor scans. These therapeutics bind to somatostatin receptors, greatly inhibiting neuropeptide release as well as other endocrine and exocrine functions of the gastrointestinal symptom. A pooled analysis suggests that octreotide or lanreotide improves symptoms in 65–72% of patients, with a biochemical response (defined as a reduction in urinary 5-HIAA) of 45–46% (Hofland et al. 2019). In addition to symptomatic relief, prospective data also suggest that these somatostatin analogs offer disease control and antitumor activity (Bongiovanni et al. 2017). Ondansetron, a 5-hydroxytryptamine-3 antagonist, is another therapy that may offer relief to patients experiencing carcinoid syndrome. In particular, ondansetron has been found to be most effective for diarrhea (Wymenga et al. 1998), including in patients that have symptoms refractory to somatostatin analogs (Kiesewetter et al. 2019; Kiesewetter and Raderer 2013).

5.3 Radionuclides

While somatostatin analogs may have some antitumoral properties, the addition of peptide receptor radionuclides such as ^{177}lutetium (Lu)-DOTATATE may further benefit patients with somatostatin receptor-positive tumors. ^{177}Lu-DOTATATE was demonstrated in the randomized NETTER-1 trial to offer a progression-free survival advantage in patients with well-differentiated gastroenteropancreatic tumors (Strosberg et al. 2017). Although no randomized data are available specifically for pulmonary carcinoid tumors, the high affinity of ^{177}Lu-DOTATATE for somatostatin subtype 2 receptors suggests that it may be an effective treatment in somatostatin receptor-positive tumors that have progress on somatostatin receptor antagonists (Kwekkeboom et al. 2005).

Another peptide receptor radionuclide, ^{90}yttrium(Y)-edotreotide, has demonstrated a statistically significant improvement in carcinoid symptoms (63–74%) in cases refractory to somatostatin analogs (Waldherr et al. 2002; Bushnell Jr et al. 2010). While response rates to ^{90}Y-edotreotide in two prospective studies of patients with bronchial or gastroenteropancreatic tumors were low (4–23%), the proportions of patients deriving clinical benefit (i.e., stable disease) were high (67–92%) (Waldherr et al. 2002; Bushnell Jr et al. 2010).

5.4 Chemotherapy

Currently, there is no role for adjuvant chemotherapy in the setting of localized pulmonary carcinoid tumors. Guidelines from the NCCN do not recommend adjuvant chemotherapy in patients with localized disease (National Comprehensive Cancer Network 2020). For patients with locally advanced presentation (stage IIIA) amenable to surgical resection, adjuvant chemotherapy may be considered in the setting of atypical (intermediate-grade) tumors that have more aggressive characteristics such as poorly differentiated histology, higher Ki-67, or increased mitotic index. Chemotherapy should be considered in patients with locally advanced disease that is not amenable to surgical resection (stage IIIA–C), in those with metastatic disease, or in those who have progressed through initial therapy (Marty-Ané et al. 1995; Caplin et al. 2015). Etoposide and a platinum agent are the two most commonly used regimens. Response rates in patients with metastatic pulmonary carcinoid tumors have been found to range from 20% to 23% (Chong et al. 2014; Wirth et al. 2004). Temozolomide with or without capecitabine is another regimen that is gaining popularity due to a potentially higher clinical benefit in patients with advanced disease, with response rates up to 30% in retrospective series (Chong et al. 2014; Ekeblad et al. 2007; Al-Toubah et al. 2020). Prior chemotherapeutic regimens tested include adriamycin, doxorubicin, cyclophosphamide, oxaliplatin, streptozotocin, and 5-fluorouracil; however, these have fallen out of favor due to lack of response or high toxicities (Bukowski et al. 1987; Engstrom et al. 1984; Walter et al. 2016; Moertel and Hanley 1979).

5.5 Targeted Therapy

Everolimus is a rapamycin derivative that selectively inhibits mTORC1, thereby affecting cell proliferation. It can be considered in patients with advanced, symptomatic pulmonary carcinoids. The RAD001 In Advance Neuroendocrine Tumors-2 (RADIANT-2) trial was a phase III double-blinded, randomized trial in which 429 patients with functional neuroendocrine tumors received either everolimus or placebo. All patients received octreotide long-acting repeatable (LAR). This study found a significant improvement in median progression-free survival (16.4 months versus 11.3 months, HR 0.77, 95% CI 0.59–1.00, $P = 0.026$) (Pavel et al. 2011). Secondary analysis of the 44 patients with lung neuroendocrine tumors demonstrated an increase in progression-free survival in patients receiving everolimus, although not significant (13.6 versus 3.6, HR 0.72; 95% CI 0.31–1.68, $P = 0.23$) (Fazio et al. 2013). Everolimus can also be considered as a first-line therapy for progressive, well-differentiated, and nonfunctional pulmonary neuroendocrine tumors in the unresectable, locally advanced, or metastatic settings. The RADIANT-4 trial was a phase III, double-blinded trial in which patients were randomized to receive everolimus with supportive care versus placebo with supportive care. The study enrolled 302 patients with lung or gastrointestinal neuroendocrine tumors. Across all tumor types, everolimus demonstrated an improved progression-free survival versus the placebo (11.0 months versus 3.9 months, HR 0.48, 95% CI 0.35–0.67, $P < 0.00001$) (Yao et al. 2016). The results of this trial led to approval of everolimus as a first-line therapy for advanced, nonfunctional neuroendocrine tumors in February 2016 by the United States Food and Drug Administration. A later subset analysis of the RADIANT-4 trial examined the 90 patients with pulmonary carcinoid tumors and demonstrated the benefit of everolimus over placebo with respect to progression-free survival (9.2 months versus 3.6 months, HR 0.50, 95% CI 0.28–0.88) (Fazio et al. 2018). Notably, the rates of adverse events were low: stomatitis (11%), hyperglycemia (10%), and infection (8%).

Bevacizumab and sunitinib are two other therapies that are being explored in phase III trials. Neuroendocrine tumors have been found to be highly vascular with elevated levels of expression of angiogenic markers such as vascular endothelial growth factor (VEGF) (Scoazec 2013). Phase II data have demonstrated mixed rates of response and toxicity (Kulke et al. 2008; Yao et al. 2008; Chan et al. 2012; Hobday et al. 2007). A phase III trial (SWOG S0518) of interferon alfa-2b versus bevacizumab in patients with advanced neuroendocrine tumors receiving depot octreotide did not demonstrate any improvement in progression-free survival between the arms. At this time, inhibitors of angiogenesis are not recommended by the NCCN (National Comprehensive Cancer Network 2020).

Several basket trials have been conducted to test immunotherapy agents in patients with cancers of neuroendocrine derivation (Maggio et al. 2020). Although data are limited with respect to immunotherapy treatments in patients with pulmonary carcinoid, some findings are available. KEYNOTE-028 enrolled 471 patients with programmed death ligand 1 (PD-L1)-positive, advanced solid tumors, of which 25 patients had carcinoid tumors (9 pulmonary carcinoids). Patients were treated with pembrolizumab until disease progression or toxicity. The 25 patients with carcinoid tumors demonstrated a 12% objective response rate as well as progression-free survival and overall survival of 27% and 65%, respectively, at 12 months (Ott et al. 2018).

The safety profile of immunotherapy treatment in these patients demonstrated toxicities requiring hospitalization in 8 patients; however, only 1 of 25 patients needed to stop therapy due to adverse events (Mehnert et al. 2020). Out of the patients screened for the study, only 21% of those with carcinoid tumors were found to express PD-L1 (Mehnert et al. 2020).

5.6 Radiation Therapy

Owing to the relative rarity of bronchopulmonary carcinoid tumors, there have been no prospective studies examining the utility of radiation therapy (RT) in the definitive, adjuvant, or palliative settings. These limitations must be carefully taken into account when performing clinical decision-making for these neoplasms; as a result, multidisciplinary coordination is essential.

Definitive RT is generally utilized for the indications of medical/surgical inoperability (or in a minority of cases, patient refusal of surgery) and/or if the risk of progression with observation is deemed high enough to warrant intervention. Definitive local therapy using RT is effective for pulmonary carcinoids (Table 2), and results of the available evidence show appropriate rates of local or locoregional control, with few high-grade adverse events when utilizing modern conformal RT techniques.

As part of definitive therapy, disease that is localized, of reasonable size, and not involving the major airways may safely undergo stereotactic body RT (SBRT, also known as stereotactic ablative radiotherapy). This has replaced conventionally fractionated or hypofractionated RT for early-stage NSCLC (Onishi et al. 2007) and small cell lung cancer (Verma et al. 2017) on account of the patient convenience, cost-effectiveness, as well as high biologically effective dose (BED) delivered, resulting in high rates of local control. There are few studies of primary SBRT for pulmonary carcinoids, but the existing small-volume data illustrate high rates of local control (Colaco and Decker 2015; Singh et al. 2019). Likewise, the limited quality and quantity of retrospective data suggest that SBRT is associ-

Table 2 Patients treated with definitive radiotherapy

First author (reference)	Year	# of patients	Treatments used	RT details	Chemo details	Local control rate	Survival	Key conclusions
Wirth (2004)	2004	8 (44%) typical 10 (56%) atypical	14 (78%) chemo alone 3 (17%) concurrent chemo-RT 1 (6%) chemo → chemo-RT	54 Gy in 2 patients, 46 Gy in 1 patient, no info for 1 patient	Median 3.5 cycles 13 (72%) patients treated with etoposide-based regimen 14 (77%) patients received combination	22% (OS)	Median OS 20 months	Response rates with chemo or chemo-RT are less than those of small cell lung cancers
Colaco (2015)	2015	2 (50%) typical 2 (50%) atypical	All SBRT (100%)	54 Gy/3 fx in 2 patients, 50 Gy/5 fx in 2 patients	N/A	100% at last follow-up of 14.6 months	Not reported	SBRT may offer an effective alternative for inoperable patients
Singh (2019)	2019	9 (90%) typical 1 (10%) atypical	All SBRT (100%)	Median dose 50 Gy (range, 40–60 Gy) in 5–10 fractions Median BED 100 Gy (range, 75–115.5)	N/A	100% at last follow-up	Median OS 27.1 months	SBRT/hypofractionated RT are promising local therapies for inoperable disease with favorable outcomes and without significant long-term morbidity
Wegner (2019a)	2019	154 (10%) typical cT1-2N0M0	Conventionally fractionated RT (45%) or SBRT (55%)	84 patients received SBRT: median 50 Gy (IQR, 50–55 Gy) in 4 fractions (IQR 4–5 fractions) 70 patients received conventionally fractionated RT: median 54 Gy (IQR 50–60) in 24 fractions (IQR 5–33)	10 (6%) patients received chemo	–	Median survival longer in patients receiving SBRT vs. conventional fractionation: 65 months vs. 58 months (P = ss)	National Cancer Database analysis. SBRT for early-stage bronchopulmonary carcinoid has increased over time and is associated with better survival than conventionally fractionated RT

Percentages may add to less than or more than 100% in several cases due to missing information or multiple procedures conducted for patients

ated with superior survival as compared to conventional fractionation (Wegner et al. 2019a); whether this is due to retrospective selection biases or driven by increased local control from the higher BED of SBRT remains unknown. Conservatively interpreted, it is unlikely that outcomes following SBRT are any worse than conventional fractionation.

SBRT for pulmonary carcinoids should proceed based on the fundamental principles of SBRT for other intrathoracic neoplasms. These include accounting for respiratory motion using one of a variety of techniques (e.g., respiratory gating, four-dimensional computed tomography simulation), small target margins (e.g., 5 mm), RT treatment planning aiming to achieve a sharp dose drop-off between the tumor and surrounding organs at risk (OARs), higher quality patient immobilization techniques, and daily image guidance.

The particular dose and fractionation regimen should be carefully assessed based on tumor size and location. Even for small-volume disease, cases exceeding tolerance limits for central mediastinal OARs such as the tracheobronchial tree or esophagus should not be treated with SBRT and instead converted into a hypofractionated ablative approach if feasible (e.g., 60–70 Gy in 8–10 fractions), or more modest hypofractionation. The minimum effective BED for SBRT is considered to be 100 Gy_{10} based on NSCLC data (Onishi et al. 2007), but it is unclear whether this should be extrapolated to pulmonary carcinoids. As a result, although a BED of at least 100 Gy_{10} can be readily delivered in most cases given the plethora of evidence validating its safety, clinicians can also consider regimens with BED <100 Gy_{10} if dose constraints to normal OARs cannot meet the accepted standards.

Definitive RT in a conventionally or mildly hypofractionated manner should similarly follow the principles of other intrathoracic neoplasms. This includes delineating gross disease, followed by an expansion to account for subclinical parenchymal/nodal spread (the magnitude of the expansion being largely based on individual/institutional practice). The role of elective nodal irradiation in these neoplasms is unclear but is generally not recommended as an extrapolation from NSCLC (Rosenzweig et al. 2007). An additional expansion to account for patient setup uncertainties is then placed, the size of which also depends on several factors such as individual/institutional practice, whether respiratory motion has been addressed or not, and the quality of available image guidance. The prescription dose for more advanced cases of bronchopulmonary carcinoids remains without consensus. In a national review of conventional fractionation for these tumors, the interquartile range of prescribed doses ranged from 50 to 60 Gy (Wegner et al. 2019a). In general, however, prescribed doses should reflect the tumor size, histology, and overall subjectively deemed risk of local failure. Either three-dimensional conformal RT (3D CRT) or intensity-modulated RT (IMRT) is recommended, noting that in the NSCLC setting the use of IMRT reduces the rate of severe pneumonitis (Chun et al. 2017). Whether the use of a lower prescription dose and/or the presence of a smaller volume of disease obviates the need for IMRT for pulmonary carcinoids is currently unclear.

Adjuvant RT (Table 3) for these neoplasms is highly controversial, and its necessity (or lack thereof) relates to patterns of failure data without RT. For completely resected typical carcinoids, local failure is relatively low (8% in a study by Kaplan et al. (2003)), so the utility of adjuvant RT for these cases is the lowest. Conversely, the rate of local failure in atypical carcinoids can be high (e.g., 23% in the aforementioned study). However, the utility of adjuvant RT in that setting must be carefully weighed against the risk of developing distant metastasis (also 23% from the same study).

Common indications for postoperative RT in NSCLC include positive surgical margins and/or mediastinal nodal (N2) involvement. It remains unclear whether those indications (based on non-randomized data) should be extrapolated to pulmonary carcinoids. In less proliferative neoplasms such as pulmonary carcinoids, the presence of a positive surgical margin and/or nodal involvement may not be as clinically consequential as they are for NSCLC. Additionally,

Table 3 Patients treated with adjuvant radiotherapy or chemotherapy

First author (reference)	Year	# of patients	Treatments used	Surgery details	RT details	Chemo details	Local control rate	Survival	Key conclusions
Beasley (2000)	2000	106 (100%) atypical	Surgery ± chemo ± RT	56 (52%) lobectomy 16 (15%) pneumonectomy 12 (11%) wedge resection 7 (7%) bilobectomy 5 (5%) bronchial biopsy 1 (1%) sleeve resection	Adjuvant: 13 (12%) patients	Adjuvant: 12 (11%) patients	–	5-year OS 61% 10-year OS 35% 15-year OS 28%	Higher mitotic rate, tumor size ≥3.5 cm, female sex, and presence of rosettes are independent predictors of survival
Carretta (2000)	2000	36 (82%) typical 3 (7%) atypical 5 (11%) LCNEC	Surgery ± chemo ± RT	32 (73%) lobectomy 3 (7%) bilobectomy 3 (7%) segmentectomy 3 (7%) bronchoplastic procedures 1 (2%) pneumonectomy	Adjuvant: 5 (11%) patients (median 56 Gy, range 45–58 Gy)	Adjuvant: 1 (2%) patient	–	Typical: 5-year OS 93% Atypical/LCNEC: 5-year OS 70%	Node-positive patients fare worse; however, role of adjuvant therapy remains unclear

(continued)

Table 3 (continued)

First author (reference)	Year	# of patients	Treatments used	Surgery details	RT details	Chemo details	Local control rate	Survival	Key conclusions
Kaplan (2003)	2003	144 (70%) typical	Surgery ± chemo-RT, chemo-RT alone	No details provided	Typical: 12 (8%) adjuvant chemo-RT, 2 (1%) chemo-RT only		Typical 5-year: 92%	Typical: 5-year DSS: 79% 10-year DSS: 63% 20-year DSS: 39%	Atypical patients have higher rates of locoregional and distant metastasis; postoperative combined chemo-RT is recommended
		62 (30%) atypical			Atypical: 19 (31%) adjuvant chemo-RT		Atypical 5-year: 77%	Atypical: 5-year DSS: 60% 10-year DSS: 37% 20-year DSS: 28%	
Divisi (2005)	2005	26 (62%) typical	Surgery ± chemo ± RT	30 (71%) lobectomy 6 (14%) wedge resection 5 (12%) bilobectomy 1 (2%) pneumonectomy	7 (44%) atypical stage III patients combination of chemo, RT, or both		–	Typical: 3-year OS 100% 5-year OS 96%	Long-term survival is possible with complete surgical resection
		16 (38%) atypical						Atypical: 3-year OS 81% 5-year OS 68%	
Kyriss (2006)	2006	97 (87%) typical	Surgery ± pre-op chemo ± adjuvant RT	79 (71%) lobectomy 16 (14%) bilobectomy 8 (7%) pneumonectomy 5 (5%) segmental resection 2 (2%) sleeve resection 1 (1%) exploratory thoracotomy	Adjuvant: 5 (5%) pN2 patients (mediastinal RT to 60Gy)	Neoadjuvant: 2 (2%) patients (suspected small cell at initial diagnosis)	–	Typical 5-year OS 94% Typical 10-year OS 84%	Patients who undergo radical oncologic resection with mediastinal lymphadenectomy have very good survival
		14 (13%) atypical						Atypical 5-year OS 92% Atypical 10-year OS 62%	

		Surgery ± RT						
Garcia-Yuste (2007)	2007	569 (86%) typical	374 (57%) lobectomy or bilobectomy 66 (10%) bronchoplastic procedure 66 (10%) wedge or segmental resection 63 (10%) pneumonectomy 9 (1%) sleeve resection	Adjuvant: 19 (3%) pN2 patients with mediastinal RT	N/A	—	Typical 5-year OS 97%, 100% with N+ disease	Nodal involvement and histological subtype are strongest prognostic factors
		92 (14%) atypical					Atypical 5-year OS: 78%, 60% with N+ disease	
Han (2013)	2013	12 atypical (100%)	Surgery: 6 (50%) Surgery + chemo: 3 (25%) Surgery + RT: 2 (17%) Surgery + chemo-RT: 1 (8%)	All (100%) lobectomy or pneumonectomy with mediastinal nodal dissection	Adjuvant RT to operative bed	Etoposide + cisplatin or paclitaxel + carboplatin	92%	Atypical: 5-year OS 64%	Mitotic count is an important prognostic indicator. Atypical carcinoid is prone to distant metastatic relapse
Cañizares (2014)	2014	127 atypical (100%)	Surgery: 107 (84%) Surgery + chemo: 11 (9%) Surgery + RT: 6 (5%) Surgery + chemo-RT: 3 (2%)	77 (61%) lobectomy 22 (17%) pneumonectomy 14 (11%) wedge resection 12 (9%) bilobectomy 2 (2%) bronchial resection	No details provided	No details provided	92% at last follow-up	Atypical: 5-year OS 80%	Sublobar resection is independently linked to locoregional recurrence

(continued)

Table 3 (continued)

First author (reference)	Year	# of patients	Treatments used	Surgery details	RT details	Chemo details	Local control rate	Survival	Key conclusions
Okoye (2014)	2014	57 (90%) typical	Surgery: 52 (83%) Other (radiation and/or chemo and/or octreotide): 11 (17%)	23 (37%) lobectomy 6 (10%) wedge resection 6 (10%) pneumonectomy 6 (10%) bilobectomy 4 (6%) sleeve resection 4 (6%) lobectomy with sleeve resection 2 (3%) segmentectomy 1 (2%) segmentectomy with sleeve resection	7 (11%) patients with chest-directed RT (59.4/33, 50/5, 54/30, 35/14, 40/5, 40/20)	Mixed regimens: carboplatin + etoposide, capecitabine + temozolomide	88% at 5 years	Typical: 5-year OS 95% 10-year OS 87% 5-year EFS 88% 10-year EFS 80%	Extended mediastinal dissection should be performed for central tumors, clinically aggressive, or atypical carcinoids. Nonsurgical therapies rarely achieve long-term disease control
		6 (10%) atypical						Atypical: 5-year EFS 50%	
Nussbaum (2015)	2015	4612 (100%) typical	Surgery ± chemo	All (100%) lobectomy	Not reported	37 (6%) of 629 N+ patients	–	5-year OS with chemo 69% for 82% without	National Cancer Database analysis. Adjuvant chemotherapy is not associated with improved survival in patients who undergo lobectomy
Steuer (2015)	2015	441 (100%) atypical	341 (77%) surgery 54 (12%) RT	247 (56%) lobectomy or bilobectomy 59 (13%) wedge resection 16 (4%) pneumonectomy 13 (3%) segmental resection	Not reported	Data not available	–	1-year OS 86% 3-year OS 67% RT hazard ratio Univariable 2.44 (P = ss) Multivariable: 1.42 (P = ns)	SEER analysis. Adjuvant RT was associated with increased risk of death on univariable analysis, likely reflecting higher risk population

Hobbins (2016)	2016	1341 total (unable to differentiate histology)	Observation vs. surgery ± chemo ± RT	80% surgery	4% RT	6% chemo	—	1-year OS 92% 3-year OS 85%	UK National Lung Cancer Audit. One in five patients presented with metastatic disease. Surgery for early disease is associated with favorable prognosis
Cusumano (2017)	2017	159 (82%) typical	Surgery ± chemo ± RT	Typical: 86 (54%) lobectomy 25 (16%) sleeve lobectomy 22 (14%) segmentectomy 13 (8%) bilobectomy 10 (8%) wedge resection 3 (2%) pneumonectomy	Neoadjuvant RT in 1 (1%) typical patient	Neoadjuvant chemo in 2 (1%) typical and 1 (3%) atypical patient	—	Typical: 5-year OS 97% 10-year OS 88%	Surgery confers acceptable results, which mainly depend on subtype, nodal status, and SUVmax
		36 (18%) atypical		Atypical: 21 (58%) lobectomy 5 (14%) sleeve lobectomy 4 (11%) bilobectomy 3 (8%) segmentectomy 2 (6%) pneumonectomy 1 (3%) wedge resection		Adjuvant chemo in 4 (3%) typical and 7 (19%) atypical patients		Atypical: 5-year OS 78% 10-year OS 68%	

(continued)

Table 3 (continued)

First author (reference)	Year	# of patients	Treatments used	Surgery details	RT details	Chemo details	Local control rate	Survival	Key conclusions
Cattoni (2017)	2017	240 (100%) typical	Surgery ± induction therapy or adjuvant therapy	113 (47%) lobectomy 47 (19%) wedge resection 34 (14%) sleeve lobectomy 18 (8%) bilobectomy 18 (8%) segmentectomy 2 (1%) pneumonectomy	4 (2%) patients with induction therapy, 1 (~0%) patient with adjuvant therapy. Details not provided		–	5-year OS 94%	Prognostic survival model presented with significant differences between classes
Anderson (2017)	2017	581 (100%) atypical	Surgery ± chemo	All (100%) pneumonectomy or lobectomy	N/A	Adjuvant chemo in 18% (4% for pN0 and 41% for pN+)	–	Node negative: 1-year OS 97% 5-year OS 82% Node positive: 1-year OS 99% 5-year OS 60%	National Cancer Database analysis. Adjuvant chemo in pN0 and pN+ disease conferred no survival advantage
Kneuertz (2018)	2018	2893 (87%) atypical 442 (13%) atypical	Surgery ± chemo ± RT ± chemo-RT	84% lobectomy/ bilobectomy, 8% pneumonectomy, 8% sublobar resection	Adjuvant chemo-RT in 51 (2%) patients, chemo alone in 94 (3%) patients, RT alone in 26 (1%) patients		–	Typical: N0 5-year OS 93% N+ 5-year OS 88% Atypical: N0 5-year OS 87% N+ 5-year OS 58%	National Cancer Database analysis. 1 in 5 patients had nodal involvement at diagnosis. Large tumor size predicts for nodal involvement
Herde (2018)	2018	47 (80%) typical 12 (20%) atypical	Surgery ± chemo ± RT ± chemo-RT	35 (59%) lobectomy 19 (32%) wedge resection/ segmentectomy or sublobectomy 1 (2%) pneumonectomy	Adjuvant chemo-RT in 5 (8%) patients, adjuvant RT in 1 (2%) patient, palliative RT in 1 (2%) patient, palliative chemo in 1 (2%) patient		–	5-year OS 80% 10-year OS 100% In patients with complete remission, DFS 98%	Surgical resection is adequate for most typical carcinoid patients. Adjuvant chemo or RT may be considered for atypical tumors with adverse pathological features

| Wegner (2019b) | 2019 | 662 (100%) atypical (533 stage I–II, 129 stage III) | Surgery ± chemo ± RT ± chemo-RT | 605 (91%) lobectomy 57 (9%) pneumonectomy | Adjuvant RT in 8% | Adjuvant chemo in 16% | – | 5-year OS with observation: 57% 5-year OS with adjuvant therapy: 50% | National Cancer Database analysis. No survival benefit observed with adjuvant therapy, even in stage III disease |

Percentages may add to less than or more than 100% in several cases due to missing information or multiple procedures conducted for patients the potential benefit of adjuvant RT must be carefully weighed against the risk of treatment-related toxicities, which are not trivial in the postoperative setting and are associated with poorer survival with adjuvant RT for NSCLC (PORT Meta-analysis Trialists Group 1998). More conformal techniques and substantially improved image guidance in the modern era may lead to a lower risk of severe morbidity and mortality as compared to historical publications. However, that does not diminish the necessity to thoughtfully weigh the potential benefits of adjuvant RT with these potential disadvantages.

There have been few comparative studies examining the clinical utility of adjuvant RT for these tumors. A study of atypical carcinoid tumors utilizing the US National Cancer Database did not demonstrate a difference in overall survival with adjuvant RT, even for stage III disease (Wegner et al. 2019b); however, potential differences in local or locoregional control could not be ascertained therein. Accordingly, neither the NCCN recommendations (National Comprehensive Cancer Network 2020) nor the guidelines from the North American Neuroendocrine Tumor Society (Phan et al. 2010) suggest routine delivery of adjuvant RT for either typical or atypical carcinoids, largely owing to the lack of robust data supporting its utility.

If adjuvant RT is pursued (presumably, mostly for atypical cases with or without nodal involvement), principles should follow those of postoperative RT for NSCLC. On account of the NSCLC data suggesting potentially severe toxicities, IMRT is recommended whenever feasible, although there are no high-quality data demonstrating that there are fewer toxicities with IMRT as compared to 3D CRT in the postoperative NSCLC setting. Generally, the surgical stump as well as the involved nodal station are delineated using information from preoperative imaging (i.e., the initial extent of disease), the operative report, and the simulation imaging (e.g., for surgical clips). A margin to account for patient setup uncertainties is applied (planning target volume), the magnitude of which depends on the same factors mentioned above for the definitive setting (most often, 0.3–1.0 cm). Only conventional fractionation is endorsed in the postoperative setting, and prescription doses should follow those for NSCLC (45–54 Gy, by weighing pathologic factors and the extent of existing disease with the potential for RT-related adverse events).

Lastly, palliative RT for typical or atypical carcinoids should be performed in a manner similar to other disease sites. Palliative RT for these neoplasms is effective, with over 80% of reported cases from small series achieving a clinical benefit and/or pain relief (Chakravarthy and Abrams 1995; Ameer et al. 2005). This is also true for pain relief from normal RT regimens (most commonly, 20–30 Gy in 5–10 fractions, or a single fraction of 8 Gy) in the setting of bone metastases from metastatic carcinoid (Warren and Gould 1990; Zuetenhorst et al. 2002; Nguyen and Ram 2006).

In summary, RT for bronchopulmonary carcinoids is often extrapolated from the NSCLC literature. In the absence of high-quality data to guide treatment, strong multidisciplinary management is imperative. In the definitive setting, SBRT for localized disease not involving the main airways may be effective and convenient for patients; for all other cases, conventional or mild hypofractionation may be most appropriate. Adjuvant RT is not routinely recommended but may be considered for well-selected higher risk cases. RT is an excellent treatment for palliation of symptoms.

6 Prognosis

The outcomes following surgical based therapy for pulmonary carcinoids are generally favorable. Based on a systematic review in the contemporary era (Reuling et al. 2019), it is estimated that the 5- and 10-year disease-free survival rates for typical carcinoids are 83–100% and 73–95%, respectively, although for atypical cases it is considerably lower (44–87% and 24–71%, respectively). The 5- and 10-year overall survival rates are 82–100% and 60–100% for typical cases, respectively, and 50–95% and 38–75% for atypical cases, respectively.

In addition to histology (i.e., typical or atypical), nodal involvement is a major prognostic factor (Steuer et al. 2015; Kneuertz et al. 2018). However, whereas the poor prognosis of atypical histology with lymph nodal metastasis has been corroborated (Kneuertz et al. 2018), some have questioned whether lymph nodal involvement in typical carcinoids carries meaningful prognostic value (Cardillo et al. 2004; Johnson et al. 2011). Tumor size has been reported in several studies to be associated with prognosis. However, it is unclear if this is independently prognostic or if increasing tumor size merely correlates with greater nodal involvement, the prognostic value of which has been extensively validated (Steuer et al. 2015; Kneuertz et al. 2018). Genomic alterations such as those seen in *MEN1* are hypothesized to confer poorer prognosis (Simbolo et al. 2017; Swarts et al. 2014). Lastly, some have proposed that female gender and high mitotic rates are also prognostic factors, but these have not been well validated (Beasley et al. 2000).

Treatment-related prognostic factors are largely limited to whether oncologic surgery was performed (the administration of adjuvant therapy is not a well-corroborated prognostic factor). However, as mentioned above, whether the extent of resection (surgical technique) is a true prognostic factor in pulmonary carcinoids remains controversial. Some studies have demonstrated that sublobar approaches are not prognostic for typical cases even when stratified for the disease stage (Huang et al. 2018), but others have shown that sublobar resection is associated with inferior outcomes (Aydin et al. 2011; Cañizares et al. 2014). This discordance is due to limitations in the quality (largely retrospective) and quantity (given that this is a rare neoplasm) of data.

Lastly, general oncologic prognostic factors would intuitively still apply to this neoplasm, such as age, performance status, and other comorbidities. These are essential to consider despite the generally good outcomes of pulmonary carcinoids, mainly because patients may die of other nononcologic causes without evidence of tumor progression or recurrence.

References

Al-Toubah T, Morse B, Strosberg J (2020) Capecitabine and temozolomide in advanced lung neuroendocrine neoplasms. Oncologist 25(1):e48–e52

Ameer F et al (2005) Bronchial carcinoid presenting with abdominal pain. J Coll Physicians Surg Pak 15(8):498–499

Anderson KL Jr et al (2017) Adjuvant chemotherapy does not confer superior survival in patients with atypical carcinoid tumors. Ann Thorac Surg 104(4):1221–1230

Aydin E et al (2011) Long-term outcomes and prognostic factors of patients with surgically treated pulmonary carcinoid: our institutional experience with 104 patients. Eur J Cardiothorac Surg 39(4):549–554

Beasley MB et al (2000) Pulmonary atypical carcinoid: predictors of survival in 106 cases. Hum Pathol 31(10):1255–1265

Bhansali A et al (2002) Acromegaly: a rare manifestation of bronchial carcinoid. Asian Cardiovasc Thorac Ann 10(3):273–274

Bongiovanni A et al (2017) Outcome analysis of first-line somatostatin analog treatment in metastatic pulmonary neuroendocrine tumors and prognostic significance of (18)FDG-PET/CT. Clin Lung Cancer 18(4):415–420

Bukowski RM et al (1987) A phase II trial of combination chemotherapy in patients with metastatic carcinoid tumors. A Southwest Oncology Group Study. Cancer 60(12):2891–2895

Bushnell DL Jr et al (2010) 90Y-edotreotide for metastatic carcinoid refractory to octreotide. J Clin Oncol 28(10):1652–1659

Cañizares MA et al (2014) Atypical carcinoid tumours of the lung: prognostic factors and patterns of recurrence. Thorax 69(7):648–653

Caplin ME et al (2015) Pulmonary neuroendocrine (carcinoid) tumors: European Neuroendocrine Tumor Society expert consensus and recommendations for best practice for typical and atypical pulmonary carcinoids. Ann Oncol 26(8):1604–1620

Cardillo G et al (2004) Bronchial carcinoid tumors: nodal status and long-term survival after resection. Ann Thorac Surg 77(5):1781–1785

Carretta A et al (2000) Diagnostic and therapeutic management of neuroendocrine lung tumors: a clinical study of 44 cases. Lung Cancer 29(3):217–225

Cattoni M et al (2017) External validation of a prognostic model of survival for resected typical bronchial carcinoids. Ann Thorac Surg 104(4):1215–1220

Chakravarthy A, Abrams RA (1995) Radiation therapy in the management of patients with malignant carcinoid tumors. Cancer 75(6):1386–1390

Chan JA et al (2012) Prospective study of bevacizumab plus temozolomide in patients with advanced neuroendocrine tumors. J Clin Oncol 30(24):2963–2968

Chong S et al (2007) Integrated PET/CT of pulmonary neuroendocrine tumors: diagnostic and prognostic implications. AJR Am J Roentgenol 188(5):1223–1231

Chong CR et al (2014) Chemotherapy for locally advanced and metastatic pulmonary carcinoid tumors. Lung Cancer 86(2):241–246

Chun SG et al (2017) Impact of intensity-modulated radiation therapy technique for locally advanced non-small-cell lung cancer: a secondary analysis of the NRG Oncology RTOG 0617 Randomized Clinical Trial. J Clin Oncol 35(1):56–62

Colaco RJ, Decker RH (2015) Stereotactic radiotherapy in the treatment of primary bronchial carcinoid tumor. Clin Lung Cancer 16(2):e11–e14

Cusumano G et al (2017) Surgical resection for pulmonary carcinoid: long-term results of multicentric study-the importance of pathological N status, more than we thought. Lung 195(6):789–798

Dasari A et al (2017) Trends in the incidence, prevalence, and survival outcomes in patients with neuroendocrine tumors in the United States. JAMA Oncol 3(10):1335–1342

Divisi D, Crisci R (2005) Carcinoid tumors of the lung and multimodal therapy. Thorac Cardiovasc Surg 53(3):168–172

Ekeblad S et al (2007) Temozolomide as monotherapy is effective in treatment of advanced malignant neuroendocrine tumors. Clin Cancer Res 13(10):2986–2991

Engstrom PF et al (1984) Streptozocin plus fluorouracil versus doxorubicin therapy for metastatic carcinoid tumor. J Clin Oncol 2(11):1255–1259

Fazel P et al (2008) The ectopic adrenocorticotropic hormone syndrome in carcinoid tumors. Proc (Bayl Univ Med Cent) 21(2):140–143

Fazio N et al (2013) Everolimus plus octreotide long-acting repeatable in patients with advanced lung neuroendocrine tumors: analysis of the phase 3, randomized, placebo-controlled RADIANT-2 study. Chest 143(4):955–962

Fazio N et al (2018) Everolimus in advanced, progressive, well-differentiated, non-functional neuroendocrine tumors: RADIANT-4 lung subgroup analysis. Cancer Sci 109(1):174–181

Feldman JM (1985) Increased dopamine production in patients with carcinoid tumors. Metabolism 34(3):255–260

Feldman JM, Plonk JW, Cornette JC (1974) Serum prostaglandin F2α concentration in the carcinoid syndrome. Prostaglandins 7(6):501–506

Ferguson MK (2000) et al. Long-term outcome after resection for bronchial carcinoid tumors. 18(2):156–161

Fernandez-Cuesta L et al (2014) Frequent mutations in chromatin-remodelling genes in pulmonary carcinoids. Nat Commun 5:3518

Ferolla P et al (2009) Tumorlets, multicentric carcinoids, lymph-nodal metastases, and long-term behavior in bronchial carcinoids. J Thorac Oncol 4(3):383–387

Fiala P et al (2003) Bronchial carcinoid tumors: long-term outcome after surgery. Neoplasma 50(1):60–65

Filosso PL et al (2019) Anatomical resections are superior to wedge resections for overall survival in patients with stage 1 typical carcinoids. Eur J Cardiothorac Surg 55(2):273–279

Fink G et al (2001) Pulmonary carcinoid: presentation, diagnosis, and outcome in 142 cases in Israel and review of 640 cases from the literature. Chest 119(6):1647–1651

García-Yuste M et al (2007) Typical and atypical carcinoid tumours: analysis of the experience of the Spanish Multi-centric Study of Neuroendocrine Tumours of the Lung. Eur J Cardiothorac Surg 31(2):192–197

Gustafsen J, Boesby S, Man WK (1988) Histamine in carcinoid syndrome. Agents Actions 25(1–2):1–3

Halperin DM et al (2017) Frequency of carcinoid syndrome at neuroendocrine tumour diagnosis: a population-based study. Lancet Oncol 18(4):525–534

Han B et al (2013) Clinical outcomes of atypical carcinoid tumors of the lung and thymus: 7-year experience of a rare malignancy at single institute. Med Oncol 30(1):479

Hassan MM et al (2008) Risk factors associated with neuroendocrine tumors: a U.S.-based case-control study. Int J Cancer 123(4):867–873

Hemminki K, Li X (2001) Incidence trends and risk factors of carcinoid tumors: a nationwide epidemiologic study from Sweden. Cancer 92(8):2204–2210

Herde RF et al (2018) Primary pulmonary carcinoid tumor: a long-term single institution experience. Am J Clin Oncol 41(1):24–29

Hobbins S et al (2016) Patient characteristics, treatment and survival in pulmonary carcinoid tumours: an analysis from the UK National Lung Cancer Audit. BMJ Open 6(9):e012530

Hobday TJ et al (2007) MC044h, a phase II trial of sorafenib in patients (pts) with metastatic neuroendocrine tumors (NET): A Phase II Consortium (P2C) study. J Clin Oncol 25(18_Suppl):4504

Hofland J et al (2019) Management of carcinoid syndrome: a systematic review and meta-analysis. Endocr Relat Cancer 26(3):R145–r156

Huang Y et al (2018) Assessment of the prognostic factors in patients with pulmonary carcinoid tumor: a population-based study. Cancer Med 7(6):2434–2441

Jiang Y, Hou G, Cheng W (2019) The utility of 18F-FDG and 68Ga-DOTA-Peptide PET/CT in the evaluation of primary pulmonary carcinoid: a systematic review and meta-analysis. Medicine 98(10):e14769

Johnson R et al (2011) Histology, not lymph node involvement, predicts long-term survival in bronchopulmonary carcinoids. Am Surg 77(12):1669–1674

Kaplan B et al (2003) Outcomes and patterns of failure in bronchial carcinoid tumors. Int J Radiat Oncol Biol Phys 55(1):125–131

Kayani I et al (2009) A comparison of 68Ga-DOTATATE and 18F-FDG PET/CT in pulmonary neuroendocrine tumors. J Nucl Med 50(12):1927–1932

Kiesewetter B, Raderer M (2013) Ondansetron for diarrhea associated with neuroendocrine tumors. N Engl J Med 368(20):1947–1948

Kiesewetter B et al (2019) Oral ondansetron offers effective antidiarrheal activity for carcinoid syndrome refractory to somatostatin analogs. Oncologist 24(2):255–258

Kim JT et al (2015) Differential expression and tumorigenic function of neurotensin receptor 1 in neuroendocrine tumor cells. Oncotarget 6(29):26960–26970

Kneuertz PJ et al (2018) Incidence and prognostic significance of carcinoid lymph node metastases. Ann Thorac Surg 106(4):981–988

Krug S et al (2016) Acromegaly in a patient with a pulmonary neuroendocrine tumor: case report and review of current literature. BMC Res Notes 9:326

Kulke MH, Mayer RJ (1999) Carcinoid tumors. N Engl J Med 340(11):858–868

Kulke MH et al (2008) Activity of sunitinib in patients with advanced neuroendocrine tumors. J Clin Oncol 26(20):3403–3410

Kuyumcu S et al (2012) Somatostatin receptor scintigraphy with 111In-octreotide in pulmonary carcinoid tumours correlated with pathological and 18FDG PET/CT findings. Ann Nucl Med 26(9):689–697

Kwekkeboom DJ et al (2005) Overview of results of peptide receptor radionuclide therapy with 3 radiolabeled somatostatin analogs. J Nucl Med 46 Suppl 1:62s–6s

Kyriss T et al (2006) Carcinoid lung tumors: long-term results from 111 resections. Thorac Surg Sci 3:Doc03

Leoncini E et al (2016) Risk factors for neuroendocrine neoplasms: a systematic review and meta-analysis. Ann Oncol 27(1):68–81

Machuca TN et al (2010) Surgical treatment of bronchial carcinoid tumors: a single-center experience. Lung Cancer 70(2):158–162

Maggio I et al (2020) Landscape and future perspectives of immunotherapy in neuroendocrine neoplasia. Cancers (Basel) 12(4):832

Marty-Ané CH et al (1995) Carcinoid tumors of the lung: do atypical features require aggressive management? Ann Thorac Surg 59(1):78–83

Mehnert JM et al (2020) Pembrolizumab for the treatment of programmed death-ligand 1-positive advanced carcinoid or pancreatic neuroendocrine tumors: results from the KEYNOTE-028 study. Cancer 126(13):3021–3030

Mezzetti M et al (2003) Assessment of outcomes in typical and atypical carcinoids according to latest WHO classification. Ann Thorac Surg 76(6):1838–1842

Modlin IM, Lye KD, Kidd M (2003) A 5-decade analysis of 13,715 carcinoid tumors. Cancer 97(4):934–959

Moertel CG, Hanley JA (1979) Combination chemotherapy trials in metastatic carcinoid tumor and the malignant carcinoid syndrome. Cancer Clin Trials 2(4):327–334

Musi M et al (1998) Bronchial carcinoid tumours: a study on clinicopathological features and role of octreotide scintigraphy. Lung Cancer 22(2):97–102

National Comprehensive Cancer Network (2020) Neuroendocrine and adrenal tumors (Version 2.2020). https://www.nccn.org/professionals/physician_gls/pdf/neuroendocrine.pdf. Accessed 24 Jul 2020

Nguyen BD, Ram PC (2006) Bronchopulmonary carcinoid tumor and related cervical vertebral metastasis with PET-positive and octreotide-negative scintigraphy. Clin Nucl Med 31(2):101–103

Nussbaum DP et al (2015) Defining the role of adjuvant chemotherapy after lobectomy for typical bronchopulmonary carcinoid tumors. Ann Thorac Surg 99(2):428–434

Okereke IC et al (2016) Outcomes after surgical resection of pulmonary carcinoid tumors. J Cardiothorac Surg 11:35

Okoye CC et al (2014) Divergent management strategies for typical versus atypical carcinoid tumors of the thoracic cavity. Am J Clin Oncol 37(4):350–355

Onishi H et al (2007) Hypofractionated stereotactic radiotherapy (HypoFXSRT) for stage I non-small cell lung cancer: updated results of 257 patients in a Japanese multi-institutional study. J Thorac Oncol 2(7 Suppl 3):S94–S100

Ott PA et al (2018) T-cell–inflamed gene-expression profile, programmed death ligand 1 expression, and tumor mutational burden predict efficacy in patients treated with pembrolizumab across 20 cancers: KEYNOTE-028. J Clin Oncol 37(4):318–327

Pavel ME et al (2011) Everolimus plus octreotide long-acting repeatable for the treatment of advanced neuroendocrine tumours associated with carcinoid syndrome (RADIANT-2): a randomised, placebo-controlled, phase 3 study. Lancet 378(9808):2005–2012

Pelosi G et al (2014) Ki-67 antigen in lung neuroendocrine tumors: unraveling a role in clinical practice. J Thorac Oncol 9(3):273–284

Phan AT et al (2010) NANETS consensus guideline for the diagnosis and management of neuroendocrine tumors: well-differentiated neuroendocrine tumors of the thorax (includes lung and thymus). Pancreas 39(6):784–798

Pikin O (2017) et al. Two-stage surgery without parenchyma resection for endobronchial carcinoid tumor. 104(6):1846–1851

PORT Meta-analysis Trialists Group (1998) Postoperative radiotherapy in non-small-cell lung cancer: systematic review and meta-analysis of individual patient data from nine randomised controlled trials. Lancet 352(9124):257–263

Ramirez RA et al (2017) Prognostic factors in typical and atypical pulmonary carcinoids. Ochsner J 17(4):335–340

Rea F et al (2007) Outcome and surgical strategy in bronchial carcinoid tumors: single institution experience with 252 patients. Eur J Cardiothorac Surg 31(2):186–191

Reuling EMBP et al (2019) Endobronchial and surgical treatment of pulmonary carcinoid tumors:

a systematic literature review. Lung Cancer 134: 85–95

Rosenzweig KE et al (2007) Involved-field radiation therapy for inoperable non-small-cell lung cancer. J Clin Oncol 25(35):5557–5561

Rugge M et al (2008) Bronchopulmonary carcinoid: phenotype and long-term outcome in a single-institution series of Italian patients. Clin Cancer Res 14(1):149–154

Sadowski SM et al (2018) Nationwide multicenter study on the management of pulmonary neuroendocrine (carcinoid) tumors. Endocr Connect 7(1):8–15

Scanagatta P et al (2004) Cushing's syndrome induced by bronchopulmonary carcinoid tumours: a review of 98 cases and our experience of two cases. Chir Ital 56(1):63–70

Schrevens L et al (2004) Clinical-radiological presentation and outcome of surgically treated pulmonary carcinoid tumours: a long-term single institution experience. Lung Cancer 43(1):39–45

Scoazec JY (2013) Angiogenesis in neuroendocrine tumors: therapeutic applications. Neuroendocrinology 97(1):45–56

Simbolo M et al (2017) Lung neuroendocrine tumours: deep sequencing of the four World Health Organization histotypes reveals chromatin-remodelling genes as major players and a prognostic role for TERT, RB1, MEN1 and KMT2D. J Pathol 241(4):488–500

Singh D et al (2019) Inoperable pulmonary carcinoid tumors: local control rates with stereotactic body radiotherapy/hypofractionated RT with image-guided radiotherapy. Clin Lung Cancer 20(3):e284–e290

Skuladottir H et al (2002) Pulmonary neuroendocrine tumors: incidence and prognosis of histological subtypes. A population-based study in Denmark. Lung Cancer 37(2):127–135

Soga J, Yakuwa Y (1999) Bronchopulmonary carcinoids: an analysis of 1,875 reported cases with special reference to a comparison between typical carcinoids and atypical varieties. Ann Thorac Cardiovasc Surg 5(4):211–219

Steuer CE et al (2015) Atypical carcinoid tumor of the lung: a surveillance, epidemiology, and end results database analysis. J Thorac Oncol 10(3):479–485

Stolz A et al (2015) Long-term outcomes and prognostic factors of patients with pulmonary carcinoid tumors. Neoplasma 62(3):478–483

Strosberg J et al (2017) Phase 3 trial of 177Lu-dotatate for midgut neuroendocrine tumors. N Engl J Med 376(2):125–135

Swarts DR et al (2014) MEN1 gene mutation and reduced expression are associated with poor prognosis in pulmonary carcinoids. J Clin Endocrinol Metab 99(2):E374–E378

Travis WD et al (1998) Survival analysis of 200 pulmonary neuroendocrine tumors with clarification of criteria for atypical carcinoid and its separation from typical carcinoid. Am J Surg Pathol 22(8):934–944

Travis WD et al (2008) The IASLC Lung Cancer Staging Project: proposals for the inclusion of bronchopulmonary carcinoid tumors in the forthcoming (seventh) edition of the TNM Classification for Lung Cancer. J Thorac Oncol 3(11):1213–1223

Travis WD et al (2015) The 2015 World Health Organization classification of lung tumors: impact of genetic, clinical and radiologic advances since the 2004 classification. J Thorac Oncol 10(9):1243–1260

Verma V et al (2017) Multi-institutional experience of stereotactic ablative radiation therapy for stage I small cell lung cancer. Int J Radiat Oncol Biol Phys 97(2):362–371

Waldherr C et al (2002) Tumor response and clinical benefit in neuroendocrine tumors after 7.4 GBq (90) Y-DOTATOC. J Nucl Med 43(5):610–616

Walter T et al (2016) Evaluation of the combination of oxaliplatin and 5-fluorouracil or gemcitabine in patients with sporadic metastatic pulmonary carcinoid tumors. Lung Cancer 96:68–73

Warren WH, Gould VE (1990) Long-term follow-up of classical bronchial carcinoid tumors. Clinicopathologic observations. Scand J Thorac Cardiovasc Surg 24(2):125–130

Wegner RE et al (2019a) Stereotactic body radiation therapy versus fractionated radiation therapy for early-stage bronchopulmonary carcinoid. Lung Cancer Manag 8(3):Lmt14

Wegner RE et al (2019b) The role of adjuvant therapy for atypical bronchopulmonary carcinoids. Lung Cancer 131:90–94

Wirth LJ et al (2004) Outcome of patients with pulmonary carcinoid tumors receiving chemotherapy or chemoradiotherapy. Lung Cancer 44(2):213–220

Wymenga AN et al (1998) Effects of ondansetron on gastrointestinal symptoms in carcinoid syndrome. Eur J Cancer 34(8):1293–1294

Yao JC et al (2008) Targeting vascular endothelial growth factor in advanced carcinoid tumor: a random assignment phase II study of depot octreotide with bevacizumab and pegylated interferon alpha-2b. J Clin Oncol 26(8):1316–1323

Yao JC et al (2016) Everolimus for the treatment of advanced, non-functional neuroendocrine tumours of the lung or gastrointestinal tract (RADIANT-4): a randomised, placebo-controlled, phase 3 study. Lancet 387(10022):968–977

Zhong C-X et al (2012) Long-term outcomes of surgical treatment for pulmonary carcinoid tumors: 20 years' experience with 131 patients. Chin Med J (Engl) 125(17):3022–3026

Zuetenhorst JM et al (2002) Evaluation of (111) In-pentetreotide, (131)I-MIBG and bone scintigraphy in the detection and clinical management of bone metastases in carcinoid disease. Nucl Med Commun 23(8):735–741

Part IX

Treatment-Related Toxicity

Hematological Toxicity in Lung Cancer

Francesc Casas, Diego Muñoz-Guglielmetti, Gabriela Oses, Carla Cases, and Meritxell Mollà

Contents

1	Introduction	908
2	Hematological Toxicity in Chemotherapy	908
3	Hematological Toxicity in Radiotherapy	910
4	Hematologic Toxicity After Combined Chemo- and Radiotherapy	911
5	Preventive or Support Treatment of Hematologic Toxicity After Concurrent ChRT in Lung Cancer	914
5.1	Neutropenia	914
5.2	Anemia	916
5.3	Thrombocytopenia	917
6	Hematological Toxicity After New Biomarker-Based Targeted Therapies in Stage IV NSCLC	918
	References	919

Abstract

The toxicity of tumor cells after chemotherapy (Ch) and radiotherapy (RT), administered alone or in combination, is dose dependent. Aggression to the bone marrow, which is expressed by a reduction in circulating blood cells, is often the main dose-limiting toxicity in the treatment of lung cancer due to the risks of anemia, bleeding, and infection.

Prophylactic treatment with granulocyte colony-stimulating factors (G-CSF) or biosimilars is available to reduce the risk of Ch-induced neutropenia/febrile neutropenia.

The American Society of Clinical Oncology (ASCO) made recommendations (level of evidence II) on the treatment of anemia with erythropoiesis-stimulating agents (ESA). For patients with Ch-induced anemia, the committee recommended starting ESA when hemoglobin (Hb) approaches 10 g/dL, to increase the Hb level and decrease transfusions. A recent phase III study demonstrated the definitive positive impact of darbepoetin r-HuEPO (DARB). DARB was not inferior to placebo for OS and PFS and was superior to placebo for transfusion for Hb ≤8.0 g/dL.

In the last decade, systemic therapy for stage IV NSCLC has been selected for the presence of specific biomarkers. All of these patients should undergo molecular testing for programmed death ligand 1 (PD-L1) protein expression and mutations. The hematologic

F. Casas (✉) · M. Mollà
Thoracic Unit, Radiation Oncology Department, Hospital Clínic i Universitari, Barcelona, Spain
e-mail: fcasas@clinic.cat; molla@clinic.cat

D. Muñoz-Guglielmetti · G. Oses · C. Cases
Radiation Oncology Department, Hospital Clínic i Universitari, Barcelona, Spain
e-mail: munozgugli@gmail.com; oses@clinic.cat; cases@clinic.cat

toxicity of these molecules is considered a rare toxicity (frequency <1%) but can be very significant.

1 Introduction

In this chapter, normal bone marrow (BM) physiology is presented followed by a synthesis of current knowledge about the toxicity of these two treatments (Ch and RT), either alone or in combination. Later, supportive treatments and management of these side effects are discussed. Finally, we will finish with the hematological toxicity (HT) of biomarker-directed therapies and new empirical treatment regimens in metastatic lung cancer (LC).

The toxicity of tumor cells after ChRT, administered alone or in combination, is dose dependent. Aggression to the BM is expressed by a reduction in circulating blood cells and is often the main dose-limiting toxicity due to the risks of anemia, bleeding, and infection. The strategies aimed at protecting the hematopoietic cells or the stroma of BM from death induced by treatment, as well as the acceleration of hematopoiesis after treatment, would theoretically allow more intensive treatments in LC, reducing the associated risks mentioned before. To know the true impact of the treatment, either individually or combined in a sequential or concomitant way, and act accordingly, it is necessary to know the structure and function of the BM as an organ. Thus, pluripotent stem cells replicate and differentiate into lymphoid or myeloid lines through a complex process regulated by a network of hematopoietic growth factors and by cellular interactions. The cascade through myeloid differentiation leads to erythrocytes, platelets, granulocytes, and macrophages, while lymphoid differentiation leads to T and B cells. Families of growth factors (or cytokines) that control these processes of replication and differentiation have been identified. Hematopoietic progenitor cells and their daughter cells are enveloped in a stroma of endothelial cells, adventitious cells, fibroblasts, macrophages, and fat cells in the sinus of the BM. This microscopic medium provides physical support and direction of the development of the replication process. Furthermore, the topographic distribution of the BM is especially relevant to know possible local effects of RT in the treatment of LC. The most functional and important locations are the pelvis, the vertebrae (these two represent 60% of the total BM), as well as the ribs, sternum, skull, scapulae, and proximal portions of the femur and humerus. It is important to remember that hematopoietic stem cells are also found in the spleen and peripheral bleeding (Plowman et al. 1991).

BM dysfunction in neoplastic processes can be due to different etiologies:

1. Depletion or direct damage to hematopoietic stem cells
2. Functional or structural damage to the stroma or microcirculation
3. Lesion of other helper cells that have a regulatory or hemostasis function

The consequences of the aggression of cytotoxic and radiotherapeutic treatment to BM must be understood in the context of the mechanisms previously described. However, it may be difficult to elucidate the most important variables due to limitations in the evaluation, both of the structure and of the function of the BM. Peripheral determination of blood cells fails to demonstrate the true extent of BM suppression or tolerance to additional cytotoxic therapy, mainly due to the BM ability to temporarily compensate for insult. To evaluate quantitative and functional aspects of BM cultures of progenitor cells, histopathological studies (aspirate and BM biopsy) and determination by radioisotopes or stromal cell cultures can be performed, although to a limited extent.

2 Hematological Toxicity in Chemotherapy

Myelosuppression caused directly by Ch depends not only on the agent used, but also on individual patient factors, such as age, previous pathologies, and general condition. Important factors in relation to the type of Ch administered are the dose, the interval between the doses, the route of administration, and the use of one or more antitumor agents. On the other hand, the site of action of the antineoplastic drug within the cell cycle also seems to influence myelosuppression.

The damage is the result of a depletion of the total number of stem cells (the stem cell pool) with a pattern of delayed myelosuppression that occurs when peripheral blood cells die and cannot be replaced. Ch myelotoxicity results in a decrease in blood cell production rather than an immediate elimination of peripheral cells (Ratain et al. 1990).

Due to differences in the half-life of peripheral blood cells, myelosuppressive drugs first result in leukopenia followed by thrombocytopenia, the former being generally more severe than the latter. Therefore, the neutrophil and platelet nadir is normally found between 7 and 15 days after drug administration. For most compounds, neutropenia and thrombocytopenia are reversible and not cumulative. In addition to direct cytotoxicity at the progenitor cell level, erythrocytes have a longer half-life, so the mechanism involved may be direct hemolysis after administration or a decrease in endogenous erythropoietin production secondary to renal failure due to cisplatin (CDDP) (Pivot et al. 2000). Pluripotent stem cells are protected from the toxic effects of Ch due to their slow proliferation.

Ch-induced febrile neutropenia (FN) is a life-threatening complication of cancer treatments, when it presents with infection and sepsis. It is seen most frequently during the initial cycles of myelosuppressive therapy (Timmer-Bonte et al. 2005). FN is defined as an absolute neutrophil count (ANC) of $<0.5 \times 10^9/L$, or $<1.0 \times 10^9/L$ that is predicted to fall below $0.5 \times 10^9/L$ in 48 h, associated with fever or clinical signs of sepsis (Crawford et al. 2010). As a consequence of FN, delays in antitumor treatment and dose reduction can occur, which can negatively affect tumor control (Khan et al. 2008). For instance, poor outcomes in cancer patients have been attributed to the failure in the delivery of planned Ch regimens for LC (Lyman 2009).

Early recognition of patients at risk of complications from FN can be achieved using risk indices such as the one developed by the Multinational Association for Supportive Care in Cancer (MASCC) (De Souza Viana et al. 2008). Using the MASCC score, patients with 21 or more points are considered high-risk FN. Identifying patients at risk for bacteremia facilitates the appropriate initiation of antibiotics (Klastersky et al. 2010).

Patient-related risk factors should be evaluated in the overall risk assessment for FN before each cycle of Ch is administered. Special attention should be paid to high-risk elderly patients (65 years and older). Other risk factors that can influence the risk of FN include advanced stages of the disease, previous episodes of FN, lack of use of G-CSF, and absence of antibiotic prophylaxis. The risk of FN associated with Ch regimens should be taken into account when assessing the need for prophylactic intervention. In recent years, the Clinical Index of Stable Febrile Neutropenia (CISNE) (Table 1) has been emerging as a very useful prognostic score for predicting serious complications in outpatients with solid tumors and episodes of stable FN. The CISNE score identifies six variables associated with serious complications and classifies patients into three prognostic classes: low risk (0 points), intermediate risk (1–2 points), and high risk (3 points or more). The results of a multicenter validation study suggest that the CISNE score may be more accurate than the MASCC score (Carmona-Bayonas et al. 2015).

On the other hand, new Ch regimens associated with targeted agents have been shown to improve OS. This is the case with the addition of cetuximab or bevacizumab to Ch in patients with

Table 1 Clinical Index of Stable Febrile Neutropenia (CISNE) score

Characteristics	Points
ECOG-PS ≥ 2	2
Stress-induced hyperglycemia	2
Chronic obstructive pulmonary disease	1
Chronic cardiovascular disease	1
Mucositis National Cancer Institute ≥ 2	1
Monocytes <200 per μ/L	1

NSCLC (Pirker et al. 2009; Reck et al. 2009). A higher incidence of FN has been reported in patients receiving bevacizumab and Ch compared to Ch alone (Sandler et al. 2006).

The elevated risk of FN should be considered when using certain Ch regimens, such as the combination of docetaxel with carboplatin (CB) (Milward et al. 2003). One of the main toxicity factors for a certain Ch agent is the pharmacodynamic interaction when combined with other anticancer drugs. One of the general principles for combining different drugs is that they must have different limiting toxicity, although a sum of these myelotoxic effects generally occurs. However, there is an exception to this rule; it is the case of the combination of paclitaxel with CB: paclitaxel decreases platelet toxicity of CB in relation to a nonpharmacokinetic mechanism (Calvert et al. 1999).

The most common Ch regimens currently used in NSCLC include combinations of CDDP or CB with other drugs (gemcitabine, vinorelbine, paclitaxel, docetaxel). All have been shown to have similar efficacy in stage IV, although the observed toxicities, including HT, differ between them (Schiller et al. 2002). These combinations of Ch cause grade 3 and 4 neutropenia in a range of 40–70%, with FN in less than 10%. Grade 3 and 4 platelet toxicity has been observed in 1–55% of patients, with the combination of CDDP and gemcitabine increasing the percentage of thrombocytopenia (Cardenal et al. 1999). Patients with CB-based Ch were more likely to experience thrombocytopenia (Luo et al. 2011). Regarding anemia, the percentages vary between 10% and 30%, being the regimens based on CDDP and gemcitabine or vinorelbine, which produced a higher percentage of patients with anemia (Kelly et al. 2001).

The sequence of administration is also a relevant factor. An increase in myelotoxicity has been reported when CDDP is administered before paclitaxel. Platelet toxicity is not prominent in regimens that include paclitaxel associated with CB, suggesting that paclitaxel could protect. The combination of CDDP and etoposide (ET) produces less neutropenia than cyclophosphamide, doxorubicin, and vincristine (CAV), although with more anemia (Fukuoka et al. 1991). The HT profile with the combination of ET and CB is similar to that found with CDDP, except that it presents a higher percentage of thrombocytopenia.

It is important to note the possible HT of pemetrexed. This is a multidirectional antimetabolite that inhibits several key folate-dependent enzymes in the thymidine and purine biosynthetic pathways, including thymidylate synthase. It is currently approved for use in patients with NSCLC and malignant mesothelioma. The appearance of HT from this new drug, which can produce life-threatening complications during the early phase of development, prompted the urgent need to identify possible predictive factors for these HT. An association was found between elevated plasma homocysteine (HC) concentration, which is indicative of impaired folate functional status, and an increased risk of HT from pemetrexed (Kao et al. 2010).

The decrease in the incidence of toxicity after vitamin supplementation confirms the importance of the above. But this correlation between folate functional status and vitamin supplementation is not observed in other CDDP-based Ch regimens, as it is in Ch regimens with pemetrexed (Minchom et al. 2014). However, further studies might be necessary to increase the rate of successful supplementation and to test the biomarker potential of HC levels after supplementation to predict Ch-induced neutropenia in CDDP-based regimens. This is because post hoc analysis of this randomized clinical trial (RCT) showed that patients in the successfully supplemented arm (9/36 = 25%) had less neutropenic toxicity (0% vs. 69%; $p = 0.02$) compared to patients who received no supplements.

3 Hematological Toxicity in Radiotherapy

In the case of irradiation in the LC, the acute toxicity of BM depends on the irradiated volume and the radiation dose and its rate. Although compensatory mechanisms are primarily relevant to understanding long-term effects, some of the effects are acute. Thus, when limited volumes are irradiated to BM, such as 10–15%, the remaining bone marrow responds by increasing the progenitor cell population. That is why BM, as an organ as a whole, is capable of regenerating the previously irradiated area through a compensatory effect to satisfy the needs of hematopoiesis, avoiding acute toxicity. This compensatory phenomenon can be observed by factors (CSF) of the cell stroma that suggest the involvement of a humoral mechanism.

It has been shown that there is an extensive communication and compensation network in the BM after the assault with RT, and this can be summarized as follows:

1. Regeneration in the field of irradiation
2. Hyperactivity in nonirradiated regions
3. Extension of the BM production function in previously inactive areas (Tubiana et al. 1979)

This repairing or compensatory capacity of the BM makes the RT-induced BM toxicity in LC difficult to observe clinically. However, exclusive irradiation using standard fractionation produces a subclinical but quantifiable HT, which we will describe in more depth later when we move to combination therapy (ChRT) and compare the resulting myelotoxicity using RCT studies related to RT alone as a reference.

4 Hematologic Toxicity After Combined Chemo- and Radiotherapy

The selective action of Ch agents for different hematopoietic cell populations determines the temporal consequences of BM tolerance to RT after Ch. Furthermore, when using wide irradiation fields before Ch, the expected tolerance is lower. This may be due not only to the suppression or ablation of certain segments or portions of the BM, but also to the increased sensitivity of the unexposed areas of the BM that, at that time, are in a period of hyperactivity. This situation occurs in the case of sequential treatments of RT and Ch, further complicating the issue of combined treatments. In the case of small cell lung cancer (SCLC), one study is worth highlighting (Abrams et al. 1985). These authors randomized 42 patients to receive Ch alone or in combination with thoracic RT. In the group that received the combination treatment, an increase in HT was observed as well as in the circulating number of progenitor cells, suggesting that the toxicity of the concomitant treatment is additive. It was found that:

(a) The combination of Ch with thoracic RT produces more HT during the irradiation period than when Ch is administered alone.
(b) This increase in HT may be explained by a toxicity that is generally subclinical, although measurable, of thoracic RT when administered alone.
(c) The potential HT induced by irradiation itself may vary in relation to the time, the volume of treatment, the irradiated region, and the treatment fields used. In other words, the greater the volume treated and the greater the amount of cardiac circuit and BM involved in the irradiated fields, the greater the toxicity.

In recent decades, it has been observed that both the timing of the administration of RT (early or late) in the concurrent combined treatment and the fractionation (accelerated hyperfractionation versus standard fractionation) have a relevant role in the development of HT in patients with SCLC. In one RCT (Murray et al. 1993), a group of patients were randomized to early concurrent RT (in the 3rd week) versus late concurrent RT (in the 15th week). It was observed that although the differences between neutropenia and thrombocytopenia greater than or equal to grade 3 were not statistically significant, grade 3 anemia was higher in the late RT arm ($p < 0.03$).

In an RCT (Jeremic et al. 1997), 107 patients received daily low doses of Ch plus early hyperfractionated RT (weeks 1–4) simultaneously with Ch versus late RT (weeks 6–9), without finding statistically significant differences in HT. In the same year, the EORTC group (Gregor et al. 1997) published an RCT of patients with limited-stage

SCLC comparing sequential ChRT with alternating treatment, reporting that the latter regimen was as effective as sequential administration, but caused higher rates of HT grade 3 and 4. Another RCT (Turrisi et al. 1999) compared concurrent Ch with hyperfractionated RT versus the same concomitant Ch with standard fractionated RT, observing greater toxicity in the hyperfractionated treatment. Finally, the RCT of concurrent versus sequential ChRT (Takada et al. 2002) also observed a higher HT in the concurrent arm.

Finally, in the clinical trials on SCLC that address issues related to RT, it is important to highlight the CONVERT study (Concurrent Once-Daily Versus Twice-Daily Radiotherapy) (Faivre-Finn et al. 2017) that provides us with new information on HT secondary to the RT of more limited fields, on the technology currently used, and on different fractionation schemes. Between April 7, 2008, and November 29, 2013, 547 patients were enrolled in an RCT and assigned to receive concurrent ChRT twice daily or concurrent ChRT once daily. With a median follow-up of 45 months (IQR 35–58), the median overall survival (OS) was 30 months (95% CI 24–34) in the twice-daily group versus 25 months (95% CI 21–31) in the other group. The most common grade 3–4 adverse event for toxicity secondary to Ch was neutropenia (197 [74%] of 266 patients in the twice-daily group versus 170 [65%] of 263 in the once-daily group). Most toxicities were similar between the two groups, except for the grade 4 neutropenia rate, which was significantly higher in the RT twice-daily arm (129 [49%] vs. 101 [38%]; $p = 0.05$). This RCT seems to demonstrate that limited RT fields (involved fields) and 3D and/or IMRT techniques can have a significant impact on the development of HT.

In the early 1990s, a series of RCTs in NSCLC were conducted that evaluated both the effectiveness and toxicity of concurrent or sequential ChRT versus RT alone. Three hundred and fifty-three patients were randomized (Le Chevalier et al. 1991) to receive 65 Gy of exclusive RT versus RT at the same dose, preceded by three cycles of vindesine, lomustine, CDDP, and cyclophosphamide. In the exclusive RT group, three times less of HT was observed than in the combined therapy group.

Another study randomized (Dillman et al. 1990) 155 patients to receive two cycles of CDDP and vinblastine followed by 60 Gy of RT versus RT alone at the same dose. Although HT was not fully explained in this study, neutropenic infection was found to be more prevalent in patients receiving Ch, with twice the number of hospital admissions due to serious infections compared to patients receiving RT alone.

In a later study (Trovo et al. 1992), 173 patients with stage III NSCLC received 45 Gy versus CDDP 6 mg/m^2 daily concurrently with RT at the same dose as the other group. The HT of combined treatment was only slightly higher than that of RT alone. In 1993, 331 patients received 56 Gy administered by split-course versus the same RT schedule plus CDDP 30 mg/m^2 administered each week of RT, versus the same total dose of RT administered continuously with a daily dose of CDDP 6 mg/m^2 during RT (Schaake-Koning et al. 1992). Grade 3–4 HT was observed to be four times higher in the RT plus weekly CDDP group compared to RT alone and twice as high in the concurrent treatment with daily CDDP versus weekly CDDP.

In another RCT (Sause et al. 1995) of patients with stage III NSCLC, the patients who underwent sequential ChRT had a longer survival than the group who underwent exclusive hyperfractionated RT or normofractionated RT. However, grade 3 or higher neutropenia was observed in 50% of the combined treatment patients and was absent in the other two arms of the study. In another RCT (Jeremic et al. 1996), 169 patients were randomized to receive hyperfractionated RT at 1.2 Gy/2 times daily up to a total dose of 64.8 Gy versus the same dose of RT plus 100 mg of CB on days 1 and 2, and 100 mg of ET on days 1 and 3 of each week of RT, compared to a third group in which the same RT was administered plus 200 mg of CB administered on days 1 and 2, and 100 mg of ET on days 1 and 5 of the first, third, and fifth weeks of RT. Greater toxicity was observed in the combined treatment group, especially in the second treatment arm.

After observing a greater efficacy with sequential treatment of ChRT, but with a higher incidence of HT than with exclusive RT, the next step was to demonstrate that HT with concurrent treatment would be higher than with sequential treatment. In an RCT (Furuse et al. 1999), 320 patients with stage III NSCLC were assigned to receive concurrent ChRT with CDDP, vindesine, and mitomycin plus 56 Gy given in a split-course (28 Gy followed by a rest period of 10 days, and then repeated) versus the same Ch schedule plus sequential RT of 56 Gy. A greater immunosuppression was observed in the concurrent treatment arm.

Along the same lines, a second RCT compared concurrent (group A) versus sequential (group B) ChRT with CDDP and vinorelbine in locally advanced NSCLC (Zatloukal et al. 2004). Grade 3 or 4 toxicity was more frequent in arm A, with a significantly higher incidence of leukopenia (53% versus 19%, $p = 0.009$). However, in the concurrent ChRT arm, an increase in OS was observed.

The combination of concurrent treatment of ChRT with weekly paclitaxel at a dose of 60 mg/m^2 versus RT alone after induction Ch in inoperable stage IIIA or IIIB NSCLC has also been investigated (Huber et al. 2006). Ch induction was well tolerated, presenting 3.8% grade 3 or 4 leukopenia (2.1% grade 4). HT was equivalent in the RT-alone group and in ChRT, with no grade 3 or 4 toxicity.

Cancer and Leukemia Group B (CALGB), in a randomized phase II study (Vokes et al. 2002) of CDDP with gemcitabine or paclitaxel or vinorelbine as induction Ch followed by concomitant ChRT for stage IIIB NSCLC, studied efficacy and tolerance of these treatments. HT was presented separately for induction Ch and for concomitant ChRT treatment. In the first, grade 3–4 granulocytopenia was observed in 50% of patients in all three treatment arms. However, in the gemcitabine group, 25% of the patients also had grade 3 and 4 thrombocytopenia. In concurrent treatment, important differences were found in the three study treatment groups. Patients treated with gemcitabine and paclitaxel developed grade 3 and 4 granulocytopenia in 51% and 53%, respectively. However in the vinorelbine group, this HT was observed in 27% of the patients. In addition, platelet toxicity was found to be higher (50%) in the group concurrent with gemcitabine. Subsequently, the CALGB developed another RCT (Vokes et al. 2007) where 366 patients were randomly assigned to arm A, which involved immediate concurrent ChRT with CB area under the concentration-time curve (AUC) of 2 and administered paclitaxel 50 mg/m^2 weekly for 66 Gy of chest RT, or arm B, involving two cycles of CB AUC 6 and paclitaxel 200 mg/m^2 given every 21 days followed by identical ChRT. They found no differences in survival between both arms. Treatment adverse events during induction Ch in arm B included grade 3 and 4 granulocytopenia in 18% and 20% of patients, respectively. Neutropenia increased significantly in arm B, reflecting the cumulative effect of induction Ch.

Another RCT (Hanna et al. 2008) demonstrated that consolidation with docetaxel after CDDP/ET and concurrent RT results in greater toxicity, without increasing survival compared to CDDP/ET and concurrent RT in patients with unresectable stage III NSCLC. 10.9% of the patients receiving docetaxel experienced NF, and 28.8% of the patients were hospitalized during the docetaxel versus 8.1% in the observation arm. 5.5% died from complications secondary to docetaxel.

In recent years, three major RCTs have been conducted on radical ChRT in unresectable stage III NSCLC with secondary HT results to treatment.

The first was the RTOG 0617 study (Bradley et al. 2015), which aimed to compare OS after 60 Gy (standard dose), 74 Gy (high dose), 60 Gy plus cetuximab, or 74 Gy plus cetuximab. All patients also received Ch with paclitaxel and CB simultaneously. Two weeks after ChRT, consolidation Ch was administered. The median OS was 28.7 months for group A and 20.3 months for group B (HR 1.38, 95% CI 1.09–1.76, $p = 0.004$). The median OS in patients who received cetuximab was 25.0 months (95% CI 20.2–30.5) compared with 24.0 months (19.8–28.6) in those who did not receive cetuximab (HR 1.07, 95% CI 0.84–1.35, $p = 0.29$). Anemia grade 3 and 4 was similar between cetuximab plus 74 Gy and cetuximab plus 60 Gy groups (9% and 0% vs. 5% and

1%, respectively). Similar results were observed in grade 3 and 4 lymphopenia: arm A presented 8% and 0%, while arm B had 12% and 2%, respectively. Grade 3 and 4 thrombocytopenia was found in 6% and 2% in arm A versus 10% and 6% in arm B, respectively.

The second was the PROCLAIM study (Senan et al. 2016) that evaluated OS with concurrent ChRT with pemetrexed/CDDP followed by consolidation pemetrexed (arm A) versus concurrent ChRT with CDDP/ET followed by consolidation Ch with doublet without pemetrexed (arm B). Group A was not superior to group B in terms of OS with a median of 26.8 versus 25.0 months (HR 0.98, 95% CI 0.79–1.20, $p = 0.831$). Group A had a significantly lower incidence of any grade 3–4 drug-related adverse event (64.0% vs. 76.8%; $p = 0.001$), including neutropenia (24.4% vs. 44.5%; $p = 0.001$).

The third study, the PACIFIC trial (Antonia et al. 2017), has produced a paradigm shift in the treatment of unresectable locally advanced stage III NSCLC. This phase III study compared the anti-programmed death ligand 1 antibody durvalumab as consolidation therapy with placebo in patients with stage III NSCLC who did not have disease progression after two or more cycles of platinum-based ChRT. The total HT was not specified in detail, but grade 3–4 anemia in each arm was close to 3%. In the first published OS analysis (Antonia et al. 2017), with a median follow-up of 25.2 months, the OS at 24 months was 66.3% (95% CI, 61.7–70.4) with durvalumab compared to 55.6% (95% CI, 48.9–61.8) in the placebo group ($p = 0.005$). Updated analyses confirm these results with a median follow-up of 4 years (Antonia et al. 2018).

5 Preventive or Support Treatment of Hematologic Toxicity After Concurrent ChRT in Lung Cancer

5.1 Neutropenia

Prophylactic treatment with granulocyte colony-stimulating factors (G-CSF) is available to reduce the risk of Ch-induced neutropenia. FN is a life-threatening complication of myelosuppressive therapy that often may require hospitalization and may result in interruptions of the Ch regimen planned. Known risk factors for FN allow clinicians to stratify patient risk and initiate G-CSF prophylaxis. The strongest evidence supporting the use of G-CSF to prevent FN comes from three level I meta-analyses (Lyman et al. 2002; Bohlius et al. 2008; Kuderer et al. 2007). The latter presented information from 13 RCTs and 3122 patients with lymphoma or solid tumors, where G-CSF was used in conjunction with standard Ch, resulting in a significant reduction in early mortality.

However, G-CSF prophylaxis varies greatly in clinical practice, both at the time of administration and in the patients to whom it is offered. In 2005, the European Organization for Research and Treatment of Cancer (EORTC) created a European Guidelines Working Group to review the available evidence and its recommendations for the appropriate use of G-CSF in adult patients receiving Ch (Aapro et al. 2006), updating in 2010 (Aapro et al. 2011). They recommend assessing advanced age (greater than or equal to 65 years) and total neutrophil count as adverse risk factors related to the patient and assessing the risk of FN before administering each cycle of Ch (Table 2). It is important that after an episode of FN, patients receive G-CSF prophylaxis in subsequent cycles. There are Ch schemes that are considered high risk (>20%) or intermediate risk (10–20%) of FN. In high-risk regimens, prophylaxis with G-CSF is still recommended. In intermediate-risk regimens, patient-related risk factors that may increase the overall risk of FN should be carefully considered. Previously, a small level II study suggested a tendency for improved long-term survival in patients with favorable-prognosis SCLC receiving VICE Ch (vincristine-ifosfamide-CB-ET) plus G-CSF compared with Ch alone (Woll et al. 1995). Furthermore, a harmful effect with the use of this cytokine has been observed in patients with intrathoracic stage SCLC who were treated with concomitant ChRT, as well as in extrathoracic stages treated with high doses of Ch (Adams et al. 2002). In 1996, the American Society of Clinical

Table 2 Common Ch regimens associated with intermediate or high risk of FN

Malignancy	FN risk factory (%)	Chemotherapy regimen
Small cell lung cancer	>20	Doxorubicin/cyclophosphamide/etoposide Topotecan Ifosfamide/carboplatin/etoposide Vincristine/ifosfamide/carboplatin/etoposide
	10–20	Cyclophosphamide/doxorubicin/vincristine Etoposide/carboplatin Topotecan/cisplatin Tirapazamine/cisplatin/etoposide/irradiation Cisplatin/vincristine/doxorubicin/etoposide
	<10	Cyclophosphamide/doxorubicin/vincristine Paclitaxel/carboplatin
Non-small cell lung cancer	>20	Docetaxel/carboplatin Etoposide/cisplatin Cisplatin/vinorelbine/cetuximab
	10–20	Vinorelbine/ifosfamide/gemcitabine Paclitaxel/cisplatin Docetaxel/cisplatin Vinorelbine/cisplatin
	<10	Paclitaxel/carboplatin Gemcitabine/cisplatin Bevacizumab/paclitaxel/carboplatin

Oncology (ASCO) recommended to avoid the use of G-CSF in patients who had received concomitant ChRT. Four years later, ASCO specified that the use of G-CSF should be avoided in patients with ChRT if the mediastinum had been irradiated (Ozer et al. 2000) as in the case of LC, due to a significant increase in grade 3–4 thrombocytopenia and excess deaths due to pulmonary toxicity. However, the CONVERT trial provided more information on concomitant mediastinal RT and G-CSF administration (Sheikh et al. 2011). Thirty-eight patients with limited-stage SCLC were randomized to receive RT once daily (66 Gy in 33 fractions) or twice daily (45 Gy in 30 fractions) concurrently with CDDP and ET, plus G-CSF as primary or secondary prophylaxis or as a therapeutic measure during an episode of FN. Thirteen (34%) patients received G-CSF at the same time as RT. With a median follow-up of 16.9 months, no treatment-related deaths were observed. Seven (54%) patients experienced grade 3–4 thrombocytopenia and 5 (38%) experienced grade 3–4 anemia. Thirty-one percent required platelet transfusions. No bleeding episodes were observed. There were no cases of grade 3–4 acute pneumonitis. These data suggest that with modern three-dimensional (3D) conformal RT, G-CSF administration at the same time as ChRT does not increase the risk of pulmonary toxicity, but it does increase the risk of thrombocytopenia.

Antibiotic prophylaxis to prevent infection and its related complications in cancer patients at risk of developing neutropenia is controversial (Cullen et al. 2005). Two meta-analyses (Gafter-Gvili et al. 2005; Herbst et al. 2009) and one systematic review (van de Wetering et al. 2005) indicated that the evidence is too limited to allow conclusions to be drawn about the relative advantage of antibiotics over primary prophylaxis with G-CSF. Antibacterial prophylaxis has resulted in substantial reductions in infection-related mortality in neutropenic patients and is recommended for high-risk patients. The results of a meta-analysis of 52 trials of neutropenic patients with primarily hematologic malignancies demonstrated the efficacy of fluoroquinolones (FQ) in preventing bacterial infections without an increase in resistant organisms (Gafter-Gvili et al. 2007). Levofloxacin is the recommended FQ according to national guidelines. High-dose levofloxacin (500–750 mg) has a broader scope of coverage compared to ciprofloxacin or moxifloxacin, by covering pseudomonas, other gram-negative rods, and some gram-positive pathogens. Nevertheless, in certain high-risk patients with clear predictors of a worse prognosis (e.g., sepsis, pneumonia, fungal infections), the use of G-CSF in conjunction with antibiotics may be justified (Bennett et al. 1999). In 2002, a systematic review of RCTs conducted on the role of G-CSF in the treatment of SCLC was published (Berghmans et al. 2002).

Twelve studies were eligible; they were divided into three groups: (1) maintenance of dose intensity when Ch was administered in conventional doses and time intervals (seven trials); (2) accelerated Ch with an increase in dose intensity by reducing the delay between Ch cycles (five trials); and (3) Ch concentration in a shorter overall duration time with a smaller number of cycles (one trial). The results of the review were negative for all strategies: in the maintenance group, the administration of G-CSF was associated with a detrimental effect on OS; in the accelerated group, no significant impact on response rate or OS was found; and concentrated Ch was associated with no difference in response rate and reduced OS.

In patients receiving first-line Ch for advanced NSCLC, Ch-induced neutropenia is associated with significantly longer OS (Di Maio et al. 2005). Adjuvant Ch after radical surgery has become a standard treatment for early-stage NSCLC. CDDP-based Ch has been used in all recent clinical trials, showing a significant advantage for treatment compared to observation (Douillard et al. 2006). But despite the significant HT of these Ch regimens, the incidence of FN is notably less than 20%, and thus primary G-CSF prophylaxis is not recommended according to guidelines (Winton et al. 2005). Regarding the use of daily G-CSF versus pegylated G-CSF once per cycle, additional evidence has emerged since the publication of the latest EORTC guidelines. In addition, more filgrastim biosimilar molecules have been approved. These developments highlight the need to reevaluate the current evidence and update existing guidelines regarding the prophylactic use of G-CSF. The efficacy of standard and pegylated agents in the prophylaxis of FN is well established in terms of decreased risk of FN, severity and duration of FN episodes, and changes in Ch administration, without sustained evidence of superiority of either of these formulations (Wingard and Elmongy 2009). Following the expiration of the filgrastim patent in Europe in 2006, the European Medicines Agency has approved several biosimilar agents. A biosimilar biological medicine or Biosimilar is a version of an already authorized biochemical medicine with demonstrated similarity in physicochemical characteristics, efficacy, and safety, based on a comprehensive comparability exercise. MONITOR-GCSF was an international, multicenter, prospective, observational, open-label, pharmacoepidemiological study of 1447 cancer patients treated with myelosuppressive Ch in a total of 6213 cycles and who received prophylaxis with Zarzio®, one of the biosimilar agents of filgrastim (Gascon et al. 2016). LC was the second most frequent solid neoplasm in the study, with 466 patients (32.2%) of the total cohort. According to the EORTC guidelines, 56.6% of patients received prophylaxis correctly, 17.4% received over-prophylaxis, and 26.0% under-prophylaxis. The following incidence rates were recorded: Ch-induced grade 4 neutropenia 13.2% and 3.9% of cycles; 5.9% of the patients developed FN and in 1.4% of the cycles; hospitalizations secondary to FN in 6.1% of patients and in 1.5% of cycles; Ch alterations due to FN in 9.5% of patients and in 2.8% of cycles; and composite outcomes index 22.3% of patients and in 6.7% of cycles. In conclusion, the clinical and safety results of this biosimilar are within the range of historically reported data for the original filgrastim, underlining the clinical efficacy and safety of the biosimilar in daily clinical practice.

5.2 Anemia

Anemia, another known consequence of BM toxicity, has a multifactorial etiology that includes inadequate production of erythropoietin in response to the alteration of normal Hb levels. This anomaly is accentuated by Ch. On the other hand, the recombinant human erythropoietin (r-HuEPO) has been used to improve the anemia seen in cancer patients by increasing the number of erythroid progenitors in both the bone marrow and the peripheral blood.

Several large community studies have shown that epoetin alfa effectively corrects anemia and improves quality of life in anemic cancer patients receiving Ch (Kosmidis et al. 2005). However, the contribution of r-HuEPO to the outcome of curative cancer treatment has been controversial (Macktay et al. 2007; Bohlius et al. 2009). A safety analysis in an RCT suggested a decrease in OS in patients with advanced NSCLC treated with r-HuEPO (Wright et al. 2007). ASCO has made recommendations with a level of evidence of II on the treatment of anemia with r-HuEPO (Rizzo et al. 2008). For patients with Ch-induced anemia, the Committee continues to recommend initiating an erythropoiesis-stimulating agent (ESA) in cases where Hb values approach or fall below 10 g/dL, thereby increasing Hb and decreasing indications for transfusion.

In a prospective phase II trial (Casas et al. 2003), the impact of the use of r-HuEPO on the maintenance of Karnofsky and Hb levels was studied in patients with LC who received concomitant treatment with ChRT after one cycle of induction Ch (11 SCLC and 40 NSCLC). In addition to finding a beneficial impact of the administration of r-HuEPO on the general status and Hb levels, it was also found to be a prognostic factor for OS in the multivariate analysis, together with classical factors such as weight loss, final improvement in Hb, SCLC histology, and, finally, Hb levels greater than 10 g/dL before ChRT.

A recent phase III noninferiority study (Gascón et al. 2020) has concluded on the positive impact of r-HuEPO, in this case with darbepoetin (DARB), on OS and PFS in anemic patients with NSCLC treated to a 12.0 g/dL Hb ceiling. Patients with stage IV NSCLC who were expected to receive two or more cycles of myelosuppressive Ch and Hb ≤11.0 g/dL were randomized 2:1 to 500 µg of blinded DARB or placebo every 3 weeks. The primary endpoint was OS, and the secondary endpoints were PFS and incidence of transfusions or Hb ≤8.0 g/dL from week 5 to the end of the efficacy treatment period. A total of 1680 patients received DARB and 836 placebo. DARB was not inferior to placebo for OS and PFS, and DARB significantly reduced odds of transfusion or Hb ≤8.0 g/dL. The objective tumor response was similar between the arms, and the incidence of serious adverse events (AE) was 31.1% in both arms.

5.3 Thrombocytopenia

Thrombopoietin (TPO), a factor synthesized for the stimulation of platelets with the intention of preventing bleeding problems after myelosuppressive Ch, is still under evaluation. TPO, a key physiological regulator of platelet production, has been found to be the most potent thrombopoietic cytokine studied to date. Unfortunately, the clinical development of recombinant human thrombopoietin has faced challenges related to the biology of TPO, observing a delayed platelet response peak and the presence of neutralizing antibodies against the pegylated molecule (Vadhan-Raj et al. 2005). A Cochrane review (Zhang et al. 2017) concludes that the available evidence is not sufficient to support the use of TPO-RAs to prevent Ch-induced thrombocytopenia (CIT) or to prevent recurrence of CIT in patients with solid tumors.

In addition to the development of specific cytokines for the production and secretion of different hematological cells, trials are currently being carried out with molecules such as glutathione on different methods of prevention of BM toxicity. Glutathione has been shown to be an effective chemoprotectant against CDDP-induced toxicity. Although the majority of experience is in ovarian cancer, RCTs in other types of tumors such as LC and head and neck tumors have shown a lower HT in patients who received glutathione (Schmidinger et al. 2000).

Other drugs, such as amifostine, have also shown a reduction in HT in RCTs that include LC patients treated with concomitant ChRT (Antonadou et al. 2003). However, in another RCT (Movsas et al. 2005) and in a phase II trial (Han et al. 2008), both in LC, amifostine was associated with a higher incidence of FN, so it does not seem useful to prevent the HT.

The use of intensity-modulated RT (IMRT) is another way to reduce BM toxicity using RT alone or in combination with Ch. This technique has been shown to significantly reduce radiation doses to critical tissues (Lujan et al. 2003). With the planning of IMRT, the volume of radiation in the BM at the thoracic level and in the cardiac circulation can be reduced, which allows reducing the irradiation on the blood cells both in RT alone and combined with Ch.

Finally, it is possible to monitor or even predict the occurrence of leukopenia or thrombocytopenia during the course of fractionated local RT using the variation in plasma concentration of the Flt-3 ligand as a biomarker for RT-induced BM damage (Huchet et al. 2003).

6 Hematological Toxicity After New Biomarker-Based Targeted Therapies in Stage IV NSCLC

In the last decade, year after year, systemic therapy for stage IV NSCLC was selected according to the presence of specific biomarkers. All patients with stage IV NSCLC should undergo molecular testing for the mutations and expression of the programmed death ligand 1 (PD-L1). Molecular alterations that predict response to treatment (e.g., EGFR mutations, ALK rearrangements, ROS1 rearrangements, and BRAF V600E mutations) are present in approximately 30% of these patients. Targeted therapy for these disorders improves PFS compared to Ch. Tyrosine kinase inhibitors such as gefitinib, erlotinib, and afatinib improve PFS in patients with EGFR mutations. In patients with overexpression of ALK protein, the response rate was significantly better with crizotinib, a tyrosine kinase inhibitor (TKI), compared to the combination of Ch-based pemetrexed and CDDP or CB (74% vs. 45%, respectively; $p < 0.001$) and PFS (median 10.9 months vs. 7.0 months; $p < 0.001$) (Rosell et al. 2012). With the new generations of TKI, these agents have been improved. In patients without biomarkers indicating susceptibility to specific targeted therapies, regimens containing immune checkpoint inhibitors (ICIs), either as monotherapy or in combination with Ch, are superior to Ch alone.

These advances in biomarker-based therapy have led to improvements in OS. For example, the 5-year OS currently exceeds 25% in patients with tumors that have high PD-L1 expression (tumor proportion score $\geq 50\%$) and 40% in patients with ALK-positive tumors (Arbour and Riely 2019). Any degree of lymphopenia and thrombocytopenia (63% and 54%, respectively) can be found after the administration of anti-EGFR, but severe toxicity is rare. The same occurs with anti-ALK targeted therapy, with some degree of anemia observed in 62% of patients, but without serious toxicities.

ICIs have radically changed the prognosis of several cancers with lasting responses. Cytotoxic T lymphocyte antigen 4 (CTLA-4), programmed cell death 1 (PD-1), and programmed cell death ligand 1 (PD-L1) represent ICIs that can be used as monotherapy or in combination with other agents .The toxicity profiles of ICIs differ from the side effects of cytotoxic agents, presenting new toxicities such as adverse events related to the immune system. Normally, these toxicities can occur in all organs. However, the main organs affected are the skin, digestive tract, liver, lungs, endocrine, and rheumatological systems. HT is considered as a rare toxicity with a frequency of 1%, but it can be very serious. Isolated cases of disseminated intravascular coagulation, acquired hemophilia, idiopathic thrombocytopenic purpura, and autoimmune hemolytic anemia (AHA) have been reported after ICI treatment. These occurred more frequently in patients treated for Hodgkin's lymphoma (Durrechou et al. 2020). In a recent article (Tanios et al. 2019) with 68 cases of AHA associated with ICI, they found 24 cases in patients with LC. Eighteen cases were due to nivolumab, five were due to pembrolizumab, and one was associated with atezolizumab. ICIs are believed to cause random activation of the immune system resulting in the formation of autoantibodies, activation of T-cell clones, and decreased function of regulatory T cells. AHA, although rare, is not the only hematologic complication of ICIs. Several cases of autoimmune neutropenia, thrombocytopenia, and even pancytopenia have recently been published (Tokumo et al. 2018). Even in cases of combined treatments with Ch and ICIs for patients with metastatic NSCLC, the combination of CB, paclitaxel, atezolizumab (Socinski et al. 2018), and bevacizumab can produce an infrequent severe FN in 9% of cases. Treatment of immunotoxicity usually involves corticosteroid therapy or use of immunomodulators. In cases of HT due to ICIs, oral or intravenous (IV) corticosteroids are usually used, as well as G-CSF in cases of neutropenia. In refractory cases, IV immunoglobulins or cyclosporine treatment can be used. A complete blood count is essential to identify abnormalities before each infusion of treatment, although hematologic irregularities may not be identified with these tests. For those patients who develop toxicity with ICIs, and who are not candidates to receive other treatments for different reasons, early and adequate management of toxicity could allow resuming treatment with ICI.

References

Aapro MS, Cameron DA, Pettengell R, Bohlius J, Crawfor J, Ellis M et al (2006) EORTC guidelines for the use of granulocyte–colony stimulating factor to reduce the incidence of chemotherapy induced febrile neutropenia in adult patients with lymphomas and solid tumours. Eur J Cancer 42:2433–2453. https://doi.org/10.1016/j.ejca.2006.05.002

Aapro MS, Bohlius J, Cameron DA, Dal Lago L, Donnelly JP, Kearney N et al (2011) 2010 update of EORTC guidelines for the use of granulocyte-colony stimulating factor to reduce the incidence of chemotherapy-induced febrile neutropenia in adult patients with lymphoproliferative disorders and solid tumours. Eur J Cancer 10.1016/j.ejca.2010.10.013(47):8–32

Abrams RA, Lichter AS, Bromer RH, Minna JD, Cohen MH, Deisseroth AB (1985) The hematopoietic toxicity of regional radiation therapy. Correlations for combined modality therapy with systemic chemotherapy. Cancer 55:1429–1435. https://doi.org/10.1002/1097-0142(19850401)55:7<1429::aid-cncr2820550702>3.0.co;2-4

Adams JR, Lyman GH, Djubegovic B, Feinglass J, Bennett CL (2002) G-CSF as prophylaxis of febrile neutropenia in SCLC. Review of findings from 13 studies of cost-effectiveness, evidence-based guidelines, patterns of care and surveys of ASCO members. Expert Opin Pharmacother 3:1273–1281. https://doi.org/10.1517/14656566.3.9.1273

Antonadou D, Throuvalas N, Petridis A, Bolanos N, Sagriotis A, Synodinou M (2003) Effect of amifostine on toxicities with radiochemotherapy in patients with locally advanced non-small-cell lung cancer. Int J Radiat Oncol Biol Phys 57:402–408. https://doi.org/10.1016/s0360-3016(03)00590-x

Antonia SJ, Villegas A, Daniel D, Vicente D, Murakami S, Hui R et al (2017) Durvalumab after chemoradiotherapy in stage III non-small-cell lung cancer. N Engl J Med 377(20):1919–1929. https://doi.org/10.1056/NEJMoa1709937

Antonia SJ, Villegas A, Daniel D, Vicente D, Murakami S, Hui R et al (2018) Overall survival with durvalumab after chemoradiotherapy in stage III NSCLC. N Engl J Med. https://doi.org/10.1056/NEJMoa1809697

Arbour KC, Riely GJ (2019) Systemic therapy for locally advanced and metastatic non-small cell lung cancer: a review. JAMA 322(8):764–774. https://doi.org/10.1001/jama.2019.11058

Bennett CL, Weeks JA, Somerfield MR, Feinglass J, Smith TJ (1999) Use of hematopoietic colony-stimulating factors: comparison of the 1994 and 1997 American Society of Clinical Oncology surveys regarding ASCO Clinical Practice Guidelines. Health Services Research Committee of the American Society of Clinical Oncology. J Clin Oncol 17:3676–3681. https://doi.org/10.1200/JCO.1999.17.11.3676

Berghmans T, Paesmans M, Lafitte JJ, Mascaux C, Meert AP, Sculier JP (2002) Role of granulocyte and granulocyte–macrophage colony-stimulating factors in the treatment of small-cell lung cancer: a systematic review of the literature with methodological assessment and meta-analysis. Lung Cancer 37:115–123. https://doi.org/10.1016/S0169-5002(02)00082-X

Bohlius J, Herbst C, Reiser M, Schwarzer G, Engert A (2008) Granulopoiesis-stimulating factors to prevent adverse effects in the treatment of malignant lymphoma (Review). Cochrane Database Syst Rev (4):CD003189. https://doi.org/10.1002/14651858.CD003189.pub4

Bohlius J, Scmindlin K, Brillant C, Schwarzer G, Trelle S, Seindenfeld J et al (2009) Recombinant human erythropoiesis-stimulating agents and mortality in patients with cancer: a meta-analysis of randomized trials. Lancet 373:1532–1542. https://doi.org/10.1016/S0140-6736(09)60502-X

Bradley JD, Paulus R, Komaki R, Masters G, Blumenschein G, Schild S et al (2015) Standard-dose versus high-dose conformal radiotherapy with concurrent and consolidation carboplatin plus paclitaxel with or without cetuximab for patients with stage IIIA or IIIB non-small-cell lung cancer (RTOG 0617): a randomised, two-by-two factorial phase 3 study. Lancet Oncol 16:187–199. https://doi.org/10.1016/S1470-2045(14)71207-0]

Calvert AH, Ghokul S, Al Azraqui A, Wright J, Lind M, Bailey N et al (1999) Carboplatin and paclitaxel, alone and in combination: dose escalation, measurements of renal function, and role of the p53 tumor suppressor gene. Semin Oncol 26:676–684

Cardenal F, Lopez-Cabrerizo MP, Anton A, Alberola V, Massuti B, Carrato A et al (1999) Randomized phase III study of gemcitabine-cisplatin versus etoposide-cisplatin in the treatment of locally advanced or metastatic non-small-cell lung cancer. J Clin Oncol 17:12–18. https://doi.org/10.1200/JCO.1999.17.1.12

Carmona-Bayonas A, Jimenez-Fonseca P, Viriziuela Echaburu J, Antonio M, Font C, Biosca M et al (2015) Prediction of serious complications in patients with seemingly stable febrile neutropenia: validation of the clinical index of stable febrile neutropenia in a prospective cohort of patients from the FINITE study. J Clin Oncol 33(5):465–471. https://doi.org/10.1200/JCO.2014.57.2347

Casas F, Viñolas N, Ferrer F, Farrús B, Gimferrer JM, Agustí C, Belda J, Luburich P (2003) Improvement in performance status after erythropoietin treatment in lung cancer patients undergoing concurrent chemoradiotherapy. Int J Radiat Oncol Biol Phys 55:116–124. https://doi.org/10.1016/s0360-3016(02)03823-3

Crawford J, Caserta C, Roila F (2010) Hematopoietic growth factors ESMO clinical practice guidelines for the applications. Ann Oncol 21(Suppl 5):v248–v251. https://doi.org/10.1093/annonc/mdq195

Cullen M, Steven N, Billingham L, Gaunt C, Hastings M, Simmonds P et al (2005) Antibacterial prophylaxis after chemotherapy for solid tumors and lymphomas. N Engl J Med 353:988–998. https://doi.org/10.1056/NEJMoa050078

De Souza Viana L, Serufo JC, da Costa Rocha MO, Nogueira Costa R, Carlos Duarte R (2008) Performance of a modified MASCC index score for identifying low-risk febrile neutropenic cancer patients. Support Care Cancer 16:841–846. https://doi.org/10.1007/s00520-007-0347-3

Di Maio M, Gridelli C, Gallo C, Shepherd F, Piantedosi FV, Cigolari S et al (2005) Chemotherapy-induced neutropenia and treatment efficacy in advanced non-small-cell lung cancer: a pooled analysis of three randomized trials. Lancet Oncol 6:669–677. https://doi.org/10.1016/S1470-2045(05)70255-2

Dillman RO, Seagren SL, Propert KJ, Guerra J, Eaton WL, Perryet MC et al (1990) A randomized trial of induction chemotherapy plus high-dose radiation versus radiation alone in stage III non-small cell lung cancer. N Engl J Med 323:940–945. https://doi.org/10.1056/NEJM199010043231403

Douillard JY, Rosell R, De Lena M, Carpagnano F, Ramlau R, Gonzáles-Larriba JL et al (2006) Adjuvant vinorelbine plus cisplatin versus observation in patients with completely resected stage IB-IIIA non-small-cell lung cancer (Adjuvant Navelbine International Trialist Association [ANITA]): a randomised controlled trail. Lancet Oncol 7:719–727. https://doi.org/10.1016/S1470-2045(06)70804-X

Durrechou Q, Domblides C, Sionneau B, Lefort F, Quivy A, Ravaud A et al (2020) Management of immune checkpoint inhibitor toxicities. Cancer Manag Res 12:9139–9158. https://doi.org/10.2147/CMAR.S218756

Faivre-Finn C, Snee M, Ashcroft L, Appel W, Barlesi F, Bhatnagar A et al (2017) Concurrent once-daily versus twice-daily chemoradiotherapy in patients with limited-stage small-cell lung cancer (CONVERT): an open-label, phase 3, randomised, superiority trial. Lancet Oncol 18:1116–1125. https://doi.org/10.1016/S1470-2045(17)30318-2

Fukuoka M, Furuse K, Saijo N, Nishiwaki Y, Ikegami H, Tamura T et al (1991) Randomized trial of cyclophosphamide, doxorubicin, and vincristine versus cisplatin and etoposide versus alternation of these regimens in small cell lung cancer. J Natl Cancer Inst 83:885–891. https://doi.org/10.1093/jnci/83.12.855

Furuse K, Fukuoka M, Kawahara M, Nishikawa H, Takada Y, Kudoh S et al (1999) Phase III study of concurrent versus sequential thoracic radiotherapy in combination with mitomycin, vindesine and cisplatin in unresectable stage III non-small-cell lung cancer. J Clin Oncol 17:2692–2699. https://doi.org/10.1200/JCO.1999.17.9.2692

Gafter-Gvili A, Fraser A, Paul M, Leibovici L (2005) Meta-analysis: antibiotic prophylaxis reduces mortality in neutropenic patients. Ann Intern Med 142:977–995. https://doi.org/10.7326/0003-4819-142-12_part_1-200506210-00008

Gafter-Gvili A, Paul M, Fraser A, Leivibovici L (2007) Effect of quinolone prophylaxis in afebrile neutropenic patients on microbial resistance: systematic review and meta-analysis. J Antimicrob Chemother 59:5–22. https://doi.org/10.1093/jac/dkl425

Gascon P, Aapro M, Ludwig H, Bokemeyer C, Boccadoro M (2016) Treatment patterns and outcomes in the prophylaxis of chemotherapy-induced (febrile) neutropenia with biosimilar filgrastim (the MONITOR-GCSF study). Support Care Cancer 24:911–925. https://doi.org/10.1007/s00520-015-2861-z

Gascón P, Nagarkar R, Šmakal M, Syrigos KN, Barrios CH, Cárdenas Sánchez J et al (2020) A randomized, double-blind, placebo-controlled, phase III noninferiority study of the long-term safety and efficacy of darbepoetin alfa for chemotherapy-induced anemia in patients with advanced non-small cell lung cancer. J Thorac Oncol 15(2):190–202. https://doi.org/10.1016/j.jtho.2019.10.005

Gregor A, Drings P, Burghouts J, Postmus PE, Morgan D, Sahmoud T (1997) Randomized trial of alternating versus sequential radiotherapy/chemotherapy in limited-disease patients with small-cell lung cancer: a European Organization for Research and Treatment of Cancer Lung Cancer Cooperative Group Study. J Clin Oncol 15:2840–2849. https://doi.org/10.1200/JCO.1997.15.8.2840

Han HY, Han J-Y, Yu SY, Pyo HR, Kim HY, Cho KH, Lee DH et al (2008) Randomized phase 2 study of subcutaneous amifostine versus epoetin-alfa given 3 times weekly during concurrent chemotherapy and hyperfractionated radiotherapy for limited-disease small cell lung cancer. Cancer 113:1623–1631. https://doi.org/10.1002/cncr.23790

Hanna N, Neubauer M, Yiannoutos C, McGarry R, Arsenau J, Ansari R et al (2008) Phase III study of cisplatin, etoposide, and concurrent chest radiation with or without consolidation docetaxel in patients with inoperable stage III non-small-cell lung cancer: The Hoosier Oncology Group and U.S. Oncology. J Clin Oncol 35:5755–5760. https://doi.org/10.1200/JCO.2008.17.7840

Herbst C, Naumann F, Kruse EB, Monsef I, Bohlius J, Schulzet H et al (2009) Prophylactic antibiotics or G-CSF for the prevention of infections and improvement of survival in cancer patients undergoing chemotherapy. Cochrane Database Syst Rev CD007107. https://doi.org/10.1002/14651858.CD007107.pub2

Huber RM, Flentje M, Scmindt M, Pöllinger B, Gosse H, Wilner J, Ulm K (2006) Simultaneous chemoradiotherapy compared with radiotherapy alone after induction chemotherapy in inoperable stage IIIA or IIIB non-small-cell lung cancer: study CTRT99/97 by the Bronchial Carcinoma Therapy Group. J Clin Oncol 24(27):4397–4404. https://doi.org/10.1200/JCO.2005.05.4163

Huchet A, Belkacemi Y, Frick J, Prat M, Muresan-Kloos I, Altan D et al (2003) Plasma Flt-3 ligand concentration correlated with radiation-induced bone marrow damage during local fractionated radiotherapy. Int J Radiat Oncol Biol Phys 57:508–515. https://doi.org/10.1016/s0360-3016(03)00584-4

Jeremic B, Shibamoto Y, Acimovic L, Milisavljevic S (1996) Randomized trial of hyperfractionated radiation therapy with or without concurrent chemotherapy for stage III non-small-cell lung cancer. J Clin Oncol 13:452–458. https://doi.org/10.1200/JCO.1996.14.4.1065

Jeremic B, Shibamoto Y, Acimovic L, Milisavljevic S (1997) Initial versus delayed accelerated hyperfractionated radiation therapy and concurrent chemotherapy in limited small-cell lung cancer: a randomized study. J Clin Oncol 15:893–900. https://doi.org/10.1200/JCO.1997.15.3.893

Kao SCH, Phan VH, Clarke SJ (2010) Predictive markers for haematological toxicity of pemetrexed. Curr Drugs. Targets 11(1):48–57. https://doi.org/10.2174/138945010790031072

Kelly K, Crowley J, Bunn PA, Presant CA et al (2001) Randomized phase III trial of paclitaxel plus carboplatin versus vinorelbine plus cisplatin in the treatment of patients with advanced non-small-cell lung cancer: a southwest oncology group trial. J Clin Oncol 19:3210–3218. https://doi.org/10.1200/JCO.2001.19.13.3210

Khan S, Dhadda A, Fyfe D, Sundar S (2008) Impact of neutropenia on delivering planned chemotherapy for solid tumours. Eur J Cancer Care (Engl) 17:19–25. https://doi.org/10.1111/j.1365-2354.2007.00797.x

Klastersky J, Awada A, Paesmans M, Aoun M (2010) Febrile neutropenia: a critical review of the initial management. Crit Rev Oncol Hematol 78(3):185–194. https://doi.org/10.1016/j.critrevonc.2010.03.008

Kosmidis P, Krzakowski M, ECAS Investigators (2005) Anemia profiles in patients with lung cancer: what have we learned from the European Cancer Anaemia Survey (ECAS). Lung Cancer 50:401–412. https://doi.org/10.1016/j.lungcan.2005.08.004

Kuderer NM, Dale DC, Crawford J, Lyman GH (2007) Impact of primary prophylaxis with granulocyte colony-stimulating factor on febrile neutropenia and mortality in adult cancer patients receiving chemotherapy: a systematic review. J Clin Oncol 25:3158–3167. https://doi.org/10.1200/JCO.2006.08.8823

Le Chevalier T, Arraigada R, Quoix E, Ruffie P, Martin M, Tarayre M et al (1991) Radiotherapy alone versus combined chemotherapy and radiotherapy in nonresectable non-small-cell lung cancer. First analysis of a randomized trial in 353 patients. J Natl Cancer Inst 83:417–423. https://doi.org/10.1093/jnci/83.6.417

Lujan AE, Mundt AJ, Yamada SD, Rotmensch J, Roeske JC (2003) Intensity-modulated radiotherapy as a means of reducing dose to bone marrow in gynecologic patients receiving whole pelvic radiotherapy. Int J Radiar Oncol Biol Phys 57:515–521. https://doi.org/10.1016/s0360-3016(00)00771-9

Luo J, Lear SJ, Xu Y, Zheng D (2011) Comparison of cisplatin and carboplatin based third-generation chemotherapy in 1014 Chinese patients with advanced non-small-cell lung cancer. Med Oncol 28(4):1418–1424. https://doi.org/10.1007/s12032-010-9575-3

Lyman GH (2009) Impact of chemotherapy dose intensity on cancer patient outcomes. J Natl Compr Canc Netw 7(1):99–108. https://doi.org/10.6004/jnccn.2009.0009

Lyman GH, Kuderer NM, Djulbegovic B (2002) Prophylactic granulocyte colony-stimulating factor in patients receiving dose-intensive cancer chemotherapy: a meta-analysis. Am J Med 112:406–411. https://doi.org/10.1016/s0002-9343(02)01036-7

Macktay M, Pajak TF, Suntharalingam M, Shenouda G, Hershock D, Strippet DC et al (2007) Radiotherapy with or without erythropoietin for anemic patients with head and neck cancer: a randomized trial of the Radiation Therapy Oncology Group (RTOG 99-03). Int J Radiat Oncol Biol Phys 69:1008–1017. https://doi.org/10.1016/j.ijrobp.2007.04.063

Milward MJ, Boyer MJ, Lehnert M, Clarke S, Rischin D, Goh D-C et al (2003) Docetaxel and carboplatin is an active regimen in advanced non-small-cell lung cancer: a phase II study in Caucasian and Asian patients. Ann Oncol 10.1093/annonc/mdg118(14):449–454

Minchom AR, Saksornchai K, Bhosle J, Gunapala R, Puglisi M, Lu SK (2014) An unblinded, randomised phase II study of platinum-based chemotherapy with vitamin B12 and folic acid supplementation in the treatment of lung cancer with plasma homocysteine blood levels as a biomarker of severe neutropenic toxicity. BMJ Open Respir 1(1):e000061. https://doi.org/10.1136/bmjresp-2014-000061

Movsas B, Scott C, Langer C, Werner-Wasik M, Nicolaou N, Komaki R et al (2005) Randomized trial of amifostine in locally advanced non-small-cell lung cancer patients receiving chemotherapy and hyperfractionated radiation: Radiation Therapy Oncology Group trial 98-01. J Clin Oncol 145:2145–2154. https://doi.org/10.1200/JCO.2005.07.167

Murray N, Coy P, Pater JL, Hodson I, Arnold A, Zee BC et al (1993) Importance of timing for thoracic irradiation in the combined modality treatment of limited-stage SCLC. J Clin Oncol 11:336–344. https://doi.org/10.1200/JCO.1993.11.2.336

Ozer H, Armitage JO, Bennet CL, Crawford J, Demetri GD, Pizzo PA et al (2000) 2000 update of recommendations for the use of hematopoietic colony-stimulating factors: evidence-based, clinical practice guidelines. J Clin Oncol 18:3558–3585. https://doi.org/10.1200/JCO.2000.18.20.3558

Pirker R, Pereira JR, Szczesna A, Pavel JV, Krzakowski M, Ramlau R, Vynnychenko I et al (2009) Cetuximab plus chemotherapy in patients with advanced non-small-cell lung cancer (FLEX): an open-label randomized phase III trial. Lancet 373:1525–1531. https://doi.org/10.1016/S0140-6736(09)60569-9

Pivot X, Guardiola E, Etienne M, Thys A, Foa C, Otto J et al (2000) An analysis of potential factors allowing an individual prediction of cisplatin-induced anemia. Eur J Cancer 36:852–857. https://doi.org/10.1016/s0959-8049(00)00010-1

Plowman PN, McElwain T, Meadows A (1991) Complications of cancer management, 1st edn. Butterworth-Heinemann, Oxford

Ratain MJ, Schilsky RL, Conley BA, Egorin MJ (1990) Pharmacodynamics in cancer therapy. J Clin Oncol 8:1739–1753. https://doi.org/10.1200/JCO.1990.8.10.1739

Reck M, von Pawel J, Zatlooukal P, Ramlau R, Gorbounova V, Hirsh V et al (2009) Phase III trial of cisplatin plus gemcitabine with either placebo or bevacizumab as first-line therapy for nonsquamous non-small-cell lung cancer: AVAil. J Clin Oncol 27:1227–1234. https://doi.org/10.1200/JCO.2007.14.5466

Rizzo JD, Somerfiweld MR, Hagerty KL, Seindenfeld J, Bohlius J et al (2008) Use of epoetin and darbopetin in patients with cancer: 2007 American Society of Clinical Oncology/American Society of Hematology Clinical Practice Guideline Update. J Clin Oncol 26:132–149. https://doi.org/10.1200/JCO.2007.14.3396

Rosell R, Carcereny E, Gervais R, Vergnenegre A, Massuti B, Felip E, et al; Spanish Lung Cancer Group in collaboration with Groupe Français de Pneumo-Cancérologie and Associazione Italiana Oncologia Toracica (2012) Erlotinib versus standard chemotherapy as first-line treatment for European patients with advanced EGFR mutation-positive non-small-cell lung cancer (EURTAC): a multicentre, open-label, randomised phase 3 trial. Lancet Oncol 13(3):239–246. https://doi.org/10.1016/S1470-2045(11)70393-X

Sandler A, Gray R, Perry MC, Brahmer J, Schiller JH, Dowlati A et al (2006) Paclitaxel–carboplatin alone or with bevacizumab for non-small-cell lung cancer. N Engl J Med 355:2542–2550. https://doi.org/10.1056/NEJMoa061884

Sause WT, Scott C, Taylor S, Livingston R, Komaki R, Emami B et al (1995) Radiation Therapy Oncology Group (RTOG) 88-08 and Eastern Cooperative Oncology Group (ECOG) 4588: preliminary results of a phase III trial in regionally advanced, unresected non-small cell lung cancer. J Natl Cancer Inst 87:198–205. https://doi.org/10.1093/jnci/87.3.198

Schaake-Koning C, van der Bogaert W, Dalesio O, Festen J, Hoogenhout J, van Houtte P et al (1992) Effects of concomitant cisplatin and radiotherapy on inoperable non-small-cell lung cancer. N Engl J Med 326:524–530. https://doi.org/10.1056/NEJM199202203260805

Schiller JH, Harrington D, Belani CP, Langer C, Sandler A, Krook J et al (2002) Comparison of four chemotherapy regimens for advanced non-small-cell lung cancer. N Engl J Med 346:92–98. https://doi.org/10.1056/NEJMoa011954

Schmidinger M, Budinsky AC, Wenzel C, Piribauer M, Brix R, Kautzky M et al (2000) Glutathione in the prevention of cisplatin induced toxicities. A prospectively randomized pilot trial in patients with head and neck cancers and non-small cell lung cancer. Wien Klin Wochenschr 28:617–623

Senan S, Brade A, Wang L-H, Vansteenkiste J, Dakhil S, Biesma B et al (2016) PROCLAIM: randomized phase III trial of pemetrexed-cisplatin or etoposide-cisplatin plus thoracic radiation therapy followed by consolidation chemotherapy in locally advanced nonsquamous non-small-cell lung cancer. J Clin Oncol 34:953–962. https://doi.org/10.1200/JCO.2015.64.8824

Sheikh H, Colaco R, Lorigan P, Blackhall F, Califano R, Ashcroft L et al (2011) Use of G-CSF during concurrent chemotherapy and thoracic radiotherapy in patients with limited-stage small-cell lung cancer safety data from a phase II trial. Lung Cancer 74(1):75–79. https://doi.org/10.1016/j.lungcan.2011.01.020

Socinski MA, Jotte RM, Cappuzzo F, Orlandi F, Stroyakovskiy D, Nogami Y (2018) Atezolizumab for first-line treatment of metastatic nonsquamous NSCLC. N Engl J Med 378(24):2288–2301. https://doi.org/10.1056/NEJMoa1716948

Takada M, Fukuoka M, Kawahara M, Sugiura T, Yokoyama A, Yokota S et al (2002) Phase III study of concurrent versus sequential thoracic radiotherapy in combination with cisplatin and etoposide for limited-stage small-cell lung cancer: results of the Japan Clinical Oncology Group Study 9104. J Clin Oncol 20:3054–3060. https://doi.org/10.1200/JCO.2002.12.071

Tanios GE et al (2019) Autoimmune hemolytic anemia associated with the use of immune checkpoint inhibitors for cancer: 68 cases from the Food and Drug Administration database and review. Eur J Haematol 102(2):157–162. https://doi.org/10.1111/ejh.13187. Epub 2018 Nov 29

Timmer-Bonte JN, de Boo TM, Smith HJ, Biesma B, Wilschut FA, Cheragwandi SA et al (2005) Prevention of chemotherapy–induced febrile neutropenia by prophylactic antibiotics plus or minus granulocyte colony-stimulating factor in small-cell lung cancer: a Dutch Randomized Phase III study. J Clin Oncol 23:7994–7984. https://doi.org/10.1200/JCO.2004.00.7955

Tokumo K, Masuda T, Miyama T, Miura S, Yamaguchi K, Sakamoto S et al (2018) Nivolumab-induced severe pancytopenia in a patient with lung adenocarcinoma. Lung Cancer 119:21–24. https://doi.org/10.1016/j.lungcan.2018.02.018

Trovo MG, Minatel E, Franchin G, Boccieri MG, Nascimben O, Bolzicco G et al (1992) Radiotherapy versus radiotherapy enhanced by cisplatin in stage III non-small cell lung cancer. Int J Radiat Oncol Biol Phys 254:11–15. https://doi.org/10.1016/0360-3016(92)91014-e

Tubiana M, Frindel E, Croizat H (1979) Effects of radiation on bone marrow. Pathol Biol 27:326–334

Turrisi AT, Kim K, Blum R, Sause WT, Livingston RB, Komaki R et al (1999) Twice-daily compared with once-daily thoracic radiotherapy in limited small-cell lung cancer treated concurrently with cisplatin and etoposide. N Engl J Med 340:265–271. https://doi.org/10.1056/NEJM199901283400403

Vadhan-Raj S, Cohen V, Bueso-Ramos C (2005) Thrombopoietic growth factors and cytokines. Curr Hematol Rep 4:137–144

Van de Wetering MD, de Witte MA, Kremer LC, Offringa M, Scholten HJPM, Caron HM (2005) Efficacy of oral prophylactic antibiotics in neutropenic afebrile oncology patients: a systematic review of randomised controlled trials. Eur J Cancer 41:1372–1382. https://doi.org/10.1016/j.ejca.2005.03.006

Vokes EE, Rendón JE, Crawford J, Leopold KA, Perry MC, Miller AA et al (2002) Randomized phase II study of cisplatin with gemcitabine or paclitaxel or vinorelbine as induction chemotherapy followed by concomitant chemoradiotherapy for stage IIIB non-small-cell lung cancer: cancer and leukemia group B study 9431. J Clin Oncol 20:4191–4198. https://doi.org/10.1200/JCO.2002.03.054

Vokes EE, Herdon JE, Kelley MJ, Cichetti MG, Ramnath N, Neill H et al (2007) Induction chemotherapy followed by chemoradiotherapy compared with chemoradiotherapy alone for regionally advanced unresectable stage III NSCLC: Cancer and Leukemia Group B. J Clin Oncol 13:1698–1704. https://doi.org/10.1200/JCO.2006.07.3569

Wingard JR, Elmongy M (2009) Strategies for minimizing complications of neutropenia: prophylactic myeloid growth factors or antibiotics. Crit Rev Oncol Hematol 72:144–154. https://doi.org/10.1016/j.critrevonc.2009.01.003

Winton T, Livingston R, Johnson D, Rigas J, Rigas J, Johnston M, Butts C et al (2005) Vinorelbine plus cisplatin vs. observation in resected non-small-cell lung cancer. N Engl J Med 352:2589–2597. https://doi.org/10.1056/NEJMoa043623

Woll PJ, Hodgetts J, Lomax L, Bildet F, Cour-Chabernaud V, Thacher N et al (1995) Can cytotoxic dose-intensity be increased by using granulocyte colony-stimulating factor? A randomized controlled trial of lenograstim in small-cell lung cancer. J Clin Oncol 13:652–659. https://doi.org/10.1200/JCO.1995.13.3.652

Wright JR, Ung YC, Julian JA, Pritchard KI, Whelan TJ, Smith C et al (2007) Randomized, double-blind, placebo-controlled trial of erythropoietin in non-small-cell lung cancer with disease-related anemia. J Clin Oncol 25:1027–1032. https://doi.org/10.1200/JCO.2006.07.1514

Zatloukal P, Petruzelka L, Zemanova M, Havel L, Janku F, Judas L et al (2004) Concurrent versus sequential chemoradiotherapy with cisplatin and vinorelbine in locally advanced non-small cell lung cancer: a randomized study. Lung Cancer 46:87–98. https://doi.org/10.1016/j.lungcan.2004.03.004

Zhang X, Chuai Y, Nie W, Wang A, Dai G (2017). Thrombopoietin receptor agonists for prevention and treatment of chemotherapy-induced thrombocytopenia in patients with solid tumours. Cochrane Database Syst Rev 2017(11):CD012035. https://doi.org/10.1002/14651858.CD012035.pub2

Radiation Therapy-Induced Lung and Heart Toxicity

Soheila F. Azghadi and Megan E. Daly

Contents

1 Introduction 925
2 **Lung Toxicity** 926
2.1 Pathophysiology of Radiation-Induced Pneumonitis 926
2.2 Contributing Patient-Related Risk Factors 927
2.3 Radiation Treatment-Related Risk Factors 928
2.4 Tumor Factors 930
2.5 Systemic Treatment Risk Factors for Lung Injury 930
2.6 Heart Toxicity 934
2.7 Treatment of Cardiac Toxicity 936
3 **Conclusions** 936
References 936

1 Introduction

Radiation therapy is an essential treatment modality for the treatment of thoracic malignancies and plays a crucial role in the treatment of both non-small cell (NSCLC) and small cell lung cancer (SCLC). In lung cancer patients, radiation therapy is used as a curative-intent treatment for nonmetastatic disease, with or without other modalities such as surgery and systemic therapies. Radiation also plays a crucial role in the noncurative setting, improving quality of life and survival in the metastatic setting. The Cancer Treatment & Survivorship Facts & Figures (2019–2021) by the American Cancer Society has shown that 31% of patients with stage I–II non-small cell lung cancer, 53% of patients with stage III NSCLC, and 41% of patients with stage IV NSCLC receive radiation therapy to the chest either as a single modality or combined with surgery and/or systemic therapy (Miller et al. 2019).

Historically, the radiation was delivered with two-dimensional (2D) technique. However, in the recent years, the new radiation delivery technology and modality such as intensity-modulated radiation therapy (IMRT), stereotactic body radiation therapy (SBRT), and three-dimensional conformal radiation therapy (3D CRT) have been developed to conform the radiation dose to the tumor and spare the adjacent organs at risk (OARs).

Despite these advancements in radiation delivery, adverse effects are still common due to the

S. F. Azghadi · M. E. Daly (✉)
Department of Radiation Oncology, University of California Davis Comprehensive Cancer Center, Sacramento, CA, USA
e-mail: medaly@ucdavis.edu

unavoidable dose to surrounding structures. Toxicity to the heart and lungs is among the most feared and potentially lethal complications of thoracic radiation. Furthermore, concurrent or adjuvant systemic therapies have shown to accentuate some of the adverse heart and lung events caused by radiation therapy. In this chapter, we review the pathophysiology, risk factors, treatment, and prevention of radiation-induced heart and lung toxicity following thoracic radiation therapy for lung cancer.

2 Lung Toxicity

2.1 Pathophysiology of Radiation-Induced Pneumonitis

Radiation-induced lung injury (RILI) encompasses any lung toxicity induced by radiation therapy (RT) and can manifest acutely as radiation pneumonitis (RP) and/or chronically as radiation pulmonary fibrosis (RF). Radiation causes damage to both epithelial and endothelial cells, leading to interruption of alveolar function and evoking an inflammatory response which leads to increase in vascular permeability and cytokine release. DNA damage and generation of reactive oxygen species (ROS) are two mechanisms of radiation-induced normal tissue damage (Azzam et al. 2012). The alveolar epithelium consists of pneumocytes type I and II. Type II cells are precursors of type I and constitute 10% of alveolar epithelial cells, and type I cells constitute 90% of the alveolar epithelium. Type II cells are responsible for secretion of the pulmonary surfactant, which regulates the alveolar-surface tension. After radiation, the sensitive type I cells are lost, and it takes about 4 weeks for the type II cells to drive the reepithelialization of the alveolus (Kasper and Haroske 1996; Giuranno et al. 2019).

In the acute phase, within minutes to hours after radiation therapy, intracellular signaling pathways are triggered leading to altered gene expression and release of cytokines and growth factors such as tumor necrosis factor-alpha (TNF-alpha), interleukin-1 (IL-1), interleukin-6 (IL-6), and basic fibroblast growth factor (βFGF) among others, causing vascular congestion and type I pneumocyte apoptosis (Kouloulias et al. 2013; Jack et al. 1996). This is followed by the second wave of events 6–8 weeks after radiation therapy including further overexpression of transforming growth factor-beta 1 (TGF-β1), oxidative damage to the DNA, hypoxia, and decreased lung perfusion (Wang et al. 2017a).

Additionally, radiation ionizes water molecules leading to generation of reactive oxygen species such as superoxide, hydrogen peroxide, and hydroxyl radicals that are responsible for about 60% of the damage inflicted (Tak and Park 2009; Terasaki et al. 2011; Zhao and Robbins 2009). These reactive oxygen species can directly damage nuclear DNA and mitochondrial DNA and damage organelles, provoking inflammation and apoptosis (Imlay 2013; Schieber and Chandel 2014; Kim et al. 2014; Liu and Chen 2017). In response, hypoxia-inducible factor (HIF) 1α and 2α are activated to counteract these effects. This in turn leads to the activation of cytokines and growth factors including vascular epithelial growth factor (VEGF) that promotes endothelial cell proliferation (Giuranno et al. 2019). Additionally, the enhanced HIF-1-regulated transcript enhances endothelial cell radioresistance (Moeller et al. 2004).

Clinically, patients may experience shortness of breath, increased oxygen requirement, cough, or fever as manifestations of RP, an acute and reversible event in RILI. Clinical symptoms typically manifest 3–12 weeks following radiation, primarily as a result of proliferation of type II pneumocytes, alveolar secretion of a fibrin-rich exudate, alveolar collapse, narrowing of the pulmonary capillaries, and microvascular thrombosis (Iyer and Jhingran 2006). Most patients, however, develop only radiological signs of RP without symptoms (Giuranno et al. 2019). Radiation-induced pulmonary fibrosis can occur 6 months after radiation therapy and is characterized by extensive collagen deposits in the pulmonary interstitial and alveolar regions, increased myofibroblasts, and overall reduced lung volume (Hanania et al. 2019).

2.2 Contributing Patient-Related Risk Factors

Overall, approximately 5–20% of patients develop RP after receiving chest radiotherapy (Giuranno et al. 2019), although this percentage is markedly influenced by the setting and disease stage of the patient undergoing treatment, with much higher rates of pneumonitis noted in patients treated for larger fields for locally advanced disease. The risk of RP is influenced by many patient- and disease-related factors. Patient-specific factors including sex and age, smoking history, underlying lung conditions, and genetics are among confounding factors contributing to the development of RILI. On average, older patients have a lower functional lung status and a great preponderance of other comorbid conditions affecting the lungs and are at higher risk of developing symptomatic (grade ≥ 2) RP (Briere et al. 2016). Specifically, age 70 and above has been shown to be an independent predictor for both grade ≥ 2 (odds ratio 1.99) and grade ≥ 3 RP (odds ratio 8.9) (Dang et al. 2014). The effect of sex on developing RILI is unclear (Kong and Wang 2015). In general, women have smaller lung volumes than men; therefore, women have smaller volume spared from 5 Gy (V5), which puts them at higher risk of developing radiation pneumonitis. On the other hand, women develop autoimmune diseases more often than men, which may theoretically increase their risk of developing RILI. A study by Giuranno et al. showed that in 148 patients with lung cancer treated with chemoradiation, women were significantly at higher risk of developing RILI than men (15% vs. 4%), and gender was a predictor of developing $G \geq 2$ lung toxicity (Giuranno et al. 2019). However, this finding has not been confirmed in subsequent studies.

In contrast to correlation of smoking and developing lung cancer, smoking paradoxically appears in some studies to have a protective role against acute RILI (Kong and Wang 2015; Senzer 2002; Jin et al. 2009; Vogelius and Bentzen 2012). The frequency of $G \geq 3$ RP is higher in remote former smokers in comparison to the recent former smokers and current smokers (Hildebrandt et al. 2010). In a large retrospective cohort study, analyzing 576 patients with stage III NSCLC treated with concurrent chemoradiation, radiation-induced pneumonitis was significantly higher in nonsmokers in comparison to smokers (37% vs. 14%) (Jin et al. 2009). It has been hypothesized that lungs damaged by smoking are less sensitive to radiation due to nonfunctional airspaces and nonvital lung parenchyma (Monson et al. 1998). Exposure of the lung to chemicals in tobacco destroys normal lung tissue, inducing the replacement of normal elastic fibers with fibrotic scars. Furthermore, smoking causes immunosuppression, causing reduced cytokines and immune response (Gokula et al. 2013). Hypoxia caused by carbon monoxide in smokers' lungs may result in less reactive oxygen species (ROS) and thus less lung DNA and tissue damage (Gokula et al. 2013). Despite this potential association with reduced RILI, tobacco consumption should be strongly discouraged in cancer patients.

Approximately 40–70% of patients with lung cancer have underlying chronic obstructive pulmonary disease (COPD) and/or interstitial lung disease (ILD) which are independent prognostic factors for cancer mortality and are associated with increased risk of developing pneumonitis (OR 22.6) (Ozawa et al. 2015). Patients with pre-existing lung disease are at higher risk of developing RILI by exacerbating inflammation and destruction of the remaining normal parenchyma (Li et al. 2017; Zhou et al. 2017; Li et al. 2018). A study by Rancati et al. found in their cohort that patients with underlying COPD undergoing thoracic radiation therapy had 24.1% more lung toxicity in comparison to patients with no COPD (Rancati et al. 2003). Interstitial lung disease (ILD) is a particularly robust risk factor for RILI, with most studies showing a markedly increased risk of high-grade or even fatal lung toxicity

(Goodman et al. 2020). One cohort study with 537 patients treated with radiation for early-stage NSCLC including 39 with interstitial changes on imaging found an odds ratio of 5.81 for the development of grade 2+ pneumonitis (Glick et al. 2018). In aggregate, the data suggest that radiation should be used with great caution in patients with preexisting ILD, particularly symptomatic ILD.

Genetic variations in genes involved in DNA damage repair, inflammation, and oxidative stress pathways may either exacerbate or ameliorate RILI (Arroyo-Hernández et al. 2021). Single nucleotide polymorphism (SNP) has been associated with differences in radiosensitivity. Mainly, SNPs affect cell survival, DNA damage response, and DNA repair genes. SNPs in ATM, IL-1, IL-8, TGF-beta, TNF, and VEGF all are associated with increased risk of RILI (Hildebrandt et al. 2010; Akulevich et al. 2009).

2.3 Radiation Treatment-Related Risk Factors

In the last two decades, radiation delivery and treatment planning have evolved significantly. Historically, radiation therapy was delivered via conventional 2D techniques in which a few radiation beams were used based on plain radiographs to delineate anatomic landmarks. Use of 2D radiation therapy resulted in relatively heterogenous treatment plans and required larger margins to avoid geographic miss of the tumor, resulting in irradiation of a larger volume of normal tissue outside of the targeted tumor (Benveniste et al. 2019).

In the recent years, significant improvements have occurred in radiation delivery by incorporating CT-based planning to allow three-dimensional conformal delivery (3D CRT) with multiple intersecting beams to limit dose to surrounding structures. Subsequent developments included intensity-modulated radiation therapy (IMRT) and an inverse-planned technique using dynamic multileaf collimation to sculpt dose around convex and concave targets (Fig. 1a). A secondary analysis of the phase III randomized RTOG 0617 trial, which allowed both 3D CRT and IMRT, found that IMRT was associated with less grade 3+ pneumonitis (7.9% vs. 3.5%, $p = 0.039$) (Chun et al. 2017). Stereotactic body radiation therapy (SBRT) is another modern planning technique that uses highly conformal planning techniques coupled with careful immobilization, motion management, and onboard imaging to deliver high dose per fraction treatments with sharp dose falloff, greatly limiting dose to surrounding normal tissue (Benveniste et al. 2019) (Fig. 1b). SBRT has become a standard of care for treating patients with early-stage, node-negative, medically inoperable non-small cell lung cancer (Shields 1993) and is also used to treat limited metastatic sites.

In general, RILI has been reported in up to about 20% of patients receiving thoracic radiotherapy (van Sörnsen de Koste et al. 2001; Prezzano et al. 2019), with lung dosimetric parameters serving as the greatest predictive factor. Quantitative analysis of normal tissue effects in the clinic (QUANTEC) was a collaborative effort to summarize the existing literature on 3D dose and volume effects in normal tissues with outcome data and provide clinical guidance to practitioners on prudent dose volume limits for use in the clinic (Bentzen et al. 2010). The QUANTEC paper devoted to RILI, while acknowledging the challenges of providing firm dose limits in the setting of variable risk tolerance, suggests limiting the combined mean lung dose to $\leq$20–23 Gy and lung V20 to $\leq$30–35% with conventional fractionation in order to limit pneumonitis risk to <20% (Marks et al. 2010).

A large body of retrospective literature has attempted to define specific risk thresholds for pneumonitis associated with specific dosimetric parameters among patients undergoing conventionally fractionated chemoradiation for locally advanced lung cancer. Among the most comprehensive of such studies is an individual patient data meta-analysis that included 836 patients treated with concurrent chemoradiation for locally advanced NSCLC. In their cohort, the overall rate of symptomatic pneumonitis was 29.8%, and 1.9% of patients experienced fatal

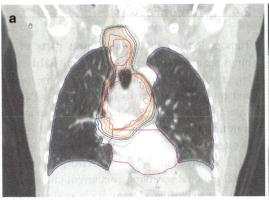
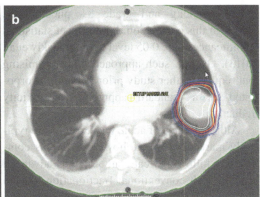

Fig. 1 (**a**) Intensity-modulated radiation therapy (IMRT) uses inverse planning modulate dose, allowing for convex and concave dose distributions. Shown here is a patient with stage IIIB NSCLC treated with concurrent chemoradiation with IMRT. IMRT allows minimization of dose delivered to the heart and lungs. (**b**) Stereotactic body radiation therapy (SBRT) uses highly conformal treatment planning to create steep dose gradients around the tumor. Advanced imaging techniques are used for planning and localization to limit the necessary margins of the tumor. In this figure, a T2N0M0 NSCLC of the left lower lobe treated with SBRT is shown. The tumor abuts the heart, and the isodose line is modulated to minimize dose to the heart

lung toxicity. The lung V20 was predictive of symptomatic pneumonitis, with an odds ratio of 1.03 per 1% increase ($p = 0.008$). In their dataset, the mean lung dose was not statistically significantly predictive in the multivariable model, although it was predictive in univariable modeling (Palma et al. 2013).

An additional substantial body of predominantly retrospective literature has attempted to define safe lung dose volume constraints to minimize the risk of RILI. A large number of dose volume parameters have been identified as predictive of pneumonitis in addition to the traditionally used mean lung dose and lung V20. In a retrospective cohort study by Han et al., the incidence of $G \geq 2$ RP was 31.7% in patients with NSCLC treated with concurrent chemoradiation. Their univariate analysis showed that V5 > 41%, V20 > 24%, and MLD > 13 Gy were significantly associated with RILI regardless of radiation delivery technique (Han et al. 2015). Another retrospective study by Robnett et al. found that MLD and patient performance status were the two most significant predictors of developing RILI in their cohort (Robnett et al. 2000). In another retrospective study by Hernando et al., MLD >10 Gy was significantly associated with increased risk of RP (Hernando et al. 2001).

Other studies have shown that V20 and V30 are associated with RILI (Han et al. 2015; Fay et al. 2005). In general, MLD has been reported as the best predictor of RP grade ≥ 3 (Harder et al. 2016).

There is also interest in the concept of functional lung-sparing approaches to radiation in the thorax, under the assumption that lung function may be preferentially spared by limiting dose to more highly functioning regions of the lung, particularly in patients with significant emphysema who may have swaths of low-functioning or nonfunctioning lung. Although this approach remains investigational, several studies have suggested potential benefits to the type of treatment. Functional lung can be defined based on a range of novel imaging techniques, including 4D CT ventilation imaging (Palma et al. 2013; Yamamoto et al. 2016), single photon emission computed tomography (Lee and Park 2020), and hyperpolarized helium magnetic resonance imaging (Hoover et al. 2014). While prospective studies are ongoing, preliminary retrospective analyses suggest that dose to functional lung correlates to high-grade pneumonitis. Vinogradskiy and colleagues analyzed pretreatment 4D CT ventilation maps for 96 lung cancer patients and found a correlation between dose to functional lung and grade 3+ pneumonitis, although this correlation did not meet statistical significance at the 0.05 level (Vinogradskiy et al. 2013). Overall, such approaches are promising but require further study prior to being incorporated as a standard approach for toxicity reduction.

Although rates of acute pneumonitis are typically markedly lower following SBRT as compared to following treatment of locally advanced disease with conventional fractionation, due to the typically smaller volume of irradiated lung with SBRT, both acute and late RILI are still observed in patients treated with lung SBRT. The HYTEC analysis was an effort through the American Association of Physicists in Medicine's working group on the biological effects of SBRT that analyzed 97 studies evaluating lung toxicity following SBRT. They found that there was no clear "tolerance dose volume level," but that symptomatic RILI was low after SBRT with a mean combined lung dose of ≤8 Gy for 3–5 fraction treatments and total lung V20 <10–25% (Kong et al. 2021). Another large, pooled analysis of 88 studies including 7752 patients treated with lung SBRT identified a 9.1% incidence of grade 2+ pneumonitis and 1.8% rate of grade 3+ pneumonitis. In their analysis, older age and larger tumor size correlated to higher rates of pneumonitis in patients treated with SBRT, and mean lung dose was associated with increased risk of pneumonitis (Zhao et al. 2016). Scheduling considerations may impact the risk of pneumonitis as well, although the implications are far less clear than those for dosimetric considerations. SBRT has historically been delivered on nonconsecutive days, based on the practice of early prospective studies, although consecutive schedules are also used in some clinical practices. A recent multi-institutional analysis comparing the impact of fractionation showed that patients receiving daily treatments experienced significantly more grade ≥2 toxicity than patients undergoing every-other-day treatment (Verma et al. 2017). However, another retrospective analysis found no toxicity difference between consecutive and nonconsecutive treatments (Alite et al. 2016).

2.4 Tumor Factors

Tumors located in the mid-lower parts of the lungs are at higher risk of developing RILI due to larger volume of treatment because of the motion and higher perfusion in these regions. Patients with a higher tumor volume usually have a more significant lung and surrounding radiated volume (Kong and Wang 2015; Vogelius and Bentzen 2012; Zhang et al. 2012). In a retrospective study of 60 patients receiving concurrent chemoradiation, the risk of developing RP was significantly higher in tumors located at the base of the lobe (70%) in comparison to tumors located at the upper lobes (20%) (Mehta 2005). In another study, it was shown that the incidence of RP was higher following radiation to tumors located in the posterior central and peripheral regions in comparison to anterior regions (Seppenwoolde et al. 2004). These differences in risk of developing RP based on the tumor location are thought to be mainly because of the better perfusion, ventilation, and oxygenation of the lower/posterior regions (Kong and Wang 2015). There is no clear association between the tumor histology and RILI development.

2.5 Systemic Treatment Risk Factors for Lung Injury

2.5.1 Neoadjuvant Chemotherapy

Neoadjuvant chemotherapy is no longer the standard of care for patients planned to undergo concurrent chemoradiation, but is used preoperatively for some patients who may ultimately receive thoracic radiation, either postoperatively or when planned surgery is aborted. Neoadjuvant chemotherapy is also occasionally used in an attempt to reduce the target volumes for bulky tumors when standard dose constraints cannot be achieved. In this setting, neoadjuvant chemotherapy should theoretically reduce the PTV size and the accompanying risk of RILI. The results of a retrospective study evaluating the reduction risk of RP in patients with NSCLC after receiving induction chemotherapy showed that patients had a 20% reduction in tumor volume, which translated into

5% reduction in the risk of RILI (Amin et al. 2013). However, in a prospective study by Mao et al., induction chemotherapy was associated with increased risk of RP, probably due to the prior radiosensitizing contribution of chemotherapy (Mao et al. 2007). A large individual patient data meta-analysis of 836 patients with locally advanced NSCLC treated with concurrent chemoradiation did not find that the use of neoadjuvant chemotherapy increased the risk of pneumonitis.

2.5.2 Concurrent Thoracic Chemoradiation

Receipt of concurrent chemotherapy with thoracic radiation therapy has been shown to increase lung toxicity, with some chemotherapy agents providing greater risks. In a large individual patient data meta-analysis, patients receiving concurrent carboplatin/paclitaxel had a markedly enhanced risk of symptomatic pneumonitis as compared to other concurrent regimens (OR 3.33, $p < 0.001$) (Palma et al. 2013; Park and Kim 2013), likely due to the radiosensitizing effects of concurrent Taxol. Furthermore, the results of this meta-analysis identified increased risk of radiation pneumonitis in patients receiving concurrent as compared to sequential chemotherapy (OR 1.6) (Palma et al. 2013). Pneumonitis was a dose-limiting toxicity in patients with locally advanced NSCLC who received gemcitabine twice weekly in a phase I study (Blackstock et al. 2001), and concurrent gemcitabine has generally been abandoned as a concurrent systemic agent for lung cancer due to synergistic toxicity. Other studies have demonstrated that patients receiving irinotecan are at higher risk of developing grade ≥2 RP compared with those who did not (56% vs. 14%) (Palma et al. 2013; Yamada et al. 1998).

2.5.3 Radiation Therapy and Immunotherapy

Other systemic therapies in use for lung cancer may also enhance the risk of RILI when used either concurrently or sequentially with radiation. Immune checkpoint inhibitors targeting the programmed death ligand 1 (PD-L1) and programmed death 1 (PD-1) interaction have emerged as important components of treatment for both stage III and stage IV NSCLC and are under investigation in early-stage disease. The phase III randomized PACIFIC trial identified a significant survival benefit to the addition of consolidation durvalumab, a PD-1 inhibitor, following definitive concurrent chemoradiation for stage III NSCLC, creating a new standard of care (Antonia et al. 2018). Immunotherapy is also used either as monotherapy or in combination with chemotherapy for metastatic NSCLC who may receive thoracic radiation for symptom control or as consolidation. Pneumonitis is a known complication of checkpoint inhibitors, raising concerns for the possibility of synergistic toxicity. Pneumonitis due to immunotherapy is derived from a direct cytotoxic effect, oxidative stress, and mainly immune-mediated injury. A meta-analysis of severe immune-related adverse events in trials incorporating programmed death 1 (PD1) and programmed death ligand 1 (PD-L1) has shown that pneumonitis was among the common causes of G5 toxicity (Wang et al. 2019). The analysis of phase I/II trials with combined immunotherapy and thoracic radiation has shown that the combination is safe in the short term with no evidence of an overt increase in high-grade toxicities (Verma et al. 2018a, b). In the sequential setting, rates of any-grade pneumonitis on PACIFIC were 33.9% with durvalumab and 24.8% with placebo, and grade 3–4 pneumonitis in 3.4% of durvalumab-treated patients and 2.6% of patients receiving placebo (Antonia et al. 2017).

Retrospective analyses have also analyzed the synergistic effects of consolidative durvalumab following thoracic chemoradiation. Shaverdian et al. performed a study on patients with stage III NSCLC who received concurrent chemoradiation followed by durvalumab. In this study, the authors incorporated three models (QUANTEC, Appelt, and Thor) to predict the risk of RP in patients receiving chemoradiation and consolidative durvalumab. The investigators found that patients developed delayed onset of RP when treated with concurrent chemoradiation and durvalumab with higher incidence of RP in this group (Shaverdian et al. 2020).

Tian et al. reported a multi-institution experience regarding the safety and tolerability of lung SBRT with concurrent immune checkpoint inhibitor (ICI). Receipt of checkpoint inhibitor, planning target volume size (PTV), and lobes involved in SBRT were linked to high-grade RP. Grade ≥ 3 occurred more frequently in patients treated with a checkpoint inhibitor with SBRT as compared to SBRT alone (26.8% vs. 2.9%) (Tian et al. 2020). In aggregate, the available data suggest that the combination of checkpoint inhibitors and thoracic radiation is safe, with modest increases in pneumonitis.

2.5.4 Radiation Recall Pneumonitis

Radiation recall pneumonitis (RRP) is an acute inflammatory response confined to previously irradiated lung after the administration of various pharmacological agents (Levy et al. 2013). Taxanes and anthracyclines are the most common drugs related to RRP (Ding et al. 2011). Additionally, ICIs have been reported to be associated with higher incidence of severe RP in the irradiated lungs of previously treated NSCL patients (Antonia et al. 2018; Toi et al. 2018).

2.5.5 Diagnosis and Treatment of Radiation-Induced Lung Injury

Diagnosis of RP is a clinical diagnosis which is established by clinical suspicion or radiographic presentation and should be excluded from the most common pathologies that mimic lung toxicity including disease progression or infection. There are different grading systems used to define pneumonitis severity, clinical and radiographic findings, and treatment options. Arroyo-Hernandez et al. have summarized grading based on the criteria explained by the Radiation Therapy Oncology Group (RTOG, G1-5), the Common Terminology Criteria for Adverse Events v.5.0 (CTCAE v5.0, G1-5), and the Southwest Oncology Group Criteria (SWOG, G1-4) (Arroyo-Hernández et al. 2021).

A broad spectrum of imaging findings have been noted following RILI. Radiologic manifestations are usually confined to the irradiated regions, although nonirradiated regions can appear involved. In the acute phase, RILI manifest as ground-glass opacity, attenuation, or consolidation (Fig. 2a). In the late phase, it usually manifests as traction bronchiectasis, volume loss, and scarring (Fig. 2b) (Choi et al. 2004). Radiographic findings after SBRT are different in appearance, geographic extent, and progression

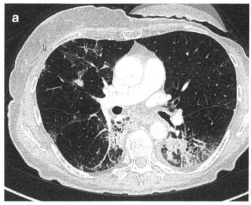
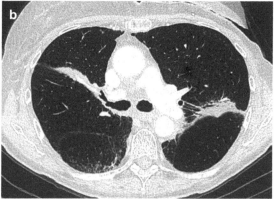
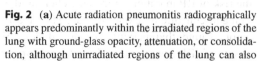

Fig. 2 (**a**) Acute radiation pneumonitis radiographically appears predominantly within the irradiated regions of the lung with ground-glass opacity, attenuation, or consolidation, although unirradiated regions of the lung can also demonstrate radiographic findings. (**b**) Late radiation fibrosis radiographically manifests as traction bronchiectasis, volume loss, and scarring within radiated regions of the lungs

timeline compared to conventional radiation therapy. Usually, SBRT-induced changes are limited to the rim of normal tissue outside the tumor and have complex shapes, which, sometimes, makes it challenging to differentiate between tumor recurrence and radiation-induced changes (Linda et al. 2011).

2.5.6 Treatment and Prevention of Radiation-Induced Lung Injury

There are several approaches sought to prevent, minimize, or delay RILI. The use of advances in patient immobilization, motion management, and onboard imaging to reduce the size of planning target margins and advanced radiation planning techniques to limit dose spillage as described previously are the most widely used and straightforward means of reducing lung injury. However, many patients due to disease distribution, location, and size may nonetheless have lung radiation dose that places them at substantial risk of RILI.

An alternative mechanism to reduce normal tissue toxicity is the use of radiation modifiers/protectors. In general, chemical/biological agents used to alter normal tissue toxicity from radiation can be broadly divided into radioprotectors which are administered prior to radiation, radiomitigators which are administered at the time of radiation, and radio-ameliorators which are administered after radiation therapy (Citrin et al. 2010). None are in routine use for preventing RILI at this time.

Amifostine is administered as a thiol prodrug, which specifically becomes dephosphorylated in normal cells. The thiol group of amifostine plays a key role in the activation of redox-sensitive transcription nuclear factor kappa-light-chain-enhancer of activated B cells (NFκB), resulting in an increased expression of superoxide dismutase 2 (SOD2), which in turn contributes to reactive oxygen species neutralization leading to normal cells to be resistant to radiation-induced DNA damage (Dziegielewski et al. 2008; Kouvaris et al. 2007; Koukourakis 2012; Murley et al. 2007). The results of a study by Hildebrandt et al. showed that patients receiving neoadjuvant amifostine experienced less RP compared to patients who did not receive neoadjuvant amifostine (0 vs. 16%: $p < 0.02$) (Murley et al. 2007). Common side effects of amifostine include nausea, fever, hypotension, and allergic reactions in a dose-dependent manner with minimal effect in interrupting treatment (Koukourakis 2012; Bourhis et al. 2011). However, amifostine is not currently widely used due to limited clinical benefit and side effects.

Radiomitigators are administered concurrently with radiation therapy with the goal of modulating radiation-induced inflammation. Angiotensin-converting enzyme (ACE) inhibitors which are used to regulate blood pressure have shown to reduce RILI in preclinical models (Medhora et al. 2012; Prasanna et al. 2012). Prospective trials have attempted to test these drugs. Alliance MC 1221 was a pilot, blinded randomized trial testing the ACE inhibitor lisinopril in patients undergoing curative-intent thoracic radiation. Twenty-three patients enrolled. The study suggested that lisinopril was safe in this setting, but was underpowered to detect symptomatic differences. For several patient-reported outcome measures, patients treated with lisinopril noted reductions in cough, shortness of breath, and dyspnea ($p < 0.05$), although overall the study was underpowered to draw firm conclusions (Sio et al. 2019). Retrospective studies have suggested that the use of ACE inhibitors during radiation therapy may limit acute pneumonitis (Kharofa et al. 2012). However, prospective trials in this space have failed to successfully accrue patients to test this hypothesis. RTOG 0123 was a randomized phase II trial testing the ability of the ACE inhibitor captopril to alter the image of pulmonary damage following radiation therapy for lung cancer, with a primary endpoint of grade 2+ radiation-induced pulmonary toxicity within 1 year. The study was terminated early due to slow accrual, with 81 patients accrued over 50 months and 40 not randomized postradiation. Among 20 analyzable patients, grade 2+ pulmonary toxicity was 23% in patients on the control arm and 14% among patients treated with captopril, but the study was underpowered and unable to address the primary endpoint (Small Jr et al. 2018).

2.5.7 Treatment

The mainstay of treatment in acute RP consists of administrating systemic corticosteroids at high doses for symptomatic patients. Oral prednisone is generally prescribed at 1–2 mg/kg/day before tapering down over 3–12 weeks. Intravenous corticosteroids equivalent to methylprednisolone at 2–4 mg/kg/day tapered over 6 weeks are recommended for grades 3–4 RP (Jain and Berman 2018). Additionally, inhaled steroids have shown efficacy in treating RP with the highest dose deposited in the airway, thus decreasing systemic side effects (Henkenberens et al. 2016). There is not currently a role for glucocorticoid therapy in the treatment of RILI (Abratt et al. 2004). Beyond the treatment of subacute RP, no effective treatment for late RF has been identified at that time.

2.6 Heart Toxicity

The use of radiation therapy for thoracic malignancies has historically been associated with high risk of developing cardiovascular side effects. Major side effects include pericarditis, coronary artery disease (CAD), radiation-induced cardiomyopathy, vulvar dysfunction, and heart failure (Hufnagle and Goyal 2020).

Historically, the data for radiation-induced cardiac diseases has been from studies of breast cancer and Hodgkin's lymphoma, in patients with typically younger age of treatment and long expected survival. The specific applicability of findings from lymphoma and breast cancer patients to lung cancer patients much be interpreted with caution, given the greater lethality of lung cancer and older average age of patients (Speirs et al. 2017; Vojtíšek 2020). However, a significant bunch of literature now suggests that cardiac toxicity from lung cancer contributes to long-term survival in many lung cancer patients treated with radiation. Clinical manifestations of radiation-induced cardiac toxicities can occur acutely such as pericarditis (uncommon, usually transient), and pericardial effusion, or as late injuries such as coronary artery disease (CAD), congestive heart failure (CHF), arrhythmias, angina, and myocardial infarction. The chronic manifestation can occur months to years after radiation therapy (Gagliardi et al. 2010). Other risk factors associated with radiation-induced heart disease include young age, irradiation of the left side of the heart, concurrent treatment with anthracyclines, prior CAD or heart disease, or presence of other cardiovascular risk factors. In general, radiation cardiac toxicity is a chronic concern with the median time to diagnosis of 19 years (Hufnagle and Goyal 2020). However, when higher doses are delivered to the heart, as occurs in some lung cancer patients, impact on survival can be noted within 2–3 years, as noted in RTOG 0617 as described below (Chun et al. 2017).

2.6.1 Dosimetry and Treatment Factors

Radiation-induced heart damage generally occurs in a dose-dependent manner. Although higher radiation doses significantly increase the risk of radiation-induced mortality, the damaging effect can also be seen with much lower doses (Hufnagle and Goyal 2020). Recent analyses have identified cardiac dose as an important predictor of OS after chemoradiation for locally advanced NSCLC. RTOG 0617, a phase III randomized trial testing both dose escalation and addition of cetuximab, brought additional attention to the role of cardiac dose on survival in locally advanced NSCLC. Multivariable analysis of enrolled patients demonstrated that increasing whole heart V5 and V30 were predictive of increased risk of death (Bradley et al. 2015). A secondary analysis of RTOG 0617 found that the use of IMRT was associated with lower whole heart V20, V40, and V60 and that heart V40 was associated with survival in an adjusted analysis (Chun et al. 2017). Since publication of the RTOG 0617 data, a large number of additional studies have sought to validate their findings and explore the role of cardiac substructure dosimetry in survival.

Wang et al. evaluated the effect of heart toxicity in patients with NSCLC who were treated in prospective radiation dose escalation trials. They found that patients with mean heart dose (MHD) >20 Gy had significantly higher rate of cardiac events than patients with MHD <10 Gy (HR, 5.47; $p < 0.001$) or 10–20 Gy (HR, 2.76; $p = 0.03$). The differences in cardiac events were not associated with OS (MHD <10 Gy, 10–20, and >20 Gy was 50%, 40%, and 44%, respectively, $p = 0.73$) (Wang et al. 2017b). In a subsequent pooled post hoc analysis which evaluated the association between radiation dose and different cardiac subvolumes (whole heart, left ventricle, left atrium, right atrium), the results showed that pericardial events were significantly associated with whole heart V30, left atrium V30, and right atrium V30, but not left ventricle dose. Ischemic events were correlated with left ventricle V30 and whole heart V30 dose. Arrhythmia events showed borderline significance associated with right atrium V30, left atrium V30, and whole heart V30. Cardiac events were associated with decreased survival on univariable analysis (Wang et al. 2017c). Similarly, Dess et al. performed a secondary analysis of four prospective trials evaluating dose-escalated, hypofractionated radiation for stage II–III lung cancer to determine if the incidence of cardiac events was associated with cardiac dose volume parameters. Among 125 patients, the 2-year incidence of grade 3+ cardiac events was 11%, and the mean whole-heart dose was associated with an increased incidence of cardiac events (HR, 1.07/Gy; 95% CI, 1.02–1.13/Gy; $p = 0.01$), as was cardiac V5 and V30. Patients with preexisting cardiac disease had a higher risk of cardiac events after thoracic radiation (HR 2.96; 95% CI, 1.07–8.21, $p = 0.04$) (Dess et al. 2017).

In a retrospective study of 748 patients with locally advanced NSCLC treated with thoracic radiotherapy, MHD was associated with a significant increased risk of major adverse cardiac events. Additionally, MHD $\geq$10 Gy was associated with a significant increased risk of all-cause mortality in patients without preexisting coronary heart disease (CHD) (Atkins et al. 2019).

However, other studies have failed to confirm these findings. A secondary analysis of the randomized ESPATUE trial, which used neoadjuvant chemotherapy followed by hyperfractionated concurrent chemoradiation, attempted to confirm the RTOG 0617 finding that whole heart V5 is predictive of survival in 155 enrolled patients with available dosimetric data. No relationship between heart V5 and survival was identified (Guberina et al. 2017). Palma and colleagues performed a systematic review of 22 studies including 5614 patients assessing 94 unique cardiac dosimetric parameters. They were unable to identify consistent dose volume parameters associated with the overall survival in NSCLC and found that multiplicity of testing may inflate the risk of type 1 errors in the body of literature devoted to radiation-induced cardiac toxicity, and they were unable to perform a meta-analysis because most negative studies did not provide estimates of effect size (Zhang et al. 2019). Currently, the cardiac toxicity literature has rapidly expanded, but specific dose volume constraints, particularly for cardiac substructure, have not been confirmed in multiple distinct datasets.

The literature analyzing cardiac toxicity following lung SBRT is even less clear. A handful of retrospective studies have analyzed the association between cardiac dose, cardiac events, and survival following lung SBRT, with inconsistent results. Wong and colleagues analyzed 189 patients treated with lung SBRT and found that higher bilateral ventricular maximum dose was associated with worse survival (Wong et al. 2018). However, Tembukar et al. analyzed 118 patients treated with lung SBRT and assessed a variety of cardiac dose volume parameters, none of which were predictive of survival in their cohort (Tembhekar et al. 2017). In aggregate, the available literature suggests that prudent reduction of cardiac dose via optimal treatment planning should be performed, but not at the expense of target volume coverage for patients undergoing curative-intent SBRT.

2.6.2 Prevention of Cardiac Toxicity

The predominant method of limiting cardiac toxicity following thoracic radiation is, as with RILI, the use of advanced planning techniques to limit radiation dose received by the heart. Advanced techniques such as IMRT allow sculpting of radiation dose away from the heart. A secondary analysis of RTOG 0617 demonstrated that the use of IMRT reduces cardiac doses ($p < 0.05$) (Chun et al. 2017). The use of proton therapy in well-selected cases may also limit cardiac dose, though it is overall less widely available and less studied than IMRT. Anatomic maneuvers such as breath hold can reduce cardiac dose for well-selected patients with mediastinal tumors (Paumier et al. 2012), as can motion management approaches such as gating that reduce the overall size of the treated planning target volume (cite).

Currently, no pharmacologic approaches have been confirmed to prevent or limit radiation-induced cardiac toxicity. Several pharmacologic strategies are under investigation, particularly those involving ACE inhibitors, angiotensin receptor blockers, and components of the TGF beta pathway. Preclinical studies suggest that ACE inhibitors, as also noted with lung damage, can lessen radiation-induced cardiac damage (van der Veen et al. 2015). Statins have also been studied (Zhang et al. 2015). However, no approach has yet been validated in randomized human trials to prevent or limit cardiac toxicity following radiation.

2.7 Treatment of Cardiac Toxicity

Treatment of radiation-induced cardiac injury is similar to that of cardiac disease of other causes. Acute pericarditis can be treated with nonsteroidal anti-inflammatories, colchicine, and steroids, and pericardiocentesis in severe cases (Marinko 2018). Longer term cardiac injury is managed depending on the manifestation. Coronary disease can be managed with percutaneous or surgical revascularization. Valvular injury can be managed with valve replacements or repair (Borges & Kapadia, ACC). Heart failure is generally managed as other heart failure patients pharmacologically. Unfortunately, surgical outcomes are significantly worse in patients treated for radiation-induced cardiac morbidity as compared to noncardiac forms of heart pathology (Wu et al. 2013).

3 Conclusions

Radiation-induced lung and heart injuries remain critically important toxicities following thoracic radiation. Currently, preventative strategies involving avoidance of radiation dose to the heart and lungs via advanced planning techniques, motion management, and imaging guidance have had the greatest impact in limiting these toxicities. Pharmacologic prevention strategies are critically needed, and several appear promising, but have not been fully vetted in large randomized human trials. However, fears of lung and cardiac toxicity must be balanced with the lethality of many lung cancers and the potential for radiation to cure early-stage and locally advanced lung cancers and to effectively palliate symptoms, at times improving survival, in metastatic lung cancers. Treatments available for both heart and lung injury are limited, suggesting that prevention via existing radiation planning strategies and judicious patient selection is a preferable strategy.

References

Abratt RP et al (2004) Pulmonary complications of radiation therapy. Clin Chest Med 25(1):167–177

Akulevich NM et al (2009) Polymorphisms of DNA damage response genes in radiation-related and sporadic papillary thyroid carcinoma. Endocr Relat Cancer 16(2):491–503

Alite F et al (2016) Local control dependence on consecutive vs. nonconsecutive fractionation in lung stereotactic body radiation therapy. Radiother Oncol 121(1):9–14

Amin NP et al (2013) Effect of induction chemotherapy on estimated risk of radiation pneumonitis in bulky non-small cell lung cancer. Med Dosim 38(3):320–326

Antonia SJ et al (2017) Durvalumab after chemoradiotherapy in stage III non-small-cell lung cancer. N Engl J Med 377(20):1919–1929

Antonia SJ et al (2018) Overall survival with Durvalumab after chemoradiotherapy in stage III NSCLC. N Engl J Med 379(24):2342–2350

Arroyo-Hernández M et al (2021) Radiation-induced lung injury: current evidence. BMC Pulm Med 21(1):9

Atkins KM et al (2019) Cardiac radiation dose, cardiac disease, and mortality in patients with lung cancer. J Am Coll Cardiol 73(23):2976–2987

Azzam EI, Jay-Gerin JP, Pain D (2012) Ionizing radiation-induced metabolic oxidative stress and prolonged cell injury. Cancer Lett 327(1–2):48–60

Bentzen SM et al (2010) Quantitative analyses of Normal tissue effects in the clinic (QUANTEC): an introduction to the scientific issues. Int J Radiat Oncol Biol Phys 76(Suppl. 3):S3–S9

Benveniste MF et al (2019) Recognizing radiation therapy-related complications in the chest. Radiographics 39(2):344–366

Blackstock AW et al (2001) Phase I study of twice-weekly gemcitabine and concurrent thoracic radiation for patients with locally advanced non-small-cell lung cancer. Int J Radiat Oncol Biol Phys 51(5):1281–1289

Bourhis J et al (2011) Effect of amifostine on survival among patients treated with radiotherapy: a meta-analysis of individual patient data. J Clin Oncol 29(18):2590–2597

Bradley JD et al (2015) Standard-dose versus high-dose conformal radiotherapy with concurrent and consolidation carboplatin plus paclitaxel with or without cetuximab for patients with stage IIIA or IIIB non-small-cell lung cancer (RTOG 0617): a randomised, two-by-two factorial phase 3 study. Lancet Oncol 16(2):187–199

Briere TM et al (2016) Lung size and the risk of radiation pneumonitis. Int J Radiat Oncol Biol Phys 94(2):377–384

Choi YW et al (2004) Effects of radiation therapy on the lung: radiologic appearances and differential diagnosis. Radiographics 24(4):985–997. discussion 998

Chun SG et al (2017) Impact of intensity-modulated radiation therapy technique for locally advanced non-Small-cell lung cancer: a secondary analysis of the NRG Oncology RTOG 0617 Randomized Clinical Trial. J Clin Oncol 35(1):56–62

Citrin D et al (2010) Radioprotectors and mitigators of radiation-induced normal tissue injury. Oncologist 15(4):360–371

Dang J et al (2014) Risk and predictors for early radiation pneumonitis in patients with stage III non-small cell lung cancer treated with concurrent or sequential chemoradiotherapy. Radiat Oncol 9:172

Dess RT et al (2017) Cardiac events after radiation therapy: combined analysis of prospective multicenter trials for locally advanced non-small-cell lung cancer. J Clin Oncol 35(13):1395–1402

Ding X et al (2011) Radiation recall pneumonitis induced by chemotherapy after thoracic radiotherapy for lung cancer. Radiat Oncol 6:24

Dziegielewski J et al (2008) WR-1065, the active metabolite of amifostine, mitigates radiation-induced delayed genomic instability. Free Radic Biol Med 45(12):1674–1681

Fay M et al (2005) Dose-volume histogram analysis as predictor of radiation pneumonitis in primary lung cancer patients treated with radiotherapy. Int J Radiat Oncol Biol Phys 61(5):1355–1363

Gagliardi G et al (2010) Radiation dose-volume effects in the heart. Int J Radiat Oncol Biol Phys 76(Suppl. 3):S77–S85

Giuranno L et al (2019) Radiation-induced lung injury (RILI). Front Oncol 9:877

Glick D et al (2018) Impact of pretreatment interstitial lung disease on radiation pneumonitis and survival in patients treated with lung stereotactic body radiation therapy (SBRT). Clin Lung Cancer 19(2):e219–e226

Gokula K, Earnest A, Wong LC (2013) Meta-analysis of incidence of early lung toxicity in 3-dimensional conformal irradiation of breast carcinomas. Radiat Oncol 8:268

Goodman CD et al (2020) A primer on interstitial lung disease and thoracic radiation. J Thorac Oncol 15(6):902–913

Guberina M et al (2017) Heart dose exposure as prognostic marker after radiotherapy for resectable stage IIIA/B non-small-cell lung cancer: secondary analysis of a randomized trial. Ann Oncol 28(5):1084–1089

Han S et al (2015) Analysis of clinical and Dosimetric factors influencing radiation-induced lung injury in patients with lung cancer. J Cancer 6(11):1172–1178

Hanania AN et al (2019) Radiation-induced lung injury: assessment and management. Chest 156(1):150–162

Harder EM et al (2016) Pulmonary dose-volume predictors of radiation pneumonitis following stereotactic body radiation therapy. Pract Radiat Oncol 6(6):e353–e359

Henkenberens C et al (2016) Inhalative steroids as an individual treatment in symptomatic lung cancer patients with radiation pneumonitis grade II after radiotherapy—a single-centre experience. Radiat Oncol 11:12

Hernando ML et al (2001) Radiation-induced pulmonary toxicity: a dose-volume histogram analysis in 201 patients with lung cancer. Int J Radiat Oncol Biol Phys 51(3):650–659

Hildebrandt MA et al (2010) Genetic variants in inflammation-related genes are associated with radiation-induced toxicity following treatment for non-small cell lung cancer. PLoS One 5(8):e12402

Hoover DA et al (2014) Functional lung avoidance for individualized radiotherapy (FLAIR): study protocol for a randomized, double-blind clinical trial. BMC Cancer 14:934

Hufnagle JJ, Goyal A (2020) Radiation therapy induced cardiac toxicity. In: StatPearls. StatPearls Publishing, Treasure Island, FL. Copyright © 2020

Imlay JA (2013) The molecular mechanisms and physiological consequences of oxidative stress: lessons from a model bacterium. Nat Rev Microbiol 11(7):443–454

Iyer, R. and A. Jhingran, Radiation injury: imaging findings in the chest, abdomen and pelvis after therapeutic radiation. Cancer Imaging, 2006; 6(Spec No A): S131–S139

Jack CI et al (1996) Indicators of free radical activity in patients developing radiation pneumonitis. Int J Radiat Oncol Biol Phys 34(1):149–154

Jain V, Berman AT (2018) Radiation pneumonitis: old problem, new tricks. Cancers (Basel) 10(7):222

Jin H et al (2009) Dose-volume thresholds and smoking status for the risk of treatment-related pneumonitis in inoperable non-small cell lung cancer treated with definitive radiotherapy. Radiother Oncol 91(3):427–432

Kasper M, Haroske G (1996) Alterations in the alveolar epithelium after injury leading to pulmonary fibrosis. Histol Histopathol 11(2):463–483

Kharofa J et al (2012) Decreased risk of radiation pneumonitis with incidental concurrent use of angiotensin-converting enzyme inhibitors and thoracic radiation therapy. Int J Radiat Oncol Biol Phys 84(1): 238–243

Kim SR et al (2014) NLRP3 inflammasome activation by mitochondrial ROS in bronchial epithelial cells is required for allergic inflammation. Cell Death Dis 5(10):e1498

Kong FM, Wang S (2015) Nondosimetric risk factors for radiation-induced lung toxicity. Semin Radiat Oncol 25(2):100–109

Kong FS et al (2021, 110) Organs at risk considerations for thoracic stereotactic body radiation therapy: what is safe for lung parenchyma? Int J Radiat Oncol Biol Phys (1):172–187

Koukourakis MI (2012) Radiation damage and radioprotectants: new concepts in the era of molecular medicine. Br J Radiol 85(1012):313–330

Kouloulias V et al (2013) Suggestion for a new grading scale for radiation induced pneumonitis based on radiological findings of computerized tomography: correlation with clinical and radiotherapeutic parameters in lung cancer patients. Asian Pac J Cancer Prev 14(5):2717–2722

Kouvaris JR, Kouloulias VE, Vlahos LJ (2007) Amifostine: the first selective-target and broad-spectrum radioprotector. Oncologist 12(6):738–747

Lee SJ, Park HJ (2020) Single photon emission computed tomography (SPECT) or positron emission tomography (PET) imaging for radiotherapy planning in patients with lung cancer: a meta-analysis. Sci Rep 10(1):14864

Levy A et al (2013) Targeted therapy-induced radiation recall. Eur J Cancer 49(7):1662–1668

Li C et al (2017) Clinical characteristics and outcomes of lung cancer patients with combined pulmonary fibrosis and emphysema: a systematic review and meta-analysis of 13 studies. J Thorac Dis 9(12):5322–5334

Li F et al (2018) Preexisting radiological interstitial lung abnormalities are a risk factor for severe radiation pneumonitis in patients with small-cell lung cancer after thoracic radiation therapy. Radiat Oncol 13(1):82

Linda A, Trovo M, Bradley JD (2011) Radiation injury of the lung after stereotactic body radiation therapy (SBRT) for lung cancer: a timeline and pattern of CT changes. Eur J Radiol 79(1):147–154

Liu X, Chen Z (2017) The pathophysiological role of mitochondrial oxidative stress in lung diseases. J Transl Med 15(1):207

Mao J et al (2007) The impact of induction chemotherapy and the associated tumor response on subsequent radiation-related changes in lung function and tumor response. Int J Radiat Oncol Biol Phys 67(5):1360–1369

Marinko T (2018) Pericardial disease after breast cancer radiotherapy. Radiol Oncol 53(1):1–5

Marks LB et al (2010) Radiation dose-volume effects in the lung. Int J Radiat Oncol Biol Phys 76(Suppl. 3):S70–S76

Medhora M et al (2012) Radiation damage to the lung: mitigation by angiotensin-converting enzyme (ACE) inhibitors. Respirology 17(1):66–71

Mehta V (2005) Radiation pneumonitis and pulmonary fibrosis in non-small-cell lung cancer: pulmonary function, prediction, and prevention. Int J Radiat Oncol Biol Phys 63(1):5–24

Miller KD et al (2019) Cancer treatment and survivorship statistics, 2019. CA Cancer J Clin 69(5):363–385

Moeller BJ et al (2004) Radiation activates HIF-1 to regulate vascular radiosensitivity in tumors: role of reoxygenation, free radicals, and stress granules. Cancer Cell 5(5):429–441

Monson JM et al (1998) Clinical radiation pneumonitis and radiographic changes after thoracic radiation therapy for lung carcinoma. Cancer 82(5):842–850

Murley JS et al (2007) Manganese superoxide dismutase (SOD2)-mediated delayed radioprotection induced by the free thiol form of amifostine and tumor necrosis factor alpha. Radiat Res 167(4):465–474

Ozawa Y et al (2015) Impact of preexisting interstitial lung disease on acute, extensive radiation pneumonitis: retrospective analysis of patients with lung cancer. PLoS One 10(10):e0140437

Palma DA et al (2013) Predicting radiation pneumonitis after chemoradiation therapy for lung cancer: an international individual patient data meta-analysis. Int J Radiat Oncol Biol Phys 85(2):444–450

Park YH, Kim JS (2013) Predictors of radiation pneumonitis and pulmonary function changes after concurrent chemoradiotherapy of non-small cell lung cancer. Radiat Oncol J 31(1):34–40

Paumier A et al (2012) Dosimetric benefits of intensity-modulated radiotherapy combined with the deep-inspiration breath-hold technique in patients with mediastinal Hodgkin's lymphoma. Int J Radiat Oncol Biol Phys 82(4):1522–1527

Prasanna PG et al (2012) Normal tissue protection for improving radiotherapy: where are the gaps? Transl Cancer Res 1(1):35–48

Prezzano KM et al (2019) Stereotactic body radiation therapy for non-small cell lung cancer: a review. World J Clin Oncol 10(1):14–27

Rancati T et al (2003) Factors predicting radiation pneumonitis in lung cancer patients: a retrospective study. Radiother Oncol 67(3):275–283

Robnett TJ et al (2000) Factors predicting severe radiation pneumonitis in patients receiving definitive chemoradiation for lung cancer. Int J Radiat Oncol Biol Phys 48(1):89–94

Schieber M, Chandel NS (2014) ROS function in redox signaling and oxidative stress. Curr Biol 24(10):R453–R462

Senzer N (2002) A phase III randomized evaluation of amifostine in stage IIIA/IIIB non-small cell lung cancer patients receiving concurrent carboplatin, paclitaxel, and radiation therapy followed by gemcitabine and cisplatin intensification: preliminary findings. Semin Oncol 29(6 Suppl. 19):38–41

Seppenwoolde Y et al (2004) Regional differences in lung radiosensitivity after radiotherapy for non-small-cell lung cancer. Int J Radiat Oncol Biol Phys 60(3):748–758

Shaverdian N et al (2020) Radiation pneumonitis in lung cancer patients treated with chemoradiation plus durvalumab. Cancer Med 9(13):4622–4631

Shields TW (1993) Surgical therapy for carcinoma of the lung. Clin Chest Med 14(1):121–147

Sio TT et al (2019) Daily Lisinopril vs placebo for prevention of Chemoradiation-induced pulmonary distress in patients with lung cancer (Alliance MC1221): a pilot double-blind randomized trial. Int J Radiat Oncol Biol Phys 103(3):686–696

Small W Jr et al (2018) Utility of the ACE inhibitor captopril in mitigating radiation-associated pulmonary toxicity in lung cancer: results from NRG oncology RTOG 0123. Am J Clin Oncol 41(4):396–401

Speirs CK et al (2017) Heart dose is an independent Dosimetric predictor of overall survival in locally advanced non-small cell lung cancer. J Thorac Oncol 12(2):293–301

Tak JK, Park JW (2009) The use of ebselen for radioprotection in cultured cells and mice. Free Radic Biol Med 46(8):1177–1185

Tembhekar AR, Wright CL, Daly ME (2017) Cardiac dose and survival after stereotactic body radiotherapy for early-stage non-small-cell lung cancer. Clin Lung Cancer 18(3):293–298

Terasaki Y et al (2011) Hydrogen therapy attenuates irradiation-induced lung damage by reducing oxidative stress. Am J Physiol Lung Cell Mol Physiol 301(4):L415–L426

Tian S et al (2020) Lung stereotactic body radiation therapy and concurrent immunotherapy: a multicenter safety and toxicity analysis. Int J Radiat Oncol Biol Phys 108(1):304–313

Toi Y et al (2018) Association of immune-related adverse events with clinical benefit in patients with advanced non-Small-cell lung cancer treated with Nivolumab. Oncologist 23(11):1358–1365

van der Veen SJ et al (2015) ACE inhibition attenuates radiation-induced cardiopulmonary damage. Radiother Oncol 114(1):96–103

van Sörnsen de Koste J et al (2001) An evaluation of two techniques for beam intensity modulation in patients irradiated for stage III non-small cell lung cancer. Lung Cancer 32(2):145–153

Verma V et al (2017) Influence of fractionation scheme and tumor location on toxicities after stereotactic body radiation therapy for large (≥5 cm) non-Small cell lung cancer: a multi-institutional analysis. Int J Radiat Oncol Biol Phys 97(4):778–785

Verma V et al (2018a) Safety of combined immunotherapy and thoracic radiation therapy: analysis of 3 single-institutional phase I/II trials. Int J Radiat Oncol Biol Phys 101(5):1141–1148

Verma V et al (2018b) Toxicity of radiation and immunotherapy combinations. Adv Radiat Oncol 3(4):506–511

Vinogradskiy Y et al (2013) Use of 4-dimensional computed tomography-based ventilation imaging to correlate lung dose and function with clinical outcomes. Int J Radiat Oncol Biol Phys 86(2):366–371

Vogelius IR, Bentzen SM (2012) A literature-based meta-analysis of clinical risk factors for development of radiation induced pneumonitis. Acta Oncol 51(8):975–983

Vojtíšek R (2020) Cardiac toxicity of lung cancer radiotherapy. Rep Pract Oncol Radiother 25(1):13–19

Wang S et al (2017a) Plasma levels of IL-8 and TGF-β1 predict radiation-induced lung toxicity in non-small cell lung cancer: a validation study. Int J Radiat Oncol Biol Phys 98(3):615–621

Wang K et al (2017b) Cardiac toxicity after radiotherapy for stage III non-small-cell lung cancer: pooled analysis of dose-escalation trials delivering 70–90 Gy. J Clin Oncol 35(13):1387–1394

Wang K et al (2017c) Heart dosimetric analysis of three types of cardiac toxicity in patients treated on dose-escalation trials for stage III non-small-cell lung cancer. Radiother Oncol 125(2):293–300

Wang Y et al (2019) Treatment-related adverse events of PD-1 and PD-L1 inhibitors in clinical trials: a systematic review and meta-analysis. JAMA Oncol 5(7):1008–1019

Wong OY et al (2018) Survival impact of cardiac dose following lung stereotactic body radiotherapy. Clin Lung Cancer 19(2):e241–e246

Wu W et al (2013) Long-term survival of patients with radiation heart disease undergoing cardiac surgery: a cohort study. Circulation 127(14):1476–1485

Yamada M et al (1998) Risk factors of pneumonitis following chemoradiotherapy for lung cancer. Eur J Cancer 34(1):71–75

Yamamoto T et al (2016) The first patient treatment of computed tomography ventilation functional image-guided radiotherapy for lung cancer. Radiother Oncol 118(2):227–231

Zhang XJ et al (2012) Prediction of radiation pneumonitis in lung cancer patients: a systematic review. J Cancer Res Clin Oncol 138(12):2103–2116

Zhang K et al (2015) Atorvastatin ameliorates radiation-induced cardiac fibrosis in rats. Radiat Res 184(6):611–620

Zhang TW et al (2019) Is the importance of heart dose overstated in the treatment of non-small cell lung cancer? A systematic review of the literature. Int J Radiat Oncol Biol Phys 104(3):582–589

Zhao W, Robbins ME (2009) Inflammation and chronic oxidative stress in radiation-induced late normal tissue injury: therapeutic implications. Curr Med Chem 16(2):130–143

Zhao J et al (2016) Simple factors associated with radiation-induced lung toxicity after stereotactic body radiation therapy of the thorax: a pooled analysis of 88 studies. Int J Radiat Oncol Biol Phys 95(5):1357–1366

Zhou Z et al (2017) Pulmonary emphysema is a risk factor for radiation pneumonitis in NSCLC patients with squamous cell carcinoma after thoracic radiation therapy. Sci Rep 7(1):2748

Spinal Cord

Timothy E. Schultheiss

Contents

1 Introduction 941
2 Histopathology 942
3 Symptoms and Treatment 942
4 Dose-Response 943
5 Other Factors 947
6 Lumbar Cord 947
7 Hyperfractionation 948
8 Retreatment 948
9 Volume 950
10 Other Observations 951
11 Conclusions 951
References 951

Abstract

Radiation myelopathy (RM) is a potential late complication of radiation treatment for lung cancer. It can be avoided in nearly all cases by well-planned dose distributions. Outside of errors in treatment planning or delivery, the greatest risk of RM occurs when retreatments are necessary. The pathogenesis, diagnosis, and treatment are discussed along with other factors that are related to RM. A previously unpublished dose-response analysis for thoracic RM is presented. It shows that the thoracic cord has a higher tolerance to high-dose radiation than the cervical cord. However, in practical terms, the responses of the two different levels to low dose are indistinguishable.

1 Introduction

Radiation myelopathy (RM) is one of the most dramatic complications of radiation therapy. The earliest clinical reports of RM were dominated by RM of the cervical cord, possibly because of the greater difficulty in achieving curative (high) doses in thoracic diseases with the technology of the mid twentieth century, especially for large-volume treatments. With advances in technology and higher achievable thoracic doses came increases in RM of the thoracic spinal cord. Consequently, clinical reports of this injury multiplied in the literature in the 1970s and 1980s. This represents a period shortly after Co-60 machines were introduced and followed by a transition from cobalt-60 to linear accelerators. The introduction of spilt-course treatments with large doses per fraction also had an impact. It is

T. E. Schultheiss (✉)
Department of Radiation Oncology, City of Hope Medical Center, Duarte, CA, USA
e-mail: timinoregon@gmail.com

primarily from these early reports upon which our current understanding of clinical RM was built. However, we are also guided by many experimental studies of radiation injury to the spinal cord in mice, rats, guinea pigs, dogs, pigs, and monkeys. Nonetheless, unanswered questions, not approachable by animal models, remain regarding specific clinical aspects of the radiation response of the spinal cord.

2 Histopathology

Late radiation damage to a tissue or organ can be diffusely distributed over a volume closely corresponding to the irradiated volume, as in late fibrosis. Conversely, it can be focal in nature and occur at unpredictable locations within a uniformly irradiated organ. The latter is the case for radiation myelopathy. The initial lesion occurs exclusively within the white matter of the spinal cord, but its pathogenesis is complex and multifactorial. In its simplest form, the pathogenesis has two manifestations—damage expressed in the white matter parenchyma ultimately leading to a necrotic lesion via a complicated pathway *or* a lesion in the white matter that is secondary to overt vascular damage. (The white matter parenchyma is understood to include glial cells in this case.) Lesions can appear adjacent to areas that show no evidence of radiation damage but were identically irradiated. Reviews of the pathology and pathogenesis of radiation myelopathy can be found in the works from the laboratories of van der Kogel (van Der Kogel and Barendsen 1974; van der Kogel 1986), Stephens (Schultheiss et al. 1988; Stephens et al. 1989), and Hopewell (1979). It is now generally accepted that the white matter lesion results from a process initiated by direct radiation damage to the vascular endothelium (Hopewell and van der Kogel 1999).

It seems clear that in most animals, including humans, there is a vascular based lesion and a parenchymal based lesion. Zeman was the first to articulate the dual hypothesis of radiation injury of the spinal cord (Zeman 1961), but van der Kogel definitively verified this hypothesis and explored it in detail in rats (van der Kogel 1979, 1980). In his studies, the white matter lesion occurred earlier and at higher doses. Clearly, if the later lesion occurred at higher doses, it would rarely be seen. This may explain why only the parenchymal based lesion is seen in some strains.

These same general observations have been made in humans through the analysis of autopsy data (Schultheiss et al. 1984, 1988). However, the data are much more difficult to interpret since autopsy reports often reflect the status of the lesions months or years after the onset of symptoms.

In humans, latencies as short as 4 months have been observed, but these are very rare. Typically, the onset of symptoms occurs 9–48 months after the completion of treatment. There is no difference between latency in the cervical and thoracic levels of the cord. The latency in children appears to be shorter than that in the adult, but there does not seem to be much difference in tolerance. However, it is customary to respect a lower tolerance in the child. The latency is shorter at higher doses in both rodents and humans; however, this effect in humans is not strong over the therapeutic dose range.

3 Symptoms and Treatment

The progression of symptoms for thoracic radiation myelopathy is generally altered sensation in the lower extremities including numbness, tingling, and reduced sensitivity to temperature. A sensory level is sometimes seen corresponding to the irradiated spinal segment. Pain is sometimes reported, often associated with tingling. This progresses to weakness, which can be manifest as changes in gait or foot drop. Paresis, rectal and bladder incontinence, and complete paralysis may develop. Symptoms can progress rapidly, with patients sometimes presenting with paralysis. Recovery from sensory losses may occur over time, but motor deficits are less frequently recovered. Although thoracic myelopathy does not have the morbidity associated with cervical myelopathy, it can still become life-threatening as a result of secondary effects of incontinence and paralysis (Schultheiss et al. 1986a).

Although no treatment has shown long-term effectiveness (Kian Ang and Stephens 1994) at a high efficacy, there are anecdotal reports that are encouraging (Chamberlain et al. 2011). In addition, a number of potential treatment methods have been put forward (Wong et al. 2015). Bevacizumab has been associated with successful treatment of brain necrosis, and anecdotal reports of its use in RM exist. It is seen to improve radiological appearance of radiation lesions more frequently than it has shown clinical benefit (Psimaras et al. 2016). It may be more effective against brain necrosis than RM (Tye et al. 2014).

4 Dose-Response

The most widely used dose limit for the spinal cord is 45 Gy at 1.8–2 Gy per fraction. Some clinicians routinely respect an even lower dose for the spinal cord. Planning the lowest achievable dose to the spinal cord is a good policy as long as the tumor is adequately irradiated. However, it would be imprudent to compromise the tumor dose in order to limit the spinal cord to a dose of 45 Gy or less in patients for whom there is no evidence of increased radiation CNS sensitivity.

It has been reported that the dose producing a 5% rate of radiation myelopathy is between 57 and 61 Gy in conventional dose fractions (Schultheiss 1994, 2008). This is based solely on cervical RM. Wong et al. state that no case of RM had been found at Princess Margaret Hospital after 50 Gy in 25 fractions (Wong et al. 1994), although there are rare literature reports of myelopathies at this dose. The dosimetry for such reports may be uncertain. This regimen was the most common dose regimen for lung cancer treatment at PMH at the time of Wong's publication. Although it may be an unusual circumstance, cord doses of 50 Gy (or higher) in 2 Gy fractions should be considered if the tumor would be underdosed otherwise. However, it is imperative that the patient be properly informed of the risk.

The reason that dose limits given above were from clinical data that were limited to the cervical cord was that it was not possible to obtain an acceptable fit of a logistic regression to thoracic dose-response data (Schultheiss 2008). The dose-response data were collected from published studies using searches of electronic databases and further searches of references within all collected papers on RM. The search was not limited to the English language. A new approach has been taken here to address and reduce the excess dispersion in the thoracic data; that is, the analysis was limited to published reports of prospective clinical trials with specific mention of complications *or* reports where the subject of the paper was specifically RM. This restriction had the effect of reducing the variance in the observed responses for the thoracic cord by eliminating papers that only parenthetically mentioned RM. Papers were excluded if all fields were not treated daily or a single and specific dose regimen that applied to the entire cohort could not be ascertained. In these cases, the correct dosimetry could not be verified. To reiterate, reports were also excluded if RM was merely reported as part of a retrospective study on disease control because the follow-up may not have been complete or uniform. The included studies are given in Table 1 for both the cervical and thoracic levels.

The data were analyzed using logistic regression where the probability, P, of RM is given by

$$\ln\left(P/(1-P)\right) = \beta_0 + \beta_1 \cdot D + \beta_2 \cdot d \cdot D \quad (1)$$

so that the ratio of β_2/β_1 can be interpreted as the α/β ratio of the LQ model (Taylor 1990). P is the probability that a patient's tolerance is exceeded by dose D given in fraction sizes of d. The log likelihood function, L, which was maximized with respect to the unknown parameters, β, is

$$\ln(L) = \sum_{i=1}^{n} r_i \ln(g_i P_i) + (m_i - r_i)\ln(1 - g_i P_i)$$

where the effects of censoring are handled by multiplying P by the term g, which is the probability that a patient whose tolerance has been exceeded will survive to express the injury (Schultheiss et al. 1986b). (This probability can be calculated as the integral over time of the distribution of latent period times the survival func-

Table 1 Data from reports of radiation myelopathy or clinical trials with RM used in the logistic regression

Reference	Cervical (C), thoracic (T)	Total dose (Gy)	Dose per fraction (Gy)	RM cases (r_i)	Total cases (m_i)	g^a
McCunniff and Liang (1989)	C	60	2	1	17	0.929
McCunniff and Liang (1989)	C	65	1.63	0	24[b]	0.929
Abbatucci et al. (1978)	C	54	3	7	21	0.836
Atkins and Tretter (1966)	C	19	9.5	4	13	0.704
Marcus and Million (1990)	C	47.5	1.85	0	211	0.738
Marcus and Million (1990)	C	52.5	1.85	0	22[b]	0.738
Jeremic et al. (1991)	C	60	2	2	19	0.891
Jeremic et al. (1991)	C	65	1.63	0	19[b]	0.891
Kim and Fayos (1981)	C	62.8	1.93	3	109	0.531
Macbeth et al. (1996)	T	37.8	3.15	0	86	0.200
Dische et al. (1981, 1986, 1988)	T	34.1	5.68	8	87	0.260
Dische et al. (1981, 1986, 1988)	T	34.9	5.82	4	31	0.368
Hatlevoll et al. (1983)	T	18	6	8	157	0.217
Hatlevoll et al. (1983)	T	18	6	9	230	0.217
Macbeth et al. (1996)	T	17.9	8.93	3	524	0.174
Macbeth et al. (1996)	T	40.9	3.15	2	153	0.211
Macbeth et al. (1996)	T	31.5	5.25	0	36	0.200
Simpson et al. (1982)	T	36	6	1	5	0.302
Fitzgerald Jr et al. (1982)	T	41.2	4.12	6	200	0.205
Eichhorn et al. (1972)	T	69.6	2.58	8	142	0.241
Eichhorn et al. (1972)	T	58.1	3.06	2	22	0.243

[a] This factor represents the probability that a patient whose tolerance was exceeded will survive to express the injury
[b] As recommended by Berkson (1953), these cases were not included in the analysis because of having 0% response at doses lower than the lowest nonzero response

tion of the cohort.) The product gP gives the probability of *observing* a RM case for the dose regimen i (out of n). Then the observed RM incidence for the ith dose pattern is r_i/m_i.

For the initial analysis, the cervical and thoracic data were analyzed separately. The result was a good fit in each dataset as measured by the Pearson χ^2 statistic, with examination of residuals showing no concern regarding outliers and the hat matrix diagonals not showing concern regarding points that seemed excessively influential in the fit (Hosmer et al. 2013). The maximum likelihood estimates of the α/β values were 0.58 and 0.48 Gy for the cervical and thoracic levels, respectively, and the location parameters, i.e., the constants β_0, showing the expected separation of the two dose-response curves. The dose-response functions are shown in Fig. 1. Comparing this figure to the original analysis of the cervical data only (Schultheiss 2008), one can appreciate that the dose-response function is shifted slightly to higher doses. This is primarily a result of using different denominators (m_i) for two of the data points. It was judged on this reanalysis that for the McCunniff et al. data, a denominator of 17 was a better representation of the data than 12 used originally, and that for Abbatucci et al., a denominator of 21 was more correct than 15. The increase in both denominators is a result of including patients treated with smaller field sizes than in the original analysis.

In the current analysis, the recommendation of Berkson was followed that states that if there are

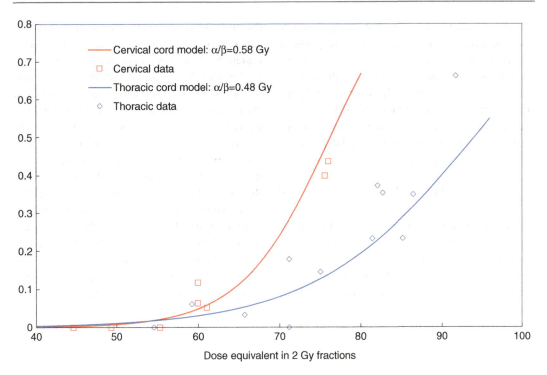

Fig. 1 Dose-response curves from logistic regression of cervical and thoracic clinical data analyzed separately. Of the three 0% responses in the cervical data, only one (Marcus and Million 1990) was used in the analysis. The dose-response parameters are given in Table 1. Since the α/β ratios for the cervical and thoracic levels differ slightly, the dose metric is not the same for both levels

multiple consecutive values of extreme responses (0 or 100%), only the ones adjacent to nonextreme responses should be used (Berkson 1953). In this analysis, only a single extreme response was used for the cervical cord, but the one with the largest number of patients in the denominator (211) was selected.

The cervical and thoracic data were pooled by adding another term, $\beta_3 \cdot \delta_T$ accounting for the level of the cord, to Eq. (1) above. The variable, δ_T, had values of 0 for the cervical and 1 for the thoracic level. Thus, e^{β_3} is the odds ratio for RM of the thoracic spinal cord relative to the cervical cord. The new analysis including the additional variable is shown in Fig. 2, and the parameter estimates are given in Table 2. Note that the weighted average of the α/β ratio found for cervical and thoracic RM found above was 0.5 Gy and was used for the pooled analysis. The empirical weights of $m_i P_i(1 - P_i)$ were used (where P is the estimated value of P).

Table 2 Dose-response parameters and fitting metrics for the logistic regression of data

Parameter	C and T separate fit	Odds ratio (OR)	Volume effect
β_0	−13.96 (C), −9.48 (T)	−10.30	−11.68
β_1 (Gy^{-1})	0.0414 (C), 0.0194 (T)	0.0254	0.0298
β_2 (Gy^{-2})	0.0709 (C), 0.0407 (T)	0.0508[a]	0.0596[a]
β_3	–	−1.115 (OR = 0.303)	–
V	–	–	0.295
LL	−46.58 (C), −208.64 (T)	−257.00	−255.93
$p(\chi^2, df)$	0.65 (C), 0.63 (T)	0.43	0.54

Note: $\alpha/\beta = \beta_2/\beta_1$
[a] α/β was constrained to be 0.5 Gy by setting $\beta_2 = 2\beta_1$

We can also pursue a mechanistic model to account for the difference between the cervical and thoracic cord rather than capturing the difference in an odds ratio. One can hypothesize that the difference between the dose-response of the two levels is due to a difference in the target volume (or the volume of targets) in the thoracic versus the cervical level. The simplest and yet a robust model for the volume effect is generally, but inexactly, called the critical element model, but it does not have any fundamental dependence on elements. It is given by

$$P(D,v) = 1 - \left[1 - P(D,1)\right]^v \quad (2)$$

where $P(D,1)$ is the probability of RM when the reference volume, for which $v = 1$, is irradiated to dose D, v is the irradiated volume relative to the reference volume, and $P(D,v)$ is the probability of RM when volume v is irradiated to dose D (Schultheiss et al. 1983). This formula is easily generalized to inhomogeneous irradiation. Equation (2) follows from applying the law of total probability to the probability of *not* inducing RM in the total spinal cord as a result of irradiating partial volumes of the cord. In this case, we can assume that the dose-responses for the thoracic and cervical levels of the cord are identical except that the thoracic cord has on average a target volume, v, relative to the cervical cord. Repeating the regression analysis, we find that the maximum likelihood estimate of the relative volume of the T-cord is 0.30. In fact, the two models for estimating the dose-response of the thoracic cord are essentially equivalent from a clinical perspective. See Fig. 2. The volume effect model has a modestly better fit.

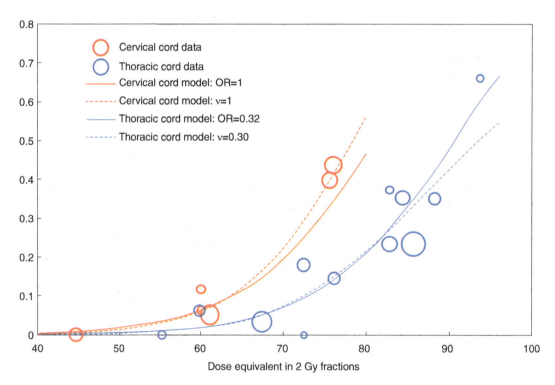

Fig. 2 Pooled dose-response analysis using two models for the thoracic response relative to the cervical response. In the first model, the thoracic response is assumed to differ only by its associated odds ratio (OR). In the second model, the difference is attributed to the relative volume, v, of targets in the thoracic cord compared to the cervical cord. The data are plotted using a bubble plot with the area of the bubbles being proportional to hat matrix diagonals for each data point. These values represent the leverage associated with the influence each point has on the regression outcome (Hosmer et al. 2013)

The above analysis is based on the historical reports of treatment protocols most of which would not be used today because of their neurotoxicity. For conventional treatments, spinal cord doses are kept well below levels that would cause a 1% complication rate. Whereas some incidence data are available at these low doses, there are not enough data to deploy in a meaningful dose-response analysis covering the low-dose region. Furthermore, cases of RM resulting from truly low doses (meaning they are not due to dose calculation errors) are likely to be a result of conditions or factors that for unknown reasons cause an increase in the radiation sensitivity of the spinal cord (Schultheiss and Stephens 1992b). Therefore, extreme caution should be used when extrapolating the results of the above analysis to regions outside the database. A reasonable approach would be to avoid any novel dose regimen for which more than a single case of RM has been reported.

5 Other Factors

Factors other than the dose schedule that affect the spinal cord tolerance, either clinically or experimentally, include irradiated volume, chemotherapeutic agents, age, oxygenation, vascular disease, concurrent disease processes, and congenital abnormalities.

There have been numerous studies of the effect of chemotherapy on the tolerance of the spinal cord, but the clinical data are mostly anecdotal (Ang et al. 1986; Bloss et al. 1991; Schultheiss 1994; van der Kogel and Sissingh 1983, 1985). With the possible exception of chemotherapeutic agents that are known to be neurotoxic, one cannot state unequivocally that chemotherapy reduces the radiation tolerance of the spinal cord. This may be especially important for those agents causing peripheral neuropathy, but not central neuropathy (St. Clair et al. 2003).

There is little evidence that thoracic level of the spinal cord differs in its intrinsic radiosensitivity from the cervical level. However, there may be extrinsic factors affecting spinal cord radiosensitivity that apply more frequently to one section of the cord than another. The thoracic cord's apparent radiosensitivity may be slightly lower (higher tolerance) simply because there is a smaller volume of white matter in the cervical cord. However, the spinal cord's dose-response is not very sensitive to changes in volume, and volume effect alone may not fully explain the difference in the incidence of radiation myelopathy in the cervical versus thoracic levels.

Dische et al. (1986) observed a dramatic effect of hemoglobin on the tolerance of the spinal cord. Furthermore, data from van den Brenk et al. (1968) and Coy and Dolman (1971) indicate that the spinal cord is sensitive to extrinsic oxygen tension. Since publications that report the incidence of thoracic radiation myelopathy come almost exclusively from studies of lung cancer, one may reasonably infer that these patients have seriously impaired oxygenation of the spinal cord, owing to a smoking history and to lung cancer. Therefore, it is possible that their spinal cord tolerance is increased due to a decrease in the oxygenation of the white matter.

6 Lumbar Cord

In rodents, the pathology and pathogenesis of the lumbar cord are inexplicably different from the thoracic and cervical levels. The dose-response and latency are generally similar, but the progression of the lesions is somewhat slower. More importantly, different regions of the nervous parenchyma are involved (Bradley et al. 1977; van Der Kogel and Barendsen 1974; van der Kogel 1977; White and Hornsey 1978). No white matter necrosis is seen in the true cord at the lumbar level as a result of radiation. The damage occurs in the nerve roots, where demyelination followed by necrosis is observed. The neurons of the irradiated nerve root ganglia remain intact, but axonal degeneration occurs outward from the irradiated region toward the neuron cell body to which the axon belongs. The work of Bradley in particular indicates that axonal degeneration seems to occur while the Schwann cells still myelinate the fibers. The inflammatory response seems limited to phagocytosis. Only pyknotic nuclei were observed in the degenerating Schwann cells, indicating that they were not stimulated into mitosis as a result of radiation.

Although the spinal cord in humans ends at the spinal levels L1–2, Schultheiss et al. found one reported autopsy case of lumbar RM in their study of 53 cases from the literature (Palmer 1972). The lesion extended from T11 to L2 with minimal necrosis but extensive demyelination. There was no examination of the nerve roots.

The different radiation response in the lumbar cord remains unexplained, and the pathogenesis has not been extensively investigated.

7 Hyperfractionation

The effect of hyperfractionation on the response of the spinal cord is not fully understood. Although the spinal cord has a high capacity for long-term repair of radiation damage, as will be discussed later, its interfraction repair is slower than many other tissues (Ang et al. 1992). Although there have not been any published reports of unexpected myelopathies occurring after two fractions per day (1.2 Gy per fraction), unanticipated myelopathies have occurred after regimens of three and four fractions per day (Dische and Saunders 1989; Wong et al. 1991), and because of a lack of data for these dose schedules, 3 and 4 fractions per day should be avoided.

In two separate publications, Jeremic has shown that 50.6 Gy in 1.1 or 50.4 Gy in 1.2 Gy fractions produced no myelopathies in either the cervical or the thoracic cord, respectively (Jeremic et al. 1998, 2001). In the adult rat, Ang et al. found that the repair was described better by a biexponential function than by a monoexponential (Ang et al. 1992). However, Ruifrok et al. found no evidence of this biexponential repair in the newborn rat (Ruifrok et al. 1992). In the rhesus monkey, no difference was observed in the response at 98.4 Gy at 1.2 Gy per fraction as compared to 84 Gy, with the responses being 8/15 versus 6/11, respectively (unpublished data).

8 Retreatment

The spinal cord has a substantial capacity for long-term recovery from subclinical radiation damage. In animals, this recovery appears to be dependent on the initial dose or level of damage and the time between the initial course of treatment and the second course of treatment. In cancer patients, the level of recovery is probably more variable and possibly dependent on intervening therapies as well.

Retreatment dose-response studies in rats have been performed by a number of authors. Generally, it appears that following a treatment of approximately 50% of the D_{50} for an untreated rat, 75% of the dose is recovered in 20 weeks, and close to 100% is recovered in a year (Wong et al. 1993a, b). In guinea pigs, Knowles found that the D_{50} for 1-year-old animals who received 10 Gy 1 day after birth was only 5% less than 1-year-old unirradiated animals (Knowles 1983). Both van der Kogel (1991) and Wong and Hao (1997) have studied the dependence of the retreatment tolerance on the initial dose and the interval between treatments. The relative steepness of the retreatment dose-response function compared to the de novo dose-response function is not certain.

Ang et al. have performed retreatment experiments on rhesus monkeys (Ang et al. 1993, 2001). Their findings indicate that about 75% of 44 Gy in 20 fractions is recovered after 1 year and nearly 100% is recovered after 3 years. Forty-four Gray represents 57% of the initial D_{50} in these animals. Thus, the primate data is in reasonable agreement with the rodent data.

The largest number of clinical cases of radiation myelopathy following retreatment was reported by Wong et al. (1994). In their 11 cases, all had single-course doses, in 2 Gy fraction equivalents, of more than 52 Gy (using an $\alpha/\beta = 0.5$ as found above). In two cases of the three cases with the lowest single-course dose, the break between courses was only 2 months and little or no repair would be expected. Thus, in all of their reported cases, either the spinal cord tolerance could have been exceeded by one of the treatment courses alone or there was insufficient time for repair between courses. The average latency following the second course of treatment was 11 months with a range of 4–25 months.

Nieder et al. (2005, 2006) used the Wong data and other sources to construct an algorithm to assess the risk of RM in retreatment of the spinal cord. The risk level was based on three factors: (1) the total ERD of the combined treatments, (2) the larger ERD of the two courses, and (3) the elapsed time between treatment courses. Note that ERD = $D[1 + d/(\alpha/\beta)]$, where D is the total dose given with fraction size d, and α/β is the α/β ratio from the LQ model. ERDs are meaningless in the abstract, i.e., without reference to the α/β, since they depend strongly on the value of α/β. This means that one cannot convert from one ERD to another by knowing the α/β value unless the dose schedule is also known.

Inventing a risk metric is a useful alternative to attempting to create a valid cohort of unrelated cases and controls that could be legitimately subjected to a regression analysis. The latter is essentially impossible. However, since Nieder et al. used an α/β value of 2 Gy instead of the much lower value that has come out of metaregression of human data, the risk may be underestimated for courses of high doses per fraction and overestimated for courses with low doses per fraction. For example, two fractions of 9 Gy followed more than 6 months later by a single fraction of 8 Gy would be considered low risk, whereas 26 × 2 Gy followed 3 years later by 8 × 1.8 Gy would be gauged as high risk. Because in the main, their algorithm seems quite reasonable, it is reproduced here:

$$\text{Risk score} = \text{Int}\left[(\text{ERD}_{total} - 110.1)/10\right]$$
$$+ 4.5 \text{ if either ERD} \geq 102\,\text{Gy}$$
$$+ 4.5 \text{ if the time between}$$
$$\text{treatments} \leq 6\,\text{months}$$

where "Int(x)" is the greatest integer in x and the total ERD is capped at 200 Gy. The risk levels are then

0–3 ⇒ low risk
4–6 ⇒ intermediate risk
≥6 ⇒ high risk

Low, intermediate, and high risks are not specifically defined, but it was stated that "low-risk patients remained free of myelopathy and 33% of intermediate-risk patients and 90% of high-risk patients developed myelopathy." Note that these percentages were not an assessment of dose-response since a true cohort was not evaluated. Thus, in nearly all circumstances, the intermediate risk level would be considered inappropriate. Some may consider even 1% a high risk of such a serious complication. Clearly, the acceptable risk depends on the context. While this tool could be considered imprecise, it captures the elements of the major components of risk in re-treating the spinal cord.

It must be emphasized that the risk score and its interpretation apply only to ERDs using $\alpha/\beta = 2$ Gy. Therefore, this algorithm cannot be used if a different value of α/β is considered more suitable. However, if one converts a dose schedule to the equivalent dose in 2 Gy fractions, then one can apply the algorithm using one's own choice of α/β. To apply the algorithm in this case, the following equation must be used:

$$\text{Risk score} = \text{Int}\left[\left(D_{2\,\text{Gy}} - 55.05\right)/5\right]$$
$$+ 4.5 \text{ if either } D_{2\,\text{Gy}} \geq 51\,\text{Gy}$$
$$+ 4.5 \text{ if the time between treatments}$$
$$\leq 6\,\text{months}$$

Then if it is believed that the original algorithm puts too little weight on high doses per fraction, a smaller value of α/β should be used to convert the dose schedules to 2 Gy per fraction equivalents.

It is clear that the spinal cord can tolerate a significant retreatment dose. The clinical decision to retreat part of the spinal cord must be based on the availability of alternative treatments, the consequences of not treating, the initial cord dose, and the interval since the initial treatment. As always, a specific and detailed informed consent is mandatory. For palliation or for treatment of cord compression, 30 Gy in 15 fractions should be given consideration if the initial treatment did not exceed

45 Gy to the cord and was given at least 9 months prior to the potential second course. Care should be taken to minimize the spinal cord volume, but radiation myelopathy is still a possibility.

9 Volume

The conventional radiation volume effect in the spinal cord is understood as a decrease in the tolerance dose as the length of irradiated cord increases. In rats, there is a striking volume effect at field sizes below 1 cm, but very little effect as the length of irradiated cord is increased beyond 1 cm (van der Kogel 1991). This volume behavior may result from the fact that the size of the lesion is not negligible compared to 1 cm. In rhesus monkeys, the volume effect is consistent with the probability model (Schultheiss et al. 1983, 1994). This model is derived using the law of total probability, where the probability of not producing a lesion in the irradiated volume is simply the product of the probabilities of not producing lesions in all subvolumes. A consequence of the model is that for steep dose-response functions, there is very little volume effect. This can explain why there is no volume effect in rats at field sizes above 1 cm.

No unequivocal volume effect for the spinal cord has been observed in humans. The reason for this is that for a specific dose regimen or clinical trials with cases of RM, for example as in a clinical trial for lung cancer, the variation in field size is not large and the sample size is too small to see any field size effect. In anecdotal radiation myelopathy reports, field size effects cannot be demonstrated because controls (patients without myelopathy) are never included. Nonetheless, it is reasonable to assume that a field size effect is operational in the radiation response of the human spinal cord. However, the increase in risk that accompanies an increase in field length is not likely to be very significant if one is operating within the limits of the conventional standard of care for cancer patients. The risk of radiation myelopathy in patients receiving conventional doses to the spinal cord is so low that no volume effect will be seen clinically at these doses.

Of more immediate concern is the risk of radiation myelopathy in patients for whom the dose varies significantly across the spinal cord. With the advent of IMRT, small portions of the cord might be irradiated to doses that would be intolerably high for the whole cord, while the remainder of the cord receives much lower doses. The first study that addressed this issue was a paper by Debus et al. where patients undergoing proton radiation therapy for base-of-skull lesions had part of their brain stems irradiated to high doses (Debus et al. 1997). They found a relative risk of 11.4 for patients for whom more than 0.9 cm^3 received 60 Gy (photon equivalent) or more. Also of significant risk on multivariate analysis was having two or more base-of-skull surgical procedures and having a diagnosis of diabetes. The maximum dose to the brain stem was not significant ($P \sim 0.09$) in this study of 348 patients.

Based on this study, one could reasonably infer that sharp dose gradient across the spinal cord can be tolerated if the maximum dose is less than 60 Gy. However, it is likely that one cannot achieve as sharp a gradient with photons as with protons. Moreover, these patients were meticulously immobilized and imaged prior to treatment. In routine practice, some dose smearing will occur as a result of setup variations. With IMRT, this smearing should be less problematic because of the care that should be taken in the positioning of these patients. Beyond stating that the spinal cord should tolerate a higher maximum dose if there is a dose gradient across the cord, it is not currently possible to give quantitative guidance related to the tolerance associated with small hotspots on the spinal cord.

In a highly cited paper, Sahgal et al. present a creative dose-response analysis of SBRT data. Nine events "were identified based on a multi-institutional and international collaboration" (Sahgal et al. 2013). In addition, 66 controls who satisfied inclusion criteria were assembled from "three experienced academic institutions," namely M.D Anderson Cancer Center, UCSF, and University of Toronto. This technique is not a cohort study, and statistical attributes of parameters estimated using logistic regression do not apply. The technique has some similarities with a case-control study, but the cases and the controls do not share common sources. Furthermore, in a case-control study, inferences regarding the location parameter of the dose-response curve are not possible when the sampling fraction of the cases or controls is not known. This means that probability estimates are not possible. Since the data were analyzed as if they were uniformly generated from a single, complete cohort, the estimates of the probability of RM are contestable. In fact, the paper states that the dose limits at low probability do not correspond with "the general understanding of radiation tolerance at the lower end of the probability spectrum." Currently, there is no dose-response function for RM following SBRT that was generated using normative statistical methods.

10 Other Observations

There are species-specific responses of the spinal cord that deserve mention. In the pig, the pathology and radiation dose-response is similar to that which is observed in other animals. The difference in the pig response is that the latent period is far shorter than is seen in other models (Hopewell and Van Den Aardweg 1992; van den Aardweg et al. 1995). In the dog, there are reactions in the meninges and the dorsal root ganglia not seen in other animals (Powers et al. 1992). Furthermore, the role of vascular response is relatively greater in the dog (Schultheiss and Stephens 1992a). In the rhesus monkey and in some rat strains, a primarily vascular lesion is infrequently seen. The reason for this in the monkey may be that these lesions occur at times longer than those for which these animals were held (24 months). In some rat strains, the reason is probably the same, with the addition that the animals' life expectancy may be of similar duration to the latency for a vascular lesion.

11 Conclusions

There is no indication that the thoracic and cervical levels of the spinal cord have different intrinsic responses. Extrinsic conditions may result in apparent differences. Differences in the survival of the cohort population may result in fewer thoracic myelopathies being observed. The morbidity of thoracic radiation myelopathy is generally lower than that for cervical myelopathy. Administration of common chemotherapeutic agents for lung cancer may reduce the radiation tolerance of the spinal cord, but no quantitative studies have demonstrated this for the most commonly used chemotherapeutic agents in lung cancer.

In the era of intensity-modulated radiation therapy, techniques for concurrent boosts of the tumor will be developed so that a cone down is no longer necessary. This will result in a lower dose per fraction to normal tissues outside the target. The effect of this decrease in the dose per fraction will be more in tissues, such as the spinal cord, whose late effects are dose limiting.

References

Abbatucci JS, DeLozier T, Quint R, Roussel A, Brune D (1978) Radiation myelopathy of the cervical spinal cord. Time, dose, and volume factors. Int J Radiat Oncol Biol Phys 4:239–248

Ang KK, Van Der Kogel AJ, Van Der Schueren E (1986) Effect of combined AZQ and radiation on the tolerance of the rat spinal cord. J Neurooncol 3:349–1346

Ang KK, Jiang GL, Guttenberger R, Thames HD, Stephens LC, Smith CD, Feng Y (1992) Impact of spinal cord repair kinetics on the practice of altered fractionation schedules. Radiother Oncol 25:287–294

Ang KK, Price RE, Stephens LC, Jiang GL, Feng Y, Schultheiss TE, Peters LJ (1993) The tolerance of primate spinal cord to re-irradiation. Int J Radiat Oncol Biol Phys 25:459–464

Ang KK, Jiang GL, Feng Y, Stephens LC, Tucker SL, Price RE (2001) Extent and kinetics of recovery of occult spinal cord injury. Int J Radiat Oncol Biol Phys 50(4):1013–1020. https://doi.org/10.1016/S0360-3016(01)01599-1

Atkins HL, Tretter P (1966) Time-dose considerations in radiation myelopathy. Acta Radiol Ther Phys Biol 5:79–94

Berkson J (1953) A statistically precise and relatively simple method of estimating the bioassay with quantal response, based on the logistic function. J Am Stat Assoc 48(263):565–599. https://doi.org/10.2307/2281010

Bloss JD, DiSaia PJ, Mannel RS, Hyden EC, Manetta A, Walker JL, Berman ML (1991) Radiation myelitis: a complication of concurrent cisplatin and

5-fluorouracil chemotherapy with extended field radiotherapy for carcinoma of the uterine cervix. Gynecol Oncol 43(3):305–307. https://doi.org/10.1016/0090-8258(91)90041-3

Bradley WG, Fewings JD, Cumming WJK, Harrison RM (1977) Delayed myeloradiculopathy produced by spinal X-irradiation in the rat. J Neurol Sci 31(1):63–82. https://doi.org/10.1016/0022-510X(77)90006-5

Chamberlain MC, Eaton KD, Fink J (2011) Radiation-induced myelopathy: treatment with bevacizumab. Arch Neurol 68(12):1608–1609. https://doi.org/10.1001/archneurol.2011.621

Coy P, Dolman CL (1971) Radiation myelopathy in relation to oxygen level. Br J Radiol 44:705–707

Debus J, Hug EB, Liebsch NJ, O'Farrel D, Finkelstein D, Efird J, Munzenrider JE (1997) Brainstem tolerance to conformal radiotherapy of skull base tumors. Int J Radiat Oncol Biol Phys 39(5):967–975

Dische S, Martin WMC, Anderson P (1981) Radiation myelopathy in patients treated for carcinoma of bronchus using a six fraction regime of radiotherapy. Br J Radiol 54(637):29–35. https://doi.org/10.1259/0007-1285-54-637-29

Dische S, Saunders MI (1989) Continuous, hyperfractionated, accelerated radiotherapy (CHART): an interim report upon late morbidity. Radiother Oncol 16(1):65–72. https://doi.org/10.1016/0167-8140(89)90071-6

Dische S, Saunders MI, Warburton MF (1986) Hemoglobin, radiation, morbidity and survival. Int J Radiat Oncol Biol Phys 12(8):1335–1337

Dische S, Warburton MF, Saunders MI (1988) Radiation myelitis and survival in the radiotherapy of lung cancer. Int J Radiat Oncol Biol Phys 15(1):75–81. https://doi.org/10.1016/0360-3016(88)90349-5

Eichhorn HJ, Lessel A, Rotte KH (1972) Einfuss verschiedener Bestrahlungsrhythmen auf Tumor- und Normalgewebe in vivo. Strahlentheraphie 146:614–629

Fitzgerald RH Jr, Marks RD Jr, Wallace KM (1982) Chronic radiation myelitis. Radiology 144(3):609–612. https://doi.org/10.1148/radiology.144.3.6808557

Hatlevoll R, Høst H, Kaalhus O (1983) Myelopathy following radiotherapy of bronchial carcinoma with large single fractions: a retrospective study. Int J Radiat Oncol Biol Phys 9(1):41–44. https://doi.org/10.1016/0360-3016(83)90206-7

Hopewell JW (1979) Late radiation damage to the central nervous system: a radiobiological interpretation. Neuropathol Appl Neurobiol 5:329–343

Hopewell JW, Van Den Aardweg GJMJ (1992) Radiation myelopathy in the pig: a model for assessing volume factors for spinal cord tolerance. In: Fortieth annual meeting of the Radiation Research Society, Salt Lake City, p 7

Hopewell JW, van der Kogel AJ (1999) Pathophysiological mechanisms leading to the development of late radiation-induced damage to the central nervous system. In: Wiegel T, Hinkelbein W, Brock M, Hoell T (eds) Controversies in neuro-oncology, Frontiers of radiation therapy and oncology, vol 33. Karger, Basel, pp 265–275

Hosmer DW, Lemeshow S, Sturdivant RX (2013) Applied logistic regression, Wiley series in probability and statistics, 3rd edn. Wiley, Hoboken, NJ

Jeremic B, Djuric L, Mijatovic L (1991) Incidence of radiation myelitis of the cervical spinal cord at doses of 5500 cGy or greater. Cancer 68(10):2138–2141. https://doi.org/10.1002/1097-0142(19911115)68:10<2138::AID-CNCR2820681009>3.0.CO;2-7

Jeremic B, Shibamoto Y, Milicic B, Acimovic L, Milisavljevic S (1998) Absence of thoracic radiation myelitis after hyperfractionated radiation therapy with and without concurrent chemotherapy for stage III nonsmall-cell lung cancer. Int J Radiat Oncol Biol Phys 40(2):343–346. https://doi.org/10.1016/S0360-3016(97)00713-X

Jeremic B, Shibamoto Y, Igrutinovic I (2001) Absence of cervical radiation myelitis after hyperfractionated radiation therapy with and without concurrent chemotherapy for locally advanced, unresectable, nonmetastatic squamous cell carcinoma of the head and neck. J Cancer Res Clin Oncol 127(11):687–691. https://doi.org/10.1007/s004320100269

Kian Ang K, Stephens LC (1994) Prevention and management of radiation myelopathy. Oncology 8(11):71–76

Kim YH, Fayos JV (1981) Radiation tolerance of the cervical spinal cord. Radiology 139:473–478

Knowles JF (1983) The radiosensitivity of the Guinea-pig spinal cord to x-rays: the effect of retreatment at one year and the effect of age at the time of irradiation. Int J Radiat Biol 44(5):433–442. https://doi.org/10.1080/09553008314551411

Macbeth FR, Wheldon TE, Girling DJ, Stephens RJ, Machin D, Bleehen NM, Lamont A, Radstone DJ, Reed NS, Bolger JJ, Clark PI, Connolly CK, Hasleton PS, Hopwood P, Moghissi K, Saunders MI, Thatcher N, White RJ (1996) Radiation myelopathy: estimates of risk in 1048 patients in three randomized trials of palliative radiotherapy for non-small cell lung cancer. Clin Oncol 8(3):176–181. https://doi.org/10.1016/S0936-6555(96)80042-2

Marcus RB, Million RR (1990) The incidence of myelitis after irradiation of the cervical spinal cord. Int J Radiat Oncol Biol Phys 19(1):3–8. https://doi.org/10.1016/0360-3016(90)90126-5

McCunniff AJ, Liang MJ (1989) Radiation tolerance of the cervical spinal cord. Int J Radiat Oncol Biol Phys 16(3):675–678. https://doi.org/10.1016/0360-3016(89)90484-7

Nieder C, Grosu AL, Andratschke NH, Molls M (2005) Proposal of human spinal cord reirradiation dose based on collection of data from 40 patients. Int J Radiat Oncol Biol Phys 61(3):851–855. https://doi.org/10.1016/j.ijrobp.2004.06.016

Nieder C, Grosu AL, Andratschke NH, Molls M (2006) Update of human spinal cord reirradiation tolerance based on additional data from 38 patients. Int J Radiat Oncol Biol Phys 66(5):1446–1449. https://doi.org/10.1016/j.ijrobp.2006.07.1383

Palmer JJ (1972) Radiation myelopathy. Brain 95:109–122

Powers BE, Beck ER, Gillette EL, Gould DH, LeCouter RA (1992) Pathology of radiation injury to the canine spinal cord. Int J Radiat Oncol Biol Phys 23(3):539–549. https://doi.org/10.1016/0360-3016(92)90009-7

Psimaras D, Tafani C, Ducray F, Leclercq D, Feuvret L, Delattre JY, Ricard D (2016) Bevacizumab in late-onset radiation-induced myelopathy. Neurology 86(5):454–457. https://doi.org/10.1212/WNL.0000000000002345

Ruifrok ACC, Kleiboer BJ, van der Kogel AJ (1992) Fractionation sensitivity of the rat cervical spinal cord during radiation retreatment. Radiother Oncol 25(4):295–300. https://doi.org/10.1016/0167-8140(92)90250-X

Sahgal A, Weinberg V, Ma L, Chang E, Chao S, Muacevic A, Gorgulho A, Soltys S, Gerszten PC, Ryu S, Angelov L, Gibbs I, Wong CS, Larson DA (2013) Probabilities of radiation myelopathy specific to stereotactic body radiation therapy to guide safe practice. Int J Radiat Oncol Biol Phys 85(2):341–347. https://doi.org/10.1016/j.ijrobp.2012.05.007

Schultheiss TE (1994) Spinal cord radiation tolerance. Int J Radiat Oncol Biol Phys 30:735–736

Schultheiss TE (2008) The radiation dose-response of the human spinal cord. Int J Radiat Oncol Biol Phys 71(5):1455–1459. https://doi.org/10.1016/j.ijrobp.2007.11.075

Schultheiss TE, Stephens LC (1992a) Pathogenesis of radiation myelopathy: widening the circle. Int J Radiat Oncol Biol Phys 23:1089–1091

Schultheiss TE, Stephens LC (1992b) Permanent radiation myelopathy. Br J Radiol 65(777):737–753

Schultheiss TE, Orton CG, Peck RA (1983) Models in radiotherapy: volume effects. Med Phys 10:410–415

Schultheiss TE, Higgins EM, El-Mahdi AM (1984) The latent period in clinical radiation myelopathy. Int J Radiat Oncol Biol Phys 10(7):1109–1115. https://doi.org/10.1016/0360-3016(84)90184-6

Schultheiss TE, Stephens LC, Peters LJ (1986a) Survival in radiation myelopathy. Int J Radiat Oncol Biol Phys 12:1765–1769

Schultheiss TE, Thames HD, Peters LJ, Dixon DO (1986b) Effect of latency on calculated complication rates. Int J Radiat Oncol Biol Phys 12:1861–1865

Schultheiss TE, Stephens LC, Maor MH (1988) Analysis of the histopathology of radiation myelopathy. Int J Radiat Oncol Biol Phys 14:27–32

Schultheiss TE, Stephens LC, Ang KK, Price RE, Peters LJ (1994) Volume effects in rhesus monkey spinal cord. Int J Radiat Oncol Biol Phys 29:67–72

Simpson JR, Perez CA, Phillips TL, Concannon JP, Carella RJ (1982) Large fraction radiotherapy plus misonidazole for treatment of advanced lung cancer: report of a phase I/II trial. Int J Radiat Oncol Biol Phys 8(2):303–308. https://doi.org/10.1016/0360-3016(82)90532-6

St. Clair WH, Arnold SM, Sloan AE, Regine WF (2003) Spinal cord and peripheral nerve injury: current management and investigations. Semin Radiat Oncol 13(3):322–332. https://doi.org/10.1016/S1053-4296(03)00025-0

Stephens LC, Ang KK, Schultheiss TE, Peters LJ (1989) Comparative morphology of radiation injury in the central nervous system. In: Radiation Research Society meeting proceedings, p 52

Taylor JM (1990) The design of in vivo multifraction experiments to estimate the alpha-beta ratio. Radiat Res 121(1):91–97

Tye K, Engelhard HH, Slavin KV, Nicholas MK, Chmura SJ, Kwok Y, Ho DS, Weichselbaum RR, Koshy M (2014) An analysis of radiation necrosis of the central nervous system treated with bevacizumab. J Neurooncol 117(2):321–327. https://doi.org/10.1007/s11060-014-1391-8

van den Aardweg GJMJ, Hopewell JW, Whitehouse EM (1995) The radiation response of the cervical spinal cord of the pig: effects of changing the irradiated volume. Int J Radiat Oncol Biol Phys 31(1):51–55

van den Brenk HAS, Richter W, Hurley RH (1968) Radiosensitivity of the human oxygenated cervical spinal cord based on analysis of 357 cases receiving 4 MeV X rays in hyperbaric oxygen. Br J Radiol 41(483):205–214

van der Kogel AJ (1977) Radiation-induced nerve root degeneration and hypertrophic neuropathy in the lumbosacral spinal cord of rats: the relation with changes in aging rats. Acta Neuropathol 39(2):139–145. https://doi.org/10.1007/BF00703320

van der Kogel AJ (1979) Late effects of radiation on the spinal cord. Dose-effect relationships and pathogenesis. PhD Thesis, University of Amsterdam, Amsterdam, Holland

van der Kogel AJ (1980) Mechanisms of late radiation injury in the spinal cord. In: Meyn RE, Withers HR (eds) Radiation biology in cancer research. Raven Press, New York

van der Kogel AJ (1986) Radiation-induced damage in the central nervous system: an interpretation of target cell responses. Br J Cancer 53(Suppl. VII):207–217

van der Kogel AJ (1991) Central nervous system radiation injury in small animal models. In: Gutin PH, Leigel SA, Sheline GE (eds) Radiation injury to the nervous system. Raven Press, New York, pp 91–111

van Der Kogel AJ, Barendsen GW (1974) Late effects of spinal cord irradiation with 300 kV X rays and 15 MeV neutrons. Br J Radiol 47(559):393–398. https://doi.org/10.1259/0007-1285-47-559-393

van der Kogel AJ, Sissingh HA (1983) Effect of misonidazole on the tolerance of the rat spinal cord to daily and multiple fractions per day of X rays. Br J Radiol 56(662):121–125. https://doi.org/10.1259/0007-1285-56-662-121

van der Kogel AJ, Sissingh HA (1985) Effects of intrathecal methotrexate and cytosine arabinoside on the radiation tolerance of the rat spinal cord. Radiother Oncol 4:239–251

White A, Hornsey S (1978) Radiation damage to the rat spinal cord: the effect of single and fractionated doses of X rays. Br J Radiol 51(607):515–523. https://doi.org/10.1259/0007-1285-51-607-515

Wong CS, Hao Y (1997) Long-term recovery kinetics of radiation damage in rat spinal cord. Int J Radiat Oncol Biol Phys 37(1):171–179

Wong CS, Minkin S, Hill RP (1993a) Re-irradiation tolerance of rat spinal cord to fractionated X-ray doses. Radiother Oncol 28(3):197–202. https://doi.org/10.1016/0167-8140(93)90058-g

Wong CS, Poon JK, Hill RP (1993b) Re-irradiation tolerance in the rat spinal cord: influence of level of initial damage. Radiother Oncol 26(2):132–138. https://doi.org/10.1016/0167-8140(93)90094-o

Wong CS, Van Dyk J, Milosevic M, Laperriere NJ (1994) Radiation myelopathy following single courses of radiotherapy and retreatment. Int J Radiat Oncol Biol Phys 30(3):575–581. https://doi.org/10.1016/0360-3016(92)90943-c

Wong CS, Van Dyk J, Simpson WJ (1991) Myelopathy following hyperfractionated accelerated radiotherapy for anaplastic thyroid carcinoma. Radiother Oncol 20(1):3–9. https://doi.org/10.1016/0167-8140(91)90105-P

Wong CS, Fehlings MG, Sahgal A (2015) Pathobiology of radiation myelopathy and strategies to mitigate injury. Spinal Cord 53(8):574–580. https://doi.org/10.1038/sc.2015.43

Zeman W (1961) Radiosensitivities of nervous tissues. Brookhaven Symp Biol 14:176–196

Radiation Therapy-Related Toxicity: Esophagus

Srinivas Raman and Meredith Giuliani

Contents

1 Pathophysiology and Clinical Picture of Esophagitis 955
1.1 Picture of Esophagitis 955
2 Evaluation of Esophagitis 957
3 Incidence of Esophagitis and Predisposing Factors 958
4 Dosimetric Factors Associated with Esophagitis 960
5 Strategies Used to Prevent or Treat Esophagitis 963
References 965

Radiation-induced esophagitis is a dose-limiting toxicity of lung cancer treatment. The majority of patients receiving concurrent chemotherapy and thoracic irradiation experience acute esophagitis. Acute esophagitis may be significant and necessitates medication for pain, intravenous fluid support, hospitalization, placement of a feeding tube in the stomach, or initiation of parenteral nutrition. Moreover, interruption of the course of radiation therapy may be required in order to permit healing of the esophageal injury or managing medical sequelae such as dehydration, acute renal failure, etc. Such treatment breaks have been demonstrated to decrease survival of patients with unresectable lung cancer. Proper prevention, diagnosis, and treatment of esophagitis are therefore essential, as it may have a direct influence on tumor control and survival.

1 Pathophysiology and Clinical Picture of Esophagitis

1.1 Picture of Esophagitis

The esophagus is lined with a convoluted squamous epithelium, with a basal cell layer, submucosa, and a layer of striated muscle fibers underneath and without surrounding serosa. In mice treated with a single fraction of radiation therapy to the thorax, evidence of damage to the esophagus was observed at a dose of 20.0 Gy, starting 3 days after radiotherapy (Phillips and Ross 1974). This included vacuolization of the basal cell layer, absence of mitosis, and submucosal edema. Some regeneration was evident by 1–2 weeks from radiotherapy, including proliferating basal cells, regenerating epithelium, and scattered areas of complete esophageal denudation. At 3 weeks, the regeneration of the esophageal lining was complete, and after 4 weeks, the appearance of the irradiated esophagus was normal. For fractionated radiotherapy doses, the LD50/28 (or radiotherapy dose causing death of 50% of the animals over 28 days) was estimated

S. Raman · M. Giuliani (✉)
Department of Radiation Oncology, University of Toronto, Toronto, ON, Canada
e-mail: srinivas.raman@rmp.uhn.ca;
Meredith.Giuliani@rmp.uhn.ca

as 57.45 Gy (in ten fractions). Radiological findings of esophageal injury were described in 30 symptomatic patients who received thoracic radiotherapy to 45–60 Gy. The most common finding was esophageal dysmotility, such as failure to complete primary peristaltic waves, non-peristaltic or tertiary contractions, or failure of distal esophageal sphincter relaxation. Smooth esophageal strictures were demonstrated in some patients, and one frank ulceration of the irradiated site was observed (Goldstein et al. 1975). Abnormal esophageal motility was noted to occur within 4–12 weeks from radiotherapy alone and as early as after 1 week of concurrent chemotherapy and radiotherapy (Lepke and Libshitz 1983). The first symptoms of acute esophagitis usually start in the second or third week of thoracic radiation therapy, corresponding to a dose of 18.0–21.0 Gy of standard fractionated radiotherapy and include a sensation of difficult swallowing (dysphagia). This may progress to painful swallowing of food and saliva (odynophagia) and later to constant pain not necessarily related to the swallowing act. In severe cases, patients may not be able to swallow at all. In patients receiving concurrent chemotherapy and thoracic radiotherapy, maximal symptoms of acute esophagitis developed within 1, 2, and 3 months from the start of radiotherapy in 19%, 32%, and 33% of the patients, respectively (Werner-Wasik et al. 2011). Patients with esophagitis require supportive management, starting with a low-acid and bland diet when the first sensation of difficulty swallowing is reported. Patients should be instructed to avoid coffee, hot beverages, spicy foods, citrus fruit and juices, tomato products, alcohol, and tobacco. In addition, a mixture of a local anesthetic (2% viscous lidocaine), coating substance (Benadryl elixir), and saline/baking soda ("Magic Mouthwash") is frequently prescribed to be taken liberally before meals to facilitate swallowing. Patients with esophagitis are also susceptible to acid reflux due to reduced lower esophageal sphincter pressure (Chowhan 1990), and therefore would benefit from proton-pump inhibitor or H2 receptor blockers.

Once symptoms progress (e.g., pain is more severe and only a soft diet is feasible), stronger oral analgesic agents should be instituted (opiates, etc.) to control pain and allow adequate oral nutrition. There should be involvement of a clinical dietician where available to assist with tailoring nutritional supplementation. High-calorie liquid oral nutritional supplements are helpful in maintaining satisfactory caloric intake and minimizing weight loss and anemia. Once adequate oral intake of fluids is impaired (as determined by dietary interview, positional changes in blood pressure and low urinary output), intravenous fluids should be instituted promptly in order to break the vicious cycle of dehydration-poor oral intake-more dehydration. A simple initial step is to give fluids intravenously on an outpatient basis while continuing thoracic radiotherapy. In some cases, placement of a gastric tube or parenteral nutrition may be necessary. If patients develop moderate to severe esophagitis limiting liquid intake, they may also require admission to hospital for intravenous hydration and electrolyte monitoring/correction. If a prolonged duration of radiation esophagitis is anticipated, a nasogastric tube, gastrostomy tube, or total parenteral nutrition may be recommended, although it is anticipated that a minority of patients will require these more invasive measures.

The speed of recovery from acute esophagitis seems related to the recovery from neutropenia induced by concurrent delivery of chemotherapy. Prolonged neutropenia prevents sufficient healing of the esophageal mucosa. This is a classic indication for a temporary suspension of radiotherapy and administration of a granulocyte stimulating factor preparation in order to shorten the neutropenic period. Short of this, thoracic radiotherapy should be continued as long as clinical judgment allows, since radiotherapy breaks are strongly associated with decreased chances of tumor control (Cox et al. 1993). Symptoms of acute esophagitis commonly persist for 1–3 weeks after the completion of radiotherapy. Late esophageal damage may subsequently develop at 3–8 months from completion of radiotherapy. It most often manifests as dysphagia to solids, caused by a permanent narrowing of the esophagus (stricture). The presence of stricture requires periodic surgical dilation of the esophagus, usually with excellent results (Choi et al. 2005).

Additionally, the course of radiotherapy may need to be halted temporarily in order to allow for healing of the esophageal lining. Treatment breaks in turn have been unequivocally demonstrated to decrease survival of patients with unresectable lung cancer (Cox et al. 1993). Steps toward prevention, prompt diagnosis, and effective treatment of radiation esophagitis may therefore have a direct impact on tumor control and overall survival.

2 Evaluation of Esophagitis

Various criteria have been used to grade acute esophagitis. "Esophagitis" is defined in Version 5.0 of National Cancer Institute's Common Terminology Criteria for Adverse Events (v5.0, CTCAE scale) as a disorder characterized by inflammation of the esophageal wall, and its grading is predominantly based on symptoms, altered diet, and need for intervention (Table 1). Grading systems such as the NCI CTCAE describe toxicity at one point in time, but they do not provide information about the length of time over which the patient experiences the symptoms of esophagitis. Esophagitis index (Werner-Wasik et al. 2002) is another measure of toxicity that is obtained by plotting the esophagitis grade over time. It may be a more comprehensive measure of normal tissue toxicity than maximum grade alone. Its calculation requires prospective accumulation of data points of toxicity over time, however, and its applicability may therefore be limited to investigational pursuits. The Radiation Therapy Oncology Group (RTOG) 98-01 study (Movsas et al. 2005) implemented other measures of esophagitis, based on physician assessment (weekly physician dysphagia log) as well as daily patient assessment of their difficulty in swallowing (patient swallowing diary).

The importance of analyzing patient-reported outcomes was highlighted in this study, which evaluated the efficacy of amifostine in preventing esophagitis in patients with stage III non-small cell lung cancer (NSCLC) undergoing chemoradiation. Although there were no statistically significant differences between the two arms in physician-assessed esophagitis, patient-reported esophagitis was significantly lower in the arm that received amifostine ($p = 0.02$). Given the potential discrepancy between these two assessments, the use of patient-reported outcomes to comprehensively measure toxicity and quality of life outcomes after cancer treatment is increasingly adopted in clinical trials. In additional to more patient-centered approaches of measuring esophageal toxicity, there has also been increasing interest in using imaging biomarkers to quantitatively assess esophagitis. For example, the geometrical expansion of the esophagus, measured on serial on-treatment CT imaging, correlated with grade 2 and 3 esophagitis endpoints in patients undergoing chemotherapy (Niedzielski et al. 2016a). Similarly, quantitative FDG PET imaging metrics have also demonstrated correlation with the incidence and severity of esophagitis in patients undergoing

Table 1 Version 5.0 of National Cancer Institute's Common Terminology Criteria for Adverse Events

	Grade 1	Grade 2	Grade 3	Grade 4	Grade 5
Dysphagia	Symptomatic, able to eat regular diet	Symptomatic and altered eating/ swallowing	Severely altered eating/swallowing; tube feeding, TPN, or hospitalization indicated	Life-threatening consequences; urgent intervention indicated	Death
Esophagitis	Asymptomatic; clinical or diagnostic observations only; intervention not indicated	Symptomatic; altered eating/ swallowing; oral supplements indicated	Severely altered eating/swallowing; tube feeding, TPN, or hospitalization indicated	Life-threatening consequences; urgent operative intervention indicated	Death

radiotherapy (Yuan et al. 2014; Mehmood et al. 2016; Niedzielski et al. 2016b).

3 Incidence of Esophagitis and Predisposing Factors

The incidence of esophagitis is related to the setting in which radiotherapy is delivered. In early-stage NSCLC, where highly conformal "stereotactic" radiotherapy is used to deliver ablative doses of radiotherapy to small target volumes, the incidence of acute esophagitis is very low, less than 5% in most series. In the CHISEL study, which prospectively compared stereotactic body radiotherapy (SBRT) and conventionally fractionated radiotherapy in peripherally located lung cancer, the rate of esophagitis was 2% in the SBRT arm, with no events of grade 3+ toxicity (Ball et al. 2019). Another institutional series from Princess Margaret reported a 3% incidence of esophageal toxicity in 632 patients who underwent SBRT to early lung cancers (Yau et al. 2018). There was only one grade 3 toxicity, and no reports of grade 4 or 5 toxicity were noted. However the risk of esophageal toxicity is elevated in patients with a central tumor location, as described in Chap. Stereotactic Ablative Radiotherapy for Early Stage Lung Cancer. The NRG Oncology/RTOG 0813 Trial evaluated the safety and efficacy of five-fraction SBRT in patients in central tumors (Bezjak et al. 2019). In this study, the rate of grade 3+ esophageal toxicity rate was approximately 3% with no reports of grade 5 esophageal events. It is believed that the risk of esophageal toxicity is even higher in patients with "ultra-central" tumors, where target volumes can directly abut or overlap the mediastinal organs at risk. Multiple institutional series have shown a higher rate of grade 3+ toxicity, median = 10% (Chen et al. 2019), and safety of this approach is being prospectively evaluated in ongoing clinical trials (e.g., NCT04375904, NCT03306680). An institutional review of 188 patients from Erasmus (Duijm et al. 2020) focused on esophagus toxicity after SBRT to central lung tumors showed an 18% incidence of esophageal toxicity and 2% incidence of high-grade toxicity.

There were also two possible treatment-related deaths from treatment. Although not explicitly stated in the manuscript, some of the patients in the series would have met the criteria for having ultra-central tumors, e.g., 9 patients had tumors directly abutting the esophagus.

In small cell lung cancer (SCLC), the development of esophagitis is of particular importance. In limited stage SCLC, patients receive radical doses of radiotherapy with concurrent chemotherapy, and since SCLC usually presents with multi-level mediastinal disease, a significant portion of the esophagus is often in the radiation field, which further increases the risk of esophageal toxicity. The data from the seminal Intergroup 0096 study, which showed improved survival with twice daily (BID) radiation, indicated a grade 3+ esophagitis rate of 27% with BID treatment (Turrisi et al. 1999). More recent data is available from the CONVERT trial, in which involved field radiotherapy was mandated, and many patients underwent intensity-modulated radiotherapy (IMRT) and positron emission tomography (PET) staging as per standard of care in the era of trial. The study showed that similar rates of toxicity in the two investigated arms (Faivre-Finn et al. 2017). The rates of grade 3+ esophagitis were 19% in both arms and lower compared to previous trials using with twice daily radiation.

Similar to limited stage SCLC, patients with locally advanced NSCLC (Stage III) undergoing definitive radiotherapy also have a significant portion of the esophagus in the radiotherapy field. The reported incidence of severe acute esophagitis (grade 3+) in patients treated with standard thoracic radiotherapy alone is 1.3%, and induction chemotherapy increases this risk slightly (Byhardt et al. 1998). Only 6% of patients receiving induction chemotherapy followed by standard radiotherapy developed severe acute esophagitis. When chemotherapy is given concurrently with thoracic radiotherapy, however, a strong radiosensitizing effect is evident. In the RTOG experience, 95% of patients receiving concurrent chemotherapy and thoracic radiotherapy experienced some degree of acute esophagitis. The highest grade of esophagitis reported was grade 1 in 20% of patients, grade 2 in 41%, grade 3 in 31%, and grade 4 in 2%. The incidence of severe esophagitis was higher (70 vs. 22%; $p < 0.0001$) in patients receiving hyperfractionated radiotherapy than in patients treated with conventional fractionation (Werner-Wasik et al. 2011). In other series, altered fractionation has been found to worsen the severity and duration of esophagitis. Ball et al. (1995) demonstrated that the duration of symptomatic esophagitis was 1.4 months in the conventional radiotherapy arm, 1.6 months in the arm given conventional radiotherapy with concurrent carboplatin, 3.2 months in the accelerated radiotherapy arm, and 2.4 months in the arm where accelerated radiotherapy was combined with concurrent carboplatin. With the continuous hyperfractionated accelerated radiation therapy (CHART) regimen, used without chemotherapy for locally advanced non-small cell lung cancer, 19% of patients experienced severe esophagitis (Saunders et al. 1997). Another altered fractionation scheme, the concomitant boost technique, resulted in a dose-limiting incidence of severe esophagitis of 33% of patients when delivered concurrently with chemotherapy (Dubray et al. 1995). It had been reported that particular agents, such as doxorubicin, cause severe primary or recall esophagitis at radiotherapy doses as low as 20.0 Gy (Boal et al. 1979). Gandara et al. (2003) reported a 20% incidence of severe acute esophagitis with radiotherapy using the cisplatin/etoposide regimen concurrently. Vokes et al. (2002) described an incidence of 52% of severe acute esophagitis (35% grade 3 and 17% grade 4 esophagitis) with concurrent gemcitabine and thoracic radiotherapy. Pulsed low dose paclitaxel (at escalating doses of 15, 20, and 25 mg/m^2 infused on Monday, Wednesday, and Friday, respectively) delivered concurrently with daily chest irradiation for radiosensitization was associated with 17% risk of grade 3 esophagitis; no grade 4 or 5 esophagitis was reported in this study (Chen et al. 2008). Other study used weekly paclitaxel 60 mg/m^2 concurrently with standard fractionated radiotherapy; the major toxicity was esophagitis, with 20% of the patients developing grade 4 esophagitis (Choy and Safran 1995). These experiences indicate that it is difficult to predict the severity of esophageal toxicity a novel chemoradiation regimen will cause. Whether the degree of esophagitis is related to scheduling of chemotherapy used (daily vs. weekly vs. every 3 weeks) is uncertain. Other factors associated with a higher risk of esophagitis include age 70 years (Langer et al. 2001), presence of dysphagia before radiotherapy initiation (Ahn et al. 2005), low pretreatment body mass index (Patel et al. 2004), and nodal stage of N2 or worse (Ahn et al. 2005). The extent of nodal involvement probably serves as a surrogate for the volume of esophagus irradiated. Despite high rates of acute esophagitis, late esophageal damage was infrequent (2% incidence) in the RTOG experience. Death due to esophagitis was practically non-existent (Werner-Wasik et al. 2011; Ahn et al. 2005) showed that the presence of acute esophageal injury was the most predictive factor for the development of late esophageal toxicity (stricture or fistula). The recent NRG/RTOG 0617 trial, comparing high-dose radiotherapy (74 Gy) vs. standard-dose radiotherapy (60 Gy), found a 21% rate of esophagitis in high-dose arm compared to 7% in the standard-dose arm. The study also showed that the development of high-grade esophagitis was independently associated with inferior survival (Bradley et al. 2015).

To summarize, the two most important factors related to the development of esophagitis are the radiation dose received to the esophagus and the use of concurrent chemotherapy. Section 4 describes the dosimetric parameters in detail. The use of concurrent chemotherapy can increase the risk of esophagitis up to sixfold, as reviewed in this meta-analysis which includes many of the trials mentioned above (Ramroth et al. 2016). Predictive factors for the development of esophagitis were also systematically reviewed in a large individual patient meta-analysis, consisting of data from 1082 patients who underwent chemoradiation for NSCLC (Palma et al. 2013). The study showed that prescription dose/fractionation, esophagus dosimetry, type of concurrent chemotherapy and stage were predictive for the development of esophagitis, but only dosimetric factors had good discrimination scores ($c > 0.60$).

In additional to conventional clinical and dosimetric parameters which can predict for esophageal toxicity, there is accruing evidence to support that patients genetic profile may modulate this risk (Guerra et al. 2012). In a multicenter prospective study from Spain and France, 247 patients undergoing radiotherapy for lung cancer were genotyped for 7 single nucleotide polymorphisms (SNPs) along the TGFB1 and HSPB1 genes, which are known to associated with cellular radio-sensitivity (Delgado et al. 2019). The study showed that rs7459185CC genotype was predictive for acute radiation-induced esophageal toxicity, and rs11466353TT/TG genotype was predictive for late radiation-induced esophageal toxicity. Further studies are required to validate these biomarkers, which could further guide the personalized delivery of radiotherapy.

4 Dosimetric Factors Associated with Esophagitis

Preclinical data suggest that doubling the length of irradiated portion of the esophagus leads to a decrease of the LD50 (dose causing the death of 50% of irradiated animals) (Michalowski and Hornsey 1986). However, the clinical evidence that esophageal toxicity is correlated to esophageal length irradiated remains controversial. Ball et al. (1995) analyzed the outcomes of 100 patients divided into three groups based on length of treatment field (<14.0, 14.0–15.9, and [16.0 cm) presumed to correlate with the length of esophagus irradiated. No relationship between treatment field length and the severity of esophagitis was observed. In Choy's analysis of 120 patients (Choy et al. 1999), there was no correlation between esophagitis grade and length of esophagus in either the primary ($p = 0.4$) or boost ($p = 0.1$) radiation fields. We studied 105 lung cancer patients treated with concurrent chemoradiotherapy or radiotherapy alone. Acute esophagitis was scored prospectively in a uniform fashion, and precise measurements of the esophageal length within each radiation field were available (Werner-Wasik et al. 2000). Again, increasing length of esophagus in the radiation field did not predict for the severity of acute esophagitis.

Recent advances in three-dimensional conformal radiation therapy (3DCRT) allow us to correlate volumetric data to organ damage rather than rely on the older estimates based on organ length (esophagus). The dosimetric study by Maguire et al. (1999) established a relationship between high-dose irradiation of the entire esophageal circumference and esophagitis risk. They reported a detailed dosimetric analysis of 91 patients treated to a median corrected dose of 78.8 Gy. The percent of esophageal volume treated to [50.0 Gy and the maximum percent of esophageal circumference treated to [80.0 Gy were significant predictors of late (but interestingly not acute) esophagitis. The concept emerging from this data was the importance of sparing portions of the esophageal circumference to limit esophageal toxicity.

The association between esophageal dose–volume histograms (DVHs) and the risk of radiation-induced esophagitis was further evaluated by several authors. These data were recently reviewed by the organ specific quantitative analysis of normal tissue effects in the clinic (QUANTEC) group (Werner-Wasik et al. 2010). In general, the data are consistent with some risk of acute esophagitis at intermediate doses of 30–50 Gy and an increasing effect for greater doses. Volumes of esophagus receiving doses higher than 50 Gy have been identified as highly statistically significantly correlated with acute esophagitis in several studies. Rates of acute grade [2 esophagitis appear to increase to over 30% as V70 exceeds 20%, V50 exceeds 40%, and V35 exceeds 50% (Fig. 1). However, due to diverse methods of reporting volumetric data (absolute volume or area, relative volume or area, and circumferential measures), no consensus for definitive dosimetric recommendations has been reached. Another confounding factor is the fact that in some studies, the entire esophagus was not delineated, making volumetric measurements difficult to interpret (Werner-Wasik et al. 2010). The entire length has to be identified (from the cricoid

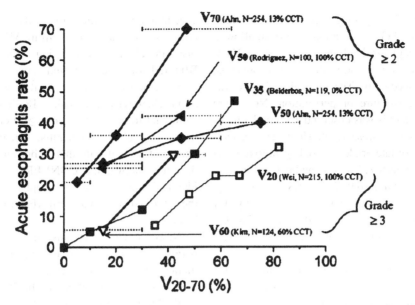

Fig. 1 Incidence of acute esophagitis according to Vx (volume receiving more than x Gy). X-axis values estimated according to range of doses reported. Each curve annotated as follows: Vdose (investigator, number of patients, percentage with concurrent chemotherapy [CCT]). Percentage of patients who received sequential chemotherapy in studies by Ahn et al. (2005), Belderbos et al. (2005), and Kim et al. (2005) was 44%, 38%, and 15%, respectively. Data for V50 (Ahn et al. 2005) at 15, 45, and 75 Gy represent reported rates of grade 2 or greater acute esophagitis plotted in dose bins at \30%, 30–60%, and [60%, respectively. Similarly, for V70 (Ahn et al. 2005), V50 (Rodríguez et al. 2009), and V60 (Kim et al. 2005), each symbol represents rates of acute esophagitis at \10% versus 11–30% versus 31–64%, and \30 versus [30%, and \30 versus [30%, respectively. Dashed horizontal lines reflect dose ranges ascribed to each data point. Upper X-axis range of greatest data point for V50 (Rodríguez et al. 2009), V50 (Ahn et al. 2005), and V60 (Kim et al. 2005), is indefinite according to data (light-gray dotted bars). Solid and open symbols represent reported rates of grade 2 or greater acute esophagitis and grade 3 or greater acute esophagitis, respectively. Thicker and thinner solid lines represent higher and lower doses of Vx, respectively (i.e., thicker line for V70 and thinner line for V20). (Reprinted from Werner-Wasik et al. (2010). Copyright (2010), with permission from Elsevier)

cartilage to the gastro-esophageal junction). Moreover, on axial computed-tomography (CT) imaging, the esophageal circumference varies significantly. This is a reflection of the swallowing act, and it does not reflect the anatomic reality of a relatively uniform circumference (Kahn et al. 2005). Therefore, conventional DVHs might not correctly reflect the partial volume dose and may be misleading. Likewise, the esophagus is slightly mobile; the cephalad, middle, and caudal esophagus can move \5, 7, and 9 mm, respectively, during normal respiration (Dieleman et al. 2007). This may introduce additional uncertainties into volumetric analyses based on planning CT scans. No specific margin recommendations can be given at the present time (Werner-Wasik et al. 2010). Recent studies evaluating escalating radiotherapy dose (standard fractionation) or hypofractionated schedules for lung cancer have been published or designed. In each situation, novel restraints had to be placed on the doses to be delivered to the normal organs in the chest such as lung, esophagus, and spinal cord.

RTOG 93-11 study evaluated the feasibility of dose escalation for patients with locally advanced non-small cell lung cancer treated with 3DCRT to the gross tumor only, without elective nodal irradiation. Maximum doses of 77.4–90.3 Gy were prescribed, depending on the percentage of the total lung receiving more than 20.0 Gy. This trial of thoracic radiotherapy alone escalated the dose to the tumor up to 90.3 Gy in group 1 (<25% of both lungs receiving [20 Gy), up to 83.8 Gy in group 2 (25–37% of lungs receiving <20 Gy), and up to 77.4 Gy in group 3 (<37% of lung receiving <20 Gy). The maximum dose allowed to 1/3 of esophageal volume was 65 Gy, to 2/3 of the volume, 58 Gy, and to the whole esophagus, 55 Gy, respectively. The clinical endpoint was esophageal stricture or perforation. No severe acute esophagitis was observed even in the highest radiotherapy dose level. However, the estimated rate of late grade [3 esophageal toxicity at 18 months was 8%, 0%, 4%, and 6% for group 1 patients receiving 70.9, 77.4, 83.8, and 90.3 Gy, respectively, and 0% and 5%, respectively, for group 2 patients receiving 70.9 and 77.4 Gy (Bradley et al. 2005), suggesting a dose–response relationship.

As described above, the risk factors for development of esophagitis were systematically reviewed in the STRIPE meta-analysis (Palma et al. 2013), which showed that increased radiation dose to the esophagus was most predictive for developing high-grade radiation esophagitis. On multivariable analysis, the esophageal volume receiving ≥60 Gy (V60) alone emerged as the best predictor of grade 2+ and 3+ esophagitis. Patients with a very low V60 <1% have a low risk of esophagitis (<5% risk of grade ≥3 toxicity), whereas a V60 above 17% conferred a high risk of esophagitis (22% of grade ≥3 toxicity). Other correlated dosimetric parameters including V50 also served as good predictors of radiation esophagitis. The recent NRG/RTOG 0617 trial, which showed that the development of high-grade esophagitis was independently associated with inferior survival (Bradley et al. 2015), recommended that mean esophageal dose be limited to 34 Gy and that the esophageal V60 should be documented for each patient. Patients in the 74 Gy arm had a higher median V60 of 25.4% compared to patients in the 60 Gy arm, where the median V60 was 11.7%.

In limited stage, SCLC patients undergoing chemoradiation to a dose of 40 Gy in 15 fractions and 45 Gy in 30 fractions, institutional series from Princess Margaret Cancer Center showed that grade 3 esophagitis was correlated with mean esophagus dose and minimum dose to the hottest 45% of the esophagus (Giuliani et al. 2015). The study showed no significant difference in toxicity profile between the two radiation doses. A similar analysis from MD Anderson institutional series comparing once daily and BID radiation did not find any difference in esophageal toxicity between the two fractionation schemes (Suzuki et al. 2018). The study did show that total radiation dose ≥60 Gy was predictive of grade 3+ esophagitis, with an 18% incidence of toxicity in this subgroup. Also, as described above, the CONVERT trial showed identical rates of grade 3+ esophagitis (19%) in the BID and once daily arm (Faivre-Finn et al. 2017).

Newer models have investigated dosimetric parameters predictive of esophagitis in proton therapy. A Lyman–Kutcher–Burman (LKB) normal tissue complication probability (NTCP) model has been proposed and the TD50 = 45 Gy for grade 2+ esophagitis (Wang et al. 2020). As described below, experience with proton therapy is limited to centers with access to these facilities, and the techniques and models will need to be externally validated before more widespread adoption.

The existing models and dose–volume parameters described above should be applied only to regimens using conventional fractionated radiotherapy regimens. In patients undergoing lung SBRT, the development of esophageal toxicity is rare, but increased in patients with central lung tumors. An institutional review of 125 patients from Memorial Sloan Kettering identified dosimetric predictors of esophageal toxicity after SBRT to central lung tumors (Wu et al. 2014). The study indicated that dose to the hottest 5 cc and Dmax of the esophagus were the best predictors of toxicity. It was recommended that the D5cc BED10 to the esophagus should be kept less than 16.8, 18.1, and 19.0 Gy for 3, 4, and 5 fractions, respectively, to keep the acute toxicity rate <20%. For more protracted SBRT schedules, the Erasmus series estimated that the probability of late high-grade toxicity is 1.1% for 8 fractions and 1.4% for 12 fractions when using the D1cc ≤40 Gy for 8 fractions and D1cc ≤48 Gy for 12 fractions (Duijm et al. 2020).

In addition to using dosimetric parameters alone to predict the esophageal toxicity, there is increasing interest in using multi-parametric models to improve the predictive capabilities for esophagitis. For example, Wijsman et al. (2015) showed that multivariable NTCP model including use of concurrent chemotherapy, esophagus Dmean, clinical tumor stage, and gender was highly predictive for grade 2+ radiation esophagitis with a AUC of 0.82. Similarly, Wang et al. (2018) investigated the use of inflammatory cytokines in predicting radiation esophagitis and showed that adding age and IL-8 to esophagus generalized equivalent uniform dose created a model with more predictive power.

5 Strategies Used to Prevent or Treat Esophagitis

Given the potential for dosimetry to impact the incidence and severity of radiation esophagitis, various approaches have been tested to optimize these parameters. Intensity-modulated radiation therapy (IMRT) seems well suited for such a purpose, with its ability to deliver concave-shaped radiotherapy dose distributions around organs at risk, such as esophagus. Grills et al. (2003) compared four different radiotherapy techniques for 18 patients with stage I–IIIB inoperable non-small cell lung cancer: IMRT, optimized 3DCRT using multiple beam angles, limited 3DCRT using 2–3 beams, and traditional radiotherapy using elective nodal irradiation to treat the mediastinum. The techniques were compared by giving each plan a tumor control probability equivalent to that of the optimized 3DCRT plan delivering 70 Gy. Using this method, IMRT and 3DCRT offered similar results with regard to the mean lung dose and the esophageal normal tissue complication probability (NTCP) in lymph node negative patients. However, IMRT reduced the lung V20 and the mean lung dose by approximately 15% and the lung NTCP by 30% when compared with 3DCRT in lymph node positive cases. The authors concluded that IMRT is beneficial in selected patients, particularly those with positive lymph nodes or those with target volumes in close proximity to the esophagus.

Moreover, in lymph node positive patients, IMRT allowed delivery of radiation doses 25–30% greater than 3DCRT while maintaining an equal probability of pulmonary and esophageal toxicity.

The potential clinical advantages of using IMRT compared to 3D CRT we investigated in a post-hoc analysis of NRG/RTOG 0617 (Chun et al. 2017). Although the study showed marginally higher esophagus doses in the 3D CRT arm, this did not translate into an observed difference in grade 3+ esophageal toxicity. In addition to planning a homogenous dose distribution to the target volumes, there has been interest in using functional imaging (18F-FDG PET) to guide dose escalation to metabolically active sites of disease and dose de-escalation to elective lymph node regions. The strategy of Imaging-based target volume reduction was formally tested in a randomized controlled trial PET-Plan, where the experimental arm received radiotherapy to the ^{18}F-FDG PET-based targets, and no elective nodal irradiation was allowed (Nestle et al. 2020). The study showed that locoregional control was non-inferior in experimental arm; however there was no difference in grade 3+ toxicity in both arms. Additional methods to limit further limit esophageal toxicity in IMRT have been investigated including a Contralateral Esophagus Sparing Technique (CEST). In this method, the esophageal wall contralateral to gross tumor is contoured as an avoidance structure to guide a steep dose falloff gradient across the esophagus, except on slices where tumor surrounded the esophagus (Al-Halabi et al. 2015). Preliminary results from a phase I study of 20 analyable patients with locally advanced lung cancer treated with chemoradiation showed a lower rate than expected rates of esophagitis, with no grade 3+ toxicities observed (Kamran et al. 2020).

The use of IMRT has been conventionally limited to localized cancers where radical doses of radiotherapy are delivered. However, there is increasing recognition that patients receiving palliative doses of radiotherapy for incurable disease may also develop esophagitis (Nieder et al. 2020). A recent randomized phase III trial,

PROACTIVE, investigated the potential of esophageal sparing IMRT in reducing esophagitis after 20 Gy in 5 fractions or 30 Gy in 10 fractions of palliative radiotherapy. Preliminary results from the study showed IMRT demonstrated a trend toward improved esophageal quality of life and reduced the incidence of symptomatic esophagitis (Louie et al. 2020).

To further optimize radiation dosimetry, the use of proton beam radiotherapy has been investigated (Chap. xxx), which allows a rapidly increasing dose at the end of the beam range (Bragg peak). Therefore, with proper distribution of proton energies, the dose can be uniform across the target volume and essentially zero deep to it. As a result, dose to the tumor can be increased, while the frequency and severity of the treatment-related toxicity could theoretically be decreased.

Early experience from MD Anderson Center showed that when proton radiation was delivered concurrently with carboplatin and paclitaxel chemotherapy, a higher dose of radiotherapy could be delivered with a very low risk of toxicity (grade 3+ pneumonitis = 2% and grade 3+ esophagitis = 5%) compared to other cohorts treated with IMRT or 3D-CRT (Sejpal et al. 2011). A subsequent randomized trial comparing passive scattering proton therapy and IMRT in LA-NSCLC did not demonstrate a difference in radiation pneumonitis or local control (Liao et al. 2018). The role of proton therapy in lung cancer is being definitively tested in NRG Oncology RTOG1308, a randomized phase 3 trial comparing 70-Gy photon radiation versus 70-Gy proton radiation, with concurrent chemotherapy (platinum-based doublet).

In addition to optimizing the technical delivery of radiotherapy, additionally strategies to limit esophagitis using a radioprotective agent have also been explored. The most well studied radioprotectant agent in in lung cancer is amifostine, which is a phosphorothioate delivered intravenously or subcutaneously prior to radiation treatment. Encouraging results reported in Phase II (Komaki et al. 2004) as well as Phase III randomized trials (Antonadou et al. 2001) led to the development of RTOG 98-01, a large cooperative group Phase III randomized study that tested the efficacy of amifostine in preventing esophagitis in non-small cell lung cancer patients receiving thoracic radiotherapy with concurrent carboplatin, paclitaxel chemotherapy (Movsas et al. 2005). Patients were randomized to receive amifostine (500 mg intravenously four times weekly, preceding the afternoon dose of radiotherapy) versus no amifostine. RTOG 98-01 showed that amifostine did not reduce severe esophagitis (30% rate with amifostine vs. 34% without), as assessed by the NCI CTCAE criteria and weekly physician dysphagia logs. Evaluation of patient diaries, however, indicated that amifostine conferred a significant reduction in swallowing dysfunction measured over time (equivalent of esophagitis index), a decrease in pain after chemoradiotherapy, and diminished weight loss in patients receiving chemoradiation (Sarna et al. 2008). Of note, only 40% of all radiotherapy fractions were "protected" by amifostine infusion in that study, and only 29% of patients received the medication according to the protocol. Further investigation of this agent is therefore justified, possibly with subcutaneous administration in order to increase the compliance and to allow higher dose intensity of amifostine. Another agent utilized to limit esophagitis is oral sucralfate. Although applied commonly in the clinic, this agent was shown not to have value in decreasing acute esophagitis in a double-blind Phase III randomized trial of 97 patients receiving thoracic radiotherapy (McGinnis et al. 1997).

An interesting approach of plasmid/liposome delivery by the human manganese superoxide dismutase transgene has been reported to be successful in prevention of radiation esophagitis in mice receiving carboplatin, paclitaxel, and thoracic radiotherapy (Stickle et al. 1999). GC4419, a superoxide dismutase mimetic, has been shown to reduce severe oral mucositis from concurrent chemoradiotherapy in head and neck cancer (Anderson et al. 2019). Its use is being investigated in reducing esophagitis in lung cancer patients undergoing chemoradiotherapy (NCT04225026).

In addition to novel pharmacological targets, the use of natural supplements has been investigated in a few trials. Based on encouraging data from head and neck clinical trials, the use of prophylactic Manuka honey was investigated in patients undergoing chemoradiation in NRG Oncology RTOG 1012 (Fogh et al. 2017). The study showed that both liquid and lozenge honey were not superior to best supportive care in preventing radiation esophagitis. More recently, the use of the oral epigallocatechin-3-gallate (EGCG) was tested in a prospective single arm and subsequent phase II randomized study (Zhao et al. 2019). The randomized study showed that prophylactic administration of EGCG was associated with decreased maximum grade of radiation esophagitis, and as well as esophagitis, pain, and dysphagia index scores. Chang et al. (2019) investigated the role of oral glutamine supplements in reducing esophagitis in a randomized study of patients undergoing chemoradiation for NSCLC. The study showed that glutamine supplements decreased the incidence of grade 2/3 radiation esophagitis, delayed the onset of esophagitis and reduced the incidence of clinically significant weight loss. However, a subsequent placebo-controlled trial did not show any benefit of glutamine for prevention of radiation-induced esophagitis (Alshawa et al. 2021).

Addressing this dose-limiting toxicity is imperative for the intensification of radiotherapy and chemotherapy protocols. Future effort is necessary in order to find effective measures to minimize or eliminate esophagitis.

References

Ahn S-J et al (2005) Dosimetric and clinical predictors for radiation-induced esophageal injury. Int J Radiat Oncol Biol Phys 61(2):335–347
Al-Halabi H et al (2015) A contralateral esophagus-sparing technique to limit severe esophagitis associated with concurrent high-dose radiation and chemotherapy in patients with thoracic malignancies. Int J Radiat Oncol Biol Phys 92(4):803–810
Alshawa A et al (2021) Effects of glutamine for prevention of radiation-induced esophagitis: a double-blind placebo-controlled trial. Invest New Drugs 39:1113–1122
Anderson CM et al (2019) Phase IIb, randomized, double-blind trial of GC4419 versus placebo to reduce severe oral mucositis due to concurrent radiotherapy and cisplatin for head and neck cancer. J Clin Oncol 37(34):3256
Antonadou D et al (2001) Randomized phase III trial of radiation treatment ± amifostine in patients with advanced-stage lung cancer. Int J Radiat Oncol Biol Phys 51(4):915–922
Ball D et al (1995) A phase III study of accelerated radiotherapy with and without carboplatin in nonsmall cell lung cancer: an interim toxicity analysis of the first 100 patients. Int J Radiat Oncol Biol Phys 31(2): 267–272
Ball D et al (2019) Stereotactic ablative radiotherapy versus standard radiotherapy in stage 1 non-small-cell lung cancer (TROG 09.02 CHISEL): a phase 3, open-label, randomised controlled trial. Lancet Oncol 20(4):494–503
Belderbos J et al (2005) Acute esophageal toxicity in non-small cell lung cancer patients after high dose conformal radiotherapy. Radiother Oncol 75(2):157–164
Bezjak A et al (2019) Safety and efficacy of a five-fraction stereotactic body radiotherapy schedule for centrally located non–small-cell lung cancer: NRG oncology/RTOG 0813 trial. J Clin Oncol 37(15):1316
Boal DK, Newburger PE, Teele RL (1979) Esophagitis induced by combined radiation and adriamycin. Am J Roentgenol 132(4):567–570
Bradley J et al (2005) Toxicity and outcome results of RTOG 9311: a phase I–II dose-escalation study using three-dimensional conformal radiotherapy in patients with inoperable non–small-cell lung carcinoma. Int J Radiat Oncol Biol Phys 61(2):318–328
Bradley JD et al (2015) Standard-dose versus high-dose conformal radiotherapy with concurrent and consolidation carboplatin plus paclitaxel with or without cetuximab for patients with stage IIIA or IIIB non-small-cell lung cancer (RTOG 0617): a randomised, two-by-two factorial phase 3 study. Lancet Oncol 16(2):187–199
Byhardt RW et al (1998) Response, toxicity, failure patterns, and survival in five Radiation Therapy Oncology Group (RTOG) trials of sequential and/or concurrent chemotherapy and radiotherapy for locally advanced non–small-cell carcinoma of the lung. Int J Radiat Oncol Biol Phys 42(3):469–478
Chang S-C et al (2019) Oral glutamine supplements reduce concurrent chemoradiotherapy-induced esophagitis in patients with advanced non small cell lung cancer. Medicine 98(8):e14463
Chen Y et al (2008) Toxicity profile and pharmacokinetic study of a phase I low-dose schedule–dependent radiosensitizing paclitaxel chemoradiation regimen for inoperable non–small-cell lung cancer. Int J Radiat Oncol Biol Phys 71(2):407–413
Chen H et al (2019) Safety and effectiveness of stereotactic ablative radiotherapy for ultra-central lung lesions: a systematic review. J Thorac Oncol 14(8):1332–1342
Choi GB et al (2005) Fluoroscopically guided balloon dilation for patients with esophageal stricture after radiation treatment. J Vasc Interv Radiol 16(12):1705–1709
Chowhan NM (1990) Injurious effects of radiation on the esophagus. Am J Gastroenterol 85(2):115–120

Choy H, Safran H (1995) Preliminary analysis of a phase II study of weekly paclitaxel and concurrent radiation therapy for locally advanced non-small cell lung cancer. Semin Oncol 22(4 Suppl 9):55

Choy H et al (1999) Esophagitis in combined modality therapy for locally advanced non-small cell lung cancer. Semin Radiat Oncol 9(2 Suppl 1):90

Chun SG et al (2017) Impact of intensity-modulated radiation therapy technique for locally advanced non–small-cell lung cancer: a secondary analysis of the NRG oncology RTOG 0617 randomized clinical trial. J Clin Oncol 35(1):56

Cox JD et al (1993) Interruptions of high-dose radiation therapy decrease longterm survival of favorable patients with unresectable nonsmall cell carcinoma of the lung: analysis of 1244 cases from 3 radiation therapy oncology group (RTOG) trials. Int J Radiat Oncol Biol Phys 27(3):493–498

Delgado BD, Enguix-Riego MV, de Bobadilla JC, Rivera DH, Gómez JM, Praena-Fernández JM, Del Campo ER, Gordillo MJ, Fernandez MD, Guerra JL (2019) Association of single nucleotide polymorphisms at HSPB1 rs7459185 and TGFB1 rs11466353 with radiation esophagitis in lung cancer. Radiot and Oncol 135:161–9.

Dieleman EMT et al (2007) Four-dimensional computed tomographic analysis of esophageal mobility during normal respiration. Int J Radiat Oncol Biol Phys 67(3):775–780

Dubray B et al (1995) Combined chemoradiation for locally advanced nonsmall cell lung cancer. J Infus Chemother 5(4):195–196

Duijm M et al (2020) Predicting high-grade esophagus toxicity after treating central lung tumors with stereotactic radiation therapy using a normal tissue complication probability model. Int J Radiat Oncol Biol Phys 106(1):73–81

Faivre-Finn C et al (2017) Concurrent once-daily versus twice-daily chemoradiotherapy in patients with limited-stage small-cell lung cancer (CONVERT): an open-label, phase 3, randomised, superiority trial. Lancet Oncol 18(8):1116–1125

Fogh SE et al (2017) A randomized phase 2 trial of prophylactic manuka honey for the reduction of chemoradiation therapy–induced esophagitis during the treatment of lung cancer: results of NRG oncology RTOG 1012. Int J Radiat Oncol Biol Phys 97(4):786–796

Gandara DR et al (2003) Consolidation docetaxel after concurrent chemoradiotherapy in stage IIIB non–small-cell lung cancer: Phase II Southwest Oncology Group Study S9504. J Clin Oncol 21(10):2004–2010

Giuliani ME et al (2015) Correlation of dosimetric and clinical factors with the development of esophagitis and radiation pneumonitis in patients with limited-stage small-cell lung carcinoma. Clin Lung Cancer 16(3):216–220

Goldstein HM et al (1975) Radiological manifestations of radiation-induced injury to the normal upper gastrointestinal tract. Radiology 117(1):135–140

Grills IS et al (2003) Potential for reduced toxicity and dose escalation in the treatment of inoperable non–small-cell lung cancer: a comparison of intensity-modulated radiation therapy (IMRT), 3D conformal radiation, and elective nodal irradiation. Int J Radiat Oncol Biol Phys 57(3):875–890

Guerra JL, Gomez D, Wei Q, Liu Z, Wang LE, Yuan X, Zhuang Y, Komaki R, Liao Z (2012) Association between single nucleotide polymorphisms of the transforming growth factor β1 gene and the risk of severe radiation esophagitis in patients with lung cancer. Radiother Oncol 105(3):299–304

Kahn D et al (2005) "Anatomically-correct" dosimetric parameters may be better predictors for esophageal toxicity than are traditional CT-based metrics. Int J Radiat Oncol Biol Phys 62(3):645–651

Kamran SC et al (2020) Phase I trial of an IMRT-based Contralateral Esophagus Sparing Technique (CEST) in locally advanced NSCLC and SCLC treated to 70 Gy. Int J Radiat Oncol Biol Phys 108(3):S104–S105

Kim TH et al (2005) Dose-volumetric parameters of acute esophageal toxicity in patients with lung cancer treated with three-dimensional conformal radiotherapy. Int J Radiat Oncol Biol Phys 62(4):995–1002

Komaki R et al (2004) Effects of amifostine on acute toxicity from concurrent chemotherapy and radiotherapy for inoperable non–small-cell lung cancer: report of a randomized comparative trial. Int J Radiat Oncol Biol Phys 58(5):1369–1377

Langer CJ et al (2001) Do elderly patients (pts) with locally advanced non-small cell lung cancer (NSCLC) benefit from combined modality therapy? A secondary analysis of RTOG 94-10. Int J Radiat Oncol Biol Phys 51(3):20–21

Lepke RA, Libshitz HI (1983) Radiation-induced injury of the esophagus. Radiology 148(2):375–378

Liao Z et al (2018) Bayesian adaptive randomization trial of passive scattering proton therapy and intensity-modulated photon radiotherapy for locally advanced non–small-cell lung cancer. J Clin Oncol 36(18):1813

Louie AV et al (2020) A phase III randomized trial of palliative radiation for advanced central lung tumors with intentional avoidance of the esophagus (PROACTIVE). Int J Radiat Oncol Biol Phys 108(3):S105–S106

Maguire PD et al (1999) Clinical and dosimetric predictors of radiation-induced esophageal toxicity. Int J Radiat Oncol Biol Phys 45(1):97–103

McGinnis WL et al (1997) Placebo-controlled trial of sucralfate for inhibiting radiation-induced esophagitis. J Clin Oncol 15(3):1239–1243

Mehmood Q et al (2016) Predicting radiation esophagitis using 18F-FDG PET during chemoradiotherapy for locally advanced non–small cell lung cancer. J Thorac Oncol 11(2):213–221

Michalowski A, Hornsey S (1986) Assays of damage to the alimentary canal. Br J Cancer Suppl 7:1

Movsas B et al (2005) Randomized trial of amifostine in locally advanced non–small-cell lung cancer patients receiving chemotherapy and hyperfractionated radiation: Radiation Therapy Oncology Group trial 98-01. J Clin Oncol 23(10):2145–2154

Nestle U et al (2020) Imaging-based target volume reduction in chemoradiotherapy for locally advanced non-small-cell lung cancer (PET-Plan): a multicentre, open-label, randomised, controlled trial. Lancet Oncol 21(4):581–592

Nieder C et al (2020) Risk factors for esophagitis after hypofractionated palliative (chemo) radiotherapy for non-small cell lung cancer. Radiat Oncol 15:1–6

Niedzielski JS et al (2016a) Objectively quantifying radiation esophagitis with novel computed tomography-based metrics. Int J Radiat Oncol Biol Phys 94(2):385–393

Niedzielski JS et al (2016b) 18F-Fluorodeoxyglucose Positron Emission Tomography can quantify and predict esophageal injury during radiation therapy. Int J Radiat Oncol Biol Phys 96(3):670–678

Palma DA, Senan S, Oberije C, Belderbos J, De Dios NR, Bradley JD, Barriger RB, Moreno-Jiménez M, Kim TH, Ramella S, Everitt S (2013) Predicting esophagitis after chemoradiation therapy for non-small cell lung cancer: an individual patient data meta-analysis. Int J Radiat Oncol Biol Phys 87(4):690–696

Patel AB et al (2004) Predictors of acute esophagitis in patients with non–small-cell lung carcinoma treated with concurrent chemotherapy and hyperfractionated radiotherapy followed by surgery. Int J Radiat Oncol Biol Phys 60(4):1106–1112

Phillips TL, Ross G (1974) Time-dose relationships in the mouse esophagus. Radiology 113(2):435–440

Ramroth J, Cutter DJ, Darby SC, Higgins GS, McGale P, Partridge M, Taylor CW (2016) Dose and fractionation in radiation therapy of curative intent for non-small cell lung cancer: meta-analysis of randomized trials. Int J Radiat Oncol Biol Phys 96(4):736–47

Rodríguez N et al (2009) Predictors of acute esophagitis in lung cancer patients treated with concurrent three-dimensional conformal radiotherapy and chemotherapy. Int J Radiat Oncol Biol Phys 73(3):810–817

Sarna L et al (2008) Clinically meaningful differences in patient-reported outcomes with amifostine in combination with chemoradiation for locally advanced non–small-cell lung cancer: an analysis of RTOG 9801. Int J Radiat Oncol Biol Phys 72(5):1378–1384

Saunders M et al (1997) Continuous hyperfractionated accelerated radiotherapy (CHART) versus conventional radiotherapy in non-small-cell lung cancer: a randomised multicentre trial. Lancet 350(9072):161–165

Sejpal S et al (2011) Early findings on toxicity of proton beam therapy with concurrent chemotherapy for nonsmall cell lung cancer. Cancer 117(13):3004–3013

Stickle RL et al (1999) Prevention of irradiation-induced esophagitis by plasmid/liposome delivery of the human manganese superoxide dismutase transgene. Radiat Oncol Investig 7(4):204–217

Suzuki R et al (2018) Twice-daily thoracic radiotherapy for limited-stage small-cell lung cancer does not increase the incidence of acute severe esophagitis. Clin Lung Cancer 19(6):e885–e891

Turrisi AT et al (1999) Twice-daily compared with once-daily thoracic radiotherapy in limited small-cell lung cancer treated concurrently with cisplatin and etoposide. N Engl J Med 340(4):265–271

Vokes EE et al (2002) Randomized phase II study of cisplatin with gemcitabine or paclitaxel or vinorelbine as induction chemotherapy followed by concomitant chemoradiotherapy for stage IIIB non–small-cell lung cancer: Cancer and Leukemia Group B study 9431. J Clin Oncol 20(20):4191–4198

Wang S et al (2018) A model combining age, equivalent uniform dose and IL-8 may predict radiation esophagitis in patients with non-small cell lung cancer. Radiother Oncol 126(3):506–510

Wang Z et al (2020) Lyman–Kutcher–Burman normal tissue complication probability modeling for radiation-induced esophagitis in non-small cell lung cancer patients receiving proton radiotherapy. Radiother Oncol 146:200–204

Werner-Wasik M et al (2000) Predictors of severe esophagitis include use of concurrent chemotherapy, but not the length of irradiated esophagus: a multivariate analysis of patients with lung cancer treated with nonoperative therapy. Int J Radiat Oncol Biol Phys 48(3):689–696

Werner-Wasik M et al (2002) Phase II: trial of twice weekly amifostine in patients with non-small cell lung cancer treated with chemoradiotherapy. Semin Radiat Oncol 12(1):34–39

Werner-Wasik M et al (2010) Radiation dose-volume effects in the esophagus. Int J Radiat Oncol Biol Phys 76(3):S86–S93

Werner-Wasik M et al (2011) Acute esophagitis and late lung toxicity in concurrent chemoradiotherapy trials in patients with locally advanced non–small-cell lung cancer: analysis of the Radiation Therapy Oncology Group (RTOG) database. Clin Lung Cancer 12(4):245–251

Wijsman R et al (2015) Multivariable normal-tissue complication modeling of acute esophageal toxicity in advanced stage non-small cell lung cancer patients treated with intensity-modulated (chemo-) radiotherapy. Radiother Oncol 117(1):49–54

Wu AJ et al (2014) Dosimetric predictors of esophageal toxicity after stereotactic body radiotherapy for central lung tumors. Radiother Oncol 112(2):267–271

Yau V et al (2018) Low incidence of esophageal toxicity after lung stereotactic body radiation therapy: are current esophageal dose constraints too conservative? Int J Radiat Oncol Biol Phys 101(3):574–580

Yuan ST et al (2014) Timing and intensity of changes in FDG uptake with symptomatic esophagitis during radiotherapy or chemo-radiotherapy. Radiat Oncol 9(1):1–6

Zhao H et al (2019) A prospective, three-arm, randomized trial of EGCG for preventing radiation-induced esophagitis in lung cancer patients receiving radiotherapy. Radiother Oncol 137:186–191

Brain Toxicity

C. Nieder

Contents

1 Introduction 969
2 Pathogenesis of Radiotherapy-Induced Brain Toxicity 970
3 Acute and Subacute Radiotherapy-Induced Brain Toxicity 973
4 Delayed or Chronic Radiotherapy-Induced Brain Toxicity 973
5 Toxicity Prevention Strategies 977
6 Treatment of Radiotherapy-Induced Brain Toxicity 979
7 Aspects of Chemotherapy-Induced Brain Toxicity 979

References 979

Abstract

Since lung cancer generally has a high, stage-, histology-, and molecular subtype-dependent propensity for brain metastases, many patients receive prophylactic or therapeutic radiotherapy to the brain and are therefore at risk of acute, subacute, or chronic side effects. Certain types of systemic treatment might also cause brain toxicity. In this chapter the different types of toxicity, the pathogenesis, and emerging prevention and treatment strategies are reviewed.

1 Introduction

Prevention and treatment of brain metastases continue to be an important issue despite considerable improvements in local and systemic therapy for lung cancer. As long as many patients are diagnosed in advanced stages of the disease, their risk for developing brain metastases is high. Up to 60% of patients with small cell lung cancer (SCLC) will be diagnosed with brain metastases at some time during the natural course of the disease. Therefore, prophylactic cranial irradiation (PCI) has historically been recommended in the majority of patients with SCLC (Rusthoven and Kavanagh 2017). Recently, magnetic resonance imaging (MRI) surveillance with deferred radiotherapy (if needed) has emerged as

C. Nieder (✉)
Department of Oncology and Palliative Medicine,
Nordland Hospital, Bodø, Norway
e-mail: Carsten.Nieder@nordlandssykehuset.no

possible strategy for patients with extensive disease who respond to systemic therapy (Takahashi et al. 2017; Nosaki et al. 2018). The second indication for brain irradiation in lung cancer is palliation of symptoms from brain metastases (in selected cases durable local control is the aim) (Nieder et al. 2019). Depending on the number of lesions, their size and location, and well-established prognostic factors (Nieder et al. 2009; Sperduto et al. 2017; Nieder et al. 2018), whole-brain radiotherapy (WBRT), open surgical resection, or stereotactic radiosurgery (SRS) may be the preferred option. Another indication is adjuvant radiotherapy after resection of brain metastases, traditionally administered to the whole brain, and now increasingly as fractionated stereotactic radiotherapy (FSRT) or SRS of the tumor bed (Brown et al. 2017). This chapter will therefore cover the normal tissue effects of both partial brain radiotherapy and WBRT to the normal adult brain. The issue of reduced tolerance in the immature brain will not be discussed, due to the fact that it is less relevant in the context of lung cancer.

The physical and technical developments and refinements over the last decades in radiation oncology have been impressive. But still, the easiest and most effective way of avoiding side effects to the normal brain is by minimizing its exposure to ionizing radiation. While individually shaped, highly conformal dose distributions can be created, and relevant structures such as hippocampus can be excluded from the high-dose regions, this does not solve the problem of the presence of normal tissue within the irradiated target volume (the result of diffuse microscopic spread, which escapes current imaging technology, and also intended coverage of surgical tracts). These considerations have long been emphasized by proponents of WBRT (Mehta 2015). Where a reduction of the irradiated volume is not feasible, further progress can only be expected from efforts directed at optimizing fractionation or widening the therapeutic window between tumor and normal tissue through modulation of the patient's responses to radiotherapy.

We will discuss the pathogenesis of radiation-induced brain toxicity, the incidence of typical side effects, risk factors, diagnostic aspects, and the role of multimodal treatment concepts in the development of side effects. Increasing evidence can be found in the literature about the influence of cytotoxic and immune modulating drugs, and the general side effects of cancer treatment, such as anemia, on the normal brain. Finally, preclinical and clinical data on the prevention and treatment of side effects will be reviewed.

2 Pathogenesis of Radiotherapy-Induced Brain Toxicity

Early evaluations of radiotherapy-induced central nervous system (CNS) toxicity date back to over 70 years ago. It is not the aim of this chapter to discuss these historical data, which have been summarized in previous reviews, for example, by van der Kogel (1986). When appropriate, data from spinal cord radiotherapy will be included in the current chapter, because of the similarity of radiation-induced changes in the brain and the spinal cord. In brief, previous experimental studies have indicated that signs of diffuse demyelination develop in animals 2 weeks after CNS radiotherapy. After approximately 2 months, remyelination processes have been observed. These early changes correspond to clinical symptoms such as Lhermitte's sign and somnolence in humans. After a variable latency period, and dependent on total dose, white matter necrosis may develop. The gray matter is less sensitive. Latency time decreases with increasing radiation dose. The most important determinants of CNS tolerance are the volume of normal tissue exposed, dose per fraction, and total dose. Overall treatment time is less important. With multiple fractions per day, incomplete repair needs to be accounted for, especially when the interfraction interval is less than 6 h.

When WBRT is being administered, the complete intracranial vascular system is exposed to ionizing radiation, although at relatively modest doses, in contrast to focal treatment where only limited parts of the blood vessels might receive a significantly higher dose. When high focal doses are combined with lower doses to a large surrounding volume, tolerance decreases, compared with the same focal treatment alone.

Significant long-term recovery has been observed after spinal cord radiotherapy. Although not experimentally tested in the same fashion, it can be assumed that the brain recovers, too. Especially with larger intervals of at least 1–2 years and when the first treatment course was not too close to tolerance, re-irradiation is now considered a realistic option (Loi et al. 2020). Experimental data from fractionated radiotherapy of rhesus monkeys suggest a recovery of up to 75% of the initial damage within 2–3 years (Ang et al. 2001).

The past few years have witnessed a significant improvement, as far as techniques are concerned, in cellular and molecular biology, resulting, for example, in a description of more and more radiobiologically relevant cellular pathways. Better methods for the identification of stem and progenitor cells have been developed. This progress has led to a better understanding of tissue responses to ionizing radiation (Schaue et al. 2012). Obviously, radiation-induced reactions of the CNS are not limited to reproductive or mitotic cell death in mature parenchymal and vascular cell populations. Apoptosis, induced by sphingomyelinase-mediated release of ceramide, has been described as an early reaction in endothelial cells within the irradiated CNS (Pena et al. 2000), as well as in oligodendrocytes (Larocca et al. 1997). Besides cell death, a large number of alterations in gene expression, transcription factor activation, and functional changes in basically every cell type examined may develop (Raju et al. 2000). Current models of radiotherapy-induced brain alterations include a cascade of complex and dynamic interactions between parenchymal cells (oligodendrocytes, astrocytes, microglia), stem and progenitor cells, and vascular endothelial cells (Tofilon and Fike 2000; Fike et al. 2009; Hanbury et al. 2015; Hladik and Tapio 2016). The latent time preceding the clinical manifestation of damage is viewed as an active phase, where cytokines and growth factors play important roles in intra- and intercellular communication (Nieder et al. 2007). Clinically recognized phenomena, such as intellectual decline, memory loss, lethargy, dysphoria, dementia, and ataxia, also suggest the possible involvement of neurons in radiotherapy-induced CNS reactions (Parihar et al. 2015). In vitro studies have demonstrated that neurons may undergo apoptosis after radiotherapy (Gobbel et al. 1998). Fractionated brain irradiation inhibited the formation of new neurons in the dentate gyrus of the hippocampus in rats (Madsen et al. 2003). Animals with blocked neurogenesis performed poorer in short-term memory tests that are related to hippocampal function. The deficit in neurogenesis is based on both the reduced proliferative capacity of progenitor cells and alterations in the microenvironment, which regulates progenitor cell fate (disruption of the microvascular angiogenesis, activation of microglia) (Monje et al. 2002, 2007).

CNS radiotherapy induces the production of inflammatory cytokines, such as tumor necrosis factor α (TNF-α) and interleukin-1 (IL-1), by microglia and astrocytes (Chiang and McBride 1991; Hayakawa et al. 1997; Betlazar et al. 2016). IL-1 release leads, via autocrine mechanisms, to further activation and proliferation of these glia cells. As shown in vivo, this cascade results in the development of astrogliosis (Chiang et al. 1993). Already 2 h after single-fraction radiotherapy to the midbrain of mice (25 Gy), TNF-α and IL-1 mRNA levels were shown to increase (Hong et al. 1995). After 24 h, the levels started returning to normal. Experimental rat brain irradiation has also been shown to induce apoptosis, which, in turn, appears to result in an increase in the number of microglial cells participating in phagocytotic reactions. Besides the cytotoxic effects of TNF-α on oligodendrocytes, for example, through induction of caspase-mediated apoptosis (Hisahara et al. 1997; Gu et al. 1999), the cytokine in vitro prevents the differentiation of O-2A progenitor cells into oligodendrocytes. Thus, compensation for radiation-induced cell loss can be impaired. TNF-α is also known to damage endothelial cells, leading to increased vascular permeability. TNF-α and IL-1 induce the expression of intercellular adhesion molecule-1 (ICAM-1) in oligodendrocytes and microvascular endothelial cells (Satoh et al. 1991; Wong and Dorovini 1992). Increased levels of ICAM-1 mRNA were detectable after midbrain irradiation with 2 Gy (Hong et al. 1995). Results of localized single-fraction treatment with 20 Gy confirm the presence of an early inflammatory response, an increased number of leukocytes, increased vascular permeability, altered integrity of endothelial tight junctions, and increased cell adhesion (Yuan et al. 2003). The exact role of such cytokines and mediators after radiotherapy with conventional fraction sizes is not well understood yet. Clearly, the cellular and molecular events during the latent phase require further research.

Studies of boron neutron capture therapy (BNCT) support the view that vascular damage is one of the crucial components of radiotherapy-induced CNS toxicity. The choice of boron compounds that are unable to cross the blood–brain barrier allows a largely selective irradiation of the vessel walls with BNCT. Nevertheless, as with conventional non-selective radiotherapy methods, spinal cord lesions (with a similar histological appearance) were induced. Latency time also was comparable between damage induced by BNCT and conventional radiotherapy (Morris et al. 1996). Additional evidence has been provided by histological examinations of rat brains after radiotherapy with 22.5 Gy or 25 Gy, resulting in reduced numbers of blood vessels and endothelial cells before manifestation of necrosis (Calvo et al. 1988). These changes are accompanied by hyperpermeability, resulting in perivascular edema and consecutive ischemic damage (Hopewell and van der Kogel 1999).

Microvascular networks, consisting of arterioles, capillaries, and venules, which impact the delivery of oxygen and nutrients to tissues and organs, are the most radiosensitive parts of the vascular system (Roth et al. 1999). Common therapeutic doses of ionizing radiation lead to functional and, later, to structural vascular damage, such as increased permeability and changes in shape and diameter, as well as in fibrous proliferation, ultimately resulting in reduced perfusion (Murphy et al. 2015). These changes develop earlier in small versus large vessels. After lower doses, structural changes are hardly ever seen. After WBRT in rats (5 fractions of 4 Gy) alterations in vessel configuration, either density or diameter, were not detected (Mildenberger et al. 1990). Interestingly, a localized significant increase of microglia was found after 6 months, possibly as a result of the loss of axons in the striatal white matter. The pattern was suggestive of vascular insufficiency in this region, which was being perfused by only few small vessels. Electron microscopy in rats 15 days after the end of conventional fractionated WBRT (40 Gy) showed increased vascular permeability without structural changes of the blood–brain barrier or astrocytes (Cicciarello et al. 1996). A follow-up examination after 90 days revealed ultrastructural changes of the microvasculature and the neuropil, as well as astrocytes with perivascular edema.

Another study (partial brain irradiation with 40 Gy or 60 Gy, or WBRT with 25 Gy in rats) showed a 15% reduction in the number of endothelial cells 24 h to 4 weeks after radiotherapy. A further reduction was seen with even longer intervals (Ljubimova et al. 1991). Kamiryo et al. showed how the latency to development of vascular damage after SRS to the parietal cortex of rat brain with a 4 mm collimator decreases from 12 months to 3 weeks with an increase in radiation dose from 50 to 75 Gy or 120 Gy (Kamiryo et al. 1996). The amount of vessel dilation, increased permeability, thickening of the vessel wall, vessel occlusion, and necrosis also increased with dose. In a different model of rat brain irradiation, time- and dose-dependent vascular alterations were also seen (dilation, wall thickening, reactive hypertrophy of neighboring astrocytes) before the development of white matter necrosis (Hopewell et al. 1989). Rubin et al. performed comprehensive MRI and histological examinations of rat brains after 2–24 weeks following high-dose, single-fraction irradiation with 60 Gy (Rubin et al. 1994). After 2 weeks, a significant increase in blood–brain permeability was observed. Partial recovery occurred after 8–12 weeks, followed by pronounced deterioration after 24 weeks when the first sites of necrosis developed. Spinal cord data suggest an increase in the release of vascular endothelial growth factor (VEGF) as a result of impaired perfusion and hypoxia signaling. Obviously, the clinically observed latent phase is characterized by persistent and increasing oxidative stress and active responses to this factor. The extreme sensitivity of the myelin membrane to oxidative damage explains the preference of radiotherapy-induced lesions for white matter.

3 Acute and Subacute Radiotherapy-Induced Brain Toxicity

As stated in the previous paragraph, acute and subacute radiotherapy-induced brain toxicity can develop within hours from the start of treatment, even if low doses are given. It is usually characterized by increased vascular permeability, edema, and demyelination, manifesting as headache, nausea, somnolence, or lethargy. However, it has been characterized as a temporary, self-limiting reaction, which responds to corticosteroid treatment (Schultheiss et al. 1995). Subacute reactions may develop 2–6 months after WBRT, resulting, for example, in lethargy, reduced vigilance and impaired cognitive performance. Most likely, such symptoms are related to a second phase of transient demyelination and blood–brain barrier disturbance. Treatment with corticosteroids again is likely to improve the patients' condition. With SRS, acute reactions are rare. They include symptomatic edema, seizures, and nausea and vomiting, especially when doses >3.75 Gy are given to the area postrema. Antiemetics, corticosteroids, and anticonvulsant drugs may be used to treat these symptoms. Temporary blood–brain barrier disturbance may result in increased contrast enhancement on computed tomography (CT) or MRI during the first few months after SRS (Knitter et al. 2018). These changes (pseudoprogression) should not be misinterpreted as tumor progression. Usually they resolve with longer follow-up. The Response Assessment in Neuro-Oncology Brain Metastases criteria were developed to guide imaging assessment (Lin et al. 2015). Research efforts in the radiomics field likely will influence response assessment in the near future (Lohmann et al. 2020). Positron emission tomography (PET) is often useful in otherwise difficult diagnostic situations, including the assessment of pseudoprogression after treatment with immune checkpoint inhibitors (Galldiks et al. 2020a). The latter drugs have rapidly changed the management of patients with stage III and IV lung cancer, as have different targeted agents for non-small cell lung cancer (NSCLC) with actionable molecular alterations. Combining these drugs with brain irradiation may increase the number of follow-up imaging studies that are difficult to interpret (Eguren-Santamaria et al. 2020; Galldiks et al. 2020b; Helis et al. 2020).

4 Delayed or Chronic Radiotherapy-Induced Brain Toxicity

Sustaining toxicity that may impair the patient's lifestyle significantly can be observed even several years after radiotherapy in the form of radionecrosis and cognitive dysfunction associated with leukoencephalopathy. Necrosis develops for the most part after 9–36 months (Keime-Guibert et al. 1998). Symptoms of radionecrosis depend on lesion localization and are comparable to tumor-related symptoms before treatment (focal neurologic deficits and seizures, speech disturbance, signs of increased intracranial pressure). CT and T1- and T2-weighted anatomic MRI are unable to firmly discriminate between hypometabolic necrosis and tumor relapse. Dynamic susceptibility contrast-enhanced MRI, magnetic resonance spectroscopy (MRS), and functional imaging by means of PET and ^{201}Tl–single photon emission computed tomography (SPECT) can provide useful additional information (Munley et al. 2001; Nakajima et al. 2009; Romagna et al. 2016). Eventually, in some cases, only histopathological examination of resection specimens can establish the diagnosis. The typical finding is coagulation necrosis in the white matter, with a largely normal appearance of the cortex. Fibrinoid necrosis and hyalinous wall thickening of blood vessels are commonly observed. The risk of radionecrosis amounts to approximately 5% within 5 years ($ED_{5/5}$) after conventional fractionated partial brain radiotherapy (one-third of the brain) with 60 Gy or WBRT with 45 Gy. The dose–response curves are quite steep. Thus, the risk increases to 10% within 5 years when a partial brain dose of 65 Gy is applied (according to data from the randomized U.S. intergroup low-grade glioma trial) and 50% when 75 Gy is given. Irradiated volume, dose per fraction, and total dose are the most important risk factors (Lawrence et al. 2010). Recent series reported radionecrosis after SRS of brain metastases in 1–6% of cases, probably dependent on brain region and vascular supply. Commonly prescribed doses are in the range of 15–20 Gy, depending on volume, technique of SRS, and use of sequential WBRT. The risk increases when more than 10 cm^3 of the normal brain receives more than 10 Gy. The optic apparatus should not receive more than 8 Gy (Mayo et al. 2010). Varlotto et al. reported the results of SRS in 137 patients with brain metastases who had a minimum follow-up of 1 year after SRS (Varlotto et al. 2003). The median marginal tumor dose was 16 Gy. NSCLC was the underlying primary tumor in 77 patients. Eleven patients developed serious side effects, such as visual loss, hemorrhage, and persistent steroid-dependent edema or necrosis necessitating surgical intervention. The actuarial incidence of such adverse events was 4% after 5 years for patients with brain metastases ≤2 cm^3 and 16% for those with larger lesions. Age and additional use of WBRT did not influence the complication rate. In a series of 156 patients with different primary tumors managed with FSRT (2–10 fractions) only 3% developed radionecrosis (all these patients were previously irradiated to the index lesion (Jimenez et al. 2017). Therapeutic intervention with corticosteroids or anticoagulants is sometimes successful (Glantz et al. 1994). Often, surgical resection is the only way to effectively improve the symptoms.

Diffuse white matter changes are frequently observed in imaging studies (Figs. 1 and 2). Fluid-attenuated inversion recovery (FLAIR) and diffusion-weighted MRI may improve visualization of white matter abnormalities. These abnormalities are not necessarily associated with clinical symptoms but often present after fractionated doses of ≥30 Gy. Neurocognitive sequelae typically manifest within 4 years of radiotherapy. In a randomized study that included patients with resected brain metastases, cognitive-deterioration-free survival was longer in patients assigned to post-operative SRS (median 3.7 months) than in patients assigned to WBRT (median 3.0 months; hazard ratio 0.47 [95% confidence interval (CI) 0.35–0.63]; $p < 0.0001$), and

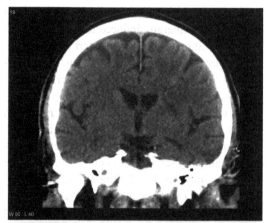

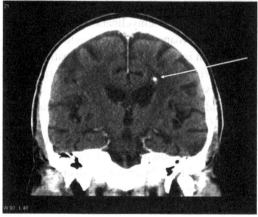

Fig. 1 Initial CT scans (top) before whole-brain radiotherapy (30 Gy in 10 fractions of 3 Gy) in a 66-year-old man with multiple brain metastases from small cell lung cancer (no previous prophylactic brain irradiation). The lower CT scan was taken 2 years later and shows moderate brain atrophy and white matter changes. In addition, periventricular calcifications (white arrow) can be seen. The patient had developed overt neurocognitive decline interfering with activities of daily living

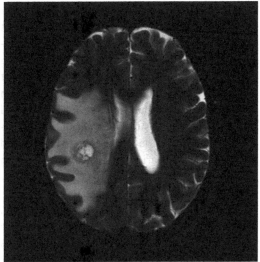

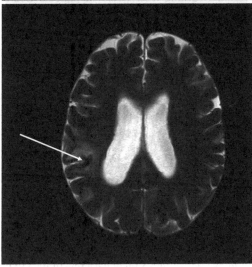

Fig. 2 Initial T2-weighted MRI scan before stereotactic radiosurgery (gamma knife, peripheral dose 20 Gy) in a 67-year-old woman with solitary brain metastasis from non-small-cell lung cancer. The lower MRI scan was taken 2.8 years later and shows focal white matter changes (white arrow). No clinical late toxicity was apparent

cognitive deterioration at 6 months was less frequent in patients who received SRS than those who received WBRT (28 [52%] of 54 evaluable patients assigned to SRS versus 41 [85%] of 48 evaluable patients assigned to WBRT; difference −33.6% [95% CI −45.3 to −21.8], $p < 0.0003$) (Brown et al. 2017). In a different randomized study without surgery (1–3 brain metastases), there was less cognitive deterioration at 3 months after SRS alone (40/63 patients [63.5%]) than when combined with WBRT (44/48 patients [91.7%]; difference, −28.2%; 90% CI, −41.9% to −14.4%; $p < 0.001$) (Brown et al. 2016). Quality of life was higher at 3 months with SRS alone, including overall quality of life (mean change from baseline, −0.1 versus −12.0 points; mean difference, 11.9; 95% CI, 4.8–19.0 points; $p = 0.001$).

Psychometric findings suggest greater vulnerability of white matter and subcortical structures, resulting in reduced processing speed, heightened distractibility, and memory impairment. Within the temporal lobe, the hippocampal formation plays a central role in short-term memory and learning (Tomé et al. 2016). These functions are related to the activity of neural stem cells. The hippocampal granule cell layer undergoes continuous renewal and restructuring. Radiotherapy can affect this sensitive cell layer leading to impaired function without overt pathological changes. Our own retrospective data from 49 patients who had received WBRT with a median dose of 30 Gy showed that 33% of patients developed mild to moderate clinical symptoms of brain toxicity (in one case, RTOG/EORTC grade III, median follow-up 10 months, median dose per fraction 3 Gy) (Nieder et al. 1999). This resulted in a Karnofsky performance status decline in 10 patients (20%). None of the PCI patients belonged to this subgroup. CT showed increasing brain atrophy and bilateral periventricular hypodensity in most patients (Fig. 1). The actuarial risk of brain atrophy was 84% after 2 years. Median time to development of this side effect was 11 months. Patients with pre-existing brain atrophy had a higher risk of further shrinkage of the brain parenchyma compared to those with normal baseline status. White matter changes were observed in 85% of surviving patients. Radiologic abnormalities did not correlate with the rate of clinical symptoms. Previous studies described such correlations for patients treated with PCI and chemotherapy for SCLC (Laukkanen et al. 1988; Johnson et al. 1990). Whether or not clinical symptoms, quality of life and radiologic abnormalities correlate, might depend on variables such as length of follow-up, methods of assessment, and severity of clinical symptoms (Witlox et al. 2020).

When evaluating radiotherapy-induced cognitive impairment, it is important to consider reference values from the normal population. A Canadian Study of Health and Aging with 9008 randomly selected men and women 65 years or older showed cognitive impairment 5 years after baseline examination in 9% and dementia in an additional 6% (Laurin et al. 2001). Decline was significantly associated with reduced physical activity. There is increasing evidence that partial brain radiotherapy alone rarely causes significant neurocognitive decline (Torres et al. 2003; Klein et al. 2021). Some authors found indications for increased toxicity when fraction size exceeded 2 Gy (Herskovic and Orton 1986; Twijnstra et al. 1987; De Angelis et al. 1989). A large study in patients with NSCLC was reported by Sun et al. (2011). Randomization between PCI (30 Gy in 15 fractions of 2 Gy) and observation was done in a group of 356 patients. PCI was associated with a significant decline in memory at 1 year (Hopkins Verbal Learning Test; recall deterioration in 26% versus 7% and delayed recall deterioration in 32 versus 5%). Three months after PCI, but not at later time points, there was also a significant deterioration in Mini-Mental-Status examination (36% versus 21%). Also, the large intergroup study that used PCI with 10 fractions of 2.5 Gy in patients with SCLC reported mild deterioration of intellectual and memory function (Le Pechoux et al. 2011). A recent review (8 different randomized trials, 8 observational studies) included 3,553 patients in total (858 NSCLC, 2695 SCLC) of which 74% received PCI (Zeng et al. 2020). Incidence of mild/moderate cognitive decline after PCI varied from 8% to 89% (grading not always provided). For those without PCI, the corresponding figure was 3–42%. Interestingly, 23–95% had baseline cognitive impairment. Risk factors were often not reported. In one of the included trials, both age (>60 years) and higher PCI dose (36 Gy) including twice-daily PCI were associated with a higher risk of cognitive decline. In one trial, white matter abnormalities were more frequent in the concurrent or sandwiched PCI arm, but without significant neuropsychological differences. One trial identified hippocampal sparing PCI to limit the neurocognitive toxicities of PCI and another reported an association between hippocampal dose volume effects and memory decline. As neurocognition was a secondary endpoint in most randomized trials, and was assessed by various instruments with often poor to moderate compliance, high-quality data is lacking (Zeng et al. 2020).

In patients who developed brain metastases, WBRT has also been shown to interfere with recall functions as measured by the Hopkins Verbal Learning Test (64% in patients treated with WBRT plus SRS as compared to 20% in those with SRS alone after 4 months, i.e., in the subacute phase) (Chang et al. 2009). Sometimes, such decline precedes radiological progression of brain metastases. In patients with impaired neurocognition before WBRT who respond to this treatment, improvements might be observed. As mentioned briefly, preclinical and clinical data suggest a role for hippocampal avoidance (HA) radiotherapy (Gondi et al. 2010, 2014; Popp et al. 2020). A recent phase III trial enrolled patients with brain metastases to HA-WBRT plus memantine or WBRT plus memantine (Brown et al. 2020). The primary end point was time to cognitive function failure, defined as decline using the reliable change index on at least one of the cognitive tests. Overall, 518 patients were randomly assigned. Risk of cognitive failure was significantly lower after HA-WBRT plus memantine versus WBRT plus memantine (adjusted hazard ratio, 0.74; 95% CI, 0.58–0.95; $p = 0.02$). This difference was attributable to less deterioration in executive function at 4 months (23% versus 40%; $p = 0.01$) and learning and memory at 6 months. Treatment arms did not differ significantly in overall survival, intracranial progression-free survival, or toxicity. At 6 months, patients who received HA-WBRT plus memantine reported less fatigue, less difficulty with remembering things, and less difficulty with speaking. Memantine was given in this study because earlier results suggested clinical benefits in the conventional WBRT setting (Brown et al. 2013; Wilke et al. 2018).

Neurocognitive dysfunction was reported to stabilize spontaneously (Van De Pol et al. 1997; Armstrong et al. 2002) or to progress over time (Johnson et al. 1990). In extreme cases, subcortical dementia may result, which often is associated with gait disturbance and incontinence. Due to the lack of effective treatment, most patients with this severe complication die after several months or a few years. Histopathologic findings include diffuse spongiosis and demyelination, as well as disseminated miliary necrosis.

Further late complications in terms of stenosis of blood vessels and moyamoya syndrome (multiple, diffuse, progressive infarctions due to occlusion of the anterior and medial cerebral arteries) have occasionally been described, mostly in patients irradiated at a younger age. Endocrine dysfunction resulting from damage to the pituitary gland or the hypothalamic region can result in hypothyroidism, amenorrhea, etc. Hearing loss is very uncommon after doses typically prescribed for lung cancer metastases.

Importantly, all types of iatrogenic neurotoxicity can only be diagnosed after comprehensive evaluation, i.e., exclusion of other causes, for example, brain metastases, leptomeningeal spread, infections, cerebral infarction, and hemorrhage. In addition, systemic metabolic disorders (hypercalcemia, hepatic failure, diabetes, changes in osmolality, etc.), alcoholic cerebellar degeneration, Wernicke-Korsakoff syndrome, paraneoplastic disorders (for example, limbic encephalitis, chorea, cerebellar degeneration, and Lambert-Eaton myasthenic syndrome in SCLC), and immune-related adverse events (Winer et al. 2018) must be considered. Besides physical and neurologic examination, blood tests, EEG, and cerebrospinal fluid diagnostic are indicated. In addition to imaging studies—for example, myelography, CT, MRI, and functional imaging—factors such as time interval between radiotherapy and diagnosis, dose per fraction, number of fractions per day, total dose, and location of the treatment fields need to be considered. In the era of multimodal treatment regimens, injury should not be attributed solely to one modality (Dietrich et al. 2015). Therefore, interdisciplinary evaluation integrating the radiobiological knowledge of radiation oncologists is mandatory when radiotherapy-induced neurotoxicity is being considered.

5 Toxicity Prevention Strategies

At present, pharmacologic or biologic prevention is not universally established, despite clinical data in favor of memantine regarding cognitive tests. Older preliminary data, e.g., from a non-randomized trial of SRS of arteriovenous malformations, suggested that patients treated with gamma linolenic [omega-6] acid had less permanent complications than those who did not receive this medication (Sims and Plowman 2001). Still, the most effective way of toxicity prevention is adherence to established dose constraints and, if necessary, reduction of fraction size and normal tissue volume, the latter, for example, by means of several high-precision techniques including HA. There is also interest in proton beam radiotherapy and FLASH radiotherapy using ultra-high dose rates, which results in normal tissue sparing in preclinical models (Montay-Gruel et al. 2019).

Several rational experimental interventions based on the pathogenetic models reviewed in this chapter have been studied. The clinical effectiveness of these putative prevention strategies has yet to be established. The prophylactic use of dexamethasone 24 h and 1 h before radiation exposure reduced the expression of TNF-α, IL-1, and ICAM-1 (Hong et al. 1995). In vitro, corticosteroids influence the function of microglial cells and inhibit their proliferation (Tanaka et al. 1997). The hyperpermeability of blood vessels could be reduced at all time points after irradiation by application of rh-MnSOD (manganese superoxide dismutase), suggesting that free oxygen radicals could be involved in the dysfunction of microvessels. Fike et al. reported that i.v. injection of α-difluoromethylornithine (DMFO), a polyamine synthesis inhibitor, starting 2 days before and continuing for 14 days after ^{125}I brachytherapy reduced the volume of radionecrosis in irradiated dog brain (Fike et al. 1994). Kondziolka et al. irradiated rats with implanted cerebral C6 glioma by SRS, either with or without i.v. administration of U-74389G, a 21-aminosteroid which is largely selective for endothelium (Kondziolka et al. 1999). The compound reduced the development of peritumoral edema and radiation-induced vascular changes in the parts of the brain that were within the region of the steep dose gradient outside the target volume. No tumor protection was observed. In general, normal tissue selectivity of prevention approaches is an important issue. Protecting tumor cells against the effects of radiation can counteract the effort towards an improved therapeutic ratio.

Other data suggest a possible role of certain growth factors with antiapoptotic effects that also influence the proliferation of stem cells, neurogenesis, and angiogenesis. Pena et al. showed that i.v. injections of basic fibroblast growth factor (FGF-2) 5 min before, immediately after and 1 h after total body irradiation in mice (1–20 Gy or 50 Gy) significantly reduced the number of apoptotic vascular and glial cells in the CNS (Pena et al. 2000). Spinal cord experiments suggested that other growth factors, such as platelet-derived growth factor (PDGF) and insulin-like growth factor-1 (IGF-1), can increase the long-term radiation tolerance by approximately 5–10% (Andratschke et al. 2005). Whether these effects result primarily from protection of the vascular system or from more widespread action is presently not known. The experiments, however, demonstrate that delayed toxicity can be prevented by early intervention at the time of radiation treatment, and they offer strategies of toxicity prevention.

The growing body of evidence linking radiation-induced brain injury with oxidative stress and/or inflammation has provided the rationale for applying proven anti-inflammatory interventions to prevent radiation-induced cognitive impairment. Older studies have tested drugs that can either attenuate inflammation or reduce chronic oxidative stress, namely peroxisome proliferator-activated (PPAR) agonists and renin angiotensin system (RAS) blockers. Given the putative role of oxidative stress/inflammation in radiation-induced brain injury, Zhao et al. (2007) tested the hypothesis that administration of the PPARγ agonist, pioglitazone (Pio), would mitigate the severity of radiation-induced cognitive impairment. Indeed, administering Pio to young adult rats starting prior to, during, and for 4 or 54 weeks after the completion of fractionated WBRT, prevented cognitive impairment measured 52 weeks post-irradiation. Promising results were also reported for the PPARα agonist fenofibrate (Greene-Schloesser et al. 2014). Robbins et al. (2009) hypothesized that blocking the brain RAS with the AT_1RA, L-158,809, would prevent or ameliorate radiation-induced cognitive impairment. As hypothesized, administering L-158,809 before, during, and for 28 or 54 weeks after fractionated WBRT prevented or ameliorated cognitive impairment observed 26 and 52 weeks post-irradiation. Moreover, giving L-158,809 before, during, and for only 5 weeks post-irradiation ameliorated the significant cognitive impairment seen 26 weeks post-irradiation.

Transplantation of stem cells or stimulation of the endogenous stem cell compartment by growth factor application might also offer exciting prospects (Smith and Limoli 2017). In principle, mature functional cells can be generated by proliferation and differentiation from stem and progenitor cells or by recovery and repair of damage in already existing cells, which then continue to survive. IGF-1 has been found to influence the restoration of neurogenesis in the adult and aging hippocampus (Lichtenwalner et al. 2001) and might thus offer interesting prospects. In another experiment, athymic nude rats subjected to head irradiation were transplanted 2 days afterward with human embryonic stem cells (hESC) into the hippocampal formation and analyzed for stem cell survival, differentiation, and cognitive function (Acharya et al. 2009). Animals receiving hESC transplantation exhibited superior performance on a hippocampal-dependent cognitive task 4 months post-irradiation, compared to their irradiated counterparts that did not receive hESCs. Significant stem cell survival was found at 1 and 4 months post-irradiation. Furthermore, cell-free alternatives to stem cells, such as extracellular vesicles (delivery vectors) passing the blood–brain barrier, which have been shown to have similar ameliorating effects in other tissues and injury models, have been proposed (Leavitt et al. 2019).

6 Treatment of Radiotherapy-Induced Brain Toxicity

Despite improvements in biologic understanding of CNS reactions, treatment options unfortunately are still limited. It is of course important to exclude other causes of CNS dysfunction, to correct any metabolic abnormality, and to optimize the treatment of endocrinological dysfunction, depression, and other comorbid conditions. A few small studies have described successful treatment of late CNS toxicity, e.g., radionecrosis, by hyperbaric oxygen treatment (HBO) (Co et al. 2019). For example, one out of seven patients with cognitive impairment at least 1.5 years after radiotherapy improved after 30 sessions of HBO (Hulshof et al. 2002). In contrast, HBO during radiotherapy can cause radiosensitization. Patients with leukoencephalopathy and moderate hydrocephalus (diagnosed by intracranial pressure monitoring) may profit from ventriculoperitoneal shunt insertion (Perrini et al. 2002). Quality of life can be improved by supportive measures (cognitive training, rehabilitation, special education, etc.). The prophylactic administration of memantine has already been discussed. For radionecrosis, therapeutic intervention with bevacizumab might offer clinical benefit (Levin et al. 2011). Previously, surgical resection often was the only way to effectively improve symptoms. As suggested from a small double-blind placebo-controlled trial intravenous bevacizumab given every 3 weeks might improve both clinical and radiological symptoms. Additional small retrospective studies support this view (Boothe et al. 2013; Bodensohn et al. 2020). More recently, laser interstitial thermal therapy (LITT) has been reported as additional therapeutic option (Hong et al. 2020).

7 Aspects of Chemotherapy-Induced Brain Toxicity

Chemotherapy can cause a variety of brain injuries. Most of these changes are temporary and reversible. Sometimes the symptoms are secondary to hyponatremia or hypomagnesemia. Posterior reversible encephalopathy syndrome can develop after systemic administration of cytotoxic drugs, including gemcitabine, cisplatin, 5-fluorouracil (5-FU), methotrexate, and paclitaxel. White matter hyperintensity from vasogenic edema can clinically result in headache, somnolence, and seizures. Symptoms can be reversed when the drugs are discontinued. Cerebellar toxicity of 5-FU is rare and mostly found in patients with a deficiency of dihydropyrimidine dehydrogenase. Cisplatin is able to induce cerebral edema and cortical blindness, as reviewed by (Sloan et al. 2003; Rajeswaran et al. 2008). Mild to moderate, typically transient neurocognitive impairment can develop after systemic chemotherapy (Dietrich et al. 2015), for example, with paclitaxel (Ahles and Saykin 2001) and cisplatin/etoposide (Whitney et al. 2008). Chronic encephalopathy also can result from chemo- or radiochemotherapy (Keime-Guibert et al. 1998). Furthermore, immune checkpoint inhibitors may cause different complications, e.g., limbic encephalitis, meningoencephalitis, and cerebellitis (Vogrig et al. 2020). Some patients developed isolated confusion and Parkinsonism. Associated autoantibodies included onconeural, astrocytic, and neuronal surface specificities. In this particular study, immune checkpoint inhibitors were withheld and corticosteroid treatment was given in all cases.

References

Acharya MM, Christie LA, Lan ML et al (2009) Rescue of radiation-induced cognitive impairment through cranial transplantation of human embryonic stem cells. Proc Natl Acad Sci U S A 106: 19150–19155

Ahles TA, Saykin A (2001) Cognitive effects of standard dose chemotherapy in patients with cancer. Cancer Investig 19:812–820

Andratschke N, Nieder C, Price RE, Rivera B, Ang KK (2005) Potential role of growth factors in diminishing radiation therapy neural tissue injury. Semin Oncol 32(Suppl. 3):S67–S70

Ang KK, Jiang GL, Feng Y, Stephens LC, Tucker SL, Price RE (2001) Extent and kinetics of recovery of occult spinal cord injury. Int J Radiat Oncol Biol Phys 50:1013–1020

Armstrong CL, Hunter JV, Ledakis GE et al (2002) Late cognitive and radiographic changes related to radiotherapy: initial prospective findings. Neurology 59:40–48

Betlazar C, Middleton RJ, Banati RB, Liu GJ (2016) The impact of high and low dose ionising radiation on the central nervous system. Redox Biol 9:144–156

Bodensohn R, Hadi I, Fleischmann DF et al (2020) Bevacizumab as a treatment option for radiation necrosis after cranial radiation therapy: a retrospective monocentric analysis. Strahlenther Onkol 196:70–76

Boothe D, Young R, Yamada Y, Prager A, Chan T, Beal K (2013) Bevacizumab as a treatment for radiation necrosis of brain metastases post stereotactic radiosurgery. Neuro-Oncology 15:1257–1263

Brown PD, Pugh S, Laack NN, Radiation Therapy Oncology Group (RTOG) et al (2013) Memantine for the prevention of cognitive dysfunction in patients receiving whole-brain radiotherapy: a randomized, double-blind, placebo-controlled trial. Neuro-Oncology 15:1429–1437

Brown PD, Jaeckle K, Ballman KV et al (2016) Effect of radiosurgery alone vs radiosurgery with whole brain radiation therapy on cognitive function in patients with 1 to 3 brain metastases: A randomized clinical trial. JAMA 316:401–409

Brown PD, Ballman KV, Cerhan JH et al (2017) Postoperative stereotactic radiosurgery compared with whole brain radiotherapy for resected metastatic brain disease (NCCTG N107C/CEC·3): a multicentre, randomised, controlled, phase 3 trial. Lancet Oncol 18:1049–1060

Brown PD, Gondi V, Pugh S, for NRG Oncology et al (2020) Hippocampal avoidance during whole-brain radiotherapy plus memantine for patients with brain metastases: Phase III trial NRG Oncology CC001. J Clin Oncol 38:1019–1029

Calvo W, Hopewell JW, Reinhold HS, Yeung TK (1988) Time- and dose-related changes in the white matter of the rat brain after single doses of X–rays. Br J Biol 61:1043–1052

Chang EL, Wefel JS, Hess KR et al (2009) Neurocognition in patients with brain metastases treated with radiosurgery or radiosurgery plus whole-brain irradiation: a randomised controlled trial. Lancet Oncol 10:1037–1044

Chiang CS, McBride WH (1991) Radiation enhances tumor necrosis factor alpha production by murine brain cells. Brain Res 566:265–269

Chiang CS, McBride WH, Withers HR (1993) Radiation-induced astrocytic and microglial responses in mouse brain. Radiother Oncol 29:60–68

Cicciarello R, D'Avella D, Gagliardi ME et al (1996) Time-related ultrastructural changes in an experimental model of whole brain irradiation. Neurosurgery 38:772–779

Co J, De Moraes MV, Katznelson R et al (2019) Hyperbaric oxygen for radiation necrosis of the brain. Can J Neurol Sci 30:1–8

De Angelis LM, Delattre JY, Posner JB (1989) Radiation induced dementia in patients cured of brain metastases. Neurology 39:789–796

Dietrich J, Prust M, Kaiser J (2015) Chemotherapy, cognitive impairment and hippocampal toxicity. Neuroscience 309:224–232

Eguren-Santamaria I, Sanmamed MF, Goldberg SB et al (2020) PD-1/PD-L1 blockers in NSCLC brain metastases: Challenging paradigms and clinical practice. Clin Cancer Res 26:4186–4197

Fike JR, Gobbel GT, Marton LJ, Seilhan TM (1994) Radiation brain injury is reduced by the polyamine inhibitor α-difluoromethylornithine. Radiat Res 138:99–106

Fike JR, Rosi S, Limoli CL (2009) Neural precursor cells and central nervous system radiation sensitivity. Semin Radiat Oncol 19:122–132

Galldiks N, Abdulla DS, Scheffler M et al (2020a) Treatment monitoring of immunotherapy and targeted therapy using ^{18}F-FET PET in patients with melanoma and lung cancer brain metastases: initial experiences. J Nucl Med 62(4):464–470. https://doi.org/10.2967/jnumed.120.248278

Galldiks N, Kocher M, Ceccon G et al (2020b) Imaging challenges of immunotherapy and targeted therapy in patients with brain metastases: response, progression, and pseudoprogression. Neuro-Oncology 22:17–30

Glantz MJ, Burger PC, Friedman AH, Radtke RA, Massey EW, Schold SC (1994) Treatment of radiation-induced nervous system injury with heparin and warfarin. Neurology 44:2020–2027

Gobbel GT, Bellinzona M, Vogt AR, Gupta N, Fike JR, Chan PH (1998) Response of postmitotic neurons to x-irradiation: Implications for the role of DNA damage in neuronal apoptosis. J Neurosci 18:147–155

Gondi V, Tomé WA, Mehta MP (2010) Why avoid the hippocampus? A comprehensive review. Radiother Oncol 97:370–376

Gondi V, Pugh SL, Tome WA et al (2014) Preservation of memory with conformal avoidance of the hippocampal neural stem-cell compartment during whole-brain radiotherapy for brain metastases (RTOG 0933): a phase II multi-institutional trial. J Clin Oncol 32:3810–3816

Greene-Schloesser D, Payne V, Peiffer AM et al (2014) The peroxisomal proliferator-activated receptor (PPAR) α agonist, fenofibrate, prevents fractionated whole-brain irradiation-induced cognitive impairment. Radiat Res 181:33–44

Gu C, Casaccia-Bonnefil P, Srinivasan A, Chao MV (1999) Oligodendrocyte apoptosis mediated by caspase activation. J Neurosci 19:3043–3049

Hanbury DB, Robbins ME, Bourland JD et al (2015) Pathology of fractionated whole-brain irradiation in rhesus monkeys (Macaca mulatta). Radiat Res 183:367–374

Hayakawa K, Borchardt PE, Sakuma S, Ijichi A, Niibe H, Tofilon PJ (1997) Microglial cytokine gene induction after irradiation is affected by morphologic differentiation. Radiat Med 15:405–410

Helis CA, Hughes RT, Glenn CW et al (2020) Predictors of adverse radiation effect in brain metastasis patients treated with stereotactic radiosurgery and immune checkpoint inhibitor therapy. Int J Radiat Oncol Biol Phys 108:295–303

Herskovic AM, Orton CG (1986) Elective brain irradiation for small cell anaplastic lung cancer. Int J Radiat Oncol Biol Phys 12:427–429

Hisahara S, Shoji S, Okano H, Miura M (1997) ICE/CED3 family executes oligodendrocyte apoptosis by tumor necrosis factor. J Neurochem 69:10–20

Hladik D, Tapio S (2016) Effects of ionizing radiation on the mammalian brain. Mutat Res 770:219–230

Hong JH, Chiang CS, Campbell IL, Sun JR, Withers HR, McBride WH (1995) Induction of acute phase gene expression by brain irradiation. Int J Radiat Oncol Biol Phys 33:619–626

Hong CS, Beckta JM, Kundishora AJ, Elsamadicy AA, Chiang VL (2020) Laser interstitial thermal therapy for treatment of cerebral radiation necrosis. Int J Hyperth 37:68–76

Hopewell JW, van der Kogel AJ (1999) Pathophysiological mechanisms leading to the development of late radiation-induced damage to the central nervous system. Front Radiat Ther Oncol 33:265–275

Hopewell JW, Calvo W, Campling D, Reinhold HS, Rezvani M, Yeung TK (1989) Effects of radiation on the microvasculature. Front Radiat Ther Oncol 23:85–95

Hulshof MC, Stark NM, van der Kleij A, Sminia P, Smeding HM, Gonzalez D (2002) Hyperbaric oxygen therapy for cognitive disorders after irradiation of the brain. Strahlenther Onkol 178:192–198

Jimenez RB, Alexander BM, Mahadevan A et al (2017) The impact of different stereotactic radiation therapy regimens for brain metastases on local control and toxicity. Adv Radiat Oncol 2:391–397

Johnson BE, Patronas N, Hayes W et al (1990) Neurologic, computed cranial tomographic, and magnetic resonance imaging abnormalities in patients with small-cell lung cancer: further follow-up of 6- to 13-year survivors. J Clin Oncol 8:48–56

Kamiryo T, Kassell NF, Thai QA, Lopes MB, Lee KS, Steiner L (1996) Histological changes in the normal rat brain after gamma irradiation. Acta Neurochir 138:451–459

Keime-Guibert F, Napolitano M, Delattre JY (1998) Neurological complications of radiotherapy and chemotherapy. J Neurol 245:695–708

Klein M, Drijver AJ, van den Bent MJ et al (2021) Memory in low-grade glioma patients treated with radiotherapy or Temozolomide. A correlative analysis of EORTC study 22033-26033. Neuro Oncol 23(5):803–811. https://doi.org/10.1093/neuonc/noaa252

Knitter JR, Erly WK, Stea BD et al (2018) Interval change in diffusion and perfusion MRI parameters for the assessment of pseudoprogression in cerebral metastases treated with stereotactic radiation. AJR Am J Roentgenol 211:168–175

Kondziolka D, Mori Y, Martinez AJ, McLaughlin MR, Flickinger JC, Lunsford LD (1999) Beneficial effects of the radioprotectant 21-aminosteroid U-74389G in a radiosurgery rat malignant glioma model. Int J Radiat Oncol Biol Phys 44:179–184

Larocca JN, Farooq M, Norton WT (1997) Induction of oligodendrocyte apoptosis by C2-ceramide. Neurochem Res 22:529–534

Laukkanen E, Klanoff H, Allan B, Graeb D, Murray N (1988) The role of prophylactic brain irradiation in limited stage small cell lung cancer: clinical, neuropsychological, and CT sequelae. Int J Radiat Oncol Biol Phys 14:1109–1117

Laurin D, Verreault R, Lindsay J, Rockwood K (2001) Physical activity and risk of cognitive impairment and dementia in elderly persons. Arch Neurol 58:498–504

Lawrence YR, Li XA, El Naqa I, Hahn CA, Marks LB, Merchant TE, Dicker AP (2010) Radiation dose-volume effects in the brain. Int J Radiat Oncol Biol Phys 76:S20–S27

Le Pechoux C, Laplanche A, Faivre-Finn C et al (2011) Clinical neurological outcome and quality of life among patients with limited small-cell cancer treated with two different doses of prophylactic cranial irradiation in the intergroup phase III trial (PCI 99-01, EORT 22003-08004, RTOG 0212 and IFCT 99-01). Ann Oncol 22:1154–1163

Leavitt RJ, Limoli CL, Baulch JE (2019) miRNA-based therapeutic potential of stem cell-derived extracellular vesicles: a safe cell-free treatment to ameliorate radiation-induced brain injury. Int J Radiat Biol 95:427–435

Levin VA, Bidaut L, Hou P et al (2011) Randomized double-blind placebo-controlled trial of bevacizumab therapy for radiation necrosis of the central nervous system. Int J Radiat Oncol Biol Phys 79:1487–1495

Lichtenwalner RJ, Forbes ME, Bennett SA, Lynch CD, Riddle DR (2001) Intracerebroventricular infusion of insulin-like growth factor-1 ameliorates the age-related decline in hippocampal neurogenesis. Neuroscience 107:603–613

Lin NU, Lee EQ, Aoyama H, Response Assessment in Neuro-Oncology (RANO) Group et al (2015) Response assessment criteria for brain metastases: proposal from the RANO group. Lancet Oncol 16:e270–e278

Ljubimova NV, Levitman MK, Plotnikova ED, Eidus LK (1991) Endothelial cell population dynamics in rat brain after local irradiation. Br J Radiol 64:934–940

Lohmann P, Galldiks N, Kocher M et al (2020) Radiomics in neuro-oncology: Basics, workflow, and applications. Methods S1046-2023(19):30317–30312

Loi M, Caini S, Scoccianti S et al (2020) Stereotactic reirradiation for local failure of brain metastases following previous radiosurgery: Systematic review and meta-analysis. Crit Rev Oncol Hematol 153:103043

Madsen TM, Kristjansen PE, Bolwig TG, Wortwein G (2003) Arrested neuronal proliferation and impaired hippocampal function following fractionated irradiation in the adult rat. Neuroscience 119:635–642

Mayo C, Martel MK, Marks LB, Flickinger J, Nam J, Kirkpatrick J (2010) Radiation dose-volume effects of optic nerves and chiasm. Int J Radiat Oncol Biol Phys 76:S28–S35

Mehta MP (2015) The controversy surrounding the use of whole-brain radiotherapy in brain metastases patients. Neuro-Oncology 17:919–923

Mildenberger M, Beach TG, McGeer EG, Ludgate CM (1990) An animal model of prophylactic cranial irradiation: histologic effects at acute, early and delayed stages. Int J Radiat Oncol Biol Phys 18:1051–1060

Monje ML, Mizumatsu S, Fike JR, Palmer TD (2002) Irradiation induces neural precursor-cell dysfunction. Nature Med 8:928–930

Monje ML, Vogel H, Masek M et al (2007) Impaired human hippocampal neurogenesis after treatment for central nervous system malignancies. Ann Neurol 62:515–520

Montay-Gruel P, Acharya MM, Petersson K et al (2019) Long-term neurocognitive benefits of FLASH radiotherapy driven by reduced reactive oxygen species. Proc Natl Acad Sci U S A 116:10943–10951

Morris GM, Coderre JA, Bywaters A (1996) Boron neutron capture irradiation of the rat spinal cord: histopathological evidence of a vascular-mediated pathogenesis. Radiat Res 146:313–320

Munley MT, Marks LB, Hardenbergh PH, Bentel GC (2001) Functional imaging of normal tissues with nuclear medicine: applications in radiotherapy. Semin Radiat Oncol 11:28–36

Murphy ES, Xie H, Merchant TE, Yu JS, Chao ST, Suh JH (2015) Review of cranial radiotherapy-induced vasculopathy. J Neuro-Oncol 122:421–429

Nakajima T, Kumabe T, Kanamori M et al (2009) Differential diagnosis between radiation necrosis and glioma progression using sequential proton magnetic resonance spectroscopy and methionine positron emission tomography. Neurol Med Chir (Tokyo) 49:394–401

Nieder C, Leicht A, Motaref B, Nestle U, Niewald M, Schnabel K (1999) Late radiation toxicity after whole-brain radiotherapy: the influence of antiepileptic drugs. Am J Clin Oncol 22:573–579

Nieder C, Andratschke N, Astner ST (2007) Experimental concepts for toxicity prevention and tissue restoration after central nervous system irradiation. Radiat Oncol 2:23

Nieder C, Bremnes RM, Andratschke NH (2009) Prognostic scores in patients with brain metastases from non-small cell lung cancer. J Thorac Oncol 4:1337–1341

Nieder C, Mehta MP, Geinitz H, Grosu AL (2018) Prognostic and predictive factors in patients with brain metastases from solid tumors: a review of published nomograms. Crit Rev Oncol Hematol 126:13–18

Nieder C, Guckenberger M, Gaspar LE et al (2019) Management of patients with brain metastases from non-small cell lung cancer and adverse prognostic features: multi-national radiation treatment recommendations are heterogeneous. Radiat Oncol 14:33

Nosaki K, Seto T, Shimokawa M, Takahashi T, Yamamoto N (2018) Is prophylactic cranial irradiation (PCI) needed in patients with extensive-stage small cell lung cancer showing complete response to first-line chemotherapy? Radiother Oncol 127:344–348

Parihar VK, Pasha J, Tran KK, Craver BM, Acharya MM, Limoli CL (2015) Persistent changes in neuronal structure and synaptic plasticity caused by proton irradiation. Brain Struct Funct 220:1161–1171

Pena LA, Fuks Z, Kolesnick RN (2000) Radiation-induced apoptosis of endothelial cells in the murine central nervous system: protection by fibroblast growth factor and sphingomyelinase deficiency. Cancer Res 60:321–327

Perrini P, Scollato A, Cioffi F, Conti R, Di Lorenzo N (2002) Radiation leukoencephalopathy associated with moderate hydrocephalus: intracranial pressure monitoring and results of ventriculoperitoneal shunting. Neurol Sci 23:237–241

Popp I, Rau S, Hintz M et al (2020) Hippocampus-avoidance whole-brain radiation therapy with a simultaneous integrated boost for multiple brain metastases. Cancer 126:2694–2703

Rajeswaran A, Trojan A, Burnand B, Giannelli M (2008) Efficacy and side effects of cisplatin- and carboplatin-based doublet chemotherapeutic regimens versus non-platinum-based doublet chemotherapeutic regimens as first line treatment of metastatic non-small cell lung carcinoma: a systematic review of randomized controlled trials. Lung Cancer 59:1–11

Raju U, Gumin GJ, Tofilon PJ (2000) Radiation-induced transcription factor activation in the rat cerebral cortex. Int J Radiat Biol 76:1045–1053

Robbins ME, Payne V, Tommasi E et al (2009) The AT_1 receptor antagonist, L-158,809, prevents or ameliorates fractionated whole-brain irradiation-induced cognitive impairment. Int J Radiat Oncol Biol Phys 73:499–505

Romagna A, Unterrainer M, Schmid-Tannwald C et al (2016) Suspected recurrence of brain metastases after focused high dose radiotherapy: can [^{18}F]FET- PET overcome diagnostic uncertainties? Radiat Oncol 11:139

Roth NM, Sontag MR, Kiani MF (1999) Early effects of ionizing radiation on the microvascular networks in normal tissue. Radiat Res 151:270–277

Rubin P, Gash DM, Hansen JT, Nelson DF, Williams JP (1994) Disruption of the blood-brain barrier as the primary effect of CNS irradiation. Radiother Oncol 31:51–60

Rusthoven CG, Kavanagh BD (2017) Prophylactic cranial irradiation (PCI) versus active MRI surveillance for small cell lung cancer: The case for equipoise. J Thorac Oncol 12:1746–1754

Satoh J, Kastrukoff LF, Kim SU (1991) Cytokine-induced expression of intercellular adhesion molecule-1 (ICAM1) in cultured human oligodendrocytes and astrocytes. J Neuropathol Exp Neurol 50:215–226

Schaue D, Kachikwu EL, McBride WH (2012) Cytokines in radiobiological responses: a review. Radiat Res 178:505–523

Schultheiss TE, Kun LE, Ang KK, Stephens LC (1995) Radiation response of the central nervous system. Int J Radiat Oncol Biol Phys 31:1093–1112

Sims EC, Plowman PN (2001) Stereotactic radiosurgery XII. Large AVM and the failure of the radiation response modifier gamma linolenic acid to improve the therapeutic ratio. Br J Neurosurg 15:28–34

Sloan AE, Arnold SM, St. Clair WH, Regine WF (2003) Brain injury: current management and investigations. Semin Radiat Oncol 13:309–321

Smith SM, Limoli CL (2017) Stem cell therapies for the resolution of radiation injury to the brain. Curr Stem Cell Rep 3:342–347

Sperduto PW, Yang TJ, Beal K et al (2017) Estimating survival in patients with lung cancer and brain metastases: An update of the Graded Prognostic Assessment for lung cancer using molecular markers (Lung-molGPA). JAMA Oncol 3:827–831

Sun A, Bae K, Gore EM et al (2011) Phase III trial of prophylactic cranial irradiation compared with observation in patients with locally advanced non-small-cell lung cancer: neurocognitive and quality-of-life analysis. J Clin Oncol 29:279–286

Takahashi T, Yamanaka T, Seto T et al (2017) Prophylactic cranial irradiation versus observation in patients with extensive-disease small-cell lung cancer: a multicentre, randomised, open-label, phase 3 trial. Lancet Oncol 18:663–671

Tanaka J, Fujita H, Matsuda S, Toku K, Sakanaka M, Maeda N (1997) Glucocorticoid- and mineralocorticoid receptors in microglial cells: the two receptors mediate differential effects of corticosteroids. Glia 20:23–37

Tofilon PJ, Fike JR (2000) The radioresponse of the central nervous system: a dynamic process. Radiat Res 153:357–370

Tomé WA, Gökhan Ş, Gulinello ME et al (2016) Hippocampal-dependent neurocognitive impairment following cranial irradiation observed in pre-clinical models: current knowledge and possible future directions. Br J Radiol 89:20150762

Torres IJ, Mundt AJ, Sweeney PJ, Castillo M, Macdonald RL (2003) A longitudinal neuropsychological study of partial brain radiation in adults with brain tumors. Neurology 60:1113–1118

Twijnstra A, Boon PJ, Lormans ACM, Ten Velde GPM (1987) Neurotoxicity of prophylactic cranial irradiation in patients with small cell carcinoma of the lung. Eur J Cancer Clin Oncol 23:983–986

Van de Pol M, Ten Velde GP, Wilmink JT, Volovics A, Twijnstra A (1997) Efficacy and safety of prophylactic cranial irradiation in patients with small cell lung cancer. J Neuro-Oncol 35:153–160

Van der Kogel AJ (1986) Radiation-induced damage in the central nervous system: an interpretation of target cell responses. Br J Cancer 53(Suppl. 7):207–217

Varlotto JM, Flickinger JC, Niranjan A, Bhatnagar AK, Kondziolka D, Lunsford LD (2003) Analysis of tumor control and toxicity in patients who have survived at least one year after radiosurgery for brain metastases. Int J Radiat Oncol Biol Phys 57:452–464

Vogrig A, Muñiz-Castrillo S, Joubert B et al (2020) Central nervous system complications associated with immune checkpoint inhibitors. J Neurol Neurosurg Psychiatry 91:772–778

Whitney KA, Lysaker PH, Steiner AR, Hook JN, Estes DD, Hanna NH (2008) Is "chemobrain" a transient state? A prospective pilot study among persons with non-small cell lung cancer. J Support Oncol 6:313–321

Wilke C, Grosshans D, Duman J, Brown P, Li J (2018) Radiation-induced cognitive toxicity: pathophysiology and interventions to reduce toxicity in adults. Neuro-Oncology 20:597–607

Winer A, Bodor JN, Borghaei H (2018) Identifying and managing the adverse effects of immune checkpoint blockade. J Thorac Dis 10(Suppl 3):S480–S489

Witlox WJA, Ramaekers BLT, Joore MA et al (2020) Health-related quality of life after prophylactic cranial irradiation for stage III non-small cell lung cancer patients: results from the NVALT-11/DLCRG-02 phase III study. Radiother Oncol 144:65–71

Wong D, Dorovini ZK (1992) Up-regulation of intercellular adhesion molecule-1 (ICAM-1) expression in primary cultures of human brain microvessel endothelial cells by cytokines and lipopolysaccharide. J Neuroimmunol 39:11–21

Yuan H, Gaber MW, McColgan T, Naimark MD, Kiani MF, Merchant TE (2003) Radiation-induced permeability and leukocyte adhesion in the rat blood–brain barrier: modulation with anti-ICAM-1 antibodies. Brain Res 969:59–69

Zeng H, Hendriks LEL, van Geffen WH, Witlox WJA, Eekers DBP, De Ruysscher DKM (2020) Risk factors for neurocognitive decline in lung cancer patients treated with prophylactic cranial irradiation: a systematic review. Cancer Treat Rev 88:102025

Zhao W, Payne V, Tommasi E et al (2007) Administration of the peroxisomal proliferator-activated receptor (PPAR)γ agonist pioglitazone during fractionated brain irradiation prevents radiation-induced cognitive impairment. Int J Radiat Oncol Biol Phys 67:6–9

Part X

Quality of Life Studies and Prognostic Factors

Patient-Reported Outcomes in Lung Cancer

Newton J. Hurst Jr, Farzan Siddiqui, and Benjamin Movsas

Contents

1 Introduction 987
2 What Is Quality of Life 988
3 How Is Quality of Life Measured 988
4 Quality-of-Life Instruments 990
5 Appropriate Instrument Selection, Timing, and Frequency of Measurements 991
6 Compliance 991
7 Analyzing QoL Data 992
8 Real-Time PRO Monitoring 992
9 Quality-of-Life Studies in Lung Cancer 993
10 Conclusions and Future Directions 995
References 995

Abstract

Despite painstaking efforts to optimize the multimodality treatment for lung cancer patients, lung cancer remains a leading cause of all cancer deaths worldwide. The quality of life (QoL) for these patients, therefore, is of utmost importance. Quality of life, a key patient-reported outcome (PRO), has garnered great interest over the last few decades and has become a key clinically meaningful endpoint in developing cancer clinical trials, especially for lung cancer. This chapter provides a review of the clinical relevance, measurement, analysis, and challenges faced when assessing PROs in lung cancer trials. Key examples of pertinent quality-of-life studies related to lung cancer and, particularly radiation therapy, are also included.

N. J. Hurst Jr
Department of Human Oncology, University of Wisconsin-Madison School of Public Health and Medicine, Madison, WI, USA
e-mail: hurst@humonc.wisc.edu

F. Siddiqui · B. Movsas (✉)
Department of Radiation Oncology, Henry Ford Cancer Institute, Detroit, MI, USA
e-mail: fsiddiq2@hfhs.org; bmovsas1@hfhs.org

1 Introduction

Historically, the efficacy of a patient's treatment, within the context of cancer clinical trials, has been assessed by clinical endpoints, such as overall and/or progression-free survival. However, increasingly, healthcare professionals are recognizing, and placing emphasis on, the improvement of the physical, emotional, and social well-being of their cancer patients to achieve greater value-based cancer care. To that end, the incorporation of patient quality of life (QoL) and patient-reported outcomes (PROs) has been vaulted to the forefront of cancer clinical trial design.

The importance of QoL information was emphasized in the mid-1980s, by both the National Cancer Institute (NCI) and the United States Food and Drug Administration (FDA). The NCI, in its 1988 Mission Statement, proposed, "research aimed at improving survival and QoL for persons with cancer is of the highest priority to the Cancer Therapy Evaluation Program (NCI, C.T.C.G.P 1988)." Likewise, the FDA made QoL an essential part of the new cancer drug approval process (Johnson and Temple 1985). Drugs such as gemcitabine, irinotecan, vinorelbine, oxycodone, mitoxantrone, and erythropoietin have been approved, at least in part, based on QoL endpoints (Leitgeb et al. 1994; Burris et al. 1997). The FDA has since gone on to provide guidance for using patient-reported outcome measures (PROMs) to support labeling claims (Center for Drug Evaluation and Research 2020). Furthermore, the 2012 FDA Safety and Innovation Act led to workshops at the FDA that incorporated patients into the drug development process (Office of the Commissioner 2019). In meetings with patients who had lung cancer, in addition to controlling their cancer, patients wished to be better informed of the effects the treatment would have on their ability to perform their daily activities and how they would affect other aspects of their QoL US Food and Drug Administration (2013). Subsequently, in 2016, the 21st Century Cures Act was passed. As directed by this legislation, the FDA created the Oncology Center of Excellence (OCE). The OCE has initiated an oncology patient-focused drug development program to identify rigorous methods to assess the patient experience that will complement existing survival and tumor-related information US Food and Drug Administration (2020). The importance of QoL information is not unique to the United States, as Europe, Canada, and several other countries have incorporated the patient experience into their regulatory decision-making (Kluetz et al. 2018).

Given the increasing emphasis on QoL and PROs in cancer, particularly in lung cancer, this chapter provides an overview of the significance, methodology, analysis, and limitations and challenges of QoL studies. Relevant examples of QoL studies in lung cancer and radiation therapy have also been included (Siddiqui et al. 2014).

2 What Is Quality of Life

The inherent subjective and abstract nature of the term "quality of life" provides a considerable challenge to defining this construct. In addition, the notion of QoL spans a broad range of an individual's feelings, beliefs, and perceptions of life. As a result, QoL remains a fluid concept, influenced by various social, physical, financial, cultural, and emotional factors. As one might expect, the QoL concept presents a challenge to objectively quantify, and this challenge is even further compounded by both the inter- and intrapatient cross-cultural as well as temporal variability (Leplège 1997). However, application of this construct in the clinic necessitates not only its definition and quantification, but also its scientific study in the realm of clinical trials. The World Health Organization (WHO) has defined QoL as "an individual's perceptions of their position in life in the context of the culture and value system where they live, and in relation to their goals, expectations, standards, and concerns. It is a broad ranging concept incorporating in a complex way a person's physical health, psychological state, level of independence, social relationships, personal beliefs and relationship to salient features of the environment Anonymous (1993)." The WHO defined health as "a state of complete physical, mental and social well-being and not merely the absence of disease."

3 How Is Quality of Life Measured

There are several considerations regarding the measurement of QoL in clinical studies. The first consideration is that of the collection of QoL reporting. Attempts to evaluate QoL by anyone other than the patient have been shown to result in significantly different reporting (Slevin et al. 1988; Watkins-Bruner et al. 1995). As such, both the NCI and FDA have recognized the importance of the collection of patient-reported outcomes (PROs). A PRO is defined as "any report of a patient's health condition, health behavior, or experience with healthcare that comes directly from the patient, without interpretation of the patient's response by a clinician or anyone else (Center for Drug Evaluation and Research 2020)." Examples of PROs include QoL, treatment preferences, symptoms, and satisfaction with care. PROs have been shown to add value to research and to complement clinician-collected data to more fully describe the health status of oncology patients (Basch et al. 2009; Damm et al. 2013). As such, the number of clinical trials, including lung cancer trials, incorporating PRO endpoints into their designs, has increased significantly (Bottomley et al. 2003; Claassens et al. 2011).

The next consideration centers on the setting(s) in which QoL should be measured within clinical trials. Financial, data management, and few human resources may limit the measurement of QoL in some trials. Moreover, some trial designs, such as those of phase I and phase II clinical trials, in which there is no comparison arm and the trial questions are focused on maximal tolerated doses and preliminary efficacy data, may limit the relevance of QoL measurement and create undue patient burden. A more meaningful arena, as described by several authors, is to measure QoL within the context of randomized clinical trials. Carolyn Gotay, for example, reported that QoL endpoints should be included into phase III randomized clinical trials (1) when QoL is considered to be the primary endpoint, such as a study comparing two palliative regimens; (2) if two treatments are expected to be equivalent in terms of efficacy (e.g., survival), such that one treatment would be considered preferable if it is associated with a relative QoL advantage; (3) if the advantage of one arm in terms of outcome may be real but nevertheless offset by increased toxicity and deterioration in QoL; and (4) if the treatments differ in short-term efficacy, but the overall failure rate is high (Gotay 2004). Similarly, Moinpour and colleagues proposed the following guidelines: (1) if the disease site is associated with a relatively poor prognosis, (2) if different treatment modalities are being compared, (3) if different treatment intensities and/or duration are being compared, and (4) if expected survival is assumed equivalent, but the QoL is expected to be different between the two regimens (Moinpour et al. 1989).

Another critical consideration is the selection of the most appropriate QoL instrument. In reviewing, testing, and validating any QoL instrument, particular attention must be placed on the reliability, validity, sensitivity, and responsiveness to change over time of the instrument (Testa and Simonson 1996). Reliability of an instrument quantifies the freedom from random error. In other words, a reliable instrument reports values that remain consistent with repeated measurement under constant conditions. Generally, an instrument reliability of 0.70 or higher is acceptable for clinical trials (Nunnaly and Bernstein 1994). Validity can be assessed in terms of content (i.e., does it address the relevant issues), construct (i.e., does it indeed measure what it claims to measure), and clinical focus (i.e., does it differentiate patient groups with differing clinical and/or sociodemographic features). Indeed, a valid test must appropriately focus on the intended target and then measure the outcome that it claims to measure. Responsiveness refers to the ability of an instrument to detect changes in an outcome over time within a particular individual or group (Husted et al. 2000). Similar to responsiveness, sensitivity is the ability of the instrument to measure true changes or differences in outcome. Both the sensitivity and responsiveness of an instrument may be affected by "ceiling" or "floor" effects when outcome scores from patient response rest at the limits of the possible score range, thus not allowing measurement of any positive or negative movement beyond the "ceiling" or "floor," respectively. Regardless of such effects, a sensitive and responsive instrument will measure stable outcomes when there is no change in outcome.

4 Quality-of-Life Instruments

There are two main types of QoL instruments: generic and disease or condition specific. Generic QoL instruments have the broadest focus and are designed to assess the general health status of individuals across a range of diagnoses. The inherent breadth of these questionnaires, however, results in their inability to account for clinical issues in site-, condition-, or treatment-specific measures. Therefore, QoL instruments have been developed that combine generic and specific measurements into one instrument. Examples of these types of instruments within oncology include the European Organization for Research and Treatment of Cancer (EORTC) Quality of Life Questionnaire Core 30 (QLQ-C30) (Aaronson et al. 1993) and the Functional Assessment of Cancer Therapy-General (FACT-G) (Cella et al. 1993). Additional disease-specific modules exist for each generic tool, such as the EORTC QLQ-Lung Cancer (QLQ-LC13) and the FACT-Lung Cancer (FACT-L) (Bergman et al. 1994; Cella et al. 1995). A recent review of phase III randomized controlled trials for non-small cell lung cancer (NSCLC) identified 46 trials that assessed QoL and that 43.5% included the EORTC QLQ-C30, 37% the EORTC QLQ-LC13, and 50% the FACT-L (Fernández-López et al. 2016).

The EORTC QLQ-C30 is a validated oncology instrument containing 30 items with scores from 0 (not at all) to 4 (very much) for items 1–28 and from 1 (very poor) to 7 (excellent) for items 29 and 30 (Aaronson et al. 1993). The instrument has been translated in over 50 languages. The QLQ-C30 assesses various elements of QoL through nine multi-item scales: five functional scales (physical, role, cognitive, emotional, and social); three symptom scales (fatigue, pain, and nausea and vomiting); and additional global health and QoL scales. In addition to the QLQ-C30, the QLQ-LC13 has been developed and validated specifically for lung cancer (Bergman et al. 1994). The QLQ-LC13 is a 13-item lung cancer-specific questionnaire that consists of one three-question subscale (dyspnea) and ten symptom items (cough, hemoptysis, sore mouth, dysphagia, peripheral neuropathy, alopecia, pain in chest, pain in shoulder, pain, and pain medication). The score of each item ranges from 0 to 100 with higher scores indicating better functioning on the QLQ-C30, but increased symptoms on the QLQ-LC13. For advanced thoracic diseases, both the EORTC QLQ-C30 and QLQ-LC13 questionnaires have been validated in the palliative setting (Nicklasson and Bergman 2007).

The FACT-G instrument is another validated tool also available in over 50 languages and consists of a 27-item questionnaire measuring physical well-being (7 items), social/family well-being (7 items), emotional well-being (6 items), and functional well-being (7 items) (Cella et al. 1993). Each item is scored from 0 to 4 with a range of 0–28 for physical, social/family, and functional well-being and 0–24 for emotional well-being and a total score range of 0–108. In addition, the FACT-L, consisting of the FACT-G and a lung cancer subscale (LCS), has been developed and validated for lung cancer (Cella et al. 1995). The FACT-L LCS is a 9-item lung cancer-specific questionnaire that assesses dyspnea, cough, weight loss, chest pain, alopecia, appetite loss, and smoking. In contrast to the EORTC QLQ-LC13, FACT-L LCS does not assess hemoptysis, sore mouth, dysphagia, or peripheral neuropathy. FACT-Trials Outcome Index, or TOI, is an abbreviated, validated component of the FACT-L QoL instrument that has been extensively used in patients with lung cancer and can be completed in under 10 min (Cella et al. 1995; Butt et al. 2005). It consists of the physical well-being (PWB), functional well-being (FWB), and the LCS described above.

The NCI has also developed PRO tools for symptom score measurement, patient-reported outcomes common terminology for criteria for adverse events (PRO-CTCAE), and patient-reported outcomes measurement information system (PROMIS). PRO-CTCAE was introduced by the NCI to add the direct patient-reported experience to the clinician-reported CTCAE (Dueck et al. 2015). This is based on a validated single-item symptom reporting system with up to four attributes for each symptom: presence/absence, frequency, severity, and/or interference with usual or daily activities (Movsas 2015). The PRO-CTCAE item bank consists of 78 symptoms relevant to cancer and its treatment, including symptoms related to immunotherapy. PROMIS measures the physical, mental, and social health of adults and children and has been supported by the NCI to ensure that PROMIS is valid for cancer patients and survivors (Garcia et al. 2007). PROMIS tools are typically multi-item questionnaires and include item banks and short forms. Many of the QoL instruments described have computer-adaptive versions.

5 Appropriate Instrument Selection, Timing, and Frequency of Measurements

Selection of the appropriate QoL instrument depends on several factors including (1) the underlying hypothesis of the trial, (2) the patient population, (3) the treatments and their toxicity profiles, and (4) the degree of resources available (Gelber and Gelber 1995). In addition, selected questionnaires must be reliable and validated. Furthermore, one should consider the burden of filling out the questionnaire, as lost or missing data results in bias.

After selection of an appropriate QoL instrument, attention must be turned to establishing the optimal timing and frequency of administration. Instrument administration varies between clinical trials and is influenced by the hypothesis and the treatment protocol of the clinical trial, the natural course of the disease, and the anticipated side effects of treatment (Osoba et al. 1996). Regardless of these factors, all clinical trials with QoL endpoints must perform a baseline QoL assessment. This baseline assessment not only is essential for the QoL analysis, but also has prognostic significance for lung cancers (Langendijk et al. 2000; Montazeri et al. 2001; Movsas et al. 2009). The baseline assessment also determines differences in pretreatment QoL in treatment groups and allows comparison to posttreatment QoL. During the course of the clinical trial, the frequency of QoL data collection must balance the cost of data collection/management and patient burden with the benefit of the additional QoL data. The frequency of collection can be directed by a time-based (e.g., at a set time after randomization) or an event-based (e.g., after a specific treatment cycle) approach. As with baseline assessment, QoL assessments at the completion of treatment and postcompletion (i.e., a few weeks to months later) are essential. Such measures afford not only the study of treatment side effects, but also, and perhaps more importantly, knowledge of the course and nature of recovery from those side effects. Such knowledge can be particularly useful in making clinical decisions and recommendations.

6 Compliance

Within health and social science research, missing data and low compliance are far too commonplace. Missing data and low compliance can lead to biased research findings as a result of decreased statistical power (Rubin 2004). Claassens et al., in a systematic review of randomized lung cancer trials, reported that trial investigators either failed (26%) or provided limited information (11%) related to missing data (Claassens et al. 2011). However, investigators are improving in this regard as a more recent systematic review demonstrated only 5% of trials failing to report the statistical methods they used to deal with missing data (van der Weijst et al. 2017). Moreover, recent oncology trials submitted to the FDA have shown high rates of compliance by patients submitting PROs (Basch 2019).

To reduce the rates of data loss and missing data and to report missing information appropriately, investigators should consider several approaches. During study design, they should examine not only the potential for missing data and attrition when calculating their trial sample size, but also how they will handle missing data (van der Weijst et al. 2017). When collecting data, members of the research team and study participants should be reminded of the importance of complete PRO data. Utilization of an electronic reporting system and having an automated or human backup data completion plan may be helpful to reduce missing data and potential institutional errors (Movsas et al. 2016; Basch 2019). Several published guidelines exist to help researchers publish unbiased and robust interpretations of their PRO data including the Consolidated Standards of Reporting Trials (CONSORT)-PRO extension checklist and the Setting International Standards in Analyzing Patient-Reported Outcomes and Quality of Life Endpoints Data (SISAQOL) Consortium Recommendations (Calvert et al. 2013; Coens et al. 2020).

7 Analyzing QoL Data

Analysis of QoL data is based fundamentally on the QoL hypothesis. This allows for the necessary incorporation of QoL measurements into the power calculation and statistical design. Past lung cancer clinical trials evaluated PRO scores over time with the calculation of mean group differences (van der Weijst et al. 2017). However, this method of analysis, while allowing for direct comparisons between arms at each time point, has the inherent weaknesses of (1) ignoring sampling hierarchy differences, (2) an inability to manage missing data, and (3) an assumption of independence of observation in repeated measures (Beacon and Thompson 1996). More appropriate methods of analysis for longitudinal studies with repeated PRO measures include mixed-effect and time-to-event modeling (Bonnetain et al. 2016; van der Weijst et al. 2017). Time-to-HRQoL score(s) deterioration (TTD), a type of time-to-event modeling, allows for the easy interpretation of results by clinicians as, similar to survival analysis, TTD analyses are reported with a hazard ratio (Bonnetain et al. 2016).

A clinically meaningful difference (CMD) refers to the smallest meaningful differences in PROs that patients perceive as important. A statistically significant difference of PRO measures between trial arms may be identified, though this may not be considered a CMD. Currently, there is insufficient reporting of CMDs within lung cancer clinical trials (Claassens et al. 2011; van der Weijst et al. 2017). Vital to reporting CMDs is determination of the range or cutoff for these differences. A commonly used rule is half a standard deviation or 5–10% of the score range in the questionnaire. More research is necessary to determine CMD cutoffs for different PRO instruments within longitudinal studies.

8 Real-Time PRO Monitoring

Evidence is increasing for the capturing of PRO data electronically (ePROs) in real time. Basch et al. have designed a Web-based symptom collection system for patients with cancer, including patients with lung cancer (Basch et al. 2007). In a trial of 766 advanced-stage cancer patients, the patients were randomized to electronic symptom monitoring and asked to report 12 common symptoms via tablet or home computers versus receiving usual care (Basch et al. 2016). Patients in the intervention arm had improved QoL, received chemotherapy for a longer period of time, had less emergency room visits, and perhaps most remarkably lived longer (median OS 31.2 months versus 26 months ($p = 0.03$)) (Basch et al. 2016, 2017).

Denis et al. have also developed a Web-based symptom monitoring tool for lung cancer patients (Denis et al. 2014). Patients with advanced non-progressive stage IIA–IV lung cancer were randomized to receive either Web-based symptom monitoring (PRO group) or standard follow-up with imaging every 3–6 months. One hundred thirty-three patients were enrolled with twelve patients ineligible. With 2 years of follow-up, median overall survival was 22.5 months in the PRO group and 14.9 months in the control group without censoring for crossover ($p = 0.03$). Censoring for crossover resulted in median overall survival of 22.5 months in the intervention group versus 13.5 months in the control group ($p = 0.005$) (Denis et al. 2014, 2019). These authors also evaluated the cost-effectiveness of an electronic symptom monitoring strategy and demonstrated that the cost of follow-up was €362 less per patient in the PRO group compared with the control group (Lizée et al. 2019). Furthermore, the PRO group was found to have an incremental cost-effectiveness ratio of €12,127 per life year gained and €20,912 per quality-adjusted life year gained (Lizée et al. 2019).

Clearly, Web-based symptom monitoring and ePRO approaches have demonstrated their value within cancer care delivery, not only with improvements in overall survival and cost-effectiveness, but also in demonstrating their potential for reduction of missing data and saving of service time (Movsas et al. 2014). An even greater opportunity for clinical cancer research may be the collection of continuous, passive, real-time assessment of activity, sleep, and physiology leveraging existing smartphone, smartwatch, and consumer wearable technology (Low 2020). In a study by Ohri et al., of 50 patients undergoing definitive chemoradiation for locally advanced non-small cell lung cancer, daily step counts were assessed using a commercially available fitness tracker (Ohri et al. 2019). The authors found that inactive subjects, those with step counts below the 25th percentile of healthy individuals, were more likely to be hospitalized during treatment (50% vs. 9% $p = 0.004$) and less likely to complete radiation therapy without a treatment break of greater than 1 week (67% vs. 97% ($p = 0.006$). Perhaps more striking were the findings of median PFS (5.3 months vs. 18.3 months, HR = 5.10, $p < 0.001$) and median overall survival (15 months vs. not reached, HR = 3.91, $p = 0.004$) (Ohri et al. 2019). This study demonstrated the feasibility and value of real-time monitoring of step counts, but it also provides a glimpse of the potential for wearable technologies to further personalize cancer care and to improve the quality of life and clinical outcomes for our patients.

9 Quality-of-Life Studies in Lung Cancer

Many lung cancer studies have incorporated QoL (Kaasa et al. 1989; Ganz et al. 1991; Langendijk et al. 2000; Maione et al. 2005; Qi et al. 2009; Movsas et al. 2009; Braun et al. 2011; Fiteni et al. 2016; Movsas et al. 2016). The following highlights some examples in the setting of locally advanced NSCLC. Global baseline QoL has consistently been shown to be predictive for longer lung cancer survival with, in general, each 10-point increase in global QoL associated with an approximate 10% increase in survival (Maione et al. 2005; Qi et al. 2009; Braun et al. 2011). PROs have also been shown to maintain their predictive power after controlling for the well-accepted clinical predictors of cancer stage, performance status, and distant metastasis (Maione et al. 2005; Quinten et al. 2009; Braun et al. 2011). Indeed, evidence continues to mount demonstrating that the prognostic information gained from PROs is distinctive, and not supplied by the standard clinical outcomes, warranting their use in clinical decision-making.

One example of QoL as a key prognostic factor for long-term survival among patients with locally advanced/inoperable non-small cell lung cancer treated with chemoradiotherapy was the RTOG 9801 randomized controlled trial (Movsas et al. 2005). This trial of 243 patients with stage II–IIIA/B inoperable non-small cell lung cancer evaluated the radioprotective effects of amifostine (AM) to reduce chemoradiotherapy-induced esophagitis and its influence on QoL and swallowing symptoms. Patients underwent treatment consisting of induction paclitaxel and carboplatin, followed by concurrent weekly paclitaxel and carboplatin with hyperfractionated RT (69.6 Gy in fractions of 1.2 Gy given twice per day). Patients were randomized at registration to either receive AM (500 mg IV) four times per week or not receive it during chemoradiotherapy. Toxicity was assessed using NCI-Common Toxicity Criteria (NCI-CTC), physician dysphagia logs (PDLs), and daily patient swallowing diaries. The EORTC-QLQ C30 and QLQ-LC13 were utilized to collect prospective QoL information. Each arm had comparable baseline demographics. The median survival rates were similar between both treatment arms (17.3 months with AM versus 17.9 months without AM, $p = 0.87$) (Movsas et al. 2005). Amifostine did not significantly reduce esophagitis grade ≥3 in patients receiving hyperfractionated chemoradiation therapy (Movsas et al. 2005). Interestingly, however, patients receiving AM reported less swallowing symptoms than those on the control arm, suggesting a potential "disconnect" between patient and clinician findings (Sarna et al. 2008). Moreover, the patient-reported baseline QoL in this study was found to be an independent prognostic factor for overall survival, superseding traditional prognostic factors, such as Karnofsky performance status and cancer stage (Movsas et al. 2009).

Another study, demonstrating the importance of QoL assessment in locally advanced NSCLC, was the RTOG 0617 (Bradley et al. 2015). This phase III randomized controlled trial enrolled unresectable stage III NSCLC patients and randomized them to receive dose-escalated radiation therapy (74 Gy versus 60 Gy) with concurrent and consolidation chemotherapy with or without cetuximab to determine whether dose-escalated radiation therapy (and/or cetuximab) improved overall survival. Overall, this trial failed to demonstrate an overall survival benefit to either radiation therapy dose escalation or cetuximab (Bradley et al. 2015). In a secondary analysis, Movsas et al. reported the results of the primary QoL hypothesis from the trial that patients on the more intensive chemoradiation arm (higher radiation dose arm) would have clinically meaningful lower quality of life as measured by the lung cancer subscale (LCS) of the FACT-TOI instrument at 3 months postcompletion of the concurrent chemoradiation therapy (Movsas et al. 2016). A total of 313 patients completed the baseline QoL assessment, with 219 (70%) of those completing the 3-month QoL assessments and 137 (57%) of the living patients completing the 12-month assessments. As hypothesized, significantly more patients in the 74 Gy radiation dose arm had significantly meaningful clinical decline in FACT-LCS at 3 months than those in the 60 Gy radiation dose arm (45% versus 30%, $p = 0.02$). Moreover, fewer patients receiving IMRT versus 3D conformal radiation therapy (3D CRT) had clinically meaningful decline in FACT-LCS at 12 months (21% versus 46%, $p = 0.03$). This finding suggests that PROs may be helpful in sorting out more subtle benefits of newer technologies. As before, on multivariate analysis, baseline QoL was highly associated with overall survival (Movsas et al. 2016).

Recently, immunotherapeutic agents have shown promise in the treatment paradigm for lung cancer. With the landmark reporting of the PACIFIC lung cancer trial results, consolidative durvalumab has become the standard of care for patients with locally advanced, unresectable NSCLC (Antonia et al. 2017, 2018). This phase III trial of nonprogressing stage III NSCLC patients was randomized, after standard chemoradiation therapy, to receive durvalumab consolidative immunotherapy every 2 weeks for up to 12 months versus a placebo. With a median follow-up time of 25.2 months and greater than 700 patients enrolled, the 24-month overall survival rate was 66.3% for the durvalumab group versus 55.6% in the placebo group ($p = 0.005$) (Antonia et al. 2018). A secondary endpoint of this trial was to assess PROs with the EORTC QLQ-C30 and the QLQ-LC13 instruments (Hui et al. 2019). Changes from baseline to 12 months were analyzed with a mixed model for repeated measures and time-to-event analyses with a 10-point or greater change from baseline deemed to be clinically relevant (Hui et al. 2019). Of eligible patients, 79% in the durvalumab group and 82% in the placebo group completed questionnaires up to week 48. Importantly, the authors found no clinically relevant improvements or deteriorations between the study arms when assessing between group differences for cough, dyspnea, chest pain, fatigue, appetite loss, physical functioning, or global health status or QoL (Hui et al. 2019). As durvalumab and other immunotherapeutic agents continue to be incorporated into a greater number of lung cancer clinical trials answering questions related to efficacy, timing, and frequency, collection of PRO and QoL endpoints will continue to be extremely valuable.

Yet, despite these examples, there is much room for improvement. Reale et al. recently published a systematic review of QoL analysis in phase III lung cancer trials published between 2012 and 2018 including 11 major journals and 122 publications and found that for 17 trials of early/locally advanced-stage NSCLC, only 7 (41.2%) reported QoL endpoints (Reale et al. 2020). They raise the concern that QoL is not assessed in many phase III lung cancer trials, a setting in which QoL should be strongly considered.

10 Conclusions and Future Directions

Lung cancer continues to remain the leading cause of cancer death worldwide (Ferlay et al. 2019). The traditional outcome measures of overall and progression-free survival and local control continue to improve with advances in our diagnostics and treatments. When considering the poor prognosis for most lung cancer patients, incorporation of PROs into clinical trials is increasingly being recognized. To this end, the Standard Protocol Items: Recommendations for Interventional Trials Statement-PRO extension (SPIRIT-PRO) (Calvert et al. 2018), the CONSORT-PRO (Calvert et al. 2013), and the SISAQOL Consortium recommendations (Coens et al. 2020) provide a framework to improve robustness and scientific reliability of PROs within clinical trials. Yet, the randomized studies by Basch et al. (2016), and Denis et al. (2014), showing a survival improvement by using real-time PROs, indicate that it is now time to move this effective strategy from the clinical oncology trial setting directly into the standard clinical oncology care setting. Moreover, oncology is now in the era of personalized medicine with lung cancer therapies particularly suited by molecular fingerprints. At the same time, we must always keep the "whole person" in mind (i.e., including PROs and patient preferences) when recommending "person"-alized medicine options (Berman et al. 2016). Indeed, fascinating data is emerging that links PROs to molecular genetic findings (Sprangers et al. 2014). The ability to properly report, analyze, interpret, and apply PRO data with relevance and validity will allow for a more informed, personalized patient discussion.

References

Aaronson NK, Ahmedzai S, Bergman B, Bullinger M, Cull A, Duez NJ, Filiberti A, Flechtner H, Fleishman SB, de Haes JC (1993) The European Organization for Research and Treatment of Cancer QLQ-C30: a quality-of-life instrument for use in international clinical trials in oncology. J Natl Cancer Inst 85(5):365–376. https://doi.org/10.1093/jnci/85.5.365

Anonymous (1993) Study protocol for the World Health Organization project to develop a Quality of Life assessment instrument (WHOQOL). Qual Life Res 2(2):153–159

Antonia SJ, Villegas A, Daniel D, Vicente D, Murakami S, Hui R, Yokoi T, Chiappori A, Lee KH, de Wit M, Cho BC, Bourhaba M, Quantin X, Tokito T, Mekhail T, Planchard D, Kim Y-C, Karapetis CS, Hiret S, Ostoros G, Kubota K, Gray JE, Paz-Ares L, de Castro Carpeño J, Wadsworth C, Melillo G, Jiang H, Huang Y, Dennis PA, Özgüroğlu M, PACIFIC Investigators (2017) Durvalumab after chemoradiotherapy in stage III non-small-cell lung cancer. N Engl J Med 377(20):1919–1929. https://doi.org/10.1056/NEJMoa1709937

Antonia SJ, Villegas A, Daniel D, Vicente D, Murakami S, Hui R, Kurata T, Chiappori A, Lee KH, de Wit M, Cho BC, Bourhaba M, Quantin X, Tokito T, Mekhail T, Planchard D, Kim Y-C, Karapetis CS, Hiret S, Ostoros G, Kubota K, Gray JE, Paz-Ares L, de Castro Carpeño J, Faivre-Finn C, Reck M, Vansteenkiste J, Spigel DR, Wadsworth C, Melillo G, Taboada M, Dennis PA, Özgüroğlu M, PACIFIC Investigators (2018) Overall survival with durvalumab after chemoradiotherapy in stage III NSCLC. N Engl J Med 379(24):2342–2350. https://doi.org/10.1056/NEJMoa1809697

Basch E (2019) High compliance rates with patient-reported outcomes in oncology trials submitted to the US Food and Drug Administration. J Natl Cancer Inst 111(5):437–439. https://doi.org/10.1093/jnci/djy183

Basch E, Artz D, Iasonos A, Speakman J, Shannon K, Lin K, Pun C, Yong H, Fearn P, Barz A, Scher HI, McCabe M, Schrag D (2007) Evaluation of an online platform for cancer patient self-reporting of chemotherapy toxicities. J Am Med Inform Assoc 14(3):264–268. https://doi.org/10.1197/jamia.M2177

Basch E, Jia X, Heller G, Barz A, Sit L, Fruscione M, Appawu M, Iasonos A, Atkinson T, Goldfarb S, Culkin A, Kris MG, Schrag D (2009) Adverse symptom event reporting by patients vs clinicians: relationships with clinical outcomes. J Natl Cancer Inst 101(23):1624–1632. https://doi.org/10.1093/jnci/djp386

Basch E, Deal AM, Kris MG, Scher HI, Hudis CA, Sabbatini P, Rogak L, Bennett AV, Dueck AC, Atkinson TM, Chou JF, Dulko D, Sit L, Barz A, Novotny P, Fruscione M, Sloan JA, Schrag D (2016) Symptom monitoring with patient-reported outcomes during routine cancer treatment: a randomized controlled trial. J Clin Oncol 34(6):557–565. https://doi.org/10.1200/JCO.2015.63.0830

Basch E, Deal AM, Dueck AC, Scher HI, Kris MG, Hudis C, Schrag D (2017) Overall survival results of a trial assessing patient-reported outcomes for symptom monitoring during routine cancer treatment. JAMA 318(2):197–198. https://doi.org/10.1001/jama.2017.7156

Beacon HJ, Thompson SG (1996) Multi-level models for repeated measurement data: application to quality of life data in clinical trials. Stat Med 15(24):2717–2732. https://doi.org/10.1002/(SICI)1097-0258(19961230)15:24<2717::AID-SIM518>3.0.CO;2-E

Bergman B, Aaronson NK, Ahmedzai S, Kaasa S, Sullivan M (1994) The EORTC QLQ-LC13: a modular supplement to the EORTC Core Quality of Life Questionnaire (QLQ-C30) for use in lung cancer clinical trials. EORTC Study Group on Quality of Life. Eur J Cancer 30A(5):635–642. https://doi.org/10.1016/0959-8049(94)90535-5

Berman AT, Rosenthal SA, Moghanaki D, Woodhouse KD, Movsas B, Vapiwala N (2016) Focusing on the "person" in personalized medicine: the future of patient-centered care in radiation oncology. J Am Coll Radiol 13(12 Pt B):1571–1578. https://doi.org/10.1016/j.jacr.2016.09.012

Bonnetain F, Fiteni F, Efficace F, Anota A (2016) Statistical challenges in the analysis of health-related quality of life in cancer clinical trials. J Clin Oncol 34(16):1953–1956. https://doi.org/10.1200/JCO.2014.56.7974

Bottomley A, Efficace F, Thomas R, Vanvoorden V, Ahmedzai SH (2003) Health-related quality of life in non-small-cell lung cancer: methodologic issues in randomized controlled trials. J Clin Oncol 21(15):2982–2992. https://doi.org/10.1200/JCO.2003.01.203

Bradley JD, Paulus R, Komaki R, Masters G, Blumenschein G, Schild S, Bogart J, Hu C, Forster K, Magliocco A, Kavadi V, Garces YI, Narayan S, Iyengar P, Robinson C, Wynn RB, Koprowski C, Meng J, Beitler J, Gaur R, Curran W, Choy H (2015) Standard-dose versus high-dose conformal radiotherapy with concurrent and consolidation carboplatin plus paclitaxel with or without cetuximab for patients with stage IIIA or IIIB non-small-cell lung cancer (RTOG 0617): a randomised, two-by-two factorial phase 3 study. Lancet Oncol 16(2):187–199. https://doi.org/10.1016/S1470-2045(14)71207-0

Braun DP, Gupta D, Staren ED (2011) Quality of life assessment as a predictor of survival in non-small cell lung cancer. BMC Cancer 11:353. https://doi.org/10.1186/1471-2407-11-353

Burris HA, Moore MJ, Andersen J, Green MR, Rothenberg ML, Modiano MR, Cripps MC, Portenoy RK, Storniolo AM, Tarassoff P, Nelson R, Dorr FA, Stephens CD, Von Hoff DD (1997) Improvements in survival and clinical benefit with gemcitabine as first-line therapy for patients with advanced pancreas cancer: a randomized trial. J Clin Oncol 15(6):2403–2413. https://doi.org/10.1200/JCO.1997.15.6.2403

Butt Z, Webster K, Eisenstein AR, Beaumont J, Eton D, Masters GA, Cella D (2005) Quality of life in lung cancer: the validity and cross-cultural applicability of the Functional Assessment of Cancer Therapy-Lung scale. Hematol Oncol Clin North Am 19(2):389–420, viii. https://doi.org/10.1016/j.hoc.2005.02.009

Calvert M, Brundage M, Jacobsen PB, Schünemann HJ, Efficace F (2013) The CONSORT Patient-Reported Outcome (PRO) extension: implications for clinical trials and practice. Health Qual Life Outcomes 11:184. https://doi.org/10.1186/1477-7525-11-184

Calvert M, Kyte D, Mercieca-Bebber R, Slade A, Chan A-W, King MT, the SPIRIT-PRO Group, Hunn A, Bottomley A, Regnault A, Chan A-W, Ells C, O'Connor D, Revicki D, Patrick D, Altman D, Basch E, Velikova G, Price G, Draper H, Blazeby J, Scott J, Coast J, Norquist J, Brown J, Haywood K, Johnson LL, Campbell L, Frank L, von Hildebrand M, Brundage M, Palmer M, Kluetz P, Stephens R, Golub RM, Mitchell S, Groves T (2018) Guidelines for inclusion of patient-reported outcomes in clinical trial protocols: the SPIRIT-PRO extension. JAMA 319(5):483–494. https://doi.org/10.1001/jama.2017.21903

Cella DF, Tulsky DS, Gray G, Sarafian B, Linn E, Bonomi A, Silberman M, Yellen SB, Winicour P, Brannon J (1993) The Functional Assessment of Cancer Therapy scale: development and validation of the general measure. J Clin Oncol 11(3):570–579. https://doi.org/10.1200/JCO.1993.11.3.570

Cella DF, Bonomi AE, Lloyd SR, Tulsky DS, Kaplan E, Bonomi P (1995) Reliability and validity of the Functional Assessment of Cancer Therapy-Lung (FACT-L) quality of life instrument. Lung Cancer 12(3):199–220. https://doi.org/10.1016/0169-5002(95)00450-f

Center for Drug Evaluation and Research (2020) Patient-reported outcome measures: use in medical product development to support labeling claims. US Food Drug Administration. https://www.fda.gov/regulatory-information/search-fda-guidance-documents/patient-reported-outcome-measures-use-medical-product-development-support-labeling-claims. Accessed 1 Sep 2020

Claassens L, van Meerbeeck J, Coens C, Quinten C, Ghislain I, Sloan EK, Wang XS, Velikova G, Bottomley A (2011) Health-related quality of life in non-small-cell lung cancer: an update of a systematic review on methodologic issues in randomized controlled trials. J Clin Oncol 29(15):2104–2120. https://doi.org/10.1200/JCO.2010.32.3683

Coens C, Pe M, Dueck AC, Sloan J, Basch E, Calvert M, Campbell A, Cleeland C, Cocks K, Collette L, Devlin N, Dorme L, Flechtner H-H, Gotay C, Griebsch I, Groenvold M, King M, Kluetz PG, Koller M, Malone DC, Martinelli F, Mitchell SA, Musoro JZ, O'Connor D, Oliver K, Piault-Louis E, Piccart M, Quinten C, Reijneveld JC, Schürmann C, Smith AW, Soltys KM, Taphoorn MJB, Velikova G, Bottomley A, Setting International Standards in Analyzing Patient-Reported Outcomes and Quality of Life Endpoints Data Consortium (2020) International standards for the analysis of quality-of-life and patient-reported outcome endpoints in cancer randomised controlled trials: recommendations of the SISAQOL Consortium. Lancet Oncol 21(2):e83–e96. https://doi.org/10.1016/S1470-2045(19)30790-9

Damm K, Roeske N, Jacob C (2013) Health-related quality of life questionnaires in lung cancer trials: a systematic literature review. Health Econ Rev 3(1):15. https://doi.org/10.1186/2191-1991-3-15

Denis F, Viger L, Charron A, Voog E, Dupuis O, Pointreau Y, Letellier C (2014) Detection of lung cancer relapse using self-reported symptoms transmitted via an internet web-application: pilot study of the sentinel follow-up. Support Care Cancer 22(6):1467–1473. https://doi.org/10.1007/s00520-013-2111-1

Denis F, Basch E, Septans A-L, Bennouna J, Urban T, Dueck AC, Letellier C (2019) Two-year survival comparing web-based symptom monitoring vs routine surveillance following treatment for lung cancer. JAMA 321(3):306–307. https://doi.org/10.1001/jama.2018.18085

Dueck AC, Mendoza TR, Mitchell SA, Reeve BB, Castro KM, Rogak LJ, Atkinson TM, Bennett AV, Denicoff AM, O'Mara AM, Li Y, Clauser SB, Bryant DM, Bearden JD, Gillis TA, Harness JK, Siegel RD, Paul DB, Cleeland CS, Schrag D, Sloan JA, Abernethy AP, Bruner DW, Minasian LM, Basch E, National Cancer Institute PRO-CTCAE Study Group (2015) Validity and reliability of the US National Cancer Institute's patient-reported outcomes version of the Common Terminology Criteria for Adverse Events (PRO-CTCAE). JAMA Oncol 1(8):1051–1059. https://doi.org/10.1001/jamaoncol.2015.2639

Ferlay J, Colombet M, Soerjomataram I, Mathers C, Parkin DM, Piñeros M, Znaor A, Bray F (2019) Estimating the global cancer incidence and mortality in 2018: GLOBOCAN sources and methods. Int J Cancer 144(8):1941–1953. https://doi.org/10.1002/ijc.31937

Fernández-López C, Expósito-Hernández J, Arrebola-Moreno JP, Calleja-Hernández MÁ, Expósito-Ruíz M, Guerrero-Tejada R, Linares I, Cabeza-Barrera J (2016) Trends in phase III randomized controlled clinical trials on the treatment of advanced non-small-cell lung cancer. Cancer Med 5(9):2190–2197. https://doi.org/10.1002/cam4.782

Fiteni F, Vernerey D, Bonnetain F, Vaylet F, Sennélart H, Trédaniel J, Moro-Sibilot D, Herman D, Laizé H, Masson P, Derollez M, Clément-Duchêne C, Milleron B, Morin F, Zalcman G, Quoix E, Westeel V (2016) Prognostic value of health-related quality of life for overall survival in elderly non-small-cell lung cancer patients. Eur J Cancer 52:120–128. https://doi.org/10.1016/j.ejca.2015.10.004

Ganz PA, Lee JJ, Siau J (1991) Quality of life assessment. An independent prognostic variable for survival in lung cancer. Cancer 67(12):3131–3135. https://doi.org/10.1002/1097-0142(19910615)67:12<3131::aid-cncr2820671232>3.0.co;2-4

Garcia SF, Cella D, Clauser SB, Flynn KE, Lad T, Lai J-S, Reeve BB, Smith AW, Stone AA, Weinfurt K (2007) Standardizing patient-reported outcomes assessment in cancer clinical trials: a patient-reported outcomes measurement information system initiative. J Clin Oncol 25(32):5106–5112. https://doi.org/10.1200/JCO.2007.12.2341

Gelber RD, Gelber S (1995) Quality-of-life assessment in clinical trials. Cancer Treat Res 75:225–246. https://doi.org/10.1007/978-1-4615-2009-2_11

Gotay CC (2004) Assessing cancer-related quality of life across a spectrum of applications. J Natl Cancer Inst Monogr (33):126–133. https://doi.org/10.1093/jncimonographs/lgh004

Hui R, Özgüroğlu M, Villegas A, Daniel D, Vicente D, Murakami S, Yokoi T, Chiappori A, Lee KH, de Wit M, Cho BC, Gray JE, Rydén A, Viviers L, Poole L, Zhang Y, Dennis PA, Antonia SJ (2019) Patient-reported outcomes with durvalumab after chemoradiotherapy in stage III, unresectable non-small-cell lung cancer (PACIFIC): a randomised, controlled, phase 3 study. Lancet Oncol 20(12):1670–1680. https://doi.org/10.1016/S1470-2045(19)30519-4

Husted JA, Cook RJ, Farewell VT, Gladman DD (2000) Methods for assessing responsiveness: a critical review and recommendations. J Clin Epidemiol 53(5):459–468. https://doi.org/10.1016/s0895-4356(99)00206-1

Johnson JR, Temple R (1985) Food and Drug Administration requirements for approval of new anticancer drugs. Cancer Treat Rep 69(10):1155–1159

Kaasa S, Mastekaasa A, Lund E (1989) Prognostic factors for patients with inoperable non-small cell lung cancer, limited disease. The importance of patients' subjective experience of disease and psychosocial well-being. Radiother Oncol 15(3):235–242. https://doi.org/10.1016/0167-8140(89)90091-1

Kluetz PG, O'Connor DJ, Soltys K (2018) Incorporating the patient experience into regulatory decision making in the USA, Europe, and Canada. Lancet Oncol 19(5):e267–e274. https://doi.org/10.1016/S1470-2045(18)30097-4

Langendijk H, Aaronson NK, de Jong JM, ten Velde GP, Muller MJ, Wouters M (2000) The prognostic impact of quality of life assessed with the EORTC QLQ-C30 in inoperable non-small cell lung carcinoma treated with radiotherapy. Radiother Oncol 55(1):19–25. https://doi.org/10.1016/s0167-8140(00)00158-4

Leitgeb C, Pecherstorfer M, Fritz E, Ludwig H (1994) Quality of life in chronic anemia of cancer during treatment with recombinant human erythropoietin. Cancer 73(10):2535–2542. https://doi.org/10.1002/1097-0142(19940515)73:10<2535::aid-cncr2820731014>3.0.co;2-5

Leplège A (1997) The problem of quality of life in medicine. JAMA 278(1):47. https://doi.org/10.1001/jama.1997.03550010061041

Lizée T, Basch E, Trémolières P, Voog E, Domont J, Peyraga G, Urban T, Bennouna J, Septans A-L, Balavoine M, Detournay B, Denis F (2019) Cost-effectiveness of web-based patient-reported outcome surveillance in patients with lung cancer. J Thorac Oncol 14(6):1012–1020. https://doi.org/10.1016/j.jtho.2019.02.005

Low CA (2020) Harnessing consumer smartphone and wearable sensors for clinical cancer research. NPJ Digit Med 3(1):1–7. https://doi.org/10.1038/s41746-020-00351-x

Maione P, Perrone F, Gallo C, Manzione L, Piantedosi F, Barbera S, Cigolari S, Rosetti F, Piazza E, Robbiati SF, Bertetto O, Novello S, Migliorino MR, Favaretto A, Spatafora M, Ferraù F, Frontini L, Bearz A, Repetto L, Gridelli C, Barletta E, Barzelloni ML, Iaffaioli RV, De Maio E, Di Maio M, De Feo G, Sigoriello G, Chiodini P, Cioffi A, Guardasole V, Angelini V, Rossi A, Bilancia D, Germano D, Lamberti A, Pontillo V, Brancaccio L, Renda F, Romano F, Esani G, Gambaro A, Vinante O, Azzarello G, Clerici M, Bollina R, Belloni P, Sannicolò M, Ciuffreda L, Parello C, Cabiddu M, Sacco C, Sibau A, Porcile G, Castiglione F, Ostellino O, Monfardini S, Stefani M, Scagliotti G, Selvaggi G, De Marinis F, Martelli O, Gasparini G, Morabito A, Gattuso D, Colucci G, Galetta D, Giotta F, Gebbia V, Borsellino N, Testa A, Malaponte E, Capuano MA, Angiolillo M, Sollitto F, Tirelli U, Spazzapan S, Adamo V, Altavilla G, Scimone A, Hopps MR, Tartamella F, Ianniello GP, Tinessa V, Failla G, Bordonaro R, Gebbia N, Valerio MR, D'Aprile M, Veltri E, Tonato M, Darwish S, Romito S, Carrozza F, Barni S, Ardizzoia A, Corradini GM, Pavia G, Belli M, Colantuoni G, Galligioni E, Caffo O, Labianca R, Quadri A, Cortesi E, D'Auria G, Fava S, Calcagno A, Luporini G, Locatelli MC, Di Costanzo F, Gasperoni S, Isa L, Candido P, Gaion F, Palazzolo G, Nettis G, Annamaria A, Rinaldi M, Lopez M, Felletti R, Di Negro GB, Rossi N, Calandriello A, Maiorino L, Mattioli R, Celano A, Schiavon S, Illiano A, Raucci CA, Caruso M, Foa P, Tonini G, Curcio C, Cazzaniga M (2005) Pretreatment quality of life and functional status assessment significantly predict survival of elderly patients with advanced non-small-cell lung cancer receiving chemotherapy: a prognostic analysis of the multicenter Italian lung cancer in the elderly study. J Clin Oncol 23(28):6865–6872. https://doi.org/10.1200/JCO.2005.02.527

Moinpour CM, Feigl P, Metch B, Hayden KA, Meyskens FL, Crowley J (1989) Quality of life end points in cancer clinical trials: review and recommendations. J Natl Cancer Inst 81(7):485–495. https://doi.org/10.1093/jnci/81.7.485

Montazeri A, Milroy R, Hole D, McEwen J, Gillis CR (2001) Quality of life in lung cancer patients: as an important prognostic factor. Lung Cancer 31(2–3):233–240. https://doi.org/10.1016/s0169-5002(00)00179-3

Movsas B (2015) Proceeding with the patient-reported outcomes (PROs) version of the common terminology criteria for adverse events. JAMA Oncol 1(8):1059–1060. https://doi.org/10.1001/jamaoncol.2015.2689

Movsas B, Scott C, Langer C, Werner-Wasik M, Nicolaou N, Komaki R, Machtay M, Smith C, Axelrod R, Sarna L, Wasserman T, Byhardt R (2005) Randomized trial of amifostine in locally advanced non-small-cell lung cancer patients receiving chemotherapy and hyperfractionated radiation: radiation therapy oncology group trial 98-01. J Clin Oncol 23(10):2145–2154. https://doi.org/10.1200/JCO.2005.07.167

Movsas B, Moughan J, Sarna L, Langer C, Werner-Wasik M, Nicolaou N, Komaki R, Machtay M, Wasserman T, Bruner DW (2009) Quality of life supersedes the classic prognosticators for long-term survival in locally advanced non-small-cell lung cancer: an analysis of RTOG 9801. J Clin Oncol 27(34):5816–5822. https://doi.org/10.1200/JCO.2009.23.7420

Movsas B, Hunt D, Watkins-Bruner D, Lee WR, Tharpe H, Goldstein D, Moore J, Dayes IS, Parise S, Sandler H (2014) Can electronic web-based technology improve quality of life data collection? Analysis of Radiation Therapy Oncology Group 0828. Pract Radiat Oncol 4(3):187–191. https://doi.org/10.1016/j.prro.2013.07.014

Movsas B, Hu C, Sloan J, Bradley J, Komaki R, Masters G, Kavadi V, Narayan S, Michalski J, Johnson DW, Koprowski C, Curran WJ, Garces YI, Gaur R, Wynn RB, Schallenkamp J, Gelblum DY, MacRae RM, Paulus R, Choy H (2016) Quality of life analysis of a radiation dose-escalation study of patients with non-small-cell lung cancer: a secondary analysis of the Radiation Therapy Oncology Group 0617 randomized clinical trial. JAMA Oncol 2(3):359–367. https://doi.org/10.1001/jamaoncol.2015.3969

Nicklasson M, Bergman B (2007) Validity, reliability and clinical relevance of EORTC QLQ-C30 and LC13 in patients with chest malignancies in a palliative setting. Qual Life Res 16(6):1019–1028. https://doi.org/10.1007/s11136-007-9210-8

Nunnaly J, Bernstein I (1994) Psychometric therapy. McGraw-Hill, New York

Office of the Commissioner (2019) Food and Drug Administration Safety and Innovation Act (FDASIA). FDA. https://www.fda.gov/regulatory-information/selected-amendments-fdc-act/food-and-drug-administration-safety-and-innovation-act-fdasia. Accessed 12 Dec 2020

Ohri N, Halmos B, Bodner WR, Cheng H, Guha C, Kalnicki S, Garg M (2019) Daily step counts: a new prognostic factor in locally advanced non-small cell lung cancer? Int J Radiat Oncol Biol Phys 105(4):745–751. https://doi.org/10.1016/j.ijrobp.2019.07.055

Osoba D, Zee B, Warr D, Kaizer L, Latreille J, Pater J (1996) Quality of life studies in chemotherapy-induced emesis. Oncology 53(Suppl 1):92–95. https://doi.org/10.1159/000227647

Qi Y, Schild SE, Mandrekar SJ, Tan AD, Krook JE, Rowland KM, Garces YI, Soori GS, Adjei AA, Sloan JA (2009) Pretreatment quality of life is an independent prognostic factor for overall survival in patients with advanced stage non-small cell lung cancer. J Thorac Oncol 4(9):1075–1082. https://doi.org/10.1097/JTO.0b013e3181ae27f5

Quinten C, Coens C, Mauer M, Comte S, Sprangers MAG, Cleeland C, Osoba D, Bjordal K, Bottomley A, EORTC Clinical Groups (2009) Baseline quality of life as a prognostic indicator of survival: a meta-analysis of individual patient data from EORTC clinical trials. Lancet Oncol 10(9):865–871. https://doi.org/10.1016/S1470-2045(09)70200-1

Reale ML, De Luca E, Lombardi P, Marandino L, Zichi C, Pignataro D, Ghisoni E, Di Stefano RF, Mariniello A, Trevisi E, Leone G, Muratori L, La Salvia A, Sonetto C, Bironzo P, Aglietta M, Novello S, Scagliotti GV, Perrone F, Di Maio M (2020) Quality of life analysis in lung cancer: a systematic review of phase III trials published between 2012 and 2018. Lung Cancer 139:47–54. https://doi.org/10.1016/j.lungcan.2019.10.022

Rubin D (2004) Multiple imputation for nonresponse in surveys. Wiley, Hoboken, NJ

Sarna L, Swann S, Langer C, Werner-Wasik M, Nicolaou N, Komaki R, Machtay M, Byhardt R, Wasserman T, Movsas B (2008) Clinically meaningful differences in patient-reported outcomes with amifostine in combination with chemoradiation for locally advanced non-small-cell lung cancer: an analysis of RTOG 9801. Int J Radiat Oncol Biol Phys 72(5):1378–1384. https://doi.org/10.1016/j.ijrobp.2008.03.003

Siddiqui F, Liu AK, Watkins-Bruner D, Movsas B (2014) Patient-reported outcomes and survivorship in radiation oncology: overcoming the cons. J Clin Oncol 32(26):2920–2927. https://doi.org/10.1200/JCO.2014.55.0707

Slevin ML, Plant H, Lynch D, Drinkwater J, Gregory WM (1988) Who should measure quality of life, the doctor or the patient? Br J Cancer 57(1):109–112. https://doi.org/10.1038/bjc.1988.20

Sprangers MAG, Thong MSY, Bartels M, Barsevick A, Ordoñana J, Shi Q, Wang XS, Klepstad P, Wierenga EA, Singh JA, Sloan JA, GeneQol Consortium (2014) Biological pathways, candidate genes, and molecular markers associated with quality-of-life domains: an update. Qual Life Res 23(7):1997–2013. https://doi.org/10.1007/s11136-014-0656-1

Testa MA, Simonson DC (1996) Assessment of quality-of-life outcomes. N Engl J Med 334(13):835–840. https://doi.org/10.1056/NEJM199603283341306

US Food and Drug Administration (2013) The voice of the patient. A series of reports from the U.S. Food and Drug Administration's (FDA's) patient-focused drug development initiative. Lung Cancer. https://www.fda.gov/downloads/drugs/newsevents/ucm464932.pdf. Accessed 3 Feb 2021

US Food and Drug Administration (2020) Patient-focused drug development program. https://www.fda.gov/about-fda/oncology-center-excellence/patient-focused-drug-development. Accessed 3 Feb 2021

van der Weijst L, Surmont V, Schrauwen W, Lievens Y (2017) Systematic literature review of health-related quality of life in locally-advanced non-small cell lung cancer: has it yet become state-of-the-art? Crit Rev Oncol Hematol 119:40–49. https://doi.org/10.1016/j.critrevonc.2017.09.014

Watkins-Bruner D, Scott C, Lawton C, DelRowe J, Rotman M, Buswell L, Beard C, Cella D (1995) RTOG's first quality of life study—RTOG 90-20: a phase II trial of external beam radiation with etanidazole for locally advanced prostate cancer. Int J Radiat Oncol Biol Phys 33(4):901–906. https://doi.org/10.1016/0360-3016(95)02002-5

Importance of Prognostic Factors in Lung Cancer

Lukas Käsmann

Contents

1   Introduction 1001
2   **Non-small Cell Lung Cancer** 1002
2.1   Tumor-Related Factors 1002
2.2   Patient-Related Factors 1006
2.3   Treatment-Related Factors 1008
2.4   Prognostic Scores 1009
3   **Small Cell Lung Cancer (SCLC)** 1009
3.1   Tumor-Related Factors 1009
3.2   Patient-Related Factors 1011
3.3   Treatment-Related Factors 1011
3.4   Prognostic Scores 1012

References 1012

L. Käsmann (✉)
Department of Radiation Oncology, University Hospital, LMU Munich, Munich, Germany
e-mail: lkaesmann@googlemail.com

1   Introduction

Lung cancer is still one of the most common types of cancer worldwide and remained the leading cause of cancer deaths, with an estimated 1.8 million deaths (18%), in 2020 (Sung et al. 2021). Also, lung cancer cases have continuously increased in the last decade with more than 2.2 million (11.4% of all incident cancers) estimated today.

Historically, lung cancer has been divided into non-small cell lung cancer (NSCLC) and small cell lung cancer (SCLC) (Zheng 2016). Both histological subtypes share molecular and cellular origins but distinguish in risk factors for their development, clinical presentation, and prognosis. Furthermore, the overall survival rate varies dramatically from stage IA1 NSCLC with a 5-year survival rate of more than 90% to stage IV with a 5-year survival rate of less than 20% (Goldstraw et al. 2016; Brierley et al. 2017). Due to the discovery of certain molecular targets, advances in medical imaging, introduction of immune checkpoint inhibition, and molecular targeted therapy, selected patients experience long-term survival without making compromises in their quality of life.

This chapter aims to clarify the heterogeneous nature of the disease and reveal important prognostic factors in order to guide physicians in clinical decision-making. Prognostic factors are defined as factors before treatment that have an impact on the patient's outcome "independently" of the received treatment. Therefore, prognostic factors may help physicians to determine the prognosis of an individual patient and contribute to personalized treatment approaches. However, numerous studies have been published regarding prognostic factors in lung cancer. Several factors such as selection bias, performance bias, publication bias, poor statistical power, and lack of external validity need to be considered in order to identify important prognostic factors. In this chapter, we present the current knowledge of prognostic factors in the treatment of lung cancer (NSCLC and SCLC) and discuss their impact in clinical decision-making—with a specific focus on multimodal treatment approaches.

2 Non-small Cell Lung Cancer

2.1 Tumor-Related Factors

2.1.1 Tumor Stage

Tumor staging using the TNM classification of malignant tumors (TNM) is a well-recognized standard for classifying the extent of spread in malignancy including lung cancer (Brierley et al. 2017). At the time of the initial diagnosis, the tumor stage is the most important predictor of survival. Within the TNM classification (see Table 1), the tumor stage is based on three categories: the T category describing the local extent of disease, the N category describing the regional lymph node involvement, and the M category describing the number and localization of distant metastases. The TNM classification is well established for aiding in treatment planning, providing information about the patient's prognosis and supporting benchmarking of cancer centers and research activities such as cancer registries. Historically, the Union for International Cancer Control (UICC) Committee on Tumor Nomenclature and Statistics accepted the tumor staging on the basis of anatomical staging in 1953. Since then, several revisions of the tumor classification and staging have been made. The latest revision is the eighth edition published in 2017 (Brierley et al. 2017). Several important changes regarding the previous classification have been introduced such as a T classification based on 1 cm increment, downstage of T descriptor including endobronchial tumor disregarding its distance from carina (T2), total and partial atelectasis/pneumonitis combined into the same T category (T2), upstage diaphragmatic infiltration (T4), and new classification concept of adenocarcinoma in situ, minimally invasive adenocarcinoma, and Pancoast tumor based on the invasion depth. In addition, extrathoracic diseases were stratified according to the number and sites of extrathoracic metastases (M1b versus M1c). Importantly, involvement of multiple pulmonary sites, including multiple primary lung cancer, separate lung cancer nodules, multiple ground-glass or lepidic lesions, and consolidation, was discussed. The eighth edition of the TNM lung staging system provides a more precise classification based on the prognostic analysis of each TNM descriptor; (Table 2) however, certain imaging interpretations still need to be clarified in terms of clinical staging. The patients' prognosis, especially when it comes to metastatic disease, highly depends on molecular alterations rather than imaging alone. As a result, one of the most important limitations of the latest TNM classification is that it has been made without considering driver oncogene and immune status. Therefore, it may be necessary to consider the presence or absence of driver oncogene and immune status as a new staging factor in future classifications and reconsider some of the existing staging and therapeutic algorithms for advanced NSCLC.

2.1.2 Tumor Volume

Several studies suggest the prognostic role of the tumor volume rather than the T category alone especially in patients with locally advanced stage or patients undergoing radiation treatment (Käsmann et al. 2018). For radiotherapy planning, the gross tumor volume (GTV) is mainly defined by computed tomography (CT). However, ^{18}F-fluorodeoxyglucose (^{18}F-FDG) PET may also be useful to define the gross tumor volume for radiation treatment planning (Nestle et al. 2020). Metabolic parameters such as maximum and peak standardized uptake values

Table 1 TNM classification for lung cancer in the eighth edition (Detterbeck et al. 2016)

Category	Stage		Brief description
T (tumor)	Tis		Carcinoma in situ
	T1		Largest diameter <3 cm, surrounded by lung tissue or visceral pleura, main bronchus is not involved
		T1a(mi)	Minimally invasive adenocarcinoma (solitary adenocarcinoma with predominantly lepidic growth pattern), <3 cm in greatest diameter with an invasive (solid on CT) portion <5 mm
		T1a	Largest diameter ≤1 cm
		T1b	Largest diameter >1 and ≤2 cm
		T1c	Largest diameter >2 and ≤3 cm
	T2		Largest diameter >3 and ≤4 cm
			Infiltration of the main bronchus regardless of the distance from the carina, but without direct invasion of the carina
			Infiltration of the visceral pleura
			Tumor-related partial atelectasis or obstructive pneumonia extending into the hilus and involving parts of the lung or the entire lung
	–	T2a	Largest diameter >4 and ≤5 cm
	–	T2b	
	T3		Largest diameter >5 but ≤7 cm
			Infiltration of thoracic wall (including parietal pleura and superior sulcus), phrenic nerve, parietal pericardium
			Additional tumor nodule in the same lobe of the lung as the primary tumor
	T4		Largest diameter >7 cm or with direct infiltration of diaphragm, mediastinum, heart, great vessels (vena cava, aorta, pulmonary artery, pulmonary vein intrapericardially), trachea, recurrent laryngeal nerve, esophagus, vertebral body, carina
			Additional tumor node in another ipsilateral lung lobe
N (lymph node involvement)	N0		No lymph node involvement
	N1		Lymph node metastasis in ipsilateral, peribronchial, and/or ipsilateral hilar location and/or intrapulmonary lymph node metastases or direct invasion of these lymph node locations
	N2		Lymph node metastasis in ipsilateral mediastinal and/or subcarinal location
	N3		Lymph node metastasis in contralateral mediastinal, contralateral hilar, ipsi- or contralateral deep cervical, supraclavicular location
M (metastasis)	M0		No distant metastasis
	M1		Distant metastasis
		• M1a	Separate tumor nodule in a contralateral lung lobe
			Pleura with nodular involvement
			Malignant pleural effusion
			Malignant pericardial effusion
		• M1b	Isolated distant metastasis in an extrathoracic organ
		• M1c	Multiple distant metastases (>1) in one or more organs

Table 2 NSCLC—tumor stages according to UICC/eighth TNM classification (Detterbeck et al. 2016)

Stage	T category	N category	M category
0	Tis	N0	M0
IA1	T1a(mi)	N0	M0
	T1a	N0	M0
IA2	T1b	N0	M0
IA3	T1c	N0	M0
IB	T2a	N0	M0
IIA	T2b	N0	M0
IIB	T1a-c	N1	M0
	T2a	N1	M0
	T2b	N1	M0
	T3	N0	M0
IIIA	T1a-c	N2	M0
	T2a-b	N2	M0
	T3	N1	M0
	T4	N0	M0
	T4	N1	M0
IIIB	T1a-b	N3	M0
	T2 a–b	N3	M0
	T3	N2	M0
	T4	N2	M0
IIIC	T3	N3	M0
	T4	N3	M0
IVA	Every T	Every N	M1a
	Every T	Every N	M1b
IVB	Every T	Every N	M1c

(SUV_{max}, SUV_{peak}), metabolic tumor volume (MTV), and total lesion glycolysis (TLG) provided by ^{18}F-FDG PET have been suggested to provide prognostic information. However, evidence is mainly based on retrospective or small prospective patient cohorts (Berghmans et al. 2008; Kaida et al. 2017; Chardin et al. 2020). A meta-analysis from 2015 included 1581 patients from 13 studies and found that MTV and TLG were significant prognostic factors in NSCLC independently from stage (Im et al. 2015). However, all included studies were of retrospective design. Larger prospective studies are warranted to investigate the role of (metabolic) tumor volumes in NSCLC.

2.1.3 Histology

Based on the 2015 WHO classification, NSCLC can be further described as adenocarcinoma (AC), squamous cell carcinoma (SCC), or poorly differentiated or undifferentiated large cell carcinoma (LCC) and accounts for 85–90% of all lung cancers (see Fig. 1). Furthermore, several rare cancer histologies can be found in the lung such as sarcomatoid carcinoma, adenosquamous carcinoma, a hybrid of adenocarcinoma and squamous cell lung cancer, and salivary gland-type lung carcinoma, which is most often found in the central airways of the lungs. The prognostic impact of lung cancer histology has been constantly under investigation (Hirsch et al. 2008). Several population-based studies found that AC is associated with improved outcome independently from tumor stage (Lu et al. 2019; Wang et al. 2020). Other studies found no correlation between histology and oncologic outcome questioning the prognostic information of histology alone in NSCLC (Maeda et al. 2011).

2.1.4 Serological Markers (Tumor Markers)

Serological markers are established in diagnostics and could be useful to differentiate between NSCLC and SCLC. Furthermore, tumor markers such as CYFRA 21-1, neuron-specific enolase (NSE), tissue polypeptide antigen (TPA), carcinoembryonic antigen (CEA), CA 125, and squamous cell carcinoma antigen (SCCAg) have been widely studied. A meta-analysis with 1990 NSCLC patients suggests that high serum CYFRA 21-1 level or high CEA level at initial diagnosis is correlated with a poor prognosis (Zhang et al. 2015b). Previously, studies found that the prognostic capability of CEA was rather low (Buccheri et al. 2004). The authors suggest combining both factors to increase the reliability of pretreatment CYFRA 21-1 and CEA. In a prospective study of 308 patients with advanced NSCLC (stage IIIB–IVC), dynamic changes of CEA, CA 125, CYFRA 21-1, and SCCAg were prognostically relevant (Zhang et al. 2015b). As a result, these tumor markers may be beneficial for monitoring treatment response of chemotherapy, chemoradiotherapy, checkpoint inhibition, or multimodal treatment. However, treatment decision-making on serological factors cannot be recommended.

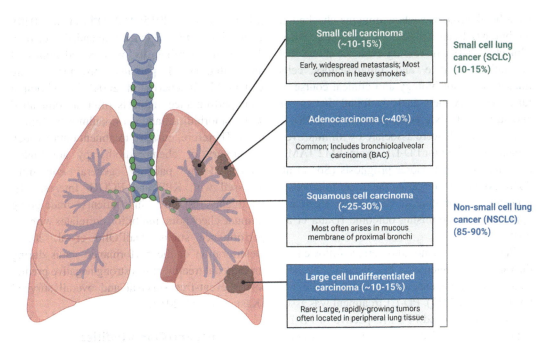

Fig. 1 Overview about lung cancer types. Adapted from "Types of Lung Cancer", by BioRender.com (2022). Retrieved from https://app.biorender.com/biorender-templates

2.1.5 Molecular and Genetic Markers

There have been numerous research studies conducted investigating molecular and genetic markers for their prognostic impact in NSCLC.

Independent prognostic factors have been identified including markers of proliferation including cell cycle regulators, angiogenesis, cellular adhesion, DNA methylation, histological features, as well as other molecular markers, which are rarely assessed in clinical routine. In addition, several molecular biomarkers have been identified with possible treatment options such as mutations in KRAS, echinoderm microtubule-associated protein like 4-anaplastic lymphoma kinase (EML4-ALK), herceptin 2 (HER2), v-raf murine sarcoma (BRAF), mesenchymal epithelial transcription factor (Met), protein kinase B (PKB/AKT1), phosphatidylinositide 3 kinase catalytic subunit (PI3KCA), neurotrophic tyrosine receptor kinase (NTRK) gene fusions, and EGFR. EGFR mutation subset can again be divided into three major categories: EGFR mutations associated with drug sensitivity, EGFR mutations associated with primary drug resistance, and EGFR mutations associated with acquired drug resistance. EGFR mutations play a pivotal role as predictive markers for EGFR TKI treatment. However, a large retrospective study found that EGFR mutations are not prognostic factors in NSCLC (Kim et al. 2013). Due to the introduction of immune checkpoint inhibition, the tumor mutational burden (TMB) characterized by the total amount of nonsynonymous mutation per mega base of DNA has been suggested to be of predictive and prognostic value. Indeed, TMB may serve as a predictive biomarker for the efficacy and clinical response, especially to PD-1/PD-L1 inhibition (Saeed and Salem 2020). Despite increasing evidence, the prognostic role of TMB has not been validated. The link between prognosis and TMB as well as underlying molecular and immune genetic mechanisms needs to be addressed in future prospective clinical trials.

2.1.6 Immune Markers

The immunological response of the host to the cancer has gained importance due to recent treatment breakthroughs such as immune checkpoint inhibition (Alsaab et al. 2017; Gandhi et al. 2018; Mok et al. 2019). Increasing evidence shows that infiltrating immune and inflammatory cells impact the tumor biology and clinical course of lung cancer. A meta-analysis found that tumor and stroma DC, NK cells, M1 TAMs, CD8+ T cells, and B cells were associated with improved prognosis, and tumor PD-L1, stromal M2 TAMs, and Treg cells had poorer prognosis (Soo et al. 2018). As a result, targeting the tumor microenvironment has become a reasonable treatment approach with promising outcome (Datta et al. 2019).

Platin-based chemoradiotherapy followed by durvalumab maintenance has become the new standard of care in unresectable stage III NSCLC (Antonia et al. 2017). PD-L1 treatment was associated with improved PFS irrespective of PD-L1 expression. Several clinical trials found PD-L1 overexpression to be associated with a poor prognosis for patients with NSCLC. Other clinical studies failed to show a relation between PD-L1 expression and prognosis (Tashima et al. 2020). In addition, a small retrospective study found that alteration of PD-L1 expression after chemoradiotherapy was associated with prognosis (Fujimoto et al. 2017). In summary, further research needs to address the prognostic role of immune markers in NSCLC.

2.2 Patient-Related Factors

2.2.1 Performance Status

Performance status assessed via Karnofsky performance scale (KPS) or Eastern Cooperative Oncology Group Performance Status (ECOG PS) represents one of the most important prognostic factors in NSCLC, aside from tumor stage. In addition, KPS and ECOG PS are used to predict tolerability to treatment and correlate with treatment response and quality of life. Until now, numerous large clinical trials and meta-analysis have confirmed the prognostic relevance of KPS and ECOG PS independently from treatment modality, e.g., chemotherapy, surgery, chemoradiotherapy, and immune checkpoint inhibition (Simmons et al. 2015; Dall'Olio et al. 2020). Utilization of ECOG is recommended over KPS due the lower reliability of KPS and improved differentiation of patients' prognosis using ECOG PS (Buccheri et al. 2004). In addition, a poor performance status is often accompanied with comorbidities and cardiopulmonary limitations. Therefore, curative treatment options such as surgery or chemoradiotherapy are highly influenced by patients' general conditions assessed with KPS and ECOG. Interestingly, treatment response in patients undergoing immune checkpoint inhibition correlates with the performance status (Dall'Olio et al. 2020). Deterioration of the performance status during multimodal treatment is a strong negative predictor of event-free survival and overall survival (Käsmann et al. 2019).

2.2.2 Age and Comorbidities

The incidence of NSCLC increases with age. As a result, more than 60% of all patients are diagnosed in the age of 60 years and older and more than 30% of all patients are ≥70 years. However, the link between patients' prognosis and age at diagnosis remains controversial. Population-based studies suggest age as an independent risk predictor for NSCLC (Chen et al. 2019). However, younger patients with an estimated improved survival have an increased risk of lymph node and distant metastases. These findings may be explained by higher treatment tolerability, compliance, and better performance status of younger patients. Several large randomized trials found that comorbidities rather than age are associated with patients' prognosis (Asmis et al. 2008). Indeed, several comorbidities should be considered for treatment allocation, prognosis, and treatment-related toxicity. Therefore, comorbidity scores have been established such as the Charlson comorbidity index (CCI), simplified comorbidity score (SCC), and age-adjusted versions of the mentioned scores. The most widely used clinical score is the CCI (Charlson et al. 1987). However, the SCC appears to be more reliable and useful (Colinet et al. 2005). Age-adapted modifications of CCI and SCC have been implemented with encouraging results regarding prognostic information. Validated comorbidity scores are available and should be considered highly prognostically relevant.

2.2.3 Gender

The importance of gender differences as modulators of tumor biology and treatment outcomes is well known in other medical disciplines, such as cardiology or endocrinology, but slowly raises more attention in oncology (Wagner et al. 2019). In NSCLC, female gender is an established independent prognostic factor for improved survival, aside from the extent of disease (Nakamura et al. 2011). In the era of immunotherapy and targeted therapy, gender differences can still be confirmed regarding outcome and therefore need to be considered for treatment and planning of clinical trials (Pinto et al. 2018). Interestingly, treatment response and outcome may be influenced by gender. A meta-analysis based on phase III randomized trials found that anti-PD-1 inhibition is more effective in male patients than women compared with chemotherapy (Pinto et al. 2018). Gender-specific oncology will receive more attention in future research and therapy. Besides prognostic relevance, the impact of gender in treatment allocation needs to be further investigated.

2.2.4 Body Composition (Weight Loss, Sarcopenia, and Obesity)

Body composition is described as the proportional distribution of different body compartments including bone, adipose tissue, and muscle. The most clinically distinct body phenotypes are obesity and sarcopenia. A higher BMI is associated with a greater risk of cancer, but patients with a higher BMI often have a paradoxically lower risk of overall mortality, a phenomenon called the "obesity paradox." In NSCLC, the positive prognostic impact of a higher BMI is discussed controversially. In a prospective patient cohort with more than 58,000 patients, a BMI ≥ 30 is associated with lower lung cancer mortality (Leung et al. 2011). Other large studies found that underweight and weight loss increased the risk for cancer-specific mortality, whereas obesity did not (Ferguson et al. 2014; Nattenmüller et al. 2017; Shepshelovich et al. 2019). In addition, being underweight is a major risk factor for sarcopenia, which is characterized by progressive and generalized loss of skeletal muscle mass and strength and correlates with physical disability, quality of life, and poorer prognosis. Several meta-analyses confirmed sarcopenia as an independent risk factor for lung cancer-related mortality independently from the tumor stage (Collins et al. 2014; Buentzel et al. 2019).

2.2.5 Laboratory, Hematologic, and Immunologic Markers

Laboratory parameters which are collected in clinical routine have several advantages as potential prognostic factors. They are usually inexpensive, easily accessible, and no additional burden for the patients as they are collected during routine tests.

Several laboratory markers have been suggested to impact patient's prognosis such as hemoglobin levels, lactate dehydrogenase (LDH), calcium, albumin, C-reactive protein, osteopontin, neutrophils, and thrombocyte and lymphocyte counts. Hemoglobin transports oxygen to the tissues and is therefore critical for oxygenation. Several clinical studies have identified intratumoral hypoxia as an important mechanism of tumor resistance, especially in patients undergoing radiotherapy. A meta-analysis found that decreased Hb had a prognostic impact on OS for patients in early-stage and advanced-stage NSCLC (Huang et al. 2018). While the heterogeneity of the included 28 studies was moderate, decreased Hb was a poor prognostic marker for OS. Other clinical studies reached similar conclusions. Furthermore, the prognostic impact of LDH is extensively investigated. It is still one of the strongest prognostic factors using laboratory markers across all stages and independent from treatment (Zhang et al. 2015a; Gong et al. 2019; Zhang et al. 2019).

Inflammation and immunologic markers gained more attention after the introduction of immune checkpoint inhibition in lung cancer. As a result, several biomarkers of systemic inflammation such as elevated C-reactive protein, reduced albumin, and high neutrophils have been evaluated for their impact on patients' prognosis. In addition, several ratios such as neutrophil-to-lymphocyte ratio (NLR), platelet-to-lymphocyte ratio (PLR), and lymphocyte-to-monocyte ratio (LMR) and systemic immune-inflammation index (SII) have been controversially discussed. Among those inflammatory ratios, the most widely recognized prognostic factor in NSCLC is the NLR. Several secondary analyses of clinical trials as well as meta-analyses found that NLR is associated with overall survival and may serve as a prognostic factor in multimodal treatment including immune checkpoint inhibition (Gu et al. 2015; Scilla et al. 2017; Jin et al. 2020).

2.3 Treatment-Related Factors

2.3.1 Clinically Resectable Disease

Radical resection remains the standard of care for resectable disease and should always be considered in early-stage NSCLC. Stereotactic body radiotherapy (SBRT) is a potential alternative treatment option to surgery, especially in patients with comorbidities or patients who decline surgery. Based on the findings of the US National Cancer Database, SBRT is superior to conventional fractionated radiation in terms of overall survival (Haque et al. 2018). In fact, SBRT achieves local control rates comparable to those of surgery with acceptable toxicity (Yahya et al. 2018). Until now, two randomized controlled trials (STARS, ROSEL) were performed in order to compare SBRT to surgical resection. However, both trials were terminated early due to slow recruitment. As a result, the published data is insufficient to demonstrate equivalence of surgery and SABR in terms of disease-free and overall survival (Chang et al. 2015). Radical resection, preferably anatomic resection with lobectomy over sublobar resection, is recommended for early-stage NSCLC. Sublobar resection is associated with increased risk of local relapse compared with lobectomy (Lackey and Donington 2013). Indeed, the highest risk of local relapse was after wedge resection. Pneumonectomy shows higher perioperative mortality rates compared to lobectomy (Martin-Ucar et al. 2002).

Completeness of resection and nodal involvement have been consistently reported as poor prognostic factors of resected NSCLC (Choi et al. 2002; Okada et al. 2005; Smeltzer et al. 2018). Multimodal treatments including surgery, radiotherapy, and chemotherapy or immune checkpoint inhibition are under investigation and may contribute to further improvements.

2.3.2 Locally Advanced Disease

In locally advanced NSCLC, performance status and tumor stage based on the TNM classification are the most important prognostic factors for survival in patients with locally advanced NSCLC. In stage III NSCLC, durvalumab maintenance treatment followed by durvalumab maintenance has become the new standard of care in unresectable stage III NSCLC (Antonia et al. 2017). Importantly, PD-L1 treatment was associated with improved PFS irrespective of PD-L1 expression. Ongoing studies investigate potential prognostic factors for survival in locally advanced NSCLC.

2.3.3 Metastatic Disease

Patients' prognosis with metastatic NSCLC is highly heterogenous due to the introduction of targeted therapy and immune checkpoint inhibition. Several biomarkers such as EGFR, KRAS, EML4-ALK, HER2, BRAF, Met, PKB/AKT1, PI3KCA, NTRK, and several more have been identified. However, conflicting data exists about their prognostic value in general. Performance status, M category, comorbidities, and weight loss have been shown to be independent prognostic factors in advanced/metastatic NSCLC. Besides localized and widely disseminated metastatic NSCLC, an intermediate stage has been described as oligometastatic disease (Hellman and Weichselbaum 1995). This stage is characterized by a limited number of metastases and a less aggressive tumor biology (Schanne et al. 2019). Several clinical trials found a survival benefit of the combination of systemic therapy and local treatment of metastases (e.g., radiotherapy and/or surgery). Oligometastatic diseases have shown to be of prognostic relevance in several clinical trials (Couñago et al. 2019). As a result, the eighth edition of the TNM classification includes, for the first time, oligometastatic disease. Metastatic patients can be divided into three categories: M1a: tumor restricted to the lung alone; M1b: single extrathoracic metastasis; and M1c: multiple extrathoracic metastases.

Besides the number of metastases, the location may play a pivotal role for prognosis. Indeed, several population-based studies found that liver metastases are associated with the poorest and lung metastases with a favorable survival (Li et al. 2019). As a result, localization should be considered as a recognized prognostic factor in the treatment of especially oligometastatic disease.

2.4 Prognostic Scores

While there are several independent prognostic factors that predict the outcome for patients with NSCLC, their value in risk stratifying for treatment allocation and personalized treatment approaches is still limited. Several prognostic scores have been developed including recognized prognostic factors such as stage, performance status, mutation status, inflammation, weight loss, tabacco consumption and comorbidities (Schild et al. 2015; Kazandjian et al. 2019; Zhang et al. 2020; Pan et al. 2021). Some of them have been validated in independent patient cohorts (Alexander et al. 2017). Other prognostic scores have been developed for specific indications such as brain metastases, spinal cord compression, or locally advanced diseases (Rades et al. 2012, 2013; Taugner et al. 2019). However, their clinical implementation is still limited and should be further validated with other datasets to confirm their utility. Nevertheless, these scores may help to tailor treatment allocation for individual patients and could identify high-risk patients for clinical trials.

3 Small Cell Lung Cancer (SCLC)

3.1 Tumor-Related Factors

3.1.1 Tumor Stage

Historically, small cell lung cancer (SCLC) has been classified into a two-stage system, limited (LD) and extensive disease (ED), using the Veterans Administration Lung Study Group (VALG) definitions. SCLC patients with a tumor confined to hemithorax of origin, mediastinum, or supraclavicular lymph nodes are considered to have limited-stage small cell lung cancer (LD-SCLC). Median survival for these patients ranges from 20 to 26 months, in contrast to 12–13 months for patients with extensive-stage SCLC (ED-SCLC) (Horn et al. 2018; Goldman et al. 2021). ED-SCLC is characterized by tumors which exceed LD-SCLC including hematogenous metastases, contralateral hilar or supraclavicular lymph nodes, and presentation of malignant pleural or pericardial effusions.

A large pooled analysis of the North Central Cancer Treatment Group found gender, age, ECOG PS, baseline creatinine levels, and number of metastatic sites as important prognostic factors in ED-SCLC (Foster et al. 2009). In contrast to LD-SCLC, only age and sex were identified as important prognostic factors.

However, the two-stage system and the definition of these categories remain controversial. With increasing utilization of the TNM classification, (Table 3) the two-stage system is becoming less important. The eighth TNM classification system seems to provide more accurate prognostic information to patients when compared to the previous TNM versions (Tendler et al. 2018). Tumor stage is an independent prognostic factor for survival in SCLC.

3.1.2 Histology

SCLC can be described as pure, combined small and large cell carcinoma and combined SCLC with squamous cell, adenocarcinoma, spindle cell, or giant cell carcinoma (Travis 2012). The frequency of mixed SCLC varies widely and

Table 3 SCLC—tumor stages according to UICC/eighth TNM classification (Nicholson et al. 2016)

Stage	T category	N category	M category
0	Tis	N0	M0
IA1	T1a(mi)	N0	M0
	T1a	N0	M0
IA2	T1b	N0	M0
IA3	T1c	N0	M0
IB	T2a	N0	M0
IIA	T2b	N0	M0
IIB	T1a–c	N1	M0
	T2a	N1	M0
	T2b	N1	M0
	T3	N0	M0
IIIA	T1a–c	N2	M0
	T2a–b	N2	M0
	T3	N1	M0
	T4	N0	M0
	T4	N1	M0
IIIB	T1a–b	N3	M0
	T2 a–b	N3	M0
	T3	N2	M0
	T4	N2	M0
IIIC	T3	N3	M0
	T4	N3	M0
IV	Every T	Every N	M1a
	Every T	Every N	M1b

depends on the tumor sample size, number of histological sections studied, types of specimen, and pathologist's interpretation. A comprehensive analysis of 100 SCLC histologies found combined SCLC in 28% of all cases with 16% combined SCLC with large cell carcinoma, 9% with adenocarcinoma, and 3% with squamous cell carcinoma (Nicholson et al. 2002). However, SCLC subtypes based on histology have no prognostic information based on the current literature (Qin and Lu 2018).

3.1.3 Serological Markers

Several serological markers have been suggested for their prognostic relevance in SCLC including neuron-specific enolase (NSE), caspase cleaved cytokeratin 19 (CYFRA 21.1), carcinoembryonic antigen (CEA), pro-gastrin-releasing peptide (proGRP), tissue polypeptide antigen (TPA), chromogranin A (cGA), and neural cell adhesion molecule (NCAM).

NSE has been tested in several clinical trials and utilized in diagnostics in order to differentiate between SCLC and NSCLC and treatment monitoring (Pinson et al. 1997). In addition, a meta-analysis found a significant correlation between NSE and survival (Tian et al. 2020). For the diagnosis of SCLC, ProGRP has also revealed high diagnostic sensitivity and specificity. While ProGRP is more sensitive than NSE for the diagnosis of SCLC, NSE is superior to ProGRP as a prognostic factor (Shibayama et al. 2001). Based on several studies, CEA and CYFRA 21-1 have correlated in univariate and multivariate analysis with survival (Pujol et al. 2003). Other studies suggest that CYFRA 21-1 is superior to CEA and NSE regarding their prognostic information (Zhang et al. 2017a). Conflicting data and limited evidence due to mainly retrospective studies need to be considered. A combination of several markers such as NSE, ProGRP, and CYFRA 21-1 may be used as a prognostic factor. However, further research needs to address the issue.

3.1.4 Molecular, Genetic, and Immune Markers

SCLC has a high load of somatic mutations due to the strong association of SCLC histology with smoking. The most common genetic alterations include the inactivation of the tumor-suppressor genes TP53 and RB1, oncogenes of the Myc family, several enzymes involved in chromatin remodeling, receptor tyrosine kinases and their downstream effectors, as well as proteins of the Notch family (Sabari et al. 2017).

Based on molecular findings, three distinct subtypes have been defined by differential expression of the neuronal basic helix–loop–helix transcription factors achaete-scute homologue-1 (ASH-1) and neurogenic differentiation factor 1 (NEUROD1) (Sabari et al. 2017). The "classic" subtype is defined by the expression of ASCL1, the "variant" subtype has been described by high expression levels of NEUROD1, and the third subtype lacks both factors. The prognostic impact of these molecular subtypes is currently under investigation.

TMB defined as the total number of nonsynonymous mutations within a tumor genome has been considered to provide prognostic information. Despite its pivotal role in predicting treatment response in patients with melanoma and NSCLC treated with immune checkpoint inhibition, the prognostic role of TMB is highly controversial. Several clinical trials found no correlation between TMB and survival (George et al. 2015; Horn et al. 2018).

The composition of the tumor microenvironment has been considered for prognostic importance in SCLC. As one of the most important factors, PD-L1 expression has been intensively investigated, and several clinical trials confirmed that increased PD-L1 expression was an unfavorable prognostic factor for SCLC. However, the correlation of PD-L1 expression and survival was stronger for NSCLC rather than SCLC (Zhang et al. 2017b).

Systemic inflammation has been evaluated as a prognostic marker of survival in several cancers. In SCLC, several immune markers or ratios such as CRP, NLR, and PLR have been investigated. Based on a meta-analysis including 16 retrospective studies, higher NLR was associated with shorter OS, whereas an association between PLR and survival could not be confirmed (Winther-Larsen et al. 2021).

3.2 Patient-Related Factors

3.2.1 Performance Status (Karnofsky and Weight Loss)

The performance status assessed with KPS or ECOG PS is an independent prognostic factor in SCLC (Sonehara et al. 2020; Friedlaender et al. 2020). The KPS describes the patient's general conditions using a comprehensive 11-point scale correlating to percentage values ranging from 100% (no evidence of disease, no symptoms) to 0% (death). ECOG OS developed by the Eastern Cooperative Oncology Group describes a patient's functional status with a simplified 6-point scale correlating to percentage values ranging from 0 (no evidence of disease, no symptoms) to 5 (death).

In addition to tumor stage and performance status, pretreatment weight loss has been identified as an adverse prognostic factor (Bremnes et al. 2003).

SCLC at initial diagnosis is often associated with tumor-related symptoms such as hemoptysis, dyspnea, superior vena cava syndrome, or neurologic symptoms due to the presence of brain metastases. Therefore, the patient's quality of life (QOL) is correlated with tumor burden. QOL is characterized as a multifactorial concept including physical, psychological, and social status and spiritual well-being. In SCLC, physical functioning and activities of daily living were most impacted (Bennett et al. 2017). However, data reporting quality of life in SCLC is still limited. Further research needs to be done in order to draw robust conclusions.

3.2.2 Age and Gender

The prognostic role of age and gender has been extensively studied in lung cancer. In SCLC, age and gender are important prognostic factors (Lim et al. 2018; Sonehara et al. 2020). Female patients with a good performance status and younger age (below 60 years) show a favorable prognosis, aside from tumor extent.

3.2.3 Laboratory, Hematologic, and Immunologic Markers

Numerous studies have investigated laboratory or immune markers as possible prognostic factors regarding survival and treatment response. The most promising factors are LDH and surrogate markers of systemic inflammation such as CRP, NLR, PLR, and mean platelet volume (MPV). Concerning laboratory markers, elevated LDH seems to be the most important adverse prognostic factor based on several clinical trials (Galvano et al. 2020). Several studies suggest NLR as an important prognostic factor regarding survival in SCLC. However, other clinical studies found no correlation between NLR and outcome (Shen et al. 2019). Further research needs to address the prognostic value of immunologic markers in SCLC.

3.3 Treatment-Related Factors

For almost 30 years, treatment of SCLC depending on tumor stage consisted of surgery, (chemo) radiotherapy, and platin-based chemotherapy. Surgical resection for cT1–2 cN0 M0 SCLC offers improved local control compared to chemoradiotherapy or chemotherapy alone (Anraku and Waddell 2006). A retrospective multicenter study found that lower tumor stage, a maximum tumor diameter of <20 mm, a history or presence of other types of cancer, and administering prophylactic cranial irradiation (PCI) are associated with improved survival (Yokouchi et al. 2015). Other studies suggested the role of PD-L1 expression and adjuvant chemotherapy in resected SCLC (Zhao et al. 2019).

In most cases with LS-SCLC, concurrent chemoradiotherapy administering etoposide and platinum-based chemotherapy represents the standard of care. Hyperfractionated twice-daily radiotherapy according to Turrisi remains the standard therapy, though conventional radiotherapy is an adequate alternative supported by randomized evidence (Turrisi et al. 1999; Faivre-Finn et al. 2017). Timing of chemoradiotherapy is known to provide prognostic relevance. Early start of chemoradiotherapy, preferably to the first or second chemotherapy cycle, is more effective compared to delayed RT or sequential chemoradiotherapy (Tjong et al. 2020). After chemoradiotherapy and treatment response with at least stable disease, prophylactic cranial irradiation (PCI) is recommended.

Platin-based chemotherapy combinations are the standard of care in ES-SCLC. Based on randomized evidence, the addition of immune checkpoint inhibition (atezolizumab and durvalumab) to established chemotherapy protocols has significantly improved the patient's prognosis. Additional research in these multimodal treatment approaches needs to be performed in order to validate classical prognostic factors in new standard therapy.

3.4 Prognostic Scores

Several prognostic scores have been developed to predict the outcome of patients with SCLC (Cerny et al. 1987; Negre et al. 2020; Winther-Larsen et al. 2021). In addition, survival score for specific indications has been introduced (Rades et al. 2012; Rades et al. 2019). However, not all of them could be validated in independent patient cohorts (Rothschild et al. 2016; Käsmann et al. 2020). Out of seven potential survival scores, only the Manchester score could be validated. However, the validation cohort was rather small with a long recruitment time, and new treatment modalities need to be assessed. In conclusion, further validation is warranted for these scores in order to support physicians aiming to create personalized treatments in SCLC.

References

Alexander M, Wolfe R, Ball D, Conron M, Stirling RG, Solomon B, MacManus M, Officer A, Karnam S, Burbury K (2017) Lung cancer prognostic index: a risk score to predict overall survival after the diagnosis of non-small-cell lung cancer. Br J Cancer 117:744

Alsaab HO, Sau S, Alzhrani R, Tatiparti K, Bhise K, Kashaw SK, Iyer AK (2017) PD-1 and PD-L1 checkpoint signaling inhibition for cancer immunotherapy: mechanism, combinations, and clinical outcome. Front Pharmacol 8:561

Anraku M, Waddell TK (2006) Surgery for small-cell lung cancer. Semin Thorac Cardiovasc Surg 18:211–216. https://doi.org/10.1053/j.semtcvs.2006.08.006

Antonia SJ, Villegas A, Daniel D, Vicente D, Murakami S, Hui R, Yokoi T, Chiappori A, Lee KH, de Wit M (2017) Durvalumab after chemoradiotherapy in stage III non-small-cell lung cancer. N Engl J Med 377:1919–1929

Asmis TR, Ding K, Seymour L, Shepherd FA, Leighl NB, Winton TL, Whitehead M, Spaans JN, Graham BC, Goss GD (2008) Age and comorbidity as independent prognostic factors in the treatment of non-small-cell lung cancer: a review of National Cancer Institute of Canada Clinical Trials Group trials. J Clin Oncol 26:54–59

Bennett BM, Wells JR, Panter C, Yuan Y, Penrod JR (2017) The humanistic burden of small cell lung cancer (SCLC): a systematic review of health-related quality of life (HRQoL) Literature. Front Pharmacol 8:339. https://doi.org/10.3389/fphar.2017.00339

Berghmans T, Dusart M, Paesmans M, Hossein-Foucher C, Buvat I, Castaigne C, Scherpereel A, Mascaux C, Moreau M, Roelandts M (2008) Primary tumor standardized uptake value (SUVmax) measured on fluorodeoxyglucose positron emission tomography (FDG-PET) is of prognostic value for survival in non-small cell lung cancer (NSCLC): a systematic review and meta-analysis (MA) by the European Lung Cancer Working Party for the IASLC Lung Cancer Staging Project. J Thorac Oncol 3:6–12

Bremnes RM, Sundstrom S, Aasebø U, Kaasa S, Hatlevoll R, Aamdal S (2003) The value of prognostic factors in small cell lung cancer: results from a randomised multicenter study with minimum 5 year follow-up. Lung Cancer 39:303–313. https://doi.org/10.1016/s0169-5002(02)00508-1

Brierley JD, Gospodarowicz MK, Wittekind C (2017) TNM classification of malignant tumours. John Wiley & Sons

Buccheri G, Ferrigno D, Barisione E, Noceti P (2004) Prognostic factors in advanced stage non-small cell lung cancer. Minerva Pneumol 43:131–142

Buentzel J, Heinz J, Bleckmann A, Bauer C, Roever C, Bohnenberger H, Saha S, Hinterthaner M, Baraki H, Kutschka I (2019) Sarcopenia as prognostic factor in lung cancer patients: a systematic review and meta-analysis. Anticancer Res 39:4603–4612

Cerny T, Anderson H, Bramwell V, Thatcher N, Blair V (1987) Pretreatment prognostic factors and scoring system in 407 small-cell lung cancer patients. Int J Cancer 39:146–149. https://doi.org/10.1002/ijc.2910390204

Chang JY, Senan S, Paul MA, Mehran RJ, Louie AV, Balter P, Groen HJ, McRae SE, Widder J, Feng L (2015) Stereotactic ablative radiotherapy versus lobectomy for operable stage I non-small-cell lung cancer: a pooled analysis of two randomised trials. Lancet Oncol 16:630–637

Chardin D, Paquet M, Schiappa R, Darcourt J, Bailleux C, Poudenx M, Sciazza A, Ilie M, Benzaquen J, Martin N (2020) Baseline metabolic tumor volume as a strong predictive and prognostic biomarker in patients with non-small cell lung cancer treated with PD1 inhibitors: a prospective study. J Immunother Cancer 8(2):e000645

Charlson ME, Pompei P, Ales KL, MacKenzie CR (1987) A new method of classifying prognostic comorbidity in longitudinal studies: development and validation. J Chronic Dis 40:373–383

Chen T, Zhou F, Jiang W, Mao R, Zheng H, Qin L, Chen C (2019) Age at diagnosis is a heterogeneous factor for non-small cell lung cancer patients. J Thorac Dis 11:2251

Choi YS, Shim YM, Kim J, Kim K (2002) Recurrence-free survival and prognostic factors in resected pN2 non-small cell lung cancer. Eur J Cardiothorac Surg 22:695–700

Colinet B, Jacot W, Bertrand D, Lacombe S, Bozonnat M, Daures J, Pujol J (2005) A new simplified comorbidity score as a prognostic factor in non-small-cell lung cancer patients: description and comparison with the Charlson's index. Br J Cancer 93:1098–1105

Collins J, Noble S, Chester J, Coles B, Byrne A (2014) The assessment and impact of sarcopenia in lung cancer: a systematic literature review. BMJ Open 4

Couñago F, Luna J, Guerrero LL, Vaquero B, Guillén-Sacoto MC, González-Merino T, Taboada B, Díaz V, Rubio-Viqueira B, Díaz Gavela AA, Marcos FJ, Del Cerro E (2019) Management of oligometastatic non-small cell lung cancer patients: current controversies and future directions. World J Clin Oncol 10:318–339. https://doi.org/10.5306/wjco.v10.i10.318

Dall'Olio FG, Maggio I, Massucci M, Mollica V, Fragomeno B, Ardizzoni A (2020) ECOG performance status≥ 2 as a prognostic factor in patients with advanced non small cell lung cancer treated with immune checkpoint inhibitors—a systematic review and meta-analysis of real world data. Lung Cancer 145:95–104

Datta M, Coussens LM, Nishikawa H, Hodi FS, Jain RK (2019) Reprogramming the tumor microenvironment to improve immunotherapy: emerging strategies and combination therapies. Am Soc Clin Oncol Educ Book 39:165–174

Detterbeck FC, Marom EM, Arenberg DA, Franklin WA, Nicholson AG, Travis WD, Girard N, Mazzone PJ, Donington JS, Tanoue LT, Rusch VW, Asamura H, Rami-Porta R (2016) The IASLC lung cancer staging project: background data and proposals for the application of TNM staging rules to lung cancer presenting as multiple nodules with ground glass or lepidic features or a pneumonic type of involvement in the forthcoming eighth edition of the TNM classification. J Thorac Oncol 11:666–680. https://doi.org/10.1016/j.jtho.2015.12.113

Faivre-Finn C, Snee M, Ashcroft L, Appel W, Barlesi F, Bhatnagar A, Bezjak A, Cardenal F, Fournel P, Harden S (2017) Concurrent once-daily versus twice-daily chemoradiotherapy in patients with limited-stage small-cell lung cancer (CONVERT): an open-label, phase 3, randomised, superiority trial. Lancet Oncol 18:1116–1125

Ferguson MK, Im HK, Watson S, Johnson E, Wigfield CH, Vigneswaran WT (2014) Association of body mass index and outcomes after major lung resection. Eur J Cardiothorac Surg 45:e94–e99

Foster NR, Mandrekar SJ, Schild SE, Nelson GD, Rowland KM, Deming RL, Kozelsky TF, Marks RS, Jett JR, Adjei AA (2009) Prognostic factors differ by tumor stage for small cell lung cancer: a pooled analysis of North Central Cancer Treatment Group trials. Cancer 115:2721–2731. https://doi.org/10.1002/CNCR.24314

Friedlaender A, Liu SV, Passaro A, Metro G, Banna G, Addeo A (2020) The role of performance status in small-cell lung cancer in the era of immune checkpoint inhibitors. Clin Lung Cancer 21:e539–e543. https://doi.org/10.1016/j.cllc.2020.04.006

Fujimoto D, Uehara K, Sato Y, Sakanoue I, Ito M, Teraoka S, Nagata K, Nakagawa A, Kosaka Y, Otsuka K (2017) Alteration of PD-L1 expression and its prognostic impact after concurrent chemoradiation therapy in non-small cell lung cancer patients. Sci Rep 7:11373

Galvano A, Peri M, Guarini AA, Castiglia M, Grassadonia A, De Tursi M, Irtelli L, Rizzo S, Bertani A, Gristina V, Barraco N, Russo A, Natoli C, Bazan V (2020) Analysis of systemic inflammatory biomarkers in neuroendocrine carcinomas of the lung: prognostic and predictive significance of NLR, LDH, ALI, and

LIPI score. Ther Adv Med Oncol 12. https://doi.org/10.1177/1758835920942378

Gandhi L, Rodríguez-Abreu D, Gadgeel S, Esteban E, Felip E, De Angelis F, Domine M, Clingan P, Hochmair MJ, Powell SF (2018) Pembrolizumab plus chemotherapy in metastatic non–small-cell lung cancer. N Engl J Med 378:2078–2092

George J, Lim JS, Jang SJ, Cun Y, Ozretić L, Kong G, Leenders F, Lu X, Fernández-Cuesta L, Bosco G, Müller C, Dahmen I, Jahchan NS, Park K-S, Yang D, Karnezis AN, Vaka D, Torres A, Wang MS, Korbel JO, Menon R, Chun S-M, Kim D, Wilkerson M, Hayes N, Engelmann D, Pützer B, Bos M, Michels S, Vlasic I, Seidel D, Pinther B, Schaub P, Becker C, Altmüller J, Yokota J, Kohno T, Iwakawa R, Tsuta K, Noguchi M, Muley T, Hoffmann H, Schnabel PA, Petersen I, Chen Y, Soltermann A, Tischler V, Choi C, Kim Y-H, Massion PP, Zou Y, Jovanovic D, Kontic M, Wright GM, Russell PA, Solomon B, Koch I, Lindner M, Muscarella LA, la Torre A, Field JK, Jakopovic M, Knezevic J, Castaños-Vélez E, Roz L, Pastorino U, Brustugun O-T, Lund-Iversen M, Thunnissen E, Köhler J, Schuler M, Botling J, Sandelin M, Sanchez-Cespedes M, Salvesen HB, Achter V, Lang U, Bogus M, Schneider PM, Zander T, Ansén S, Hallek M, Wolf J, Vingron M, Yatabe Y, Travis WD, Nürnberg P, Reinhardt C, Perner S, Heukamp L, Büttner R, Haas SA, Brambilla E, Peifer M, Sage J, Thomas RK (2015) Comprehensive genomic profiles of small cell lung cancer. Nature 524:47–53. https://doi.org/10.1038/nature14664

Goldman JW, Dvorkin M, Chen Y, Reinmuth N, Hotta K, Trukhin D, Statsenko G, Hochmair MJ, Özgüroğlu M, Ji JH, Garassino MC, Voitko O, Poltoratskiy A, Ponce S, Verderame F, Havel L, Bondarenko I, Każarnowicz A, Losonczy G, Conev NV, Armstrong J, Byrne N, Thiyagarajah P, Jiang H, Paz-Ares L, Dvorkin M, Trukhin D, Statsenko G, Voitko N, Poltoratskiy A, Bondarenko I, Chen Y, Kazarnowicz A, Paz-Ares L, Özgüroglu M, Conev N, Hochmair M, Burghuber O, Havel L, Çiçin I, Losonczy G, Moiseenko V, Erman M, Kowalski D, Wojtukiewicz M, Adamchuk H, Vasilyev A, Shevnia S, Valev S, Reinmuth N, Ji JH, Insa Molla MA, Ursol G, Chiang A, Hartl S, Horváth Z, Pajkos G, Verderame F, Hotta K, Kim S-W, Smolin A, Göksel T, Dakhil S, Roubec J, Bogos K, Garassino MC, Cornelissen R, Lee J-S, Garcia Campelo MR, Lopez Brea M, Alacacioglu A, Casarini I, Ilieva R, Tonev I, Somfay A, Bar J, Zer Kuch A, Minelli M, Bartolucci R, Roila F, Saito H, Azuma K, Lee G-W, Luft A, Urda M, Delgado Mingorance JI, Majem Tarruella M, Spigel D, Koynov K, Zemanova M, Panse J, Schulz C, Pápai Székely Z, Sárosi V, Delmonte A, Bettini AC, Nishio M, Okamoto I, Hendriks L, Mandziuk S, Lee YG, Vladimirova L, Isla Casado D, Domine Gomez M, Navarro Mendivil A, Morán Bueno T, Wu S-Y, Knoble J, Skrickova J, Venkova V, Hilgers W, Laack E, Bischoff H, Fülöp A, Laczó I, Kósa J, Telekes A, Yoshida T, Kanda S, Hida T, Hayashi H, Maeda T, Kawamura T, Nakahara Y, Claessens N, Lee KH, Chiu C-H, Lin S-H, Li C-T, Demirkazik A, Schaefer E, Nikolinakos P, Schneider J, Babu S, Lamprecht B, Studnicka M, Fausto Nino Gorini C, Kultan J, Kolek V, Souquet P-J, Moro-Sibilot D, Gottfried M, Smit E, Lee KH, Kasan P, Chovanec J, Goloborodko O, Kolesnik O, Ostapenko Y, Lakhanpal S, Haque B, Chua W, Stilwill J, Sena SN, Girotto GC, De Marchi PRM, Martinelli de Oliveira FA, Dos Reis P, Krasteva R, Zhao Y, Chen C, Koubkova L, Robinet G, Chouaid C, Grohe C, Alt J, Csánky E, Somogyiné Ezer É, Heching NI, Kim YH, Aatagi S, Kuyama S, Harada D, Nogami N, Nokihara H, Goto H, Staal van den Brekel A, Cho EK, Kim J-H, Ganea D, Ciuleanu T, Popova E, Sakaeva D, Stresko M, Demo P, Godal R, Wei Y-F, Chen Y-H, Hsia T-C, Lee K-Y, Chang H-C, Wang C-C, Dowlati A, Sumey C, Powell S, Goldman J, Zarba JJ, Batagelj E, Pastor AV, Zukin M, da Baldotto CSR, Schlittler LA, Calabrich A, Sette C, Dudov A, Zhou C, Lena H, Lang S, Pápai Z, Goto K, Umemura S, Kanazawa K, Hara Y, Shinoda M, Morise M, Hiltermann J, Mróz R, Ungureanu A, Andrasina I, Chang G-C, Vynnychenko I, Shparyk Y, Kryzhanivska A, Ross H, Mi K, Jamil R, Williamson M, Spahr J, Han Z, Wang M, Yang Z, Hu J, Li W, Zhao J, Feng J, Ma S, Zhou X, Liang Z, Hu Y, Chen Y, Bi M, Shu Y, Nan K, Zhou J, Zhang W, Ma R, Yang N, Lin Z, Wu G, Fang J, Zhang H, Wang K, Chen Z (2021) Durvalumab, with or without tremelimumab, plus platinum–etoposide versus platinum–etoposide alone in first-line treatment of extensive-stage small-cell lung cancer (CASPIAN): updated results from a randomised, controlled, open-label, phase 3 trial. Lancet Oncol 22:51–65. https://doi.org/10.1016/S1470-2045(20)30539-8

Goldstraw P, Chansky K, Crowley J, Rami-Porta R, Asamura H, Eberhardt WE, Nicholson AG, Groome P, Mitchell A, Bolejack V (2016) The IASLC lung cancer staging project: proposals for revision of the TNM stage groupings in the forthcoming (eighth) edition of the TNM classification for lung cancer. J Thorac Oncol 11:39–51

Gong T, Liu J, Jiang J, Zhai Y-F, Wu C-M, Ma C, Wen B-L, Yan X-Y, Zhang X, Wang D-M (2019) The role of lactate deshydrogenase levels on non-small cell lung cancer prognosis: a meta-analysis. Cell Mol Biol 65:89–93

Gu X-B, Tian T, Tian X-J, Zhang X-J (2015) Prognostic significance of neutrophil-to-lymphocyte ratio in non-small cell lung cancer: a meta-analysis. Sci Rep 5:1–9

Haque W, Verma V, Polamraju P, Farach A, Butler EB, Teh BS (2018) Stereotactic body radiation therapy versus conventionally fractionated radiation therapy for early stage non-small cell lung cancer. Radiother Oncol 129:264–269

Hellman S, Weichselbaum RR (1995) Oligometastases. J Clin Oncol 13:8–10. https://doi.org/10.1200/JCO.1995.13.1.8

Hirsch FR, Spreafico A, Novello S, Wood MD, Simms L, Papotti M (2008) The prognostic and predictive role of histology in advanced non-small cell lung cancer: a literature review. J Thorac Oncol 3:1468–1481

Horn L, Mansfield AS, Szczęsna A, Havel L, Krzakowski M, Hochmair MJ, Huemer F, Losonczy G, Johnson ML, Nishio M, Reck M, Mok T, Lam S, Shames DS, Liu J, Ding B, Lopez-Chavez A, Kabbinavar F, Lin W, Sandler A, Liu SV (2018) First-line Atezolizumab plus chemotherapy in extensive-stage small-cell lung cancer. N Engl J Med 379:2220–2229. https://doi.org/10.1056/NEJMoa1809064

Huang Y, Wei S, Jiang N, Zhang L, Wang S, Cao X, Zhao Y, Wang P (2018) The prognostic impact of decreased pretreatment haemoglobin level on the survival of patients with lung cancer: a systematic review and meta-analysis. BMC Cancer 18:1–15

Im H-J, Pak K, Cheon GJ, Kang KW, Kim S-J, Kim I-J, Chung J-K, Kim EE, Lee DS (2015) Prognostic value of volumetric parameters of 18 F-FDG PET in non-small-cell lung cancer: a meta-analysis. Eur J Nucl Med Mol Imaging 42:241–251

Jin J, Yang L, Liu D, Li W (2020) Association of the neutrophil to lymphocyte ratio and clinical outcomes in patients with lung cancer receiving immunotherapy: a meta-analysis. BMJ Open 10:e035031

Kaida H, Azuma K, Kawahara A, Sadashima E, Hattori S, Akiba J, Rominger A, Takamori S, Fujimoto K, Hosono M (2017) Prognostic impact of 18F-FDG PET parameters and molecular markers expression in resected non-small cell lung cancer patients. J Nucl Med 58:1047–1047

Käsmann L, Niyazi M, Blanck O, Baues C, Baumann R, Dobiasch S, Eze C, Fleischmann D, Gauer T, Giordano FA (2018) Predictive and prognostic value of tumor volume and its changes during radical radiotherapy of stage III non-small cell lung cancer. Strahlenther Onkol 194:79–90

Käsmann L, Taugner J, Eze C, Roengvoraphoj O, Dantes M, Gennen K, Karin M, Petrukhnov O, Tufman A, Belka C (2019) Performance status and its changes predict outcome for patients with inoperable stage III NSCLC undergoing multimodal treatment. Anticancer Res 39:5077–5081

Käsmann L, Abdo R, Eze C, Dantes M, Taugner J, Gennen K, Roengvoraphoj O, Rades D, Belka C, Manapov F (2020) External validation of a survival score for limited-stage small cell lung cancer patients treated with chemoradiotherapy. Lung 198:201–206. https://doi.org/10.1007/s00408-019-00312-6

Kazandjian D, Gong Y, Keegan P, Pazdur R, Blumenthal GM (2019) Prognostic value of the lung immune prognostic index for patients treated for metastatic non–small cell lung cancer. JAMA Oncol 5:1481–1485

Kim YT, Seong YW, Jung YJ, Jeon YK, Park IK, Kang CH, Kim JH (2013) The presence of mutations in epidermal growth factor receptor gene is not a prognostic factor for long-term outcome after surgical resection of non-small-cell lung cancer. J Thorac Oncol 8:171–178. https://doi.org/10.1097/JTO.0b013e318277a3bb

Lackey A, Donington JS (2013) Surgical management of lung cancer. Semin Intervent Radiol 30:133–140. https://doi.org/10.1055/s-0033-1342954

Leung CC, Lam TH, Yew WW, Chan WM, Law WS, Tam CM (2011) Lower lung cancer mortality in obesity. Int J Epidemiol 40:174–182

Li J, Zhu H, Sun L, Xu W, Wang X (2019) Prognostic value of site-specific metastases in lung cancer: a population based study. J Cancer 10:3079–3086. https://doi.org/10.7150/jca.30463

Lim JH, Ryu J-S, Kim JH, Kim H-J, Lee D (2018) Gender as an independent prognostic factor in small-cell lung cancer: Inha lung cancer cohort study using propensity score matching. PLoS One 13:e0208492. https://doi.org/10.1371/journal.pone.0208492

Lu T, Yang X, Huang Y, Zhao M, Li M, Ma K, Yin J, Zhan C, Wang Q (2019) Trends in the incidence, treatment, and survival of patients with lung cancer in the last four decades. Cancer Manage Res 11:943

Maeda R, Yoshida J, Ishii G, Hishida T, Nishimura M, Nagai K (2011) Prognostic impact of histology on early-stage non-small cell lung cancer. Chest 140:135–145

Martin-Ucar AE, Chaudhuri N, Edwards JG, Waller DA (2002) Can pneumonectomy for non-small cell lung cancer be avoided? An audit of parenchymal sparing lung surgery. Eur J Cardiothorac Surg 21:601–605. https://doi.org/10.1016/s1010-7940(02)00028-3

Mok TS, Wu Y-L, Kudaba I, Kowalski DM, Cho BC, Turna HZ, Castro G Jr, Srimuninnimit V, Laktionov KK, Bondarenko I (2019) Pembrolizumab versus chemotherapy for previously untreated, PD-L1-expressing, locally advanced or metastatic non-small-cell lung cancer (KEYNOTE-042): a randomised, open-label, controlled, phase 3 trial. Lancet 393:1819–1830

Nakamura H, Ando K, Shinmyo T, Morita K, Mochizuki A, Kurimoto N, Tatsunami S (2011) Female gender is an independent prognostic factor in non-small-cell lung cancer: a meta-analysis. Ann Thorac Cardiovasc Surg 17:469–480

Nattenmüller J, Wochner R, Muley T, Steins M, Hummler S, Teucher B, Wiskemann J, Kauczor H-U, Wielpütz MO, Heussel CP (2017) Prognostic impact of CT-quantified muscle and fat distribution before and after first-line-chemotherapy in lung cancer patients. PLoS One 12:e0169136

Negre E, Coffy A, Langlais A, Daures J-P, Lavole A, Quoix E, Molinier O, Greillier L, Audigier-Valette C, Moro-Sibilot D (2020) Development and validation of a simplified prognostic score in SCLC. JTO Clin Res Rep 1:100016

Nestle U, Schimek-Jasch T, Kremp S, Schaefer-Schuler A, Mix M, Küsters A, Tosch M, Hehr T, Eschmann SM, Bultel Y-P (2020) Imaging-based target volume reduction in chemoradiotherapy for locally advanced non-small-cell lung cancer (PET-Plan): a multicentre, open-label, randomised, controlled trial. Lancet Oncol 21(4):581–592

Nicholson SA, Beasley MB, Brambilla E, Hasleton PS, Colby TV, Sheppard MN, Falk R, Travis WD (2002) Small cell lung carcinoma (SCLC): a clinicopathologic study of 100 cases with surgical specimens. Am J Surg Pathol 26(9):1184–1197

Nicholson AG, Chansky K, Crowley J, Beyruti R, Kubota K, Turrisi A, Eberhardt WE, Van Meerbeeck J, Rami-Porta R, Goldstraw P (2016) The International Association for the Study of Lung Cancer Lung Cancer Staging Project: proposals for the revision of the clinical and pathologic staging of small cell lung cancer in the forthcoming eighth edition of the TNM classification for lung cancer. J Thorac Oncol 11:300–311

Okada M, Nishio W, Sakamoto T, Uchino K, Yuki T, Nakagawa A, Tsubota N (2005) Effect of tumor size on prognosis in patients with non–small cell lung cancer: the role of segmentectomy as a type of lesser resection. J Thorac Cardiovasc Surg 129:87–93

Pan M, Zhao Y, He J, Wu H, Pan Y, Yu Q, Zhou S (2021) Prognostic value of the Glasgow prognostic score on overall survival in patients with advanced non-small cell lung cancer. J Cancer 12:2395

Pinson P, Joos G, Watripont P, Brusselle G, Pauwels R (1997) Serum neuron-specific enolase as a tumor marker in the diagnosis and follow-up of small-cell lung cancer. Respiration 64:102–107. https://doi.org/10.1159/000196651

Pinto JA, Vallejos CS, Raez LE, Mas LA, Ruiz R, Torres-Roman JS, Morante Z, Araujo JM, Gómez HL, Aguilar A (2018) Gender and outcomes in non-small cell lung cancer: an old prognostic variable comes back for targeted therapy and immunotherapy? ESMO Open 3:e000344

Pujol J-L, Quantin X, Jacot W, Boher J-M, Grenier J, Lamy P-J (2003) Neuroendocrine and cytokeratin serum markers as prognostic determinants of small cell lung cancer. Lung Cancer 39:131–138. https://doi.org/10.1016/s0169-5002(02)00513-5

Qin J, Lu H (2018) Combined small-cell lung carcinoma. Onco Targets Ther 11:3505–3511. https://doi.org/10.2147/OTT.S159057

Rades D, Douglas S, Veninga T, Schild SE (2012) A validated survival score for patients with metastatic spinal cord compression from non-small cell lung cancer. BMC Cancer 12:1–7

Rades D, Dziggel L, Segedin B, Oblak I, Nagy V, Marita A, Schild S, Trang N, Khoa M (2013) A new survival score for patients with brain metastases from non-small cell lung cancer. Strahlenther Onkol 189:777–781

Rades D, Hansen HC, Janssen S, Schild SE (2019) Comparison of diagnosis-specific survival scores for patients with small-cell lung cancer irradiated for brain metastases. Cancer 11:233

Rothschild SI, Hagmann R, Zippelius A (2016) 92P: Validation of prognostic scores in small cell lung cancer. J Thorac Oncol 11:S96–S97. https://doi.org/10.1016/S1556-0864(16)30205-2

Sabari JK, Lok BH, Laird JH, Poirier JT, Rudin CM (2017) Unravelling the biology of SCLC: implications for therapy. Nat Rev Clin Oncol 14:549–561. https://doi.org/10.1038/nrclinonc.2017.71

Saeed A, Salem ME (2020) Prognostic value of tumor mutation burden (TMB) and INDEL burden (IDB) in cancer: current view and clinical applications. Ann Transl Med 8:575. https://doi.org/10.21037/atm-2020-75

Schanne DH, Heitmann J, Guckenberger M, Andratschke NHJ (2019) Evolution of treatment strategies for oligometastatic NSCLC patients—a systematic review of the literature. Cancer Treat Rev 80. https://doi.org/10.1016/j.ctrv.2019.101892

Schild SE, Tan AD, Wampfler JA, Ross HJ, Yang P, Sloan JA (2015) A new scoring system for predicting survival in patients with non-small cell lung cancer. Cancer Med 4:1334–1343

Scilla KA, Bentzen SM, Lam VK, Mohindra P, Nichols EM, Vyfhuis MA, Bhooshan N, Feigenberg SJ, Edelman MJ, Feliciano JL (2017) Neutrophil-Lymphocyte ratio is a prognostic marker in patients with locally advanced (Stage IIIA and IIIB) non-small cell lung cancer treated with combined modality therapy. Oncologist 22:737

Shen X-B, Wang Y, Shan B-J, Lin L, Hao L, Liu Y, Wang W, Pan Y-Y (2019) Prognostic significance of platelet-to-lymphocyte ratio (PLR) and mean platelet volume (MPV) during etoposide-based first-line treatment in small cell lung cancer patients. Cancer Manag Res 11:8965–8975. https://doi.org/10.2147/CMAR.S215361

Shepshelovich D, Xu W, Lu L, Fares A, Yang P, Christiani D, Zhang J, Shiraishi K, Ryan BM, Chen C (2019) Body Mass Index (BMI), BMI change, and overall survival in patients with SCLC and NSCLC: a pooled analysis of the international lung cancer consortium. J Thorac Oncol 14:1594–1607

Shibayama T, Ueoka H, Nishii K, Kiura K, Tabata M, Miyatake K, Kitajima T, Harada M (2001) Complementary roles of pro-gastrin-releasing peptide (ProGRP) and neuron specific enolase (NSE) in diagnosis and prognosis of small-cell lung cancer (SCLC). Lung Cancer (Amsterdam, Netherlands) 32:61–69. https://doi.org/10.1016/s0169-5002(00)00205-1

Simmons CP, Koinis F, Fallon MT, Fearon KC, Bowden J, Solheim TS, Gronberg BH, McMillan DC, Gioulbasanis I, Laird BJ (2015) Prognosis in advanced lung cancer—a prospective study examining key clinicopathological factors. Lung Cancer 88:304–309

Smeltzer MP, Faris NR, Ray MA, Osarogiagbon RU (2018) Association of pathologic nodal staging quality with survival among patients with non–small cell lung cancer after resection with curative intent. JAMA Oncol 4:80–87

Sonehara K, Tateishi K, Komatsu M, Yamamoto H, Hanaoka M (2020) Lung immune prognostic index as a prognostic factor in patients with small cell lung cancer. Thorac Cancer 11:1578–1586. https://doi.org/10.1111/1759-7714.13432

Soo RA, Chen Z, Teng RSY, Tan H-L, Iacopetta B, Tai BC, Soong R (2018) Prognostic significance of immune cells in non-small cell lung cancer: meta-analysis. Oncotarget 9:24801

Sung H, Ferlay J, Siegel RL, Laversanne M, Soerjomataram I, Jemal A, Bray F (2021) Global cancer statistics 2020: GLOBOCAN estimates of incidence and mortality worldwide for 36 cancers in 185 countries. A Cancer J Clin, CA

Tashima Y, Kuwata T, Yoneda K, Hirai A, Mori M, Kanayama M, Imanishi N, Kuroda K, Ichiki Y, Tanaka F (2020) Prognostic impact of PD-L1 expression in correlation with neutrophil-to-lymphocyte ratio in squamous cell carcinoma of the lung. Sci Rep 10:1–8

Taugner J, Käsmann L, Eze C, Dantes M, Roengvoraphoj O, Gennen K, Karin M, Petruknov O, Tufman A, Belka C (2019) Survival score to characterize prognosis in inoperable stage III NSCLC after chemoradiotherapy. Transl Lung Cancer Res 8:593

Tendler S, Grozman V, Lewensohn R, Tsakonas G, Viktorsson K, De Petris L (2018) Validation of the 8th TNM classification for small-cell lung cancer in a retrospective material from Sweden. Lung Cancer 120:75–81. https://doi.org/10.1016/j.lungcan.2018.03.026

Tian Z, Liang C, Zhang Z, Wen H, Feng H, Ma Q, Liu D, Qiang G (2020) Prognostic value of neuron-specific enolase for small cell lung cancer: a systematic review and meta-analysis. World J Surg Oncol 18:116. https://doi.org/10.1186/s12957-020-01894-9

Tjong MC, Mak DY, Shahi J, Li GJ, Chen H, Louie AV (2020) Current management and progress in radiotherapy for small cell lung cancer. Front Oncol 10:1146. https://doi.org/10.3389/fonc.2020.01146

Travis WD (2012) Update on small cell carcinoma and its differentiation from squamous cell carcinoma and other non-small cell carcinomas. Mod Pathol 25:S18–S30. https://doi.org/10.1038/modpathol.2011.150

Turrisi AT, Kim K, Blum R, Sause WT, Livingston RB, Komaki R, Wagner H, Aisner S, Johnson DH (1999) Twice-daily compared with once-daily thoracic radiotherapy in limited small-cell lung cancer treated concurrently with cisplatin and etoposide. N Engl J Med 340:265–271. https://doi.org/10.1056/NEJM199901283400403

Wagner A, Oertelt-Prigione S, Adjei A, Buclin T, Cristina V, Csajka C, Coukos G, Dafni U, Dotto G-P, Ducreux M (2019) Gender medicine and oncology: report and consensus of an ESMO workshop. Ann Oncol 30:1914–1924

Wang B-Y, Huang J-Y, Chen H-C, Lin C-H, Lin S-H, Hung W-H, Cheng Y-F (2020) The comparison between adenocarcinoma and squamous cell carcinoma in lung cancer patients. J Cancer Res Clin Oncol 146:43–52

Winther-Larsen A, Aggerholm-Pedersen N, Sandfeld-Paulsen B (2021) Inflammation scores as prognostic biomarkers in small cell lung cancer: a systematic review and meta-analysis. Syst Rev 10:40. https://doi.org/10.1186/s13643-021-01585-w

Yahya S, Ghafoor Q, Stevenson R, Watkins S, Allos B (2018) Evolution of stereotactic ablative radiotherapy in lung cancer and Birmingham's (UK) experience. Medicines (Basel) 5:77

Yokouchi H, Ishida T, Yamazaki S, Kikuchi H, Oizumi S, Uramoto H, Tanaka F, Harada M, Akie K, Sugaya F, Fujita Y, Fukuhara T, Takamura K, Kojima T, Harada T, Higuchi M, Matsuura Y, Honjo O, Minami Y, Watanabe N, Nishihara H, Suzuki H, Dosaka-Akita H, Isobe H, Nishimura M, Munakata M (2015) Prognostic impact of clinical variables on surgically resected small-cell lung cancer: results of a retrospective multicenter analysis (FIGHT002A and HOT1301A). Lung Cancer 90:548–553. https://doi.org/10.1016/j.lungcan.2015.10.010

Zhang J, Yao Y-H, Li B-G, Yang Q, Zhang P-Y, Wang H-T (2015a) Prognostic value of pretreatment serum lactate dehydrogenase level in patients with solid tumors: a systematic review and meta-analysis. Sci Rep 5:1–12

Zhang Z, Han Y, Liang H, Wang L (2015b) Prognostic value of serum CYFRA 21-1 and CEA for non-small-cell lung cancer. Cancer Med 4:1633–1638

Zhang L, Liu D, Li L, Pu D, Zhou P, Jing Y, Yu H, Wang Y, Zhu Y, He Y, Li Y, Zhao S, Qiu Z, Li W (2017a) The important role of circulating CYFRA21-1 in metastasis diagnosis and prognostic value compared with carcinoembryonic antigen and neuron-specific enolase in lung cancer patients. BMC Cancer 17:96. https://doi.org/10.1186/s12885-017-3070-6

Zhang M, Li G, Wang Y, Wang Y, Zhao S, Haihong P, Zhao H, Wang Y (2017b) PD-L1 expression in lung cancer and its correlation with driver mutations: a meta-analysis. Sci Rep 7:10255. https://doi.org/10.1038/s41598-017-10925-7

Zhang Z, Li Y, Yan X, Song Q, Wang G, Hu Y, Jiao S, Wang J (2019) Pretreatment lactate dehydrogenase may predict outcome of advanced non-small-cell lung cancer patients treated with immune checkpoint inhibitors: a meta-analysis. Cancer Med 8:1467–1473

Zhang Y-H, Lu Y, Lu H, Zhou Y-M (2020) Development of a survival prognostic model for non-small cell lung cancer. Front Oncol 10:362

Zhao X, Kallakury B, Chahine JJ, Hartmann D, Zhang Y, Chen Y, Zhang H, Zhang B, Wang C, Giaccone G (2019) Surgical resection of SCLC: prognostic factors and the tumor microenvironment. J Thorac Oncol 14:914–923. https://doi.org/10.1016/j.jtho.2019.01.019

Zheng M (2016) Classification and pathology of lung cancer. Surg Oncol Clin 25:447–468

Part XI
Technological Advances in Lung Cancer

Intensity-Modulated Radiation Therapy and Volumetric Modulated Arc Therapy for Lung Cancer

Jacob S. Parzen and Inga S. Grills

Contents

1	**Introduction**	1022
2	**Technical Aspects**	1023
2.1	Beam Modification	1023
2.2	Three-Dimensional Conformal Radiation Therapy (3D CRT)	1024
2.3	Intensity-Modulated Radiation Therapy (IMRT)	1025
2.4	Intensity-Modulated Arc Therapy (IMAT)	1025
2.5	Volumetric Modulated Arc Therapy (VMAT)	1027
3	**Potential Advantages of IMRT and VMAT: Dose Escalation and Toxicity Reduction**	1028
3.1	IMRT vs. 3D Conformal RT	1028
3.2	Toxicity and IMRT	1028
3.3	VMAT Experience	1033
4	**Treatment Planning**	1033
4.1	Simulation	1034
4.2	Target Volumes (GTV, CTV, PTV)	1034
4.3	Inverse Planning	1035
5	**Targeting and Verification**	1036
5.1	Image-Guided Radiation Therapy (IGRT)	1036
5.2	Biological Targeting with PET	1037
5.3	Treatment Verification	1037
6	**Clinical Outcomes**	1038
7	**Conclusion**	1039
	References	1043

J. S. Parzen · I. S. Grills (✉)
Department of Radiation Oncology, William Beaumont Hospital, Royal Oak, MI, USA
e-mail: Jacob.Parzen@beaumont.org; Inga.Grills@beaumont.edu

Abstract

Per 2021 American Cancer Society estimates, lung cancer has the second highest incidence and highest mortality of all malignancies in the United States. Outcomes have improved considerably over the past decade, with radiation therapy (RT) serving as a cornerstone of locoregional therapy. The technical challenges of delivering biologically effective doses of RT capable of achieving local control include accurate target definition and accounting for respiratory tumor motion, tissue heterogeneities, and normal tissue tolerance. Three-dimensional conformal radiation therapy (3D CRT) is now the minimum technical standard for treating NSCLC. Intensity-modulated radiation therapy (IMRT) and volumetrically modulated radiation therapy (VMAT), in addition to four-dimensional (4D) CT simulation and planning techniques, biological targeting via positron emission tomography (PET), and 2D and 3D image-guided delivery methods, have facilitated radiation dose escalation while respecting normal tissue tolerance of organs at risk (OAR). In patients with locally advanced disease, IMRT has demonstrated improved dosimetric and toxicity profiles when compared to 3D CRT. However, this comes at the cost of long treatment times and high integral dose. With improvements in commercial planning software and quality assurance measures, VMAT is now commonly employed to achieve the improved conformality found with IMRT along with shorter treatment times and fewer monitor units delivered. Though no randomized trials comparing 3D CRT to IMRT/VMAT have been performed, these advanced modalities should be strongly considered in patients with locally advanced disease.

1 Introduction

In the United States, 2021 estimates by the American Cancer Society suggest that lung cancer has the second highest cancer incidence, 236,000 new cases per year (trailing only breast), and highest annual cancer mortality, 132,000 deaths per year, nearly ¼ of all cancer deaths combined. However, lung cancer has also accounted for almost ½ of the total decline in cancer mortality from 2014 to 2018, likely attributable to improvements in therapy due to the lack of a corresponding shift to earlier diagnosis from increased lung cancer screening (Siegel et al. 2021).

In patients with inoperable non-small cell lung cancer (NSCLC), radiation therapy is the primary curative modality for both early-stage and locally advanced disease. Historically, delivery of radiation therapy (RT) for intrathoracic malignancies was technically challenging, and conventional radiotherapy doses and techniques yielded unacceptable results. In early-stage disease, local failure occurred in 50–70% of patients with 2-year survival under 50% using 2D treatment planning with standard fractionation (Armstrong and Minsky 1989; Dosoretz et al. 1992; Kaskowitz et al. 1993; Fang et al. 2006). In locally advanced disease treated with concurrent chemotherapy, the 2-year rate of in-field failure was greater than 30% with median survival under 19 months (Curran et al. 2011; Byhardt et al. 1995; Lee et al. 1996).

An early study from the Radiation Therapy Oncology Group (RTOG) established 60 Gy as the standard dosing in the nonoperative management of NSCLC (Perez et al. 1980). Subsequent reports from the University of Michigan, RTOG, and Memorial Sloan Kettering Cancer Center (MSKCC) showed that dose escalation was safe and feasible and offered the potential for improved local control (Bradley et al. 2005; Hayman et al. 2001; Rosenzweig et al. 2005). Across dose escalation studies, the maximum tolerated dose for standard fractionated RT without chemotherapy was approximately 83–84 Gy and with concurrent chemotherapy was 74 Gy (Bradley et al. 2010). However, the RTOG 0617 trial did not show a benefit to dose escalation to 74 Gy, and 60 Gy remains the standard of care for treatment delivered with standard fractionation (Bradley et al. 2020). In contrast, exceedingly high biological effective doses (BEDs) are now routinely administered for the treatment of stage I NSCLC by way of stereotactic body radiation therapy (SBRT), where a BED of >94–105 Gy has shown higher rates of local control (Grills et al. 2012; Wulf et al. 2005; Onishi et al. 2004). In RTOG 0236, SBRT yielded a 5-year LC rate of 80% (Timmerman et al. 2018a), and data have shown SBRT to have comparable results to sublobar (e.g., wedge) resection in terms of local and regional recurrence (Grills et al. 2010). Studies comparing SBRT and lobectomy have generally accrued poorly and thus have been unable to elucidate comparative efficacy (Chang et al. 2015). RTOG 0618, which included only operable patients, demonstrated a 2-year lobar control rate of 96% (Timmerman et al. 2018b).

Even with the advent of three-dimensional conformal radiotherapy (3D CRT), escalating to tumoricidal doses for larger tumors is highly constrained by the potential for toxicity to the spinal cord (myelitis), esophagus (esophagitis/dysphagia), and normal lung (pneumonitis). Furthermore, the amplified risk of "geographic miss" due to respiratory tumor motion is a challenge virtually unique to intrathoracic malignancies. Particularly in locally advanced disease, the advent of intensity-modulated radiation therapy (IMRT) increases the potential for dose escalation while sparing organs at risk (OARs), but requires advanced technologies to account for respiratory tumor motion such as 4D CT (four-dimensional computed tomography) to avoid tumor miss and is ideally administered using online three-dimensional image guidance for proper targeting and margin reduction.

In this chapter, we discuss technological advances beyond 3D CRT, particularly IMRT, intensity-modulated arc therapy (IMAT), and volumetric modulated arc therapy (VMAT) along with treatment planning, toxicity, and clinical outcomes associated with these modalities.

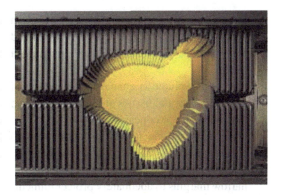

Fig. 1 A close-up photo of MLC leaves looking up into the collimator head. (Copyright © 2021, Varian Systems, Inc. All rights reserved)

2 Technical Aspects

2.1 Beam Modification

Upon exiting a treatment machine, beam modification occurs by many methods for different purposes. Custom blocks (e.g., historically lead or Cerrobend®) shape beams for target conformality, a job now replaced by the multileaf collimators (MLCs, Figs. 1 and 2), which make IMRT possible. Flattening filters improve dose homogeneity from central axis to block edge to create a uniform beam profile. Wedges confer a linear gradient of dose fluence across a beam in a single direction, whereas physical compensators manipulate dose intensity in two dimensions. Unlike wedges, compensators are custom-made for the individual patient. Irradiation with wedges and/or compensators *is* IMRT in its simplest form: radiation with heterogeneous dose fluence across the beam.

There is no universally accepted definition of IMRT. From a technical standpoint, Bortfeld described IMRT as "a radiation treatment technique with multiple beams, in which at least some of the beams are intensity-modulated and intentionally deliver a nonuniform intensity to the target. The desired dose distribution in the target is achieved after superimposing such beams from different directions. The additional degrees of freedom are utilized to achieve a better target dose conformity and/or better sparing of critical structures (Bortfeld 2006)." McDermott described IMRT as "the most technically complex development in radiation therapy in the last 25 years (McDermott and Orton 2018)."

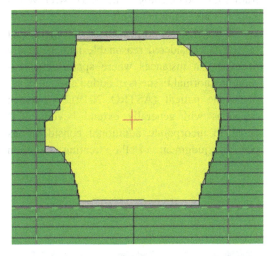

Fig. 2 An MLC portal outline (beam's-eye view) as shown on a computer display. This MLC is a tertiary system. The position of the secondary jaws is shown. There are locations where the leaves overlap the desired treatment outline and other spots where they underlap producing a "scalloped" contour. The leaf width is 1.0 cm projected to isocenter. Varian SHAPER program software. (Copyright © 2021, Varian Medical Systems, Inc. All rights reserved)

Billing definitions of IMRT are also professionally relevant. The Centers for Medicare and Medicaid Services (CMS) deems IMRT clinically indicated when at least one of the following five conditions is met:

- An immediately adjacent area has been previously irradiated, and abutting portals must be established with high precision.

- Dose escalation is planned to deliver radiation doses in excess of those commonly utilized for similar tumors with conventional treatment.
- The target volume is concave or convex, and the critical normal tissues are within or around that convexity or concavity.
- The target volume is in close proximity to critical structures that must be protected.
- The volume of interest must be covered with narrow margins to adequately protect immediately adjacent structures.

The American Society for Therapeutic Radiology and Oncology (ASTRO) IMRT Model Policy is an additional useful resource for guidance on IMRT appropriateness. It states that "IMRT is considered reasonable and medically necessary in instances where sparing the surrounding normal tissue is of added clinical benefit to the patient (ASTRO 2019)." Coverage decisions will generally extend beyond ICD codes to incorporate additional considerations per the judgment of the treating radiation oncologist.

2.2 Three-Dimensional Conformal Radiation Therapy (3D CRT)

Three-dimensional (3D) treatment planning became possible with the advent of computed tomography in the 1970s and the routine availability of computers in the 1980s. With 3D planning, target volumes and organs at risk (OARs) can be well defined, and beam shapes, directions, and energy levels can be appropriately selected to give rise to increased conformity, decreased margins, and target dose escalation with increased sparing of normal tissue. In practice, 3D CRT implies that for each given beam angle, only a *single* beam shape modifier (e.g., a Cerrobend® block or, more commonly, a single MLC portal) is allowed for each beam position. If, for example, three different blocks (beam shapes) were used at a single beam angle, the integral dose fluence from the three beams would create a map of variable dose fluence (Fig. 3), resulting in an individual IMRT beam. If an inverse planning system is used to modify the beam shape and weight for a single segment per beam, 3D plans can sometimes look more similar to those of IMRT.

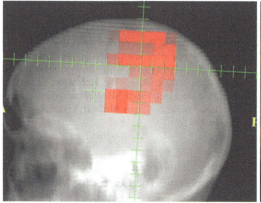
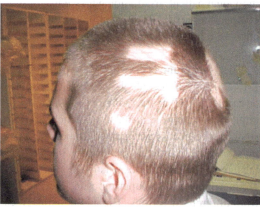

Fig. 3 Left: Intensity map of an IMRT beam superimposed on a patient digital reconstructed radiograph (DRR). Right: Radiation-induced epilation on the patient's scalp from corresponding IMRT beam intensity (left). (From McDermott and Orton, Figure 15.2, *The Physics & Technology of Radiation Therapy*, 2nd ed., © 2018)

2.3 Intensity-Modulated Radiation Therapy (IMRT)

In practice, manually cutting blocks for multiple beam segments and angles and then—in turn—manually placing each block for each segment would require great time and manual effort and create substantial potential for error. The advent of computer-generated and manipulated MLCs (Figs. 1 and 2) is what made IMRT[1] practical and logistically feasible, allowing large numbers of "segments" ("apertures"). In segmental IMRT ("static window" or "step and shoot"), the most common form, the beam turns off whenever the MLCs are in motion and is on only when the MLCs are stationary, forming a static portal. The initial beam segment for a given beam position may be the "open field" (e.g., what might be used for a 3D conformal plan). An electronic portal imaging device (EPID) routinely takes a beam's-eye-view image through this segment for target verification. Multiple "subportal" beams, with variable weights, are used to modify the initially delivered open-field beam. The resultant "IMRT beam" represents the summation of dose from all beam segments (the open portal and subportals). The IMRT beam is therefore a series of "beamlets," with each beamlet providing a different discrete intensity. At risk of oversimplification, whereas a 3D CRT beam represents a true "black-and-white" image (e.g., a beamlet is either blocked or unblocked), the IMRT beam permits many shades of gray (Figs. 4 and 5). Such heterogeneous beam intensities delivered through multiple beam angles allow dose escalation to target volumes and subvolumes (e.g., simultaneous integrated boost), organ sparing, and ultimately "dose painting" (Figs. 6 and 7) superior to 3D CRT (Brahme 1988).

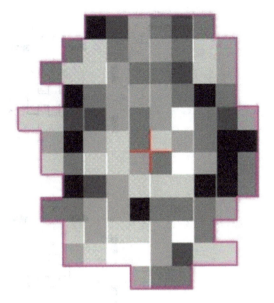

Fig. 4 An intensity map showing an IMRT beam with 1 cm × 1 cm beamlets with ten different grayscale intensity levels (white = less intense, dark = more intense). (From McDermott and Orton, Figure 15.1, *The Physics & Technology of Radiation Therapy*, 2nd ed., © 2018)

2.4 Intensity-Modulated Arc Therapy (IMAT)

Yu et al. at William Beaumont Hospital first introduced intensity-modulated arc therapy[2] (IMAT) in 1995. This was a rotational radiation therapy delivery technique in which the field shape changed dynamically as the linear accelerator

---

[1] For the purposes of this chapter, the abbreviation "IMRT" by default will henceforth refer only to fixed-field IMRT, whereby intensity-modulated beams are delivered from multiple discrete, fixed angles (using segmental or dynamic MLCs) without any gantry rotation during beam-on time, thus excluding techniques such as tomotherapy, IMAT, and VMAT. The unabbreviated term "intensity-modulated radiation therapy" may, however, confer a broader connotation.

[2] Notably, distinctions for IMAT and VMAT are not universally agreed upon. The term "arc therapy" will refer both to IMAT and VMAT. As the term "VMAT" corresponds to technological advances of IMAT, Yu et al. refer to VMAT expressly as IMAT. Further, VMAT technology has been trademarked with Elekta (VMAT™), Varian (RapidArc™), and Philips (SmartArc™) and has also been referred to as "arc-modulated radiation therapy" (AMRT). Henceforth, the terms "volumetric modulated arc therapy" and "VMAT" will refer generically to the advanced IMAT technology inclusive of variable gantry velocity and variable dose rate and exclusive of arc therapy delivered with uniform dose rate and uniform gantry velocity, which will be referred to as intensity-modulated arc therapy or "IMAT." Furthermore, tomotherapy will be considered as its own modality (not to be incorporated by default with the terms "IMRT," "arc therapy," "IMAT," or "VMAT").

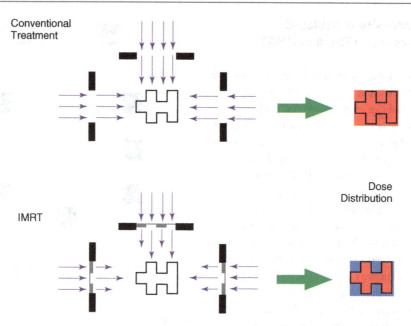

Fig. 5 Comparison of conventional RT to IMRT. Three beams are used to treat a target with an irregular shape. In the conventional treatment (upper), the jaws are used to shape the beams to correspond to the beam's-eye-view shape of the target. The resulting dose distribution is shown as homogeneous shading (upper right). With IMRT (lower), the beam is modulated in an attempt to reduce the dose to the "nooks and crannies" representative of normal tissue. The resulting heterogeneous dose distribution (lower right) shows dose reduction in these regions. (From McDermott and Orton, Figure 15.3, *The Physics & Technology of Radiation Therapy*, 2nd ed., © 2018)

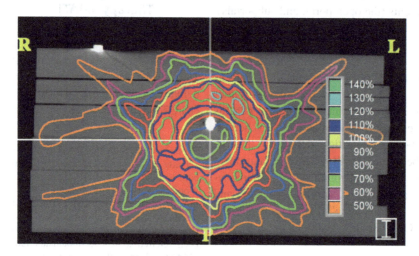

Fig. 6 The dose distribution in a geometric phantom (square slabs in virtual water) illustrating the power of IMRT. Seven gantry angles and five intensity levels were used. The target is the red annulus encompassing a cylindrical organ at risk (e.g., spinal cord). The 100% isodose line wraps tightly around both the inside and outside of the annulus giving high conformity. Dose within the target, however, is quite heterogeneous with maximum dose of 148% the prescribed dose. (From McDermott and Orton, color plate 19, *The Physics & Technology of Radiation Therapy*, 2nd ed., © 2018)

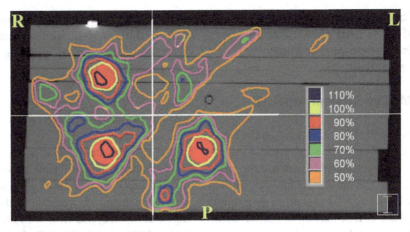

Fig. 7 The dose distribution in a geometric phantom with three targets. The targets (red) are cylinders with axes perpendicular to the page. A 7-field IMRT plan revealed high conformity with only a single isocenter (intersection of crosshairs). The maximum dose within the target is 115% the prescribed dose. (From McDermott and Orton, color plate 20, *The Physics & Technology of Radiation Therapy*, © 2010)

gantry rotated. Gantry rotational speed and dose rate were constant throughout treatment delivery. Multiple arcs with varying field shapes created an intensity-modulated arc. For treatment planning, arcs were planned using set control points: IMRT beams at incremental angles (Yu 1995; Yu et al. 1995). IMAT offered reduced treatment time and decreased MU delivery when compared to segmental IMRT. IMAT did not, however, achieve widespread use for several reasons: the arc sequencing was a lengthy process; accurate delivery was inefficient with complex fields—often multiple superimposed arcs were necessary—and available computer power and memory at the time were inadequate for dose calculations at a fine resolution. Further, support from linear accelerator control software was lacking (Otto 2008; Ramsey et al. 2001). Achievable dose distributions, however, were considered comparable to helical tomotherapy while using a standard linear accelerator (Cao et al. 2007).

2.5 Volumetric Modulated Arc Therapy (VMAT)

In pursuit of single-arc IMAT plans with ideal plan quality, Otto developed an algorithm that allowed for a variable dose rate during arc delivery referred to as volumetric modulated arc therapy (see Footnote 2) (VMAT) (Otto 2008). Industrial advances allowed the development of VMAT as a more dynamic radiation delivery method. Similar to IMAT, the beam is on during rotation of a standard linear accelerator gantry. However, the dose rate, rotational gantry speed, MLC position, and collimator angle are all dynamically modulated during RT delivery. Thus, highly conformal treatment plans can be delivered in single to multiple arcs. With VMAT, radiation treatment times can average only 1.5–3 min per 2 Gy fraction, substantially lower than required for similarly complex IMRT plans (Otto 2008). Though VMAT may be planned as a near-to-full single rotation (e.g., 340–360°) (Otto 2008; Scorsetti et al. 2010; Wolff et al. 2009; Guckenberger et al. 2009; Clark et al. 2010; Ong et al. 2010), it can also be delivered as a partial arc (e.g., 180°) (Matuszak et al. 2010; McGrath et al. 2010), dual (back-and-forth) partial arcs (Holt et al. 2011), a full + partial arc (Wolff et al. 2009), and multiple arcs, both coplanar and noncoplanar (Guckenberger et al. 2009; Clark et al. 2010). The use of multiple arcs can provide further intensity modulation or allow for more optimal normal tissue sparing and avoid spreading low dose unnecessarily to other areas of the body. The development of IMAT and its progression to VMAT are well described in a review by Yu and Tang (2011).

3 Potential Advantages of IMRT and VMAT: Dose Escalation and Toxicity Reduction

3.1 IMRT vs. 3D Conformal RT

As compared to 3D CRT, IMRT has many inherent potentially advantageous qualities. With heterogeneous beam intensities, tumor heterogeneity can be increased, allowing a higher maximum dose in the target as well as sharper dose falloff close to critical OARs, leading to normal tissue sparing (lung, esophagus, spinal cord, etc.). Schwarz et al. showed that for large concave tumors treated with IMRT, the average dose increase was as high as 35% compared to 3D CRT (Schwarz et al. 2005). The ability to spare cylindrical structures is well illustrated in Fig. 6. Figure 7 illustrates the conformity to multiple targets while using a single isocenter, a common scenario in LA-NSCLC, where tumor and nodal gross tumor volumes (GTVs) are often disjointed.

Planning studies comparing IMRT to 3D CRT have demonstrated that IMRT allows for superior coverage of the target volumes with greater sparing of OARs. In comparison to 3D CRT, Liu et al. showed that 9-field IMRT plans decreased mean lung dose (MLD) by 2 Gy and amount of lung receiving 20 Gy (lung V_{20}) by 8% (Liu et al. 2004). Grills et al. performed a systematic planning analysis comparing IMRT to two 3D CRT techniques: (1) optimized (numerous-field) 3D CRT and (2) traditional limited-field (e.g., 2–3 beams) 3D CRT. This study showed significant benefit with IMRT, particularly in node-positive patients and those with target volumes close to the esophagus. With higher mean target doses secondary to IMRT dose heterogeneity, tumor control probability (TCP) was increased 7–8%, whereas lung V_{20}, lung normal tissue complication probability (NTCP), and esophagus NTCP were reduced by approximately 15%, 30%, and 55%, respectively. For GTVs within 1.5 cm of the esophagus, IMRT reduced esophagus V_{50} by 40%. IMRT plans allowed for dose escalation of 25–30% beyond that of comparably safe 3D CRT plans (Grills et al. 2003). A comparison of 3D CRT to IMRT/VMAT with respect to critical organ dose for various planning studies is included in Table 1.

3.2 Toxicity and IMRT

Sura et al. published one of the earliest toxicity and outcome studies of patients with NSCLC treated exclusively with IMRT. This retrospective analysis included 55 patients with inoperable stage I–II ($n = 16$) and III ($n = 39$) NSCLC from 2001 to 2005 treated with 60 Gy in 2 Gy fractions at MSKCC. Toxicity was scored using a modified RTOG toxicity scoring system. The overall crude rate of any pulmonary toxicity was 13%. Acute grade 1–2 esophagitis was common (69%), but grade 3 rare (4%). All late (>4 months) esophageal toxicity was grade 1–2 and occurred in 22% of patients. Grade 2 or higher acute pulmonary toxicity rates were 18% grade 2, 11% grade 3, and 0% grade 4–5. One patient had late (>4 months) grade 3 pulmonary toxicity, and one died (grade 5 toxicity) secondary to treatment-related pneumonitis (TRP) (Sura et al. 2008).

Similarly, Jiang et al. reported on a large series of NSCLC patients treated exclusively with IMRT. Their analysis included 165 patients with stage I–II ($n = 18$) and III–IV ($n = 147$) NSCLC treated to a median of 66 Gy. Toxicity was principally assessed using the CTCAE v. 3.0. At 6 months, 11% of patients had developed grade ≥ 3 TRP_{max}, and at 12 months, 14% had developed grade ≥ 3 TRP_{max}. Two patients died from grade 5 TRP. At 12 months and 18 months, 50% and 86% of patients experienced grade ≥ 1 pulmonary $fibrosis_{max}$, respectively. Grade 3 esophagitis was rare during treatment, with a rate of only 10% by week 6 of treatment. Of the 29 patients who had grade 3 acute $esophagitis_{max}$, 3 (10%) later developed grade 2 esophageal $stricture_{max}$ and 4 (14%) later developed grade 3 esophageal $stricture_{max}$ (Jiang et al. 2012).

3.2.1 Sparing the Heart

Multiple studies have now established cardiac radiation dose as a modifiable risk factor for

Table 1 Comparison of median/mean dose to organs at risk: 3D CRT vs. IMRT/VMAT

Organ	Study	N	Patients	Parameter	3D CRT	IMRT	VMAT	Difference	p
Spinal cord	Bedford and Warrington (2009)	10	NR	D_{max}	10 Gy	–	9 Gy	−0.5 Gy	NS
	Grills et al. (2003)	9	N0	$D_{max+3mm}$	24 Gy	30 Gy	–	+5.6 Gy	–
	Grills et al. (2003)[a]	9	N2–N3	$D_{max+3mm}$	41 Gy	41 Gy	–	−0.6 Gy	–
	Lievens et al. (2011)[b]	35	N2–N3	D_{max}	47 Gy	45 Gy	–	−2.5 Gy	–
	Ong et al. (2010)	18	I	D_{max}	8 Gy	–	11 Gy	+2.9 Gy	0.014
Lungs	Lievens et al. (2011)	35	N2–N3	V_5	55%	45%	–	−10%	<0.0001
	Liu et al. (2004)	10	I–IIIB	V_5	NR	NR	–	+8.0%	0.007
	McGrath et al. (2010)[c]	21	I	V_5	NR	–	NR	4.2% RR[c]	0.03
	Murshed et al. (2004)	41	III–IV	V_5	52%	59%	–	+7%	NS
	Ong et al. (2010)[c]	18	I	V_5	18%	–	18%	+0.2%	NS
	Bedford and Warrington (2009)	10	NR	V_{10}	40%	–	34%	−5.6%	0.03
	Liu et al. (2004)	10	I–IIIB	V_{10}	NR	NR	–	−1.6%	NS
	McGrath et al. (2010)[c]	21	I	V_{10}	NR	–	NR	2.6% RR[c]	0.01
	Murshed et al. (2004)	41	III–IV	V_{10}	45%	38%	–	−7%	<0.0001
	McGrath et al. (2010)[c]	21	I	$V_{12.5}$	NR	–	NR	3.2% RR[c]	0.01
	Bedford and Warrington (2009)	10	NR	V_{20}	21%	–	24%	+2.6%	0.02
	Grills et al. (2003)[a]	9	N0	V_{20}	22%	19%	–	−2.8%	–
	Grills et al. (2003)[a]	9	N2–N3	V_{20}	29%	26%	–	−3.2%	–
	Lievens et al. (2011)	35	N2–N3	V_{20}	28%	27%	–	−1.2%	0.06
	Liu et al. (2004)	10	I–IIIB	V_{20}	NR	NR	–	−8.0%	0.005
	McGrath et al. (2010)[c]	21	I	V_{20}	NR	–	NR	4.5% RR[c]	0.02
	Murshed et al. (2004)	41	III–IV	V_{20}	35%	25%	–	−10%	<0.0001
	Ong et al. (2010)[d]	18	I	V_{20}	4.9%	–	5.4%	+0.5%	0.025
	Liu et al. (2004)	10	I–IIIB	V_{30}	NR	NR	–	−8.9%	0.005
	Liu et al. (2004)	10	I–IIIB	V_{eff}	NR	NR	–	−9.0%	0.005
	Murshed et al. (2004)	41	III–IV	V_{eff}	71 Gy	58 Gy	–	−13 Gy	<0.0001
	Bedford and Warrington (2009)	10	NR	MLD	14 Gy	–	14 Gy	+0.1 Gy	NS
	Grills et al. (2003)[a]	9	N0	MLD	13 Gy	12 Gy	–	−1.8 Gy	–
	Grills et al. (2003)[a]	9	N2–N3	MLD	18 Gy	16 Gy	–	−1.8 Gy	–
	Liu et al. (2004)	10	I–IIIB	MLD	NR	NR	–	−2.0 Gy	0.005
	Murshed et al. (2004)	41	III–IV	MLD	19 Gy	17 Gy	–	−2 Gy	<0.0001
	Lievens et al. (2011)	35	N2–N3	MLD	16 Gy	16 Gy	–	+0.1 Gy	NS
	Murshed et al. (2004)	41	III–IV	Integral Lung Dose	19 Gy	16 Gy	–	−3 Gy	<0.0001
	Grills et al. (2003)[a]	9	N0	NTCP	12%	11%	–	+1.1%	–
	Grills et al. (2003)[a]	9	N2–N3	NTCP	21%	17%	–	−3.6%	–

(continued)

Organ	Study	N	Patients	Parameter	3D CRT	IMRT	VMAT	Difference	p
Esophagus	Grills et al. (2003)[a]	9	N0	V_{50}	5%	6%	–	+0.6%	–
	Grills et al. (2003)[a]	9	N2–N3	V_{50}	26%	19%	–	–7.6%	–
	Grills et al. (2003)[a]	9	N0	Mean dose	12 Gy	12 Gy	–	–0.2 Gy	–
	Grills et al. (2003)[a]	9	N2–N3	Mean dose	27 Gy	24 Gy	–	–2.9 Gy	–
	Lievens et al. (2011)	35	N2–N3	Dmax	93 Gy	79 Gy	–	–14 Gy	<0.0001
	Grills et al. (2003)[a]	9	N0	$D_{max+3mm}$	46 Gy	43 Gy	–	–3.4 Gy	–
	Grills et al. (2003)[a]	9	N2–N3	$D_{max+3mm}$	76 Gy	74 Gy	–	–1.6 Gy	–
	Grills et al. (2003)[a]	9	N0	NTCP	5.2%	2.2%	–	–3.0%	–
	Grills et al. (2003)[a]	9	N2–N3	NTCP	41%	19%	–	–22%	–
Heart	Bedford and Warrington (2009)	10	NR	Mean dose	9.9 Gy	–	9.4 Gy	NS	–
	Grills et al. (2003)[a]	9	N0	D_{33}	8.9 Gy	9.3 Gy	–	+0.4 Gy	–
	Grills et al. (2003)[a]	9	N2–N3	D_{33}	19 Gy	20 Gy	–	+0.8 Gy	–
	Grills et al. (2003)[a]	9	N0	D_{67}	5.2 Gy	4.4 Gy	–	–0.8 Gy	–
	Grills et al. (2003)[a]	9	N2–N3	D_{67}	7 Gy	8 Gy	–	+1.5 Gy	–
	Grills et al. (2003)[a]	9	N0	D_{100}	0.3 Gy	0.6 Gy	–	+0.3 Gy	–
	Grills et al. (2003)[a]	9	N2–N3	D_{100}	0.9 Gy	1.6 Gy	–	+0.7 Gy	–
	Grills et al. (2003)[a]	9	N0	NTCP	0.1%	0%	–	–0.1%	–
	Grills et al. (2003)[a]	9	N2–N3	NTCP	20%	11%	–	–9%	–

3D CRT = 3D conformal radiation therapy, IMRT = intensity-modulated radiation therapy, VMAT = volumetric modulated radiation therapy, Difference = IMRT-3D CRT or VMAT-3D CRT, n = number of patients, D_{max} = maximum dose, V_{eff} = biologically effective volume, +3mm = volume of organ + 3mm expansion, NR = no reported data, NS = not statistically significant, I, II, III, IV = AJCC stage, N = nodal staging

[a] Both plans with equivalent tumor control probability for PTV_{GTV}. Lung dose calculations exclude gross tumor volume (GTV)
[b] Liu (2004)—both plans with dose escalation with calculations using pencil-beam algorithm
[c] Only VMAT relative (not absolute) reduction reported in this study. All variables were lower with VMAT in comparison to 3D CRT
[d] Lung volume excludes planning treatment volume (PTV)

major adverse cardiac events (MACE) and all-cause mortality (ACM) (Wang et al. 2017; Dess et al. 2017). In a planned secondary analysis of RTOG 0617 comparing those patients receiving IMRT versus 3D CRT, the use of IMRT resulted in lower heart V_{20}, V_{40}, and V_{60} ($p < 0.05$) when compared to 3D CRT. On multivariate analysis, heart V_{40} was associated with OS (HR 1.012, 95% CI 1.005–1.02, $p < 0.001$) (Chun et al. 2017). Unfortunately, actual cardiac events were not recorded on this trial, given that little was known about the potential impact of heart dose on OS for NSCLC prior to its publication.

Several subsequent studies challenged the dogma that radiation-induced heart toxicity occurs only 10 or more years following treatment, which had been observed in earlier studies of breast cancer and Hodgkin's lymphoma. A pooled analysis of 127 stage III NSCLC patients treated on prospective dose escalation trials at the University of North Carolina from 1996 to 2009 was evaluated for late cardiac events following publication of RTOG 0617 (Wang et al. 2017). On multivariate analysis, when paired with baseline World Health Organization/International Society of Hypertension score or baseline coronary artery disease, mean heart dose, heart V_5, heart V_{30}, and left ventricle V_5 were all ($p < 0.05$) associated with the development of symptomatic cardiac events (Wang). Competing risk-adjusted event rates for patients with heart mean dose <10 Gy, 10–20 Gy, and ≥20 Gy were 4%, 7%, and 21%, respectively, at 2 years. Although patients were treated with 3D CRT on this study, this study was one of the first to demonstrate significant rates of radiation-induced cardiac toxicity only 2 years following treatment. A similar analysis from the University of Michigan accumulated 125 stage II–III NSCLC patients treated from 2004 to 2013 on prospective trials, with a minority (<10%) undergoing IMRT (Dess et al. 2017). The 2-year incidence of grade ≥3 cardiac events was 11%. On multivariate analysis, preexisting heart disease (hazard ratio [HR] = 2.96, 95% confidence interval [CI] 1.07–8.21, $p = 0.04$) and higher mean heart dose (HR = 1.07/Gy, 95% CI 1.01–1.13/Gy, $p = 0.01$) were predictive of grade ≥3 cardiac events. When analyzed as a time-dependent variable, grade ≥3 cardiac events were associated with increased hazard of death (HR = 1.76, 95% CI 1.04–2.99, $p = 0.04$).

Speirs et al. evaluated 416 patients treated at Washington University/Barnes-Jewish Hospital to a median of 66 Gy between 2001 and 2015. Of note, 40% of patients underwent IMRT. IMRT was associated with decreased rates of pneumonitis ($p = 0.0007$) and cardiac toxicities ($p < 0.0001$). IMRT also decreased heart V_{15} to V_{75} relative to 3D CRT ($p \leq 0.0003$), with the largest discrepancies seen at the intermediate- to high-dose levels (≥20 Gy) (Speirs et al. 2017). Atkins et al. published the Harvard experience of 748 consecutive NSCLC patients treated to cumulative doses of 50–66 Gy. With a median follow-up of 20.4 months, the 2-year incidence of MACE was 5.8%. Mean heart dose was associated with increased risk of MACE (HR = 1.05/Gy, 95% CI 1.02–1.08, $p < 0.001$) and ACM (HR = 1.02/Gy, 95% CI 1.00–1.03, $p = 0.007$). IMRT was employed in 21.9% of patients and was associated with decreased risk of MACE on multivariate analysis (HR = 0.39, 95% CI = 0.18–0.84, $p = 0.017$) (Atkins et al. 2019). In a more recent study from the same group, cardiac substructures were manually delineated. Left anterior descending artery $V_{15} \geq 10\%$ was associated with increased risk of MACE (HR = 13.9, 95% CI 1.23–157.21, $p = 0.03$) and ACM (HR 1.58, 95% CI 1.09–2.29, $p = 0.02$), but among patients with CHD, only a left ventricle $V_{15} \geq 1\%$ was associated with increased 1-year risk of MACE (8.4% vs. 4.1%, $p = 0.046$) (Atkins et al. 2021).

Finally, Dess et al. reported on a series of 746 stage III NSCLC patients treated across a collaborative statewide consortium (Dess et al. 2020). The use of IMRT increased from 33% in 2012 to 86% in 2017 ($p < 0.001$). Usage of IMRT was associated with a lower percent of heart V_{30} (absolute reduction [AR] = 3.0%, 95% CI 0.5–5.4%) and V_{50} (AR = 3.6%, 95% CI 2.4–4.8%) and a higher percent of heart V_5 (absolute increase = 5.4%, 95% CI 0.3–10.4%). After inverse probability weighting, IMRT resulted in relative reductions in V_{40}–V_{60} of 29–48%, an increase in V_5 of 15%, and a similar mean heart dose.

The field of radiation oncology only relatively recently began strongly considering cardiac dose in advanced lung cancer planning. As such, the ideal dosimetric constraints for the heart are still in evolution. Both low and high heart doses are likely important, and while IMRT clearly reduces high cardiac doses, it may also be associated with higher low heart doses such as V_5 (Dess et al. 2020). We feel that both high and low doses are important and should be optimized and minimized whenever possible. Proton therapy, particularly intensity-modulated proton therapy (IMPT) or spot-scanning proton arc (SPArc) therapy, may ultimately prove to be the most effective method for reducing heart V_5, lung V_5, and mean heart and lung doses. RTOG 1308 includes cardiac toxicity as a primary endpoint and will hopefully be helpful in elucidating this further.

3.2.2 Sparing the Esophagus

The predominant increase in acute toxicity with concurrent over sequential chemoradiotherapy for locally advanced NSCLC is esophagitis, which can ultimately become dose limiting (Schwarz et al. 2005; Liu et al. 2004; Grills et al. 2003; Chapet et al. 2005; Murshed et al. 2004). In patients treated with 3D CRT or IMRT, Palma et al. performed an individual patient data meta-analysis to determine predictors of radiation esophagitis. They identified 1082 patients treated with a median dose of 65 Gy, with 91% of patients receiving concurrent platinum-based chemotherapy. On multivariate analysis, V_{60} of the esophagus emerged as the best predictor of grade ≥2 and ≥3 esophagitis, with the highest risk for V_{60} ≥17% (Palma et al. 2013). Multiple other studies have shown the potential for esophageal dose reduction with IMRT over 3D CRT (Liu et al. 2004; Grills et al. 2003; Murshed et al. 2004; Lievens et al. 2011). One of the planning challenges in advanced-stage NSCLC is the potential for overlap of the planning target volume for tumor or nodes with the esophagus. Chapet et al. have shown that by relaxing homogeneity constraints and using equivalent uniform dose (EUD) calculations, the planning target volume (PTV) excluding the esophagus can be dosed to higher levels with potential for better tumor control without increasing esophagus NTCP (Chapet et al. 2005, 2006). Finally, a contralateral esophagus-sparing technique utilizing IMRT has emerged, wherein the esophageal wall contralateral to the gross disease is contoured as an avoidance structure to guide a steep dose falloff across the esophagus. Early reports suggested excellent esophageal sparing, with no reported cases of grade ≥3 esophagitis in a cohort of 20 patients (Al-Halabi et al. 2015), and early prospective results similarly report favorable toxicity profiles (Kamran et al. 2020).

3.2.3 Pneumonitis: Worse with IMRT?

Although IMRT has numerous potential advantages over 3D CRT for NSCLC, IMRT plans require more monitor units (MUs) per treatment and thus have risks associated with increased total body exposure. Longer treatment times may further increase the potential for intrafraction variation. In the treatment of intrathoracic malignancies, a significant concern is the potential for increased lung toxicity—in comparison to 3D CRT—from spreading low dose throughout a larger volume of normal lung. Many studies have consistently reported the correlation between lung dose and TRP (Willner et al. 2003; Fay et al. 2005; Schallenkamp et al. 2007; Shi et al. 2010; Wang et al. 2006). In a 3D CRT dose escalation study, high-grade TRP was related to low-dose lung RT volumes: V_5, V_{10}, and V_{13} (Yorke et al. 2005). Schallenkamp et al. found V_{10} and V_{13} to be the most predictive of TRP (V_5 was not analyzed) (Schallenkamp et al. 2007). Wang's multivariate analysis of 223 patients treated with concurrent chemoradiation further supports V_5 as the strongest predictor of TRP (cutoff 42%) (Wang et al. 2006).

However, in a secondary analysis of RTOG 0617, the "low-dose bath" created by IMRT did not lead to higher rates of TRP. Though IMRT was associated with a larger lung V_5 than 3D CRT ($p < 0.001$), lung V_5 was not associated with rates of grade ≥3 TRP. Lung V_{20} was not different between groups ($p = 0.297$). Overall, IMRT was associated with a lower rate of grade ≥3 TRP (3.5% vs. 7.9%, $p = 0.039$). Similarly, Yom et al. evaluated such parameters in patients treated with IMRT ($n = 68$) as well as 3D CRT ($n = 222$) at MD Anderson, particularly predictors of grade ≥3 TRP with locally advanced NSCLC receiving concurrent chemotherapy. This study revealed a fourfold decrease in TRP with IMRT over 3D CRT (8% vs. 32%, $p = 0.002$). IMRT plans had higher V_5 (63% vs. 57%, $p = 0.011$), similar V_{10} (48% vs. 49%, $p = 0.87$), and decreased V_{15}, V_{20}, ..., V_{65} ($p < 0.05$). The 12-month incidence of TRP for IMRT-treated patients was significantly less with $V_5 \leq 70\%$ (2% vs. 21%, $p = 0.02$), suggesting a potential V_5 threshold of 70 Gy. Interestingly, however, overall rates of TRP were lower with IMRT than with 3D CRT despite higher V_5 in the IMRT group, suggesting that other factors may play a significant role in determining the risk for TRP in irradiated patients (Yom et al. 2007).

3.2.4 IMRT: Improved Quality of Life?

An additional secondary analysis of RTOG 0617 evaluated patient declines in quality of life (QOL) following treatment. Of those randomized, 360 (85%) consented to QOL evaluation, of whom 313 (88%) completed baseline QOL assessments using the Functional Assessment of Cancer Therapy (FACT)-Trial Outcome Index (TOI). At 12 months, IMRT had less clinically meaningful decline (CMD) than 3D CRT in the FACT-TOI

(36% vs. 57%, $p = 0.01$) and in the Lung Cancer Subscale (21% vs. 46%, $p = 0.003$). A notable limitation of this study was the 57% rate of QOL completion at 12 months (Movsas et al. 2016).

3.3 VMAT Experience

VMAT and IMAT offer reduced treatment times and less MUs (by about 50%) delivered compared to IMRT plans (McDermott and Orton 2018). The former may increase patient throughput. In addition, because the gantry rotates continuously and treatment is faster, there may be a lower risk for intrafraction movement. Planning studies have also shown modest dosimetric benefits to VMAT, particularly with regard to normal lung irradiation (Holt et al. 2011; Bertelsen et al. 2012; Jiang et al. 2011; Weyh et al. 2013). Bedford et al. used VMAT to replan ten NSCLC patients originally treated to 65 Gy with 3D CRT. Single-arc plans were created spanning 340° at 10° intervals. Results are included in Table 1. Notably, VMAT plans reduced lung V_{10}, though PTV coverage (93% vs. 91%, $p = 0.1$) and lung V_{20} were marginally inferior (Bedford and Warrington 2009). McGrath et al. reported on the utility of VMAT for SBRT. In this study, 21 patients previously treated with non-coplanar 3D CRT were replanned with a 180° VMAT hemi-arc, oriented to avoid contralateral lung. VMAT improved conformity (Table 2) and decreased lung V_5, V_{10}, $V_{12.5}$, and V_{20} (Table 1) with equivalent PTV coverage. Though VMAT plans resulted in marginal increases in MUs compared to single-segment DMPO plans (5.6%, $p = 0.04$), treatment time was markedly reduced (6 min vs. 12 min, $p < 0.01$) (McGrath et al. 2010). A similar planning study from the Netherlands showed that back-and-forth partial-arc VMAT plans were comparable to non-coplanar limited-segment IMRT for delivery of SBRT but required significantly less treatment time, 6.5 min vs. 23.7 min for a single 18 Gy fraction (Holt et al. 2011).

The use of VMAT has also facilitated the use of functional imaging to optimize radiation therapy planning. It is now possible to calculate regional air content, a surrogate for ventilation, in patients undergoing 4D CT simulation for motion management. Using this algorithm, VMAT planning may then achieve relative sparing of functional areas of the lung. Early results from a multi-institutional, prospective trial comparing standard VMAT plans with VMAT functional avoidance plans showed that V_{20} was decreased by an average of 3.2% for the functional avoidance plans (Vinogradskiy et al. 2018).

Table 2 Conformity comparison: 3D CRT vs. IMRT and VMAT

Study	Parameter	3D CRT	IMRT	VMAT	p
Liu et al. (2006)	CI 100%	1.5	1.3[a]	–	–
McGrath et al. (2010)	CI 95%	1.25	–	1.23	NS
McGrath et al. (2010)	CI 80%	1.93	–	1.87	0.08
Ong et al. (2010)	CI 80%	1.18	–	1.10	0.001
Ong et al. (2010)	CI 60%	2.30	–	2.11	0.001
McGrath et al. (2010)	CI 50%	5.65	–	5.19	0.01
Ong et al. (2010)	CI 40%	4.86	–	5.00	NS

CI = conformity index, CI x% = volume of x% isodose/PTV volume, NS = not statistically significant
[a] Using optimized 7-field IMRT

4 Treatment Planning

Involved field radiation therapy (tumor plus involved lymph nodes) is the accepted standard of care for definitive management in NSCLC. IMRT allows the potential for further dose escalation to the target and improved conformality and is now routinely permitted in national cooperative group research protocols. RTOG 0617 was the first RTOG protocol permitting IMRT delivery. In this two-by-two phase III randomized trial for stage IIIA–B NSCLC, RT to either 60 Gy (standard arm) or 74 Gy (dose-escalated arm) was given concurrently with carboplatin/paclitaxel with or without cetuximab followed by consolidative chemotherapy. The currently accruing RTOG 1308, which randomizes patients with stage II–IIIB NSCLC to 70 Gy (RBE) with either photon- or proton-based radiotherapy, similarly allows for either 3D CRT or IMRT on the photon arm.

4.1 Simulation

At our institution, patients are simulated supine in an alpha cradle, arms above head using 4D CT with 3 mm slices from the neck through the liver. Ten CT phases are populated to correspond to different phases of a complete respiratory cycle. PET/CT fusion—ideally with the patient in the treatment position for PET—is used in all cases for tumor and nodal target volume delineation. As treatment delay can lead to disease progression, if a staging PET has not been performed within 6–8 weeks of treatment planning, the PET is generally repeated for restaging and planning purposes (Mohammed et al. 2011a).

Though respiratory-gating and breath-hold strategies may be preferential to an adaptive image guidance strategy in a capable patient, the superiority likely only holds clinical relevance if tumor excursion is approximately 1.4 cm or greater (Hugo et al. 2007a), which is quite rare in our experience. Furthermore, 4D inverse planning has resulted in plans comparable to real-time target tracking methods (Zhang et al. 2008). Gating or breath-hold strategies are not routinely employed in our clinic, as related to the above and the difficulty for such patients who commonly have advanced emphysema complicating ease of use. We do routinely assess for the benefit of abdominal compression in patients treated with SBRT for lower lobe tumors, though its use is uncommon based on 4D CT comparisons with and without compression and patient discomfort. Thus, we have favored free-breathing treatment utilizing an "internal target volume" (ITV) approach to account for tumor motion and have implemented online image guidance to decrease PTV margins and monitor day-to-day target volume variations. Treatment planning is performed on the average-phase CT scan, which closely corresponds to the mean tumor position at the time of online cone beam CT soft tissue registration (Hugo et al. 2007b).

4.2 Target Volumes (GTV, CTV, PTV)

Per the RTOG 0617 protocol, the gross tumor volume (GTV) includes both primary tumor and clinically positive lymph nodes (short axis >1 cm on planning CT or PET SUV >3). If using an ITV approach to account for tumor motion, the GTV_{ITV} is defined as the volume encompassing the gross tumor throughout a complete respiratory cycle. The clinical target volume (CTV) includes an expansion from GTV to account for microscopic extension, defined as a 0.5–0.7 cm expansion of the entire GTV (or GTV_{ITV}). RTOG 1308 employs a CTV expansion of 0.8 cm.

At our institution, the GTV is contoured on the 3D intravenous contrast planning CT. The GTV comprises the primary tumor and clinically positive regional lymph nodes according to the combination of CT, ^{18}FDG PET/CT, and any pathological lymph node data from endobronchial ultrasound (EBUS) or mediastinoscopy. The GTV for the primary tumor is delineated on lung windows and for nodal volumes delineated on mediastinal windows. A 7 mm margin is then added to generate a CTV. The GTV and CTV are then transferred to the best matching phase CT of the 4D dataset and propagated to the remaining nine phases followed by physician verification of auto-propagation to create the IGTV and ICTV, respectively. A 7 mm margin is added to the IGTV to generate the ICTV; the ICTV is edited out of non-invaded normal tissues. Of note, a pathologic study of T1N0 adenocarcinomas suggested that a margin as small as 1.2 mm from GTV (on lung windows) to CTV may be sufficient for typical cases, but a 9 mm margin may be required to cover 90% of tumors (Grills et al. 2007).

The planning target volume (PTV) accounts for both internal tumor motion and setup error. Various methods to account for tumor motion

Table 3 CTV-to-PTV expansions: RTOG 0617[a]

	RTOG 0617				
	Free breathing	Breath hold/respiratory gating	ITV		
	No ITV	With daily imaging	No daily bone registration	With daily bone registration
Superior-inferior	**≥1.5 cm**	≥1.0 cm	≥1.0 cm	≥0.5 cm
	Motion: ≥1.0 cm			
	Setup: 0.5 cm			
Axial	**≥1.0 cm**	≥0.5 cm	≥1.0 cm	≥0.5 cm
	Motion: ≥0.5 cm			
	Setup: 0.5 cm			

RTOG = Radiation Therapy Oncology Group, Motion = internal tumor motion, ITV = internal target volume, IGRT = image-guided radiation therapy
[a] Margin in superior, inferior, anterior, and posterior directions determined according to the adaptive process

include (1) an ITV approach, (2) a maximal intensity projection (MIP) approach, (3) automatic breath hold, (4) respiratory gating, and (5) fluoroscopy. RTOG 0617 recommends fluoroscopy to assess maximal respiratory excursion when 4D CT is not available. With the various approaches to account for tumor motion, RTOG 0617 defines minimum CTV-to-PTV expansions as small as 0.5 cm in all directions—with daily bony registration and ITV planning—and up to 1.5 cm (superior-inferior) and 1.0 cm (axial) for free-breathing (non-ITV) plans (Table 3). In contrast, RTOG 1308 requires 4D CT simulation and utilizes a 5 mm PTV expansion regardless of the motion management technique.

4.3 Inverse Planning

As compared to conventional 3D CRT, which is forward planned by choosing beam angles, beam modifiers, and relative beam weights, IMRT is inversely planned by providing the treatment planning computer with a series of objectives and constraints for normal tissues and target, subsequently allowing the computer to generate segment apertures and weights and beam weights that provide the ideal fluence map for a given plan. This process is called "optimization." Older IMRT planning systems required creation of this ideal fluence map first followed by generation of deliverable segments as a second step, which is known as fluence map optimization (FMO). Contemporary software, however, allows for direct aperture optimization, where the generation of a fluence map and segments is done simultaneously considering the predefined constraints of the treatment machine, substantially shortening the required time for IMRT planning. Inverse treatment planning software takes the prescribed dose distribution and optimizes a plan by minimizing the "cost function," a function that quantifies variance from the predetermined dose volume histogram (DVH) objectives. In multicriteria optimization (MCO), unlike FMO and DAO, weights are not assigned to structures, and an ensemble of different plans are generated spanning various weights. The user can then explore the solution space to simultaneously evaluate competing plans. The major advantage of MCO is the elimination of labor-intensive manual iteration (Craft et al. 2007). Multiple guidelines exist to help define optimal normal tissue DVH constraints, and the ideal planning objectives are in constant evolution based on new toxicity data being reported on an ongoing basis. The National Comprehensive Cancer Network (NCCN) has published guidelines available online. Dose constraints utilized in RTOG 0617 and RTOG 1308 are seen in Table 4.

For arc therapy planning (either IMAT or VMAT), MLC positions must be contiguous, and incremental control points (e.g., every 6°) are used from which interval data can be interpolated. Multiple inverse planning techniques have now been developed for both single- and multiarc

Table 4 Dose constraints to organs at risk

	RTOG 0617 (60 Gy vs. 74 Gy)	RTOG 1308[a] (70 Gy [RBE])	Beaumont[b] (2 Gy/day)
Spinal cord	$D_{max} < 50.5$ Gy[c]	$D_{max} < 50$ Gy [RBE]	$D_{max} \leq 46$ Gy[c]
Lungs	(*excludes CTV*)	(*excludes CTV*)	(*excludes GTV$_{ITV}$*)
	$V_{20} \leq 37\%$ (or)	$V_{20} \leq 37\%$ (or)	$V_{20} \leq 30\%$ (and)
	$D_{mean} \leq 20$ Gy	$D_{mean} \leq 20$ Gy [RBE]	$D_{mean} \leq 20$ Gy
		$V_5 \leq 60\%$	$V_5 \leq 65\%$
Esophagus	$D_{mean} < 34$ Gy[d]	$V_{74} \leq 1.0$ cc of partial circumference	$D_{mean} < 34$ Gy
			$V_{50} \leq 30\%$
			$V_{60} \leq 17\%$
			$V_{68} \leq 2.0$ cc
			$D_{max} \leq 75$ Gy
Brachial plexus	$D_{max} < 66$ Gy	$V_{70} \leq 3.0$ cc	$V_{66} \leq 1.0$ cc
		$V_{74} \leq 1.0$ cc	
		$V_{75} \leq 0.5$ cc	
Heart	$D_{33} < 60$ Gy[e]	$V_{30} \leq 50\%$ $D_{66} < 45$ Gy	$V_{30} \leq 50\%$
	$D_{66} < 45$ Gy[e]	$V_{45} \leq 35\%$	$V_{45} \leq 35\%$
	$D_{100} < 40$ Gy[e]		$V_{50} \leq 25\%$
			$D_{max} \leq 75$ Gy
			$D_{mean} \leq 10$ Gy ideal but not to exceed 20 Gy

RBE = relative biological effectiveness, D_{max} = maximum dose, D_{mean} = mean dose, V_x = proportional volume of the region of interest receiving $\geq x$ Gy, D_y = dose delivered to $y\%$ of the region of interest
[a] Spinal cord D_{max} (0.03 cc) >52 Gy (RBE), lung V_{20} >40%, or lung D_{mean} >22 Gy (RBE) are the criteria for mandatory replanning
[b] At Beaumont, maximum dose is defined as maximum dose for contiguous volume ≥ 0.1 cc
[c] Required constraint
[d] Constraint is strongly recommended
[e] Constraint recommended but not required

treatments, facilitating VMAT planning and delivery, thereby making this treatment modality a mainstay in clinical practice (Otto 2008; Luan et al. 2008; Wang et al. 2008; Cao et al. 2009).

5 Targeting and Verification

5.1 Image-Guided Radiation Therapy (IGRT)

In an effort to accurately target disease, escalate dose, and spare organs at risk, two main targeting strategies are routinely implemented: (a) biological targeting with positron emission tomography (PET) and (b) image guidance at the machine. Four-dimensional (4D) imaging and planning techniques have further facilitated improvements in radiotherapy administration and are now standard in RTOG protocols. To elucidate the benefits of 4D technique, Harsolia et al. compared conventional 3D CRT plans—using free-breathing planning CT and fluoroscopy to assess tumor motion—to 4D techniques using combinations of 4D imaging, 4D planning, and IGRT with onboard 4D CBCT (cone beam CT) using three strategies: (1) 4D union technique, (2) 4D off-line adaptive planning with a single correction (off-line adaptive radiotherapy (ART)), and (3) 4D online adaptive planning with daily correction (online ART) (Harsolia et al. 2008). The 4D union plan used an ITV technique, defining GTV$_{ITV}$ as the union of GTV phases with 5 mm expansions for CTV and PTV. The ART process defines a probability density function (PDF) of tumor position vs. time estimated by fluoroscopy and/or 4D CT or 4D CBCT to account for tumor motion and interfraction variability of tumor location. The off-line ART process uses a single adjustment after the first week of treatment,

Table 5 Mean relative reduction compared to standard 3D CRT plan (adapted from Harsolia et al. 2008)

Parameter	3D CRT	4D union	4D off-line ART (single correction)	4D online ART (daily correction)
PTV volume	–	↓ 15%	↓ 39%	↓ 44%
Lungs V_{20} (%)	–	↓ 21%	↓ 23%	↓ 31%
Mean lung dose	–	↓ 16%	↓ 26%	↓ 31%

3D CRT = 3D conformal radiation therapy, ART = adaptive radiation therapy, PTV = planning target volume, Online ART = adaptive with daily correction, Off-line ART = adaptive plan with a single correction, V_{20} (%) = % volume of lungs excluding GTV receiving ≥20 Gy

accounting for individualized variability assessed after five fractions. The online ART process used a daily fluoroscopy-guided correction to account for daily setup error; thus, the PDF still accounted for respiratory motion, but accounted for less setup error than with the off-line technique, further decreasing the CTV-to-PTV expansion. IMRT plans decreased PTV volume, mean lung dose, and lung V_{20}, most significantly with daily online adaptive IGRT (Table 5) (Harsolia et al. 2008).

5.2 Biological Targeting with PET

18-Fluorodeoxyglucose positron emission tomography (^{18}FDG PET) is essential to all phases of radiation therapy from staging to planning to follow-up. PET has proven its role in NSCLC staging, with greater sensitivity and accuracy than CT (Dwamena et al. 1999; Gould et al. 2013). Current RTOG protocols mandate PET for appropriate staging. During treatment planning, PET helps define clinically positive lymph node regions and define tumor extent, complementary to the anatomic information provided by CT imaging alone. Early studies demonstrated that PET-to-CT (simulation/planning CT) registration can result in smaller target volumes secondary to improved GTV delineation but also upstaging, leading to increase in target volume (Giraud et al. 2001; Bradley et al. 2004; Erdi et al. 2002; Mah et al. 2002). This was confirmed on RTOG 0515, a phase II prospective trial in which patients undergoing definitive radiation therapy (≥60 Gy) were planned with CT with or without PET/CT. Among 47 evaluable patients, the GTV was statistically smaller for PET/CT-derived volumes (86.2 cc vs. 98.7 cc, $p < 0.0001$), and mean lung doses for PET/CT-derived plans were lower (17.8 Gy vs. 19 Gy, $p = 0.06$). In total, nodal contours were altered by PET/CT in 51% of patients (Bradley et al. 2012). With such biologic targeting afforded by PET, the risk of target miss can be decreased while facilitating dose escalation by shrinking treatment volume, two key goals of IMRT. For planning, the simulation acts as the primary dataset to which the CT portion of the PET/CT is merged, usually with bony registration.

PET has further been utilized to assess tumor response to radiation therapy (Mohammed et al. 2011b). Surveillance PET/CT data from Wong et al. revealed significant reduction in maximum standardized uptake value (SUV) and CT size after treatment, with relative reductions in maximal metabolic uptake greater than size reduction (62% vs. 47%, $p = 0.03$) (Wong et al. 2007). Mid-treatment PET may also identify areas of persistent metabolic activity requiring treatment intensification. Kong et al. reported a phase II multi-institutional experience of 42 patients who underwent CT and PET/CT resimulation following delivery of 40–50 Gy. The total dose to areas of persistent disease was then escalated to as high as 86 Gy in 30 fractions while limiting lung NTCP. The 2-year rates of in-field and overall locoregional control were 82% and 62% (Kong et al. 2017). RTOG 1106, which is now closed to accrual, is evaluating the feasibility and efficacy of this approach in a randomized, cooperative setting. Participating centers treated with either 3D CRT or IMRT.

5.3 Treatment Verification

With increased conformity, decreased margins, and intensity modulation comes increased dependence on quality assurance. IMRT and VMAT plans require dosimetric verification prior to

Table 6 Minimum requirements for safe delivery of IMRT (adapted from Chan et al. 2014)

4D CT simulation or equivalent
Delineation of all relevant intrathoracic organs at risk for inverse treatment planning
Model-based calculation algorithm for dose calculation
Cone beam CT target verification
End-to-end testing using a phantom/diode array prior to first clinical use
Risk assessment of interplay effects from IMRT technique and fractionation employed
Dedicated machine IMRT QA program
Patient-specific IMRT QA program including independent MU verification
Patient-specific QA of transfer of treatment plan to the treatment machine

IMRT = intensity-modulated radiation therapy, QA = quality assurance, MU = monitor unit

delivery (Ezzell et al. 2003). One method of plan validation is delivery of the plan to a phantom. Ion chambers and films are used to verify the dose and spatial dose gradient, respectively. Alternatively, individual IMRT beams can be assessed with two-dimensional (2D) arrays of diodes such as the MapCHECK® 2 (Sun Nuclear). Similarly, VMRT arcs can be assessed with arrays of diodes shaped in an acrylic cylindrical annulus, such as ArcCHECK®. Positional accuracy is assessed with imaging. Electronic portal imaging devices (EPIDs) serve to create beam's-eye-view portal images for user verification of beam position and treatment setup. Onboard imaging devices including orthogonal kV plan imaging or CBCT allow for reduced setup margins and improved clinical outcomes (Kilburn et al. 2016). Online volumetric (3D) pretreatment imaging (e.g., with online CBCT registration to the planning CT) serves as an ideal method for target verification at the time of treatment due to high rates of intrathoracic anatomical changes (Kwint et al. 2014). This is particularly important in the case of SBRT where the dose falloff between target and normal tissues is sharp and the total number of treatment fractions may be limited. We recommend online volumetric image guidance techniques daily for all patients undergoing curative thoracic radiotherapy, with a minimum of 1 day/week of 4D online verification of target motion, with daily 4D volumetric imaging for SBRT. A summary of suggested minimum requirements for safe delivery of IMRT is depicted in Table 6, adapted from Chan et al. (2014).

6 Clinical Outcomes

RTOG 0617 was a randomized phase III trial comparing 60 Gy/30 fractions (standard dose) to 74 Gy/37 fractions (high dose) with concurrent and adjuvant paclitaxel/carboplatin, with or without cetuximab, in 544 patients with unresectable stage III NSCLC. 3D CRT or IMRT was allowed, and patients were stratified by such at the time of enrollment. Surprisingly, the high-dose arm had inferior OS compared to the standard-dose arm (20.3 months vs. 28.7 months, HR 1.38, 95% CI 1.09–1.76, $p = 0.004$), and the standard-dose arm had the highest median survival reported at the time for locally advanced NSCLC (Bradley et al. 2015). Of note, on multivariate analysis, factors predicting OS included esophagitis grade, lung V_5, and heart V_5 and V_{30}. The use of IMRT was not a significant predictor for OS on multivariate analysis, although it did predict QOL improvements over 3D CRT.

A subsequent secondary analysis of RTOG 0617 compared the 53% of patients receiving 3D CRT with the 47% receiving IMRT. The technique employed was per physician discretion, and so baseline characteristics were expectedly uneven. In particular, patients receiving IMRT were more likely to have stage IIIB/N3 disease and larger PTV. Despite unfavorable baseline characteristics, 2-year rates of overall survival (OS), progression-free survival (PFS), local failure (LF), and distant metastases (DM) were not different between IMRT and 3D CRT. For IMRT patients, 2-year OS was 53.2%, 2-year PFS was 25.2%, 2-year LC was 30.8%, and 2-year DM was 45.9%. Owing to reduced heart V_{20}, V_{40}, and V_{60} and lower rate of grade ≥3 TRP (3.5% vs. 7.9%), the authors advocated for the routine use of IMRT in the treatment of locally advanced NSCLC (Chun et al. 2017).

Several retrospective studies complement the findings of RTOG 0617. The MD Anderson experience included patients with locally advanced NSCLC treated with concurrent chemoradiotherapy (mean dose 63 Gy). In the 68 patients receiving IMRT, 6- and 12-month locoregional control (LRC) was 94% and 55%, disease-free survival (DFS) 67% and 32%, and OS 79% and 57%, respectively. However, median follow-up was only 8 months (Yom et al. 2007). The same group later published an updated report of 165 patients undergoing IMRT to a median dose of 66 Gy (Jiang et al. 2012). With a median follow-up of 16.5 months, they reported 2- and 3-year local recurrence-free survival (LRFS) of 57% and 41%, DFS of 38% and 27%, distant metastasis-free survival (DMFS) of 51% and 38%, and OS of 46% and 30%, respectively.

Sura et al. similarly reported the MSKCC experience, including 55 patients with inoperable stage I–IIIB disease treated with IMRT. Median follow-up in this study was significantly longer at 21 months. Two-year LC rates were 50% (stage I–II, $n = 16$) and 58% (stage III, $n = 29$). For all patients, median DFS was 12 months, and 2-year DFS was 41%. Two-year cancer-specific survival (CSS) and OS were 63% and 57%, respectively. Survival was similar in stage I–II and stage III patients with a median of 25 months (Sura et al. 2008).

Using helical tomotherapy, a Belgian trial of hypofractionated RT (70.5 Gy, 2.35 Gy per fraction) in 40 consecutive patients with inoperable IIIA ($n = 16$) and IIIB ($n = 24$) NSCLC was reported. Patients were enrolled during 2005–2008 and permitted induction chemotherapy, but not concurrent with RT. Overall 1-year and 2-year LPFS was 66% and 50%, respectively. Median time to distant metastasis was 10.6 months, and 1-year distant metastasis-free survival (DMFS) was 43%. Median OS was 21 months vs. 12 months for IIIA and IIIB disease ($p = 0.03$) and 17 months for all patients. Two patients (5%) died of acute pulmonary toxicity; median follow-up in 14 survivors was 16 months (Bral et al. 2010).

In Scorsetti's VMAT study of 75 patients with unresectable, stage III NSCLC, patients received a mean 63.6 Gy delivered with two isocentric partial arcs. Using the RECIST (2000) (Therasse et al. 2000) criteria for assessing response to solid tumors, at 21.2 months of median follow-up, 7 (9%) had a complete response, 45 (60%) had a partial response, 9 (12%) had stable disease, and 14 (19%) had progressive disease. The 1-year and 2-year LC rates were 92% and 80% and OS rates were 80% and 39%, respectively (Scorsetti et al. 2014). A summary of outcomes for patients with LA-NSCLC treated with IMRT is seen in Table 7.

7 Conclusion

Over the past 10 years, technological advancements have brought IMRT and VMAT into routine clinical use with routine inclusion in lung RTOG protocols since 2007. In this technically challenging and prognostically poor disease, dose escalation and normal tissue sparing have been shown to be imperative for safely improving local disease control and survival while minimizing the risk for potentially severe acute and chronic toxicity. From the planning perspective, IMRT has long proven its superiority to 3D CRT for safe dose escalation in properly selected cases. The publication of a planned secondary analysis of RTOG 0617 comparing 3D CRT and IMRT confirmed the superior dosimetric and toxicity profiles afforded by IMRT. With inverse planning algorithms and quality assurance methods available, the use of VMAT has grown rapidly in the past few years. Compared to IMRT, VMAT offers the potential for shorter treatment times and less monitor units delivered. Lung cancer outcomes have improved considerably over the past 5 years. We have optimism that routine implementation of technological advances (e.g., IMRT, VMAT, 4D image guidance/planning, and potentially proton therapy) coupled with improved targeted therapies will continue to translate into significant clinical benefit for what continues to be the most common cause of cancer-related death in the United States.

Table 7 Outcomes in NSCLC treated with IMRT and VMAT

Study	n	Time	Patients	Dose (Gy) mean/median (range)	Gpf (Gy)	RT type	Chemotherapy	Follow-up median (range)	Parameter	Outcome
RTOG 0617 (Bradley et al. 2015)	228	2007–2011	Inoperable stage III	60 or 74	2	IMRT	Concurrent (100%) Consolidative (100%)	21.3 mo	Local control	2 years: 30.8%
MD Anderson (Jiang et al. 2012)	165	2005–2006	Inoperable I–IV	66 (60–76)	1.8–2.3	IMRT	Concurrent (82%)	16.5 mo	LPFS	2 years: 57% 3 years: 41%
MSKCC (Sura et al. 2008)	55	2001–2005	Inoperable stage I–IIIB	69.5 (60–90)	1.8–2.0	IMRT	Sequential (53%) Concurrent (24%)	21 mo (0–61)	Local control	2 years: 50% (stage I–II) 2 years: 58% (stage III)
MD Anderson (Yom et al. 2007)	68	2002–2005	Stage IIB–IV	63 (50.4–76)	1.8–2.0	IMRT	Induction (29%) Concurrent (100%)	8 mo (0–27)	Locoregional control	6 mo: 94% 12 mo: 55%
Milan (Scorsetti et al. 2014)	75	2009–2014	Inoperable stage III	63.6 (54–72)	2.0	VMAT	Concurrent (45%) Sequential (55%)	21.2	LC	1 year: 91% 2 years: 80%
Belgium (Bral et al. 2010)	40	2005–2008	Inoperable stage III[a]	70.5 (all)	2.35	Helical TT	Sequential (82%) Concurrent (0%) None (18%)	14 mo[a]	LPFS	1 year: 66% 2 years: 50%
Milan (Scorsetti et al. 2014)	75	2009–2014	Inoperable stage III	63.6 (54–72)	2.0	VMAT	Concurrent (45%) Sequential (55%)	21.2	RECIST (Therasse et al. 2000)	CR = 19% PR = 60% Stable disease: 12 Disease progression: 19%
RTOG 0617 (Bradley et al. 2015)	228	2007–2011	Inoperable stage III	60 or 74	2	IMRT	Concurrent (100%) Consolidative (100%)	21.3 mo	DM	2 years: 45.9%
MD Anderson (Jiang et al. 2012)	165	2005–2006	Inoperable I–IV	66 (60–76)	1.8–2.3	IMRT	Concurrent (82%)	16.5 mo	DMFS	2 years: 51% 3 years: 38%

Intensity-Modulated Radiation Therapy and Volumetric Modulated Arc Therapy for Lung Cancer

Study	N	Years	Stage	Dose (Gy)	Dose/fx	Technique	Chemo	Median FU	Endpoint	Result
Belgium (Bral et al. 2010)	40	2005–2008	Inoperable stage III	70.5 (all)	2.35	Helical TT	Sequential (82%) Concurrent (0%) None (18%)	14 mo[a]	DMFS	Median: 10.6 mo 1 year: 43%
RTOG 0617 (Bradley et al. 2015)	228	2007–2011	Inoperable stage III	60 or 74	2	IMRT	Concurrent (100%) Consolidative (100%)	21.3 mo	PFS	2 years: 25.2%
MD Anderson (Jiang et al. 2012)	165	2005–2006	Inoperable I–IV	66 (60–76)	1.8–2.3	IMRT	Concurrent (82%)	16.5 mo	DFS	2 years: 38% 3 years: 27%
MD Anderson (Yom et al. 2007)	68	2002–2005	Stage IIB–IV	63 (50.4–76)	1.8–2.0	IMRT	Concurrent (100%)	8 mo (0–27)	DFS	6 mo: 67% 12 mo: 32%
MSKCC (Sura et al. 2008)	55	2001–2005	Inoperable stage I–IIIB	69.5 (60–90)	1.8–2.0	IMRT	Sequential (53%) Concurrent (24%)	21 mo (0–61)	CSS	2 years: 63%
RTOG 0617 (Bradley et al. 2015)	228	2007–2011	Inoperable stage III	60 or 74	2	IMRT	Concurrent (100%) Consolidative (100%)	21.3 mo	OS	2 years: 53.2%
MD Anderson (Jiang et al. 2012)	165	2005–2006	Inoperable I–IV	66 (60–76)	1.8–2.3	IMRT	Concurrent (82%)	16.5 mo	OS	2 years: 46% 3 years: 30%
MSKCC (Sura et al. 2008)	55	2001–2005	Inoperable stage I–IIIB	69.5 (60–90)	1.8–2.0	IMRT	Sequential (53%) Concurrent (24%)	21 mo (0–61)	OS	Median: 25 mo 2 years: 57% 2 years: 55% (stage I–II) 2 years: 58% (stage III)
MD Anderson (Yom et al. 2007)	68	2002–2005	Stage IIB–IV	63 (50.4–76)	1.8–2.0	IMRT	Induction (29%) Concurrent (100%)	8 mo (0–27)	OS	6 mo: 79% 12 mo: 55%
Milan (Scorsetti et al. 2014)	75	2009–2014	Inoperable stage III	63.6 (54–72)	2.0	VMAT	Concurrent (45%) Sequential (55%)	21.2	OS	1 year: 80% 2 years: 39%

(continued)

Table 7 (continued)

Study	n	Time	Patients	Dose (Gy) mean/ median (range)	Gpf (Gy)	RT type	Chemotherapy	Follow-up median (range)	Parameter	Outcome
Belgium (Bral et al. 2010)	40	2005–2008	Inoperable stage III	70.5 (all)	2.35	Helical TT	Sequential (82%) Concurrent (0%) None (18%)	14 mo[a]	OS	Median: 17 mo Median: 21 mo (IIIA) Median: 12 mo (IIIB) 1 year: 65% 2 years: 27%

NSCLC = non-small cell lung cancer, IMRT = intensity-modulated radiation therapy, VMAT = volumetric modulated radiation therapy, MSKCC = Memorial Sloan Kettering Cancer Center, Gpf = Gray per fraction, mo = months, BID = twice daily, LPFS = local progression-free survival, LR = local recurrence, CR = complete remission, PR = partial remission, RR = regional recurrence, DFS = disease-free survival, DMFS = distant metastasis-free survival, CSS = cause-specific survival, OS = overall survival, TT = tomotherapy

[a] Median follow-up = 14 months in 16 survivors

References

Al-Halabi H, Paetzold P, Sharp GC, Olsen C, Willers H (2015) A Contralateral esophagus-sparing technique to limit severe esophagitis associated with concurrent high-dose radiation and chemotherapy in patients with thoracic malignancies. Int J Radiat Oncol Biol Phys 92(4):803–810

Armstrong JG, Minsky BD (1989) Radiation therapy for medically inoperable stage I and II non-small cell lung cancer. Cancer Treat Rev 16(4):247–255

ASTRO (2019) Model policies. Intensity Modulated Radiation Therapy (IMRT). https://www.astro.org/ASTRO/media/ASTRO/Daily%20Practice/PDFs/IMRTMP.pdf. Accessed 23 Feb 2021

Atkins KM, Rawal B, Chaunzwa TL, Lamba N, Bitterman DS, Williams CL, Kozono DE, Baldini EH, Chen AB, Nguyen PL, D'Amico AV, Nohria A, Hoffmann U, Aerts H, Mak RH (2019) Cardiac radiation dose, cardiac disease, and mortality in patients with lung cancer. J Am Coll Cardiol 73(23):2976–2987

Atkins KM, Chaunzwa TL, Lamba N, Bitterman DS, Rawal B, Bredfeldt J, Williams CL, Kozono DE, Baldini EH, Nohria A, Hoffmann U, Aerts H, Mak RH (2021) Association of left anterior descending coronary artery radiation dose with major adverse cardiac events and mortality in patients with non-small cell lung cancer. JAMA Oncol 7:206

Bedford JL, Warrington AP (2009) Commissioning of volumetric modulated arc therapy (VMAT). Int J Radiat Oncol Biol Phys 73(2):537–545

Bertelsen A, Hansen O, Brink C (2012) Does VMAT for treatment of NSCLC patients increase the risk of pneumonitis compared to IMRT? - a planning study. Acta Oncol 51(6):752–758

Bortfeld T (2006) IMRT: a review and preview. Phys Med Biol 51(13):R363–R379

Bradley J, Thorstad WL, Mutic S, Miller TR, Dehdashti F, Siegel BA, Bosch W, Bertrand RJ (2004) Impact of FDG-PET on radiation therapy volume delineation in non-small-cell lung cancer. Int J Radiat Oncol Biol Phys 59(1):78–86

Bradley J, Graham MV, Winter K, Purdy JA, Komaki R, Roa WH, Ryu JK, Bosch W, Emami B (2005) Toxicity and outcome results of RTOG 9311: a phase I-II dose-escalation study using three-dimensional conformal radiotherapy in patients with inoperable non-small-cell lung carcinoma. Int J Radiat Oncol Biol Phys 61(2):318–328

Bradley JD, Bae K, Graham MV, Byhardt R, Govindan R, Fowler J, Purdy JA, Michalski JM, Gore E, Choy H (2010) Primary analysis of the phase II component of a phase I/II dose intensification study using three-dimensional conformal radiation therapy and concurrent chemotherapy for patients with inoperable non-small-cell lung cancer: RTOG 0117. J Clin Oncol 28(14):2475–2480

Bradley J, Bae K, Choi N, Forster K, Siegel BA, Brunetti J, Purdy J, Faria S, Vu T, Thorstad W, Choy H (2012) A phase II comparative study of gross tumor volume definition with or without PET/CT fusion in dosimetric planning for non-small-cell lung cancer (NSCLC): primary analysis of Radiation Therapy Oncology Group (RTOG) 0515. Int J Radiat Oncol Biol Phys 82(1):435–441 e431

Bradley JD, Paulus R, Komaki R, Masters G, Blumenschein G, Schild S, Bogart J, Hu C, Forster K, Magliocco A, Kavadi V, Garces YI, Narayan S, Iyengar P, Robinson C, Wynn RB, Koprowski C, Meng J, Beitler J, Gaur R, Curran W Jr, Choy H (2015) Standard-dose versus high-dose conformal radiotherapy with concurrent and consolidation carboplatin plus paclitaxel with or without cetuximab for patients with stage IIIA or IIIB non-small-cell lung cancer (RTOG 0617): a randomised, two-by-two factorial phase 3 study. Lancet Oncol 16(2):187–199

Bradley JD, Hu C, Komaki RR, Masters GA, Blumenschein GR, Schild SE, Bogart JA, Forster KM, Magliocco AM, Kavadi VS, Narayan S, Iyengar P, Robinson CG, Wynn RB, Koprowski CD, Olson MR, Meng J, Paulus R, Curran WJ Jr, Choy H (2020) Long-term results of NRG oncology RTOG 0617: standard-versus high-dose chemoradiotherapy with or without cetuximab for unresectable stage III non-small-cell lung cancer. J Clin Oncol 38(7):706–714

Brahme A (1988) Optimization of stationary and moving beam radiation therapy techniques. Radiother Oncol 12(2):129–140

Bral S, Duchateau M, Versmessen H, Engels B, Tournel K, Vinh-Hung V, De Ridder M, Schallier D, Storme G (2010) Toxicity and outcome results of a class solution with moderately hypofractionated radiotherapy in inoperable Stage III non-small cell lung cancer using helical tomotherapy. Int J Radiat Oncol Biol Phys 77(5):1352–1359

Byhardt RW, Scott CB, Ettinger DS, Curran WJ, Doggett RL, Coughlin C, Scarantino C, Rotman M, Emami B (1995) Concurrent hyperfractionated irradiation and chemotherapy for unresectable nonsmall cell lung cancer. Results of Radiation Therapy Oncology Group 90-15. Cancer 75(9):2337–2344

Cao D, Holmes TW, Afghan MK, Shepard DM (2007) Comparison of plan quality provided by intensity-modulated arc therapy and helical tomotherapy. Int J Radiat Oncol Biol Phys 69(1):240–250

Cao D, Afghan MK, Ye J, Chen F, Shepard DM (2009) A generalized inverse planning tool for volumetric-modulated arc therapy. Phys Med Biol 54(21):6725–6738

Chan C, Lang S, Rowbottom C, Guckenberger M, Faivre-Finn C, Committee IART (2014) Intensity-modulated radiotherapy for lung cancer: current status and future developments. J Thorac Oncol 9(11):1598–1608

Chang JY, Senan S, Paul MA, Mehran RJ, Louie AV, Balter P, Groen HJ, McRae SE, Widder J, Feng L, van den Borne BE, Munsell MF, Hurkmans C, Berry DA, van Werkhoven E, Kresl JJ, Dingemans AM, Dawood O, Haasbeek CJ, Carpenter LS, De Jaeger K, Komaki R, Slotman BJ, Smit EF, Roth JA (2015) Stereotactic ablative radiotherapy versus lobectomy for operable stage I non-small-cell lung cancer: a pooled analysis of two randomised trials. Lancet Oncol 16(6):630–637

Chapet O, Thomas E, Kessler ML, Fraass BA, Ten Haken RK (2005) Esophagus sparing with IMRT in lung tumor irradiation: an EUD-based optimization technique. Int J Radiat Oncol Biol Phys 63(1):179–187

Chapet O, Fraass BA, Ten Haken RK (2006) Multiple fields may offer better esophagus sparing without increased probability of lung toxicity in optimized IMRT of lung tumors. Int J Radiat Oncol Biol Phys 65(1):255–265

Chun SG, Hu C, Choy H, Komaki RU, Timmerman RD, Schild SE, Bogart JA, Dobelbower MC, Bosch W, Galvin JM, Kavadi VS, Narayan S, Iyengar P, Robinson CG, Wynn RB, Raben A, Augspurger ME, MacRae RM, Paulus R, Bradley JD (2017) Impact of intensity-modulated radiation therapy technique for locally advanced non-small-cell lung cancer: a secondary analysis of the NRG oncology RTOG 0617 randomized clinical trial. J Clin Oncol 35(1):56–62

Clark GM, Popple RA, Young PE, Fiveash JB (2010) Feasibility of single-isocenter volumetric modulated arc radiosurgery for treatment of multiple brain metastases. Int J Radiat Oncol Biol Phys 76(1):296–302

Craft D, Halabi T, Shih HA, Bortfeld T (2007) An approach for practical multiobjective IMRT treatment planning. Int J Radiat Oncol Biol Phys 69(5):1600–1607

Curran WJ Jr, Paulus R, Langer CJ, Komaki R, Lee JS, Hauser S, Movsas B, Wasserman T, Rosenthal SA, Gore E, Machtay M, Sause W, Cox JD (2011) Sequential vs. concurrent chemoradiation for stage III non-small cell lung cancer: randomized phase III trial RTOG 9410. J Natl Cancer Inst 103(19):1452–1460

Dess RT, Sun Y, Matuszak MM, Sun G, Soni PD, Bazzi L, Murthy VL, Hearn JWD, Kong FM, Kalemkerian GP, Hayman JA, Ten Haken RK, Lawrence TS, Schipper MJ, Jolly S (2017) Cardiac events after radiation therapy: combined analysis of prospective multicenter trials for locally advanced non-small-cell lung cancer. J Clin Oncol 35(13):1395–1402

Dess RT, Sun Y, Muenz DG, Paximadis PA, Dominello MM, Grills IS, Kestin LL, Movsas B, Masi KJ, Matuszak MM, Radawski JD, Moran JM, Pierce LJ, Hayman JA, Schipper MJ, Jolly S, Michigan Radiation Oncology Quality C (2020) Cardiac dose in locally advanced lung cancer: results from a statewide consortium. Pract Radiat Oncol 10(1):e27–e36

Dosoretz DE, Katin MJ, Blitzer PH, Rubenstein JH, Salenius S, Rashid M, Dosani RA, Mestas G, Siegel AD, Chadha TT et al (1992) Radiation therapy in the management of medically inoperable carcinoma of the lung: results and implications for future treatment strategies. Int J Radiat Oncol Biol Phys 24(1):3–9

Dwamena BA, Sonnad SS, Angobaldo JO, Wahl RL (1999) Metastases from non-small cell lung cancer: mediastinal staging in the 1990s--meta-analytic comparison of PET and CT. Radiology 213(2):530–536

Erdi YE, Rosenzweig K, Erdi AK, Macapinlac HA, Hu YC, Braban LE, Humm JL, Squire OD, Chui CS, Larson SM, Yorke ED (2002) Radiotherapy treatment planning for patients with non-small cell lung cancer using positron emission tomography (PET). Radiother Oncol 62(1):51–60

Ezzell GA, Galvin JM, Low D, Palta JR, Rosen I, Sharpe MB, Xia P, Xiao Y, Xing L, Yu CX, Subcommittee I, Committee ART (2003) Guidance document on delivery, treatment planning, and clinical implementation of IMRT: report of the IMRT Subcommittee of the AAPM Radiation Therapy Committee. Med Phys 30(8):2089–2115

Fang LC, Komaki R, Allen P, Guerrero T, Mohan R, Cox JD (2006) Comparison of outcomes for patients with medically inoperable Stage I non-small-cell lung cancer treated with two-dimensional vs. three-dimensional radiotherapy. Int J Radiat Oncol Biol Phys 66(1):108–116

Fay M, Tan A, Fisher R, Mac Manus M, Wirth A, Ball D (2005) Dose-volume histogram analysis as predictor of radiation pneumonitis in primary lung cancer patients treated with radiotherapy. Int J Radiat Oncol Biol Phys 61(5):1355–1363

Giraud P, Grahek D, Montravers F, Carette MF, Deniaud-Alexandre E, Julia F, Rosenwald JC, Cosset JM, Talbot JN, Housset M, Touboul E (2001) CT and (18) F-deoxyglucose (FDG) image fusion for optimization of conformal radiotherapy of lung cancers. Int J Radiat Oncol Biol Phys 49(5):1249–1257

Gould MK, Donington J, Lynch WR, Mazzone PJ, Midthun DE, Naidich DP, Wiener RS (2013) Evaluation of individuals with pulmonary nodules: when is it lung cancer? Diagnosis and management of lung cancer, 3rd ed: American College of Chest Physicians evidence-based clinical practice guidelines. Chest 143(5 Suppl):e93S–e120S

Grills IS, Yan D, Martinez AA, Vicini FA, Wong JW, Kestin LL (2003) Potential for reduced toxicity and dose escalation in the treatment of inoperable non-small-cell lung cancer: a comparison of intensity-modulated radiation therapy (IMRT), 3D conformal radiation, and elective nodal irradiation. Int J Radiat Oncol Biol Phys 57(3):875–890

Grills IS, Fitch DL, Goldstein NS, Yan D, Chmielewski GW, Welsh RJ, Kestin LL (2007) Clinicopathologic analysis of microscopic extension in lung adenocarcinoma: defining clinical target volume for radiotherapy. Int J Radiat Oncol Biol Phys 69(2):334–341

Grills IS, Mangona VS, Welsh R, Chmielewski G, McInerney E, Martin S, Wloch J, Ye H, Kestin LL (2010) Outcomes after stereotactic lung radiotherapy or wedge resection for stage I non-small-cell lung cancer. J Clin Oncol 28(6):928–935

Grills IS, Hope AJ, Guckenberger M, Kestin LL, Werner-Wasik M, Yan D, Sonke JJ, Bissonnette JP, Wilbert J, Xiao Y, Belderbos J (2012) A collaborative analysis of stereotactic lung radiotherapy outcomes for early-stage non-small-cell lung cancer using daily online cone-beam computed tomography image-guided radiotherapy. J Thorac Oncol 7(9):1382–1393

Guckenberger M, Richter A, Krieger T, Wilbert J, Baier K, Flentje M (2009) Is a single arc sufficient in volumetric-modulated arc therapy (VMAT) for complex-shaped target volumes? Radiother Oncol 93(2):259–265

Harsolia A, Hugo GD, Kestin LL, Grills IS, Yan D (2008) Dosimetric advantages of four-dimensional adaptive image-guided radiotherapy for lung tumors using online cone-beam computed tomography. Int J Radiat Oncol Biol Phys 70(2):582–589

Hayman JA, Martel MK, Ten Haken RK, Normolle DP, Todd RF III, Littles JF, Sullivan MA, Possert PW, Turrisi AT, Lichter AS (2001) Dose escalation in non-small-cell lung cancer using three-dimensional conformal radiation therapy: update of a phase I trial. J Clin Oncol 19(1):127–136

Holt A, van Vliet-Vroegindeweij C, Mans A, Belderbos JS, Damen EM (2011) Volumetric-modulated arc therapy for stereotactic body radiotherapy of lung tumors: a comparison with intensity-modulated radiotherapy techniques. Int J Radiat Oncol Biol Phys 81(5):1560–1567

Hugo GD, Yan D, Liang J (2007a) Population and patient-specific target margins for 4D adaptive radiotherapy to account for intra- and inter-fraction variation in lung tumour position. Phys Med Biol 52(1):257–274

Hugo GD, Liang J, Campbell J, Yan D (2007b) On-line target position localization in the presence of respiration: a comparison of two methods. Int J Radiat Oncol Biol Phys 69(5):1634–1641

Jiang X, Li T, Liu Y, Zhou L, Xu Y, Zhou X, Gong Y (2011) Planning analysis for locally advanced lung cancer: dosimetric and efficiency comparisons between intensity-modulated radiotherapy (IMRT), single-arc/partial-arc volumetric modulated arc therapy (SA/PA-VMAT). Radiat Oncol 6:140

Jiang ZQ, Yang K, Komaki R, Wei X, Tucker SL, Zhuang Y, Martel MK, Vedam S, Balter P, Zhu G, Gomez D, Lu C, Mohan R, Cox JD, Liao Z (2012) Long-term clinical outcome of intensity-modulated radiotherapy for inoperable non-small cell lung cancer: the MD Anderson experience. Int J Radiat Oncol Biol Phys 83(1):332–339

Kamran SC, Yeap BY, Ulysse C, Cronin C, Bowes C, Durgin B, Khandekar MJ, Tansky JY, Keane FK, Olsen CC, Willers H (2020) Phase I trial of an IMRT-based contralateral esophagus sparing technique (CEST) in locally advanced NSCLC and SCLC treated to 70 Gy. Int J Radiat Oncol Biol Phys 108(3, Suppl):S104–S105

Kaskowitz L, Graham MV, Emami B, Halverson KJ, Rush C (1993) Radiation therapy alone for stage I non-small cell lung cancer. Int J Radiat Oncol Biol Phys 27(3):517–523

Kilburn JM, Soike MH, Lucas JT, Ayala-Peacock D, Blackstock W, Isom S, Kearns WT, Hinson WH, Miller AA, Petty WJ, Munley MT, Urbanic JJ (2016) Image guided radiation therapy may result in improved local control in locally advanced lung cancer patients. Pract Radiat Oncol 6(3):e73–e80

Kong FM, Ten Haken RK, Schipper M, Frey KA, Hayman J, Gross M, Ramnath N, Hassan KA, Matuszak M, Ritter T, Bi N, Wang W, Orringer M, Cease KB, Lawrence TS, Kalemkerian GP (2017) Effect of midtreatment PET/CT-adapted radiation therapy with concurrent chemotherapy in patients with locally advanced non-small-cell lung cancer: a phase 2 clinical trial. JAMA Oncol 3(10):1358–1365

Kwint M, Conijn S, Schaake E, Knegjens J, Rossi M, Remeijer P, Sonke JJ, Belderbos J (2014) Intra thoracic anatomical changes in lung cancer patients during the course of radiotherapy. Radiother Oncol 113(3):392–397

Lee JS, Scott C, Komaki R, Fossella FV, Dundas GS, McDonald S, Byhardt RW, Curran WJ Jr (1996) Concurrent chemoradiation therapy with oral etoposide and cisplatin for locally advanced inoperable non-small-cell lung cancer: radiation therapy oncology group protocol 91-06. J Clin Oncol 14(4):1055–1064

Lievens Y, Nulens A, Gaber MA, Defraene G, De Wever W, Stroobants S, Van den Heuvel F, Leuven Lung Cancer G (2011) Intensity-modulated radiotherapy for locally advanced non-small-cell lung cancer: a dose-escalation planning study. Int J Radiat Oncol Biol Phys 80(1):306–313

Liu HH, Wang X, Dong L, Wu Q, Liao Z, Stevens CW, Guerrero TM, Komaki R, Cox JD, Mohan R (2004) Feasibility of sparing lung and other thoracic structures with intensity-modulated radiotherapy for non-small-cell lung cancer. Int J Radiat Oncol Biol Phys 58(4):1268–1279

Liu HH, Jauregui M, Zhang X, Wang X, Dong L, Mohan R (2006) Beam angle optimization and reduction for intensity-modulated radiation therapy of non-small-cell lung cancers. Int J Radiat Oncol Biol Phys 65(2):561–572

Luan S, Wang C, Cao D, Chen DZ, Shepard DM, Yu CX (2008) Leaf-sequencing for intensity-modulated arc therapy using graph algorithms. Med Phys 35(1):61–69

Mah K, Caldwell CB, Ung YC, Danjoux CE, Balogh JM, Ganguli SN, Ehrlich LE, Tirona R (2002) The impact of (18)FDG-PET on target and critical organs in CT-based treatment planning of patients with poorly defined non-small-cell lung carcinoma: a prospective study. Int J Radiat Oncol Biol Phys 52(2):339–350

Matuszak MM, Yan D, Grills I, Martinez A (2010) Clinical applications of volumetric modulated arc therapy. Int J Radiat Oncol Biol Phys 77(2):608–616

McDermott PN, Orton CG (2018) The physics and technology of radiation therapy, 2nd edn. Medical Physics Publishing, Madison, WI

McGrath SD, Matuszak MM, Yan D, Kestin LL, Martinez AA, Grills IS (2010) Volumetric modulated arc therapy for delivery of hypofractionated stereotactic lung radiotherapy: a dosimetric and treatment efficiency analysis. Radiother Oncol 95(2):153–157

Mohammed N, Kestin LL, Grills IS, Battu M, Fitch DL, Wong CY, Margolis JH, Chmielewski GW, Welsh RJ (2011a) Rapid disease progression with delay in treatment of non-small-cell lung cancer. Int J Radiat Oncol Biol Phys 79(2):466–472

Mohammed N, Grills IS, Wong CY, Galerani AP, Chao K, Welsh R, Chmielewski G, Yan D, Kestin LL (2011b) Radiographic and metabolic response rates following image-guided stereotactic radiotherapy for lung tumors. Radiother Oncol 99(1):18–22

Movsas B, Hu C, Sloan J, Bradley J, Komaki R, Masters G, Kavadi V, Narayan S, Michalski J, Johnson DW, Koprowski C, Curran WJ Jr, Garces YI, Gaur R, Wynn RB, Schallenkamp J, Gelblum DY, MacRae RM, Paulus R, Choy H (2016) Quality of life analysis of a radiation dose-escalation study of patients with non-small-cell lung cancer: a secondary analysis of the radiation therapy oncology group 0617 randomized clinical trial. JAMA Oncol 2(3):359–367

Murshed H, Liu HH, Liao Z, Barker JL, Wang X, Tucker SL, Chandra A, Guerrero T, Stevens C, Chang JY, Jeter M, Cox JD, Komaki R, Mohan R (2004) Dose and volume reduction for normal lung using intensity-modulated radiotherapy for advanced-stage non-small-cell lung cancer. Int J Radiat Oncol Biol Phys 58(4):1258–1267

Ong CL, Verbakel WF, Cuijpers JP, Slotman BJ, Lagerwaard FJ, Senan S (2010) Stereotactic radiotherapy for peripheral lung tumors: a comparison of volumetric modulated arc therapy with 3 other delivery techniques. Radiother Oncol 97(3):437–442

Onishi H, Araki T, Shirato H, Nagata Y, Hiraoka M, Gomi K, Yamashita T, Niibe Y, Karasawa K, Hayakawa K, Takai Y, Kimura T, Hirokawa Y, Takeda A, Ouchi A, Hareyama M, Kokubo M, Hara R, Itami J, Yamada K (2004) Stereotactic hypofractionated high-dose irradiation for stage I nonsmall cell lung carcinoma: clinical outcomes in 245 subjects in a Japanese multi-institutional study. Cancer 101(7):1623–1631

Otto K (2008) Volumetric modulated arc therapy: IMRT in a single gantry arc. Med Phys 35(1):310–317

Palma DA, Senan S, Oberije C, Belderbos J, de Dios NR, Bradley JD, Barriger RB, Moreno-Jimenez M, Kim TH, Ramella S, Everitt S, Rengan R, Marks LB, De Ruyck K, Warner A, Rodrigues G (2013) Predicting esophagitis after chemoradiation therapy for non-small cell lung cancer: an individual patient data meta-analysis. Int J Radiat Oncol Biol Phys 87(4):690–696

Perez CA, Stanley K, Rubin P, Kramer S, Brady LW, Marks JE, Perez-Tamayo R, Brown GS, Concannon JP, Rotman M (1980) Patterns of tumor recurrence after definitive irradiation for inoperable non-oat cell carcinoma of the lung. Int J Radiat Oncol Biol Phys 6(8):987–994

Ramsey CR, Spencer KM, Alhakeem R, Oliver AL (2001) Leaf position error during conformal dynamic arc and intensity modulated arc treatments. Med Phys 28(1):67–72

Rosenzweig KE, Fox JL, Yorke E, Amols H, Jackson A, Rusch V, Kris MG, Ling CC, Leibel SA (2005) Results of a phase I dose-escalation study using three-dimensional conformal radiotherapy in the treatment of inoperable nonsmall cell lung carcinoma. Cancer 103(10):2118–2127

Schallenkamp JM, Miller RC, Brinkmann DH, Foote T, Garces YI (2007) Incidence of radiation pneumonitis after thoracic irradiation: dose-volume correlates. Int J Radiat Oncol Biol Phys 67(2):410–416

Schwarz M, Alber M, Lebesque JV, Mijnheer BJ, Damen EM (2005) Dose heterogeneity in the target volume and intensity-modulated radiotherapy to escalate the dose in the treatment of non-small-cell lung cancer. Int J Radiat Oncol Biol Phys 62(2):561–570

Scorsetti M, Navarria P, Mancosu P, Alongi F, Castiglioni S, Cavina R, Cozzi L, Fogliata A, Pentimalli S, Tozzi A, Santoro A (2010) Large volume unresectable locally advanced non-small cell lung cancer: acute toxicity and initial outcome results with rapid arc. Radiat Oncol 5:94

Scorsetti M, Navarria P, De Rose F, Ascolese A, Clerici E, Franzese C, Lobefalo F, Reggiori G, Mancosu P, Tomatis S, Fogliata A, Cozzi L (2014) Outcome and toxicity profiles in the treatment of locally advanced lung cancer with volumetric modulated arc therapy. J Cancer Res Clin Oncol 140(11):1937–1945

Shi A, Zhu G, Wu H, Yu R, Li F, Xu B (2010) Analysis of clinical and dosimetric factors associated with severe acute radiation pneumonitis in patients with locally advanced non-small cell lung cancer treated with concurrent chemotherapy and intensity-modulated radiotherapy. Radiat Oncol 5:35

Siegel RL, Miller KD, Fuchs HE, Jemal A (2021) Cancer statistics, 2021. CA Cancer J Clin 71(1):7–33

Speirs CK, DeWees TA, Rehman S, Molotievschi A, Velez MA, Mullen D, Fergus S, Trovo M, Bradley JD, Robinson CG (2017) Heart dose is an independent dosimetric predictor of overall survival in locally advanced non-small cell lung cancer. J Thorac Oncol 12(2):293–301

Sura S, Gupta V, Yorke E, Jackson A, Amols H, Rosenzweig KE (2008) Intensity-modulated radiation therapy (IMRT) for inoperable non-small cell lung cancer: the Memorial Sloan-Kettering Cancer Center (MSKCC) experience. Radiother Oncol 87(1):17–23

Therasse P, Arbuck SG, Eisenhauer EA, Wanders J, Kaplan RS, Rubinstein L, Verweij J, Van Glabbeke M, van Oosterom AT, Christian MC, Gwyther SG (2000) New guidelines to evaluate the response to treatment in solid tumors. European Organization for Research and Treatment of Cancer, National Cancer Institute of the United States, National Cancer Institute of Canada. J Natl Cancer Inst 92(3):205–216

Timmerman RD, Hu C, Michalski JM, Bradley JC, Galvin J, Johnstone DW, Choy H (2018a) Long-term results of stereotactic body radiation therapy in medically inoperable stage I non-small cell lung cancer. JAMA Oncol 4(9):1287–1288

Timmerman RD, Paulus R, Pass HI, Gore EM, Edelman MJ, Galvin J, Straube WL, Nedzi LA, McGarry RC, Robinson CG, Schiff PB, Chang G, Loo BW Jr, Bradley JD, Choy H (2018b) Stereotactic body radiation therapy for operable early-stage lung cancer: findings from the NRG oncology RTOG 0618 trial. JAMA Oncol 4(9):1263–1266

Vinogradskiy Y, Rusthoven CG, Schubert L, Jones B, Faught A, Castillo R, Castillo E, Gaspar LE, Kwak J, Waxweiler T, Dougherty M, Gao D, Stevens C, Miften M, Kavanagh B, Guerrero T, Grills I (2018) Interim analysis of a two-institution, prospective clinical trial of 4DCT-ventilation-based functional avoidance radiation therapy. Int J Radiat Oncol Biol Phys 102(4):1357–1365

Wang S, Liao Z, Wei X, Liu HH, Tucker SL, Hu CS, Mohan R, Cox JD, Komaki R (2006) Analysis of clinical and dosimetric factors associated with treatment-related pneumonitis (TRP) in patients with non-small-cell lung cancer (NSCLC) treated with concurrent chemotherapy and three-dimensional conformal radiotherapy (3D-CRT). Int J Radiat Oncol Biol Phys 66(5):1399–1407

Wang C, Luan S, Tang G, Chen DZ, Earl MA, Yu CX (2008) Arc-modulated radiation therapy (AMRT): a single-arc form of intensity-modulated arc therapy. Phys Med Biol 53(22):6291–6303

Wang K, Eblan MJ, Deal AM, Lipner M, Zagar TM, Wang Y, Mavroidis P, Lee CB, Jensen BC, Rosenman JG, Socinski MA, Stinchcombe TE, Marks LB (2017) Cardiac toxicity after radiotherapy for stage III non-small-cell lung cancer: pooled analysis of dose-escalation trials delivering 70 to 90 Gy. J Clin Oncol 35(13):1387–1394

Weyh A, Konski A, Nalichowski A, Maier J, Lack D (2013) Lung SBRT: dosimetric and delivery comparison of RapidArc, TomoTherapy, and IMR. J Appl Clin Med Phys 14(4):4065

Willner J, Jost A, Baier K, Flentje M (2003) A little to a lot or a lot to a little? An analysis of pneumonitis risk from dose-volume histogram parameters of the lung in patients with lung cancer treated with 3-D conformal radiotherapy. Strahlenther Onkol 179(8):548–556

Wolff D, Stieler F, Welzel G, Lorenz F, Abo-Madyan Y, Mai S, Herskind C, Polednik M, Steil V, Wenz F, Lohr F (2009) Volumetric modulated arc therapy (VMAT) vs. serial tomotherapy, step-and-shoot IMRT and 3D-conformal RT for treatment of prostate cancer. Radiother Oncol 93(2):226–233

Wong CY, Schmidt J, Bong JS, Chundru S, Kestin L, Yan D, Grills I, Gaskill M, Cheng V, Martinez AA, Fink-Bennett D (2007) Correlating metabolic and anatomic responses of primary lung cancers to radiotherapy by combined F-18 FDG PET-CT imaging. Radiat Oncol 2:18

Wulf J, Baier K, Mueller G, Flentje MP (2005) Dose-response in stereotactic irradiation of lung tumors. Radiother Oncol 77(1):83–87

Yom SS, Liao Z, Liu HH, Tucker SL, Hu CS, Wei X, Wang X, Wang S, Mohan R, Cox JD, Komaki R (2007) Initial evaluation of treatment-related pneumonitis in advanced-stage non-small-cell lung cancer patients treated with concurrent chemotherapy and intensity-modulated radiotherapy. Int J Radiat Oncol Biol Phys 68(1):94–102

Yorke ED, Jackson A, Rosenzweig KE, Braban L, Leibel SA, Ling CC (2005) Correlation of dosimetric factors and radiation pneumonitis for non-small-cell lung cancer patients in a recently completed dose escalation study. Int J Radiat Oncol Biol Phys 63(3):672–682

Yu CX (1995) Intensity-modulated arc therapy with dynamic multileaf collimation: an alternative to tomotherapy. Phys Med Biol 40(9):1435–1449

Yu CX, Tang G (2011) Intensity-modulated arc therapy: principles, technologies and clinical implementation. Phys Med Biol 56(5):R31–R54

Yu CX, Symons MJ, Du MN, Martinez AA, Wong JW (1995) A method for implementing dynamic photon beam intensity modulation using independent jaws and a multileaf collimator. Phys Med Biol 40(5):769–787

Zhang P, Hugo GD, Yan D (2008) Planning study comparison of real-time target tracking and four-dimensional inverse planning for managing patient respiratory motion. Int J Radiat Oncol Biol Phys 72(4):1221–1227

Image-Guided Radiotherapy in Lung Cancer

Julius Weng, Patrick Kupelian, and Percy Lee

Contents

1 Introduction 1049
2 Image-Guided Target Delineation Using Functional Imaging 1050
3 MRI-Guided Radiation Therapy 1051
4 Lung Tumor Motion 1052
5 Treatment Room Imaging 1053
6 Fiducial Markers 1054
References 1057

1 Introduction

The technological advances in radiation therapy over the last several decades have dramatically improved outcomes for lung cancer patients treated with radiation. In the era of two-dimensional (2D) radiation therapy, poor imaging quality during planning and treatment necessitated inclusion of a large volume of normal tissue in the treatment fields and long treatment courses delivering small doses of radiation therapy daily even for early-stage cancer. As a result, dose was limited due to toxicity, and tumor control was suboptimal. Three-dimensional (3D) conformal radiotherapy incrementally improved outcomes due to better tumor and organ spatial delineation but was still unable to account for real-time tumor motion. The advent of four-dimensional (4D) CT planning addressed this limitation by permitting the characterization of individualized tumor motion during the respiratory cycle. Further advancements in functional and anatomical imaging, precision of radiation delivery devices, and sophisticated onboard image guidance have made it possible to deliver modern-day hypofractionated radiation therapy or stereotactic body radiation therapy (SBRT) for thoracic cancers.

The main reasons for local failure after radiation therapy are (1) inadequate staging imaging to identify all areas of gross and microscopic disease; (2) geographic misses due to tumor motion as a result of respiration during treatment delivery; and (3) inadequate planned radiation dose due to nearby dose-limiting organs at risk (OARs). Image-guided radiation therapy (IGRT)

J. Weng · P. Lee (✉)
Department of Radiation Oncology, The University of Texas MD Anderson Cancer Center, Houston, TX, USA
e-mail: PercyLee@mdanderson.org

P. Kupelian
Varian Medical Systems, Inc., Palo Alto, CA, USA

based on functional planning imaging such as positron emission tomography/computed tomography (PET/CT) as well as 4D CT to account for individualized tumor and organ motion, and in-room image guidance such as stereoscopic imaging or volumetric cone beam CT (CBCT), has allowed radiation oncologists to dose-escalate radiation to the intended target while reducing dose to OARs, thereby reducing treatment-related toxicities. In medically inoperable stage I NSCLC, with very conformal SBRT approaches and IGRT, very high biological doses (up to 34 Gy in 1 fraction) can be safely delivered to peripheral tumors to achieve excellent local control (80–90%), suggesting that local control is possible when sufficiently high doses are delivered (Onishi et al. 2004; Xia et al. 2006; Timmerman et al. 2018a, b; Videtic et al. 2019).

Functional imaging such as fluorodeoxyglucose (FDG) PET/CT has become the standard of care for baseline disease staging and treatment volume delineation for radiation therapy (Bradley et al. 2004; Mac Manus and Hicks 2007; NCCN 2021; Konert et al. 2015). Most commonly, a FDG PET/CT can assist in detecting occult involved mediastinal and hilar lymph nodes less than 1 cm, distinguishing collapsed lung from tumor (Fig. 1), and identifying distant metastases. However, there are also limitations of PET-based image-guided treatment planning including poor spatial resolution (>1 cm), poor temporal resolution due to respiratory motion, and nontumor-related uptake due to inflammation. Specifically for radiotherapy planning, there are many unanswered questions such as how to best use FDG PET-guided imaging for planning.

2 Image-Guided Target Delineation Using Functional Imaging

In 3D conformal radiotherapy, delineation of the gross tumor volume (GTV) is done primarily with anatomically based CT imaging. Limitations of CT-based imaging to identify the GTV include variability in window and level settings, motion artifact, indistinct tissue boundaries between tumor and lung atelectasis that have similar density, and inability to identify pathologically involved lymph nodes less than 1 cm. By compensating for these inadequacies using excessive large margins, one adds potentially avoidable serious treatment toxicities. On the other hand, undercontouring is likely to lead to inadequate dose to the intended target and local failure due to geographic miss. For example, using CT-based treatment planning often leads to undercontouring of involved lymph nodes less than 1 cm. One study found that up to 44% of nodes involved were less than 1 cm in diameter, and 18% of patients with pathologically involved mediastinal lymph nodes did not have any nodes larger than 1 cm (Prenzel et al. 2003).

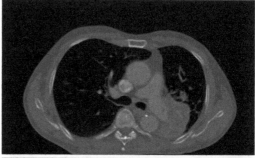
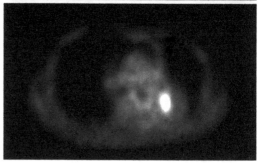

Fig. 1 (Top) Axial CT slice of a patient with medically inoperable, centrally located, stage I squamous cell carcinoma of the left lower lobe causing collapse of the left lower lobe. (Bottom) PET image of the equivalent axial slice demonstrating FDG avidity of only the tumor and not the collapsed left lower lobe. PET was used for stereotactic body radiation therapy image-guided treatment planning to target the FDG-avid tumor only

Mainly, several approaches have been proposed for defining FDG-based GTV: (1) visual interpretation of the FDG PET/CT imaging, (2) using a percentage such as 40–50% of the maximal uptake as the threshold for target delineation, or (3) using an absolute threshold such as a standard uptake value (SUV) of greater than 2.5 to segment the GTV. Despite its limitations however, the use of FDG PET/CT in radiation treatment planning has significantly improved radiation target delineation and reduced geographic misses compared to CT-based treatment planning.

Currently, investigation is ongoing to determine the utility of mid-treatment FDG PET/CT to assess responsiveness to radiation and guide adaptive radiotherapy or dose escalation to residual metabolically active tumor. A systematic review on interim FDG PET for NSCLC suggested that mid-treatment metabolic changes were prognostic for posttreatment tumor response and were associated with differences in progression-free survival and overall survival (Cremonesi et al. 2017). Kong et al. conducted a phase II clinical trial demonstrating that PET-adaptive dose escalation was feasible with improvement in local control compared to historical control (Kong et al. 2017). A similar strategy has been tested in two phase III, multi-institutional trials that have reported preliminary results. Yuan et al. compared standard 60 Gy/30 fractions to individualized PET-adaptive dose escalation ≥66 Gy/30 fractions and demonstrated an improvement of 3.5 months and 16.6 months in PFS and OS, respectively, in the intensified arm (Yuan et al. 2020). Kong et al. also compared standard fractionation to personalized PET-adaptive dose escalation and reported an 11% in-field local-regional tumor control benefit in the dose-escalated arm without an increase in toxicity (Kong et al. 2021). These studies suggest the importance of metabolic and other functional imaging for personalization of radiation therapy.

An additional area of active investigation includes the development of novel PET tracers that are specific for other biological pathways of cancer, such as hypoxia, cell proliferation, angiogenesis, apoptosis, and gene expression. These novel functional imaging tools may further assist in image-guided radiation therapy planning in the near future. Furthermore, an integrated PET/CT and linear accelerator with the goal of biology-guided radiotherapy (BgRT) is in development (Shirvani et al. 2021). In this system, PET emissions are used in real time to guide radiation delivery. A possibility in the future is to use functional information such as radioresistant subvolumes within the GTV and dose-escalated radiation using intensity-modulated radiation therapy approaches to these subvolumes.

3 MRI-Guided Radiation Therapy

Magnetic resonance imaging (MRI)-guided radiation (MRgRT) is a significant technological innovation integrating an MRI machine with a linear accelerator. There are currently two MRgRT devices that have been approved for clinical use: the ViewRay MRIdian (0.35 T and 6 mV Linac) (Mutic and Dempsey 2014) and the Elekta MR-Linac (1.5 T and 7 MV Linac) (Lagendijk et al. 2008). There are several advantages of MRgRT compared to standard CT imaging including superior soft tissue visualization particularly for chest wall invasion, superior sulcus tumors, and tumor adjacent to collapsed lung parenchyma or consolidation. Furthermore, MRgRT is capable of beam-on imaging during radiation delivery allowing for real-time monitoring of tumor and OARs without additional radiation exposure. Given these advantages, MRgRT is well suited for online adaptive therapy, which is the process of optimizing the initial radiation treatment plan based upon "anatomy of the day" obtained from daily onboard MRI imaging (Henke et al. 2016). Early data suggest that these features may increase the therapeutic ratio of radiation by reduction of OAR constraint violations and are most beneficial for tumors adjacent to multiple OARs, such as central lung tumors. Finazzi et al. conducted a retrospective study assessing the utility of adaptive therapy by comparing adaptive and nonadaptive MRgRT SBRT plans for 25 patients with central lung tumors (Finazzi et al. 2019). They found that the reoptimized adaptative plan was preferred in 92% of fractions and that adaptation improved PTV coverage in 61% of the fractions with a significant reduction of OAR doses. Henke et al. evaluated MRgRT SBRT (50 Gy in five fractions) for ultracentral lung cancer in a phase I trial of five patients (Henke et al. 2019). In this trial, four patients required at least 1 adaptive fraction, and 10 out of 25 fractions (40%) were adaptive. Of the adaptive plans, 30% were to increase PTV coverage and 70% were for constraint violations, all of which were reversed with the adaptive plans. Importantly, these treatments were well tolerated with one radiation-related grade 3 esophageal stricture reported at 15 months.

These early data suggest that MRgRT is a safe, feasible, and promising modality for tumors that have historically been challenging to treat with standard approaches. There is ongoing investigation in addressing the drawbacks of MRgRT such as optimization of motion management, development of MRI sequence for low proton density of the lungs, and dosimetric considerations of magnetic field effects on secondary electrons. Additional areas of research are the utility of functional MRI imaging sequences in improving tumor delineation, incorporation of new imaging biomarkers, and monitoring tumor response to allow for treatment intensification or de-escalation.

4 Lung Tumor Motion

Lung tumor motion is a major obstacle in accurate treatment delivery for thoracic malignancies. Respiratory-induced target motion (also known as intrafraction tumor motion) can add significant amount of geometric uncertainty to the radiation treatment. In the era of 3D conformal radiotherapy, excessively large margins were used due to uncertainty regarding the extent of the tumor motion. However, the development of 4D CT with multislice detectors and faster imaging reconstruction has facilitated the ability to obtain images while patients breathe and assess tumor and organ motion (Nehmeh et al. 2004a, b). One approach to designing individualized target volume based on the 4D CT is by contouring the lung tumor in the extreme phases of respiration (end inspiration and end expiration) during normal breathing. Another approach is using a maximum-intensity projection (MIP) image, which displays voxels with greatest intensity during the 4D CT and represents tumor position throughout the entire respiratory cycle. Using either approach, an internal gross tumor volume (iGTV) can be defined. The iGTV is defined as the gross tumor volume (GTV) plus an internal margin (IM) to account for intra- and interfractional tumor motion from respiration. Most lung tumors have a respiratory excursion of less than 5 mm. However, a minority, approximately 10%, of lung tumors move more than 10 mm, and occasionally motion of 40 mm can be seen, especially in lower lobe tumors near the diaphragm (Liu et al. 2007). The use of an iGTV allows patient-specific IM to be applied rather than population-derived values; the latter can substantially underestimate or overestimate the IM.

Tumor motion in the thorax has been assessed in multiple studies. In one study, the 3D motion of 20 lung tumors was assessed by implanting a 2 mm gold fiducial marker in or near the tumor. The 3D position of the implanted markers was determined using two in-room fluoroscopy imaging processor units. The system provided coordinates of the gold marker during beam-on and beam-off time in all directions (Seppenwoolde et al. 2002). On average, lower lobe tumor had the greatest motion in the cranial-caudal dimension (12 ± 2 mm). The lateral and anterior-posterior directions were small for both upper and lower lobe tumors (2 ± 1 mm). Since the tumor spends more time in the exhalation than in the inhalation phase, the time-averaged tumor position was closer to the exhale position. In another study, using a baseline free-breathing CT scan, the patient's couch position was fixed where each tumor showed its maximum diameter on the image. For 16 tumors, over 20 sequential CT images were taken every 2 s, with a 1-s acquisition time occurring during free breathing (Shimizu et al. 2000). In the sequential CT scanning, the tumor was not visible in the examination slice in 21% (75/357) of cases. There were statistically significant differences between lower lobe tumors (39.4%; 71/180) and upper lobe tumors (0%; 0/89; $p < 0.01$) and between lower lobe tumors and middle lobe tumors (8.9%; 4/45; $p < 0.01$) in the incidence of the disappearance of the tumor from the image. Michalski et al. evaluated the reproducibility of respiration-induced lung tumor motion by obtaining 23 pairs of 4D CT scans for 23 patients (Michalski et al. 2008). The group confirmed that the largest extent of respiration-induced motion was along the craniocaudal direction, which ranged from <0.5 to 3.59 cm. Furthermore, three patients had dissimilar respiratory-induced motion on repeated 4D CT imaging. The authors concluded that target motion reproducibility was seen in 87% of cases and advised verification of target motion during treatment. Likewise, Atkins et al. assessed the impact of tumor location on interfraction motion using daily image guidance 4D CT for 41 patients undergoing lung SBRT (Atkins et al. 2015). They found that overall interfraction motion was small (mean ≤2.5 mm); however, lower lobe tumors had a higher incidence (29%) of >5 mm motion in the craniocaudal direction.

Another aspect of tumor motion relates to its potential for deformation during the respiration cycle. Wu et al. evaluated the extent of tumor deformation, along with motion in the three dimensions for 30 patients with early-stage NSCLC (Wu et al. 2009). They evaluated the overlap index after accounting for translation-only image registration, after accounting for translation and rotation, and also after accounting for translations, rotation, and deformation. The overlap index increased only by 1.1% and 1.4%, respectively, when one accounted for rotation and rotation plus deformation. These results were independent of GTV size and motion amplitude. The authors concluded that the primary effect of normal respiration on tumor motion was the translations of tumors while tumor rotation and deformation played a minimal role.

5 Treatment Room Imaging

Most of the beneficial effects of IGRT are seen in the treatment room. As previously mentioned, due to setup uncertainty and lack of image guidance, large planning margins were traditionally added to ensure that the target is encompassed in the PTV due to setup uncertainty and tumor motion. This can lead to a substantial amount of unnecessary irradiation to normal tissue causing excessive toxicities or limiting the dose to the tumor that leads to a local recurrence. For example, adding a 0.5 cm thick shell to a spherical GTV of 4.5 cm in diameter nearly doubles its volume. Traditionally, electronic portal imaging devices (EPIDs) acquire two-dimensional orthogonal views, which were used to align and verify treatment position and isocenter (De Neve et al. 1992). Typically, the source energy of the linear accelerator with megavoltage (MV) energy was used to produce these EPIDs. This produced image of poor quality and high imaging dose while providing no soft tissue information. Alignment can be verified using EPIDs either on a daily basis or in another schedule.

Some of the limitations for onboard MV EPIDs have been overcome by the use of kilovoltage (kV) X-ray source to produce kV EPIDs. The source is offset at right angles to the gantry of the linear accelerator head, opposite to a flat-panel detector. kV EPIDs produce superior image quality over MV EPIDs while delivering a lower imaging dose to the patient. Orthogonally mounted EPIDs in room can be used to track bone and fiducial markers in real time

(Seppenwoolde et al. 2002; Shirato et al. 2000). The CyberKnife system (Accuray, Sunnyvale, CA) mounts a 6 MV miniature linear accelerator source on a robotic arm and is equipped with an in-room orthogonal EPID. The robotic arm is able to move and track a moving lung tumor by tracking either implanted fiducial markers or soft tissue correlate and make adjustments to the beam. Similarly, the ExacTrac/Novalis Body System (Brainlab AG, Heimstetten, Germany) has flat-panel detectors built in the treatment room that detects kV sources from the floor. Treatment adjustments and tracking can be performed when internal surrogate markers are used (Fig. 2). These stereoscopic IGRT approaches are particularly useful for treatment of tumors in the central nervous system or spine applications as bone is readily detected with these images in real time and are stable surrogate markers. One advantage of planar IGRT over volumetric based IGRT such as CBCT is the speed in which images are acquired and adjustments can be made. For both Accuray and Brainlab systems, an automated 2D/3D co-registration algorithm is applied to align a 3D CT patient dataset with 2 kV images. When properly calibrated such that the exact positions of the kV tubes and detectors are known with respect to the machine's isocenter, it is possible to generate DRRs from planning CT at the same positions as the kV images are acquired and compare with the acquired kV images. An automated registration algorithm based on gradient correlation is used, and corresponding shifts in three dimensions are derived.

Volumetric treatment room imaging has greatly improved the precision of radiation delivery permitting the delivery of frameless SBRT (Sonke et al. 2009) and potentially reducing toxicities such as radiation pneumonitis (Yegya-Raman et al. 2018). 2D EPID images can be reconstructed into a 3D CBCT, which facilitates a more comprehensive assessment of tumor location and correction for positional errors. However, 3D CBCT is susceptible to scatter that limits tissue contrast, and, therefore, tumor delineation can be challenging if differences in tissue density are not large. There continue to be developments in CBCT reconstruction algorithms, such as iterative CBCT, that may improve tissue contrast and further increase the accuracy of IGRT (Gardner et al. 2019). Due to the time required to acquire CBCT images, 3D CBCT suffers from significant motion artifacts. To account for respiratory motion, 2D EPID images can be binned with each phase of the respiratory cycle to create a 4D CBCT. 4D CBCT particularly improves visualization of very mobile small tumors and tumors located in close proximity to the diaphragm (Sweeney et al. 2012). An additional method of volumetric IGRT is CT-on-rails, which integrates a diagnostic CT scanner to rails that allow imaging of the patient while they are on the treatment table. Compared to CBCT, CT-on-rails has superior tissue contrast and spatial resolution with a more rapid image acquisition time (Glide-Hurst et al. 2021).

6 Fiducial Markers

For planar IGRT systems to be able to gate or track the tumor during radiation treatment, radiopaque markers need to be implanted in or near the intended target. The fiducial markers act as internal radiologic landmarks and are assumed to move with a constant relationship to the targeted tumor during therapy. The main disadvantage of using a marker-based system for IGRT is the risk of complications such as pneumothorax, bleeding, or infection. A secondary disadvantage is the delay in the therapy in order for the markers to be placed and stabilized in the patient's body. For the thorax, marker implantation can be done either transcutaneously or transbronchially. One study reported marker implantation in 15 patients performed transcutaneously and eight patients transbronchially (Kupelian et al. 2007). Eight of the 15 transcutaneous implants developed pneumothoraces, 6 of which required the placement of a chest tube. None of the patients who underwent transbronchial implantation developed pneumothorax. The authors concluded that in their patient population with many elderly patients with emphysema, transcutaneous marker implantation led to a high complication rate compared to the

Image-Guided Radiotherapy in Lung Cancer

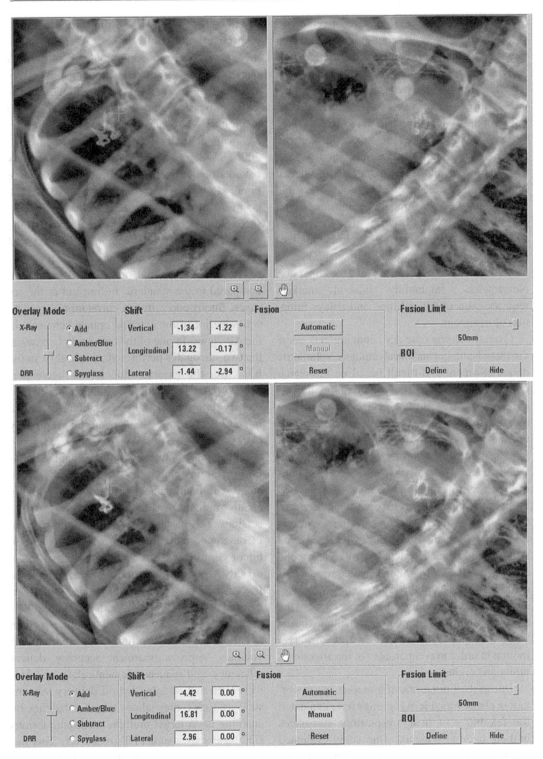

Fig. 2 (Top) DRR to kV matching using spine anatomy using paired oblique stereoscopic imaging in the treatment room. (Bottom) DRR to kV matching using implanted fiducial markers in the left upper lobe lung tumor during image-guided SBRT

transbronchial approach. Kothary et al. reported a similar study of percutaneous fiducial implantation in 132 patients (139 implants) (Kothary et al. 2009). Of the 139 implantations, 44 were in the lung. Pneumothoraces were seen in 20 of 44 lung implantations (45%); a chest tube was required in only 7 of the 44 lung implantations (16%). Of the 139 implantations, 133 were successful with six procedures leading to marker migration (4.3%). The authors concluded that percutaneous fiducial implantation is safe and effective with acceptable risks similar to conventional percutaneous organ biopsy. Thus, it would appear that the risk of complications from percutaneous marker implantation is high depending on the patient population as well as the experience of the operator. Nevertheless, implanting fiducial markers requires extra effort and time and delays initiation of treatment.

Overall stereoscopic kV imaging has some distinct advantages and disadvantages. Volumetric data assessment is difficult based on the planar images. The system will always require an internal surrogate to identify the target and track or gate the treatment, be it bony anatomy or radiopaque markers. Complications from marker implantation and marker migration after implantations are always valid concerns. The limitations of the planar imaging, however, are compensated by the simultaneous stereoscopic image acquisitions allowing for six degrees of freedom positioning assessment, especially when combined with a robotic couch system (Novalis) or robotic arm (CyberKnife), which makes the process efficient and faster than obtaining volumetric imaging. Also, this system operates independent of the treatment allowing image acquisition during treatment and real-time assessment of target motion in order to compensate for intrafractional tumor and organ motion.

Due to the limitations of a marker-based system in planar based IGRT, groups have evaluated the feasibility of using respiratory surrogates without internal fiducials. One study evaluated the feasibility for markerless tracking of lung tumors in SBRT (Richter et al. 2010). EPID movies were acquired during SBRT treatment given to 40 patients with 49 lung targets and retrospectively analyzed via 4D CT and EPID in the superior-inferior direction for intra- and interfractional variations. Tumor visibility was sufficient for markerless tracking in 47% of the EPID movies. Another study compared two respiratory surrogates for gated lung radiotherapy without internal fiducials (Korreman et al. 2006). Video clips were acquired after six patients had fiducial markers implanted in lung tumors to be used for image-guided SBRT. The positions of the markers in the clips were measured within the video frames and used as the standard for tumor volume motion. Two external surrogates, a fluoroscopic image correlation surrogate and an external optical surrogate, were compared to the standard. In four out of the six cases, fluoroscopic image correlation surrogate was superior to the external optical surrogate in the AP views. In one of the remaining two cases, the two surrogates performed comparably. In the last case, the external fiducial surrogate performed best. The authors concluded that fluoroscopic gating based on correlations of native image features may be adequate for respiratory gating.

In summary, advances in image-guided radiation therapy over the last several decades have enabled radiation oncologists to deliver highly ablative radiation doses in single or few treatment sessions. This has led to a dramatic improvement in outcomes including a vast improvement in tumor control and a reduction in normal tissue toxicity. Current innovations under development for better imaging before, during, and after treatment include 5D CT, MR-guided radiation therapy, and 4D CBCT, which will continue to allow radiation oncologists to further reduce treatment volumes, improve treatment accuracy, deliver efficiency, and reduce treatment-related morbidity. Functional imaging hybrid delivery systems such as BgRT may allow tumor debulking by enabling us to target multiple metastatic lesions simultaneously using PET-guided RT. This has the potential for radiation oncology to expand its reach and offer benefit to patients with metastatic disease.

References

Atkins KM, Chen Y, Elliott DA et al (2015) The impact of anatomic tumor location on inter-fraction tumor motion during lung stereotactic body radiation therapy (SBRT). J Radiosurg SBRT 3(3):203–213

Bradley J, Thorstad WL, Mutic S et al (2004) Impact of FDG-PET on radiation therapy volume delineation in non–small-cell lung cancer. Int J Radiat Oncol Biol Phys 59(1):78–86

Cremonesi M, Gilardi L, Ferrari ME et al (2017) Role of interim 18F-FDG-PET/CT for the early prediction of clinical outcomes of non-small cell lung cancer (NSCLC) during radiotherapy or chemo-radiotherapy. A systematic review. Eur J Nucl Med Mol Imaging 44(11):1915–1927

De Neve W, Van den Heuvel F, De Beukeleer M et al (1992) Routine clinical on-line portal imaging followed by immediate field adjustment using a tele-controlled patient couch. Radiother Oncol 24(1):45–54

Finazzi T, Palacios MA, Spoelstra FOB et al (2019) Role of on-table plan adaptation in MR-guided ablative radiation therapy for central lung tumors. Int J Radiat Oncol Biol Phys 104(4):933–941

Gardner SJ, Mao W, Liu C et al (2019) Improvements in CBCT image quality using a novel iterative reconstruction algorithm: a clinical evaluation. Adv Radiat Oncol 4(2):390–400

Glide-Hurst CK, Lee P, Yock AD et al (2021) Adaptive radiation therapy (ART) strategies and technical considerations: a state of the art review from NRG oncology. Int J Radiat Oncol Biol Phys 109:1054. http://www.sciencedirect.com/science/article/pii/S0360301620344096

Henke L, Kashani R, Yang D et al (2016) Simulated online adaptive magnetic resonance-guided stereotactic body radiation therapy for the treatment of oligometastatic disease of the abdomen and central thorax: characterization of potential advantages. Int J Radiat Oncol Biol Phys 96(5):1078–1086

Henke LE, Olsen JR, Contreras JA et al (2019) Stereotactic MR-guided online adaptive radiation therapy (SMART) for ultracentral thorax malignancies: results of a phase 1 trial. Adv Radiat Oncol 4(1):201–209

Konert T, Vogel W, MacManus MP et al (2015) PET/CT imaging for target volume delineation in curative intent radiotherapy of non-small cell lung cancer: IAEA consensus report 2014. Radiother Oncol 116(1):27–34

Kong F-M, Ten Haken RK, Schipper M et al (2017) Effect of midtreatment PET/CT-adapted radiation therapy with concurrent chemotherapy in patients with locally advanced non-small-cell lung cancer: a phase 2 clinical trial. JAMA Oncol 3(10):1358–1365

Kong FM, Hu C, Machtay M, Haken RT, Xiao Y, Matuszak M, Hirsh V, Pryma D, Siegel BA, Gelblum D, Hayman J, Robinson C, Loo Jr BW, Videtic GMM, Faria SL, Ferguson C, Dunlap N, Kundapu V, Paulus R, Bradley J (2021) Results of RTOG1106/ACRIN9969: a randomized phase II trial of individualized adaptive radiotherapy using mid-treatment FDG-PET/CT and modern technology in locally advanced non-small cell lung cancer (NSCLC). Paper presented at the annual meeting of the International Association for the Study of Lung Cancer Virtual meeting platform 2021

Korreman S, Mostafavi H, Le Q-T, Boyer A (2006) Comparison of respiratory surrogates for gated lung radiotherapy without internal fiducials. Acta Oncol 45(7):935–942

Kothary N, Heit JJ, Louie JD et al (2009) Safety and efficacy of percutaneous fiducial marker implantation for image-guided radiation therapy. J Vasc Interv Radiol 20(2):235–239

Kupelian PA, Forbes A, Willoughby TR et al (2007) Implantation and stability of metallic fiducials within pulmonary lesions. Int J Radiat Oncol Biol Phys 69(3):777–785

Lagendijk JJW, Raaymakers BW, Raaijmakers AJE et al (2008) MRI/linac integration. Radiother Oncol 86(1):25–29

Liu HH, Balter P, Tutt T et al (2007) Assessing respiration-induced tumor motion and internal target volume using four-dimensional computed tomography for radiotherapy of lung cancer. Int J Radiat Oncol Biol Phys 68(2):531–540

Mac Manus MP, Hicks RJ (2007) Impact of PET on radiation therapy planning in lung cancer. Radiol Clin North Am 45(4):627–638. v

Michalski D, Sontag M, Li F et al (2008) Four-dimensional computed tomography-based interfractional reproducibility study of lung tumor intrafractional motion. Int J Radiat Oncol Biol Phys 71(3):714–724

Mutic S, Dempsey JF (2014) The ViewRay system: magnetic resonance–guided and controlled radiotherapy. Semin Radiat Oncol 24(3):196–199

NCCN (2021) Clinical practice guidelines. Non-small cell lung cancer (Version 3.2021)

Nehmeh SA, Erdi YE, Pan T et al (2004a) Four-dimensional (4D) PET/CT imaging of the thorax: 4D PET/CT. Med Phys 31(12):3179–3186

Nehmeh SA, Erdi YE, Pan T et al (2004b) Quantitation of respiratory motion during 4D-PET/CT acquisition. Med Phys 31(6):1333–1338

Onishi H, Araki T, Shirato H et al (2004) Stereotactic hypofractionated high-dose irradiation for stage I non-small cell lung carcinoma: clinical outcomes in 245 subjects in a Japanese multiinstitutional study. Cancer 101(7):1623–1631

Prenzel KL, Mönig SP, Sinning JM et al (2003) Lymph node size and metastatic infiltration in non-small cell lung cancer. Chest 123(2):463–467

Richter A, Wilbert J, Baier K, Flentje M, Guckenberger M (2010) Feasibility study for markerless tracking of lung tumors in stereotactic body radiotherapy. Int J Radiat Oncol Biol Phys 78(2):618–627

Seppenwoolde Y, Shirato H, Kitamura K et al (2002) Precise and real-time measurement of 3D tumor motion in lung due to breathing and heartbeat, measured during radiotherapy. Int J Radiat Oncol

Biol Phys 53(4):822–834. https://doi.org/10.1016/s0360-3016(02)02803-1

Shimizu S, Shirato H, Kagei K et al (2000) Impact of respiratory movement on the computed tomographic images of small lung tumors in three-dimensional (3D) radiotherapy. Int J Radiat Oncol Biol Phys 46(5):1127–1133. https://doi.org/10.1016/s0360-3016(99)00352-1

Shirato H, Shimizu S, Kunieda T et al (2000) Physical aspects of a real-time tumor-tracking system for gated radiotherapy. Int J Radiat Oncol Biol Phys 48(4):1187–1195

Shirvani SM, Huntzinger CJ, Melcher T et al (2021) Biology-guided radiotherapy: redefining the role of radiotherapy in metastatic cancer. Br J Radiol 94(1117):20200873

Sonke J-J, Rossi M, Wolthaus J, van Herk M, Damen E, Belderbos J (2009) Frameless stereotactic body radiotherapy for lung cancer using four-dimensional cone beam CT guidance. Int J Radiat Oncol Biol Phys 74(2):567–574

Sweeney RA, Seubert B, Stark S et al (2012) Accuracy and inter-observer variability of 3D versus 4D cone-beam CT based image-guidance in SBRT for lung tumors. Radiat Oncol 7(1):81

Timmerman RD, Hu C, Michalski JM et al (2018a) Long-term results of stereotactic body radiation therapy in medically inoperable stage I non-small cell lung cancer. JAMA Oncol 4(9):1287–1288

Timmerman RD, Paulus R, Pass HI et al (2018b) Stereotactic body radiation therapy for operable early-stage lung cancer. JAMA Oncol 4:1263. https://doi.org/10.1001/jamaoncol.2018.1251

Videtic GM, Paulus R, Singh AK et al (2019) Long-term follow-up on NRG oncology RTOG 0915 (NCCTG N0927): a randomized phase 2 study comparing 2 stereotactic body radiation therapy schedules for medically inoperable patients with stage I peripheral non-small cell lung cancer. Int J Radiat Oncol Biol Phys 103(5):1077–1084

Wu J, Lei P, Shekhar R, Li H, Suntharalingam M, D'Souza WD (2009) Do tumors in the lung deform during normal respiration? An image registration investigation. Int J Radiat Oncol Biol Phys 75(1):268–275

Xia T, Li H, Sun Q et al (2006) Promising clinical outcome of stereotactic body radiation therapy for patients with inoperable Stage I/II non-small-cell lung cancer. Int J Radiat Oncol Biol Phys 66(1):117–125

Yegya-Raman N, Kim S, Deek MP et al (2018) Daily image guidance with cone beam computed tomography may reduce radiation pneumonitis in unresectable non-small cell lung cancer. Int J Radiat Oncol Biol Phys 101(5):1104–1112

Yuan S, Yu Q, Wang S et al (2020) Individualized adaptive radiotherapy versus standard radiotherapy with chemotherapy for patients with locally advanced non-small cell lung cancer: a multicenter randomized phase III clinical trial CRTOG1601. Int J Radiat Oncol Biol Phys 108(3):S105

Heavy Particles in Non-small Cell Lung Cancer: Protons

Charles B. Simone II

Contents

1　Introduction 1060
2　Rationale for Proton Therapy 1060
3　Modalities of Proton Treatment 1061
4　Challenges with Proton Therapy 1062
5　Early-Stage Non-small Cell Lung Cancer 1063
6　Locally Advanced Non-small Cell Lung Cancer 1065
7　Reirradiation 1068
8　Small Cell Lung Cancer 1069
9　Conclusions 1069
References 1070

C. B. Simone II (✉)
New York Proton Center, New York, NY, USA
e-mail: csimone@nyproton.com

Abstract

Radiation therapy is a primary treatment modality for a variety of presentations of lung cancer, but thoracic radiotherapy can be associated with significant morbidities. Due to its unique physical properties, proton therapy can allow for significant dosimetric advantage for patients with lung cancer, reducing unnecessary irradiation doses to critical thoracic structures such as the lungs, esophagus, and heart while optimizing dose to the intended tumor volume. Compared with traditional photon therapy, the dose reductions to normal tissues achievable with proton therapy in select patients can achieve significantly fewer high-grade toxicities, more safely deliver dose escalation, more adequately treat bulky tumors adjacent to critical structures, improve the therapeutic ratio of trimodality therapy, and offer a new chance of cure following locoregional recurrence after prior radiotherapy. Passively scattered and pencil beam scanning proton therapy are discussed, with pencil beam scanning affording greater dose conformality and potentially superior clinical outcomes. Proton therapy has an increasingly well-demonstrated role in the treatment of both early-stage and locally advanced non-small cell lung cancer that is detailed in this chapter. Proton therapy also has emerging roles for other thoracic malignancies, including small cell lung cancer, esophageal cancer, thymic tumors, malignant pleural mesothelioma, and cardiac malignancies. Prospective randomized evidence is emerging supporting its use as a standard treatment to optimize thoracic radiotherapy.

1 Introduction

In addition to its long-standing role in palliating or preventing symptoms for advanced lung cancer (Simone and Jones 2013), radiation therapy has well-established roles for lung cancer in the treatment of early-stage disease most typically for patients who are medically inoperable or who decline surgical resection (Videtic et al. 2017; Chang et al. 2015), in the treatment of locally advanced disease where it is delivered with chemotherapy as a definitive treatment modality (Curran et al. 2011) or before (Edelman et al. 2017) or after (Robinson et al. 2015) surgery as part of trimodality therapy, and increasingly in the treatment of oligometastatic or oligoprogressive disease (Gomez et al. 2019).

Despite significant improvements in modern-day radiotherapy with techniques like intensity-modulated radiation therapy (IMRT), the incorporation of daily image guidance, and the increased utilization of techniques that can account for and even mitigate tumor motion seen during respiration of thoracic malignancies, photon radiation therapy can still be associated with significant risks of normal tissue toxicities. As the dose of radiation therapy that is needed to optimize the chance for cure often exceeds the tolerance of surrounding normal tissues, traditional radiation modalities can lead to high-grade morbidities and even mortality from treatment (Simone 2017; Verma et al. 2017a). Risk of radiation-induced injury to the lungs is often dose limiting and can lead to potentially life-threatening pneumonitis and quality-of-life-limiting pulmonary fibrosis. Radiation esophagitis can lead to significant weight loss, failure to thrive, and worse oncology outcomes. Irradiation to the heart can lead to major cardiac events and decreased overall survival. Approaches to reduce normal tissue toxicities during thoracic radiotherapy are needed.

2 Rationale for Proton Therapy

Proton therapy may allow for a reduction of these morbidities in select patients due to its unique physical properties (Terasawa et al. 2009; Levin et al. 2005). In contrast to photons and electrons, both of which deposit most of their energy close to the patient surface and deliver lower doses of radiotherapy at the depth where the primary lung tumor or sites of nodal metastases are, the physical properties of proton therapy allow for energy to be deposited at a specific depth referred to as the Bragg peak. At this depth, the majority of proton dose is deposited across a very narrow range, with very little to no dose received by normal structures beyond the Bragg peak (Gerweck and Kozin 1999). As a result, normal tissues distal to the target volume can receive less or even no irradiation relative to photon therapy. These unique physical properties have been shown to reduce toxicities and even improve outcomes over traditional radiation therapy, including IMRT, across a number of solid malignancies (Baumann et al. 2019; Xiang et al. 2020), including head and neck cancers (Patel et al. 2014; Romesser et al. 2016), spinal tumors (Zhou et al. 2018), esophageal cancer (Lin et al. 2017a, 2020), liver tumors (Sanford et al. 2019), prostate cancer (Hoppe et al. 2014), a variety of pediatric malignancies (Kahalley et al. 2020), and recurrent tumors (Verma et al. 2017b).

Proton therapy is particularly well suited for the treatment of lung cancer and other thoracic malignancies (Simone and Rengan 2014). Proton therapy can reduce dose to normal critical structures in the chest, including the lungs, heart, esophagus, spinal cord, and brachial plexus. Reduced normal tissue dose, especially to the lungs, heart, and esophagus, can lead to a reduction in both acute and late radiation-induced toxicities. Proton therapy may also more safely allow for dose escalation (Roelofs et al. 2012), which, when delivered safely, can improve local tumor control. By reducing the contributing toxicity burden, proton therapy may be an optimal modality to deliver trimodality therapy in combination with surgery and systemic therapy, and it has the potential to increase the therapeutic ratio of trimodality therapy (Wang et al. 2013), which can improve progression-free survival. Furthermore, proton therapy can similarly widen the therapeutic ratio of reirradiation and more safely allow for a repeat course of radiotherapy in patients who have a local or regional recurrence of their disease.

3 Modalities of Proton Treatment

Unlike photon therapy that is used with traditional radiotherapy, proton therapy uses charged proton particles produced from either cyclotrons or synchrotrons, which accelerates particles to approximately two-thirds of the speed of light. Proton therapy planning and delivery are often broadly categorized as passively scattered proton therapy and active scanning proton therapy (often termed pencil beam scanning proton therapy) (Simone and Jones 2013). Both proton modalities employ a single, monoenergetic (high energy ~250 MeV) proton beam that is often just 4 mm in cross-sectional beam diameter (or spot size) and disperse the protons to the intended target volume, yet there are important differences between these modalities (Diwanji et al. 2017).

Passive scattering, sometimes referred to as first-generation proton therapy, is most ideally suited for tumors with relatively simple geometry. Passive scattering employs physical scatterers to scatter protons so that a large, bulky non-small cell lung cancer (NSCLC) can be treated from a more limited 4 mm spot size. The beam energy produced from the proton accelerators (cyclotron or synchrotron) can be modified using a carbon double-wedge energy selection system to reduce the high proton energy, which can produce a maximum energy that enables protons to stop at the distal edge of a tumor. Apertures, often made of brass, are used to shape the beam to accommodate irregularly shaped tumors. In order to fully treat the thickness of a tumor, protons need to be dispersed in a plane parallel to the beam entry. Further, in order to disperse proton dose in the plane of the beam, the particles would need to stop at different depths and thus have different Bragg peaks. As such, it is necessary to replace a monoenergetic proton beam with a beam containing proton particles with multiple different energies. This is achieved using a range-modulator wheel, which spreads out the distance that protons stop across a treatment field, achieving what is termed a spread-out Bragg peak. Compensators are additionally often used to modify differences in dose deposition in the deepest portion of the tumor (Diwanji et al. 2017).

Pencil beam scanning is a more modern and increasingly more ubiquitous proton technology. This modality, like passive scattering, can allow for a reduction or elimination of exit dose beyond the tumor, but unlike passive scattering, this proton technique can increase the dose conformality to the dose and better protect normal tissues, especially since passive scattering is unable to achieve dose conformality to the proximal edge of the target volume (Diwanji et al. 2017). From a narrow, monoenergetic beam, pencil beam scanning creates a broader target coverage. Pencil beam scanning employs a system of magnets to deflect the beam, allowing protons to be delivered across the entire cross section of the target. While the distribution of particles in the plane parallel to the direction of the beam is similar between passive scattering and pencil beam scanning, instead of using a range-modulator wheel, pencil beam scanning uses a series of wedges (termed an energy selection system) to degrade the energy in a sequential, stepwise way, allowing radiation dose to be painted across a tumor volume layer by layer (Liu and Chang 2011).

Since each layer with pencil beam scanning is able to have independent sets of spots, both the distal and proximal edges of dose are able to be conformed specifically to a given target volume. This important property has been shown to allow for reduced doses to critical normal tissues adjacent to the tumor volume when delivering pencil beam scanning relative to passive scattering proton therapy (Lin et al. 2015). Pencil beam scanning additionally does not require beam-specific apertures or compensators, which add to treatment costs and in-room treatment time (Diwanji et al. 2017). Pencil beam scanning can also enable the delivery of intensity-modulated proton therapy (IMPT), which allows multiple fields to be used with heterogeneous dose in each field that, when added together, can provide a homogenous dose distribution to the target volume. This is akin to IMRT with photons but has the significant added benefit of the Bragg peak phenomena and lack of exit dose.

4 Challenges with Proton Therapy

The benefit in normal tissue sparing with proton therapy comes at the cost of increased treatment uncertainty, particularly in the range of the proton beam and in respiratory motion. Unlike with photon therapy, proton therapy has range uncertainty caused by uncertainty in Hounsfield units (HUs) of computed tomography (CT) images, as well as the values of stopping powers, which must be accounted for. This is not trivial, since these range uncertainties can alter the proton range and dose distribution, which, when not appropriately considered, can result in potential underdosing of the target volume and/or overdosing of critical structures. Further uncertainties that arise from setup errors and/or intrafractional organ motion from respiration or even cardiac motion can also blur the dose gradient from target volume to normal tissue, result in changes in tissue densities, influence the range of proton beam, and result in differences in proton dose distribution (Chang et al. 2017a). Still further, interfractional organ motion or other anatomical changes from 1 day to the next add more potential sources of uncertainty. These include the development or resolution of a pleural effusion, re-expansion of a lung, tumor response change in target volume, weight fluctuations, central port placement, or other variations that can arise over the course of up to a 6- or 7-week treatment. Furthermore, the pronounced change in tissue density between the chest wall, lung parenchyma, tumor, mediastinal structures, and spine can have a significant impact on proton dose distribution (Lomax 2008).

A variety of techniques can be used to overcome these potential barriers, increasing the certainty and benefits of proton therapy when treating thoracic and other tumors that move from respiration during treatment delivery. Margins are added to target volumes to account for uncertainties and ensure that tumor volumes are not underdosed. Motion encompassment techniques are used, such as accounting for motion from respiration using a 4D CT, and motion mitigation techniques are also used, such as breath hold, active breathing control or coaching, forced shallow breathing such as through abdominal compression, respiratory gating, and dynamic tumor tracking (Molitoris et al. 2018, 2019; Chang et al. 2016a; Lin et al. 2017b). Daily volumetric imaging can identify anatomical changes during treatment (Veiga et al. 2016). Regular verification quality assurance CT simulations can be performed over the treatment course to assess for dose distribution changes and can facilitate adaptive replanning to ensure that tumor volume and normal tissue doses are optimized throughout treatment (Chang et al. 2017a; Verma et al. 2018). Additionally, treatment beams can be selected that are more likely to be impervious to daily anatomical changes and/or changes in tissue density along the beam path.

Of note, uncertainties are more pronounced when delivering pencil beam scanning proton therapy, and especially IMPT. First, since individual fields can be highly modulated with IMPT, changes along the beam path of a single beam can have greater dose distribution effects than for passive scattering proton therapy (Dowdell et al. 2016). Second, when using pencil beam scanning to treat tumors that move, as is routine for thoracic malignancies, there can be an interplay effect that may result in the misplacement of individual spots relative to the planned positions of those spots that have been perturbed by motion (Lomax 2008; Shan et al. 2020). This interplay effect may be most apparent when delivering only a few treatment fractions, such as is commonly delivered for stereotactic body radiation therapy (SBRT) (Chang et al. 2017a; Kang et al. 2017). Interplay effects, however, can be mitigated through dose fractionation that can abrogate extremes of motion that may be seen during a single fraction (Poulsen et al. 2018), allowing IMPT to achieve its full potential to optimally deliver radiotherapy to challenging thoracic malignancies. Furthermore, delivering a portion of the planned fractional proton dose over multiple scanning of the target volume instead of delivering the entire treatment fraction dose to each spot in just one round of scanning, a technique termed "repainting," can further smear out any motion and interplay effects (Zhou et al. 2018; Kang et al. 2017; Poulsen et al. 2018).

5 Early-Stage Non-small Cell Lung Cancer

Among early-stage NSCLC patients who are medically inoperable or who refuse surgery, radiation therapy is the long-established standard of care. While historically this was delivered with conventional fractionation, SBRT delivering a large radiation dose per fraction using four-dimensional targeting has emerged as the treatment of choice to manage these patients to reduce toxicities and improve local control and even overall survival (Chang et al. 2016b; Simone and Dorsey 2015; Ball et al. 2019; Choi and Simone 2019), especially when delivered with a biological effective dose of at least 100 Gy (Onishi et al. 2004). However, significant treatment-related toxicities are associated with photon-based SBRT lesions in close proximity to the proximal bronchial tree, esophagus, and great vessels (Timmerman et al. 2006; Senthi et al. 2013). Furthermore, larger node-negative lesions are more challenging to treat with photon-based SBRT, and some reports show that with standard SBRT dosing the local control precipitously declines for patients more than 1 year out from treatment (Verma et al. 2017c).

Proton-based SBRT and hypofractionation may provide an optimal means to protect important critical thoracic structures, especially for large or centrally located lesions, without the need to compromise dose coverage of the tumor volume (Fig. 1). With the increasing utilization of SBRT in patients receiving systemic therapy (Gomez et al. 2019; Simone et al. 2015), proton therapy may more safely allow for the delivery of these hypofractionated treatments when delivered with chemotherapy, targeted therapy, or immunotherapy, especially by reducing the volume of lung receiving unnecessary irradiation. Multiple dosimetric studies have demonstrated a

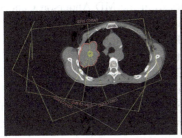 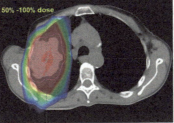 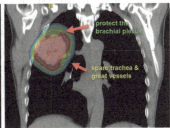

Fig. 1 Proton therapy for early-stage non-small cell lung cancer. Patient with a 7.3 cm cT4N0M0 non-small cell lung cancer determined to be medically inoperable and who refused surgery planned for treatment with definitive radiation therapy. Due to the large tumor size, extensive chest wall abutment, proximity to the proximal bronchial tree, and desire to avoid excessive right breast and brachial plexus incidental reirradiation due to the patient's history of prior right-breast radiotherapy, proton therapy was delivered. Proton therapy allowed for reduced doses to mediastinal structures and to the breast and brachial plexus, minimized dose to the chest wall, and allowed for dose escalation to a prescription of 60 Gy (CGE) in 5 fractions. (Left) Axial slice demonstrating the gross disease (contoured in red) and the proton beam arrangement (four-field plan). (Middle) Axial slice with color wash showing 50% of the prescribed dose (blue) to Dmax of 107.1% of the prescription (red). (Right) Coronal slice with color wash showing 50% of the prescribed dose (blue) to Dmax of 107.1% (red) and optimal sparing of the central airway and great vessels, as well as minimizing reirradiation of the brachial plexus

benefit in reducing dose to lungs, esophagus, spinal cord, and heart with protons compared with photons for early-stage NSCLC (Wang et al. 2009; Macdonald et al. 2009; Wink et al. 2018).

An early prospective study on the use of proton therapy to treat early-stage NSCLC was conducted by investigators at Loma Linda over 20 years ago, demonstrating 2-year disease-free survival (DFS) of 86%, with good local control of 87% and minimal toxicity among 27 stage I patients (Bush et al. 1999). These investigators then conducted a phase II trial of proton hypofractionated radiotherapy for early-stage NSCLC patients who were medically inoperable or declined surgery. Following an initial publication of the first 68 patients accrued (Bush et al. 2004), the investigators then reported on their cohort of 111 patients treated to 51, 60, or 70 Gy (CGE) in 10 fractions. An improvement in the overall survival was seen among patients receiving higher radiation doses (4-year overall survival: 18% vs. 32% vs. 51%, $p = 0.006$). Notably, no treatment-related adverse events of grade 2 or higher, including pneumonitis, were seen in this cohort, and the local control of T1 peripheral tumors was 96% at 4 years (Bush et al. 2013).

Numerous prospective reports on hypofractionated proton therapy for early-stage NSCLC have been reported from investigators in Japan. An early retrospective report from investigators at the University of Tsukuba published a prospective study of 21 stage I NSCLC patients treated most commonly to 60 Gy (CGE) in 10 fractions. At 2 years, the overall survival was 74%, the cause-specific survival (CSS) was 86%, and the local progression-free survival was 95%, respectively, with no grade ≥3 toxicities observed (Hata et al. 2007). Another prospective study of 55 medically inoperable early-stage NSCLC patients treated to 66 Gy (CGE) in 10 fractions to peripheral lesions ($n = 41$) or 72.6 Gy (CGE) in 22 fractions to central lesions ($n = 17$) showed quite impressive 2-year outcomes, with the overall survival rate of 97.8%, the progression-free survival (PFS) rate of 88.7%, and the local control rate of 97% (Nakayama et al. 2010). An updated report from the University of Tsukuba investigators on 80 prospectively enrolled early-stage patients demonstrated 5-year overall survival rate of 65.8% and 5-year PFS rate of 52.5%, and only 1 of 80 patients developed grade 3 pneumonitis (1.3%) (Kanemoto et al. 2014).

Investigators from the National Cancer Center Hospital East reported on 37 patients treated initially on a phase I dose escalation trial. The trial was terminated early due to symptomatic radiation pneumonitis seen in patients treated to 94 Gy (CGE), although patients treated to 80 Gy in 4 Gy fractions (CGE) or to 88 Gy in 4.4 Gy fractions (CGE) had limited toxicity, and at 2 years, the cohort PFS rate was 80% and overall survival rate was 84% (Nihei et al. 2006). In a report by Iwata and colleagues, 57 patients were treated to 60 Gy (CGE) in 10 fractions or 80 Gy (CGE) in 20 fractions for early-stage NSCLC. At 3 years, the local control rates were 83% for 80 Gy (CGE) and 81% for 60 Gy (CGE) (Iwata et al. 2010). These investigators then reported on a cohort of larger node-negative tumors (T2a–T2b), and a 4-year overall survival rate of 58% was reported (Iwata et al. 2013). In another study of 56 patients with stage I NSCLC treated to 66 Gy (CGE) in 10 fractions for peripheral lesions or 80 Gy (CGE) in 25 fractions for central lesions, the 3-year rates of overall survival, PFS, and local control were 81.3%, 73.4%, and 96%, respectively, with no grade 4 or 5 toxicities and only two patients with grade 3 toxicities (Makita et al. 2015).

Investigators from the MD Anderson Cancer Center (MDACC) and Massachusetts General Hospital (MGH) have led multiple recent impactful reports on the use of proton therapy for early-stage NSCLC. In their combined phase I–II prospective dose-escalated proton study of 35 early-stage NSCLC patients, the 5-year rates of overall survival and local control were 28% and 85%, respectively, with no grade 4 or 5 toxicities and only one patient with grade 3 pneumonitis (Chang et al. 2017b). MGH investigators reported on proton SBRT delivered to a median dose of 45 Gy (CGE) in 10–16 Gy (CGE) fractions for 15 high-risk patients with 20 stage I NSCLC lesions, with most of the cohort having interstitial lung disease, multiple primary tumors, or prior thoracic radiotherapy. The 2-year local control rate was 100%, with an 86% rate of survival at 2 years and only a single patient with a grade ≥3 toxicity (grade 3 pneumonitis) (Westover et al. 2012).

The first randomized trial comparing proton versus photon SBRT for early-stage NSCLC was conducted by MDACC investigators. Their phase II study was closed early due to poor accrual, although this study reinforced the feasibility of proton SBRT to achieve excellent outcomes with a modest toxicity profile. Both arms achieved excellent 3-year local control (88% photons, 90% protons), while the overall survival was higher with proton therapy (not reached at a median follow-up of 32 months vs. 28 months), and no patient in either arm developed a grade ≥3 acute toxicity (Nantavithya et al. 2018).

Additionally, a recent meta-analysis reaffirmed the potentials of proton hypofractionation for early-stage NSCLC. That analysis compared 72 photon SBRT studies to 9 proton hypofractionated studies. Despite proton therapy treating larger (2.92 cm vs. 2.41 cm, $p = 0.02$) and more advanced T-stage tumors ($p = 0.01$), the 5-year OS was significantly longer with proton therapy on univariate analysis (60% versus 41.3%, $p = 0.005$). Furthermore, the 3-year local control was improved with proton therapy on multivariate analysis ($p = 0.03$). Patients treated with proton therapy also had fewer grade 3–5 toxicities (4.8% versus 6.9%, $p = 0.05$), including fewer grade ≥3 radiation pneumonitis (0.9% versus 3.4%, $p = 0.001$), at the expense of an increase in grade ≥3 chest wall toxicity (1.9% versus 0.9%, $p = 0.03$) (Chi et al. 2017).

6 Locally Advanced Non-small Cell Lung Cancer

Currently, the standard of care for patients with inoperable locally advanced NSCLC is chemotherapy given concurrently with radiation therapy to a dose of 60–70 Gy (Curran et al. 2011; Bradley et al. 2015; Perez et al. 1982; National Comprehensive Cancer Network 2021). Dose escalation with photon therapy, while an attractive treatment approach to attempt to improve local control and overall survival, has been shown to be deleterious, with a survival decrement compared with more standard radiation doses likely driven by an excess in treatment-related toxicities, including major cardiac events, which are associated with radiation dose to the heart and overall survival (Bradley et al. 2015; Speirs et al. 2016; Dess et al. 2017).

The dosimetric benefits in reducing irradiation dose to normal tissues—including the lungs, heart, esophagus, and spinal cord—with proton therapy compared with photon therapy for locally advanced NSCLC are well established (Chang et al. 2006; Nichols et al. 2011; Stuschke et al. 2012; Kesarwala et al. 2015) (Fig. 2), and there is a growing body of evidence that these dosimetric benefits translate into improved clinical outcomes.

One of the earliest phase II trials on the use of proton therapy for locally advanced NSCLC, now published over a decade ago by investigators from MDACC, reported on proton therapy to 74 Gy (CGE) delivered concurrently with chemotherapy (Chang et al. 2011). Unlike the findings of RTOG 0617, where this same dose with photon therapy was associated with excess morbidity and a deleterious effect on survival (Bradley et al. 2015), when delivered to a cohort of 44 locally advanced patients with proton therapy, the toxicities were quite low, with 11% developing grade 3 esophagitis, only 2% with grade 3 pneumonitis, and no grade 4–5 toxicities. Furthermore, clinical outcomes were quite good, with a median overall survival of 29.4 months and low rates of local failure (Chang et al. 2011).

Similar findings were reported by investigators from the University of Florida, with no acute grade 3 toxicities and only one late grade 3 gastrointestinal and one late grade 3 pulmonary toxicity among 14 patients treated to 74–80 Gy (CGE) with proton therapy and concurrent chemotherapy (Hoppe et al. 2016). These results were further supported in a prospective cohort of 15 patients with stage III NSCLC treated with chemotherapy to 74 Gy (CGE) to the primary tumor and 66 Gy (CGE) to lymph nodes, with grade 3 esophagitis in one patient and late grade 3 pneumonitis in one patient (Oshiro et al. 2014). These early prospective findings suggest that dose escalation might be more feasible when

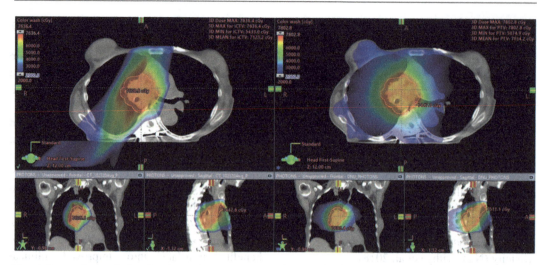

Fig. 2 Proton therapy for locally advanced non-small cell lung cancer. Patient with a history of early-stage NSCLC status post- and prior to lobectomy 8 years earlier now with a morphologically distinct new cT4N2M0 locally advanced non-small cell lung cancer with multistation nodal disease. She was determined not to be a surgical candidate due to mediastinal invasion and was recommended for definitive chemoradiotherapy. Due to her prior lobectomy and desire to spare the remaining normal lung, as well as her extensive nodal involvement, proton therapy was delivered. Proton therapy allowed for reduced doses to the lungs, heart, and esophagus as well as dose escalation to a prescription of 70 Gy (CGE) in 35 fractions. Proton dose entrance through the spine was intentionally avoided to reduce uncertainties given the patient's prior history of complete spinal fusion. Images depict color wash showing 20 Gy (blue) up to Dmax of 76.36 Gy (CGE) for protons and 78.03 Gy for photons (red). Comparison plans between proton therapy delivered with pencil beam scanning (left panel of three CT views) and photon therapy delivered with volumetric modulated arc radiotherapy (right panel of three CT views)

limiting doses to critical normal tissues, which can be more easily achieved with proton therapy for locally advanced NSCLC.

In a separate MDACC report on two separate phase II trials, 62 patients with stage III NSCLC treated with proton therapy who were matched to case-controlled patients treated with 3D conformal radiation therapy (3DCRT) and IMRT were found to have significantly lower pulmonary and esophageal toxicity rates (Sejpal et al. 2011). MDACC also reported long-term outcomes of concurrent proton therapy and chemotherapy in a large cohort of 134 patients with stage II–III NSCLC (84% stage III). The median overall survival was 30.4 months for stage III patients, with one patient experiencing grade 4 esophagitis, six reporting grade 3 esophagitis, and two with grade 3 pneumonitis (Nguyen et al. 2015). Similarly, long-term results of their prospective phase II study showed a median overall survival of 26.5 months, with only 16% developing a local recurrence at a median follow-up of 4.7 months (Chang et al. 2017c).

Dose escalation afforded by the ability of proton therapy to protect normal tissues may be particularly beneficial in patients who are not candidates for or refuse chemotherapy. A retrospective analysis of 35 patients with locally advanced NSCLC treated to a median dose of 72.6 Gy (CGE) alone reported an overall survival of 81.8% at 1 year and 58.9% at 2 years, with no grade 3 toxicities (Nakayama et al. 2011). A similar retrospective analysis of 27 locally advanced NSCLC patients, of whom 11 received sequential chemotherapy, treated to a median dose of 77 Gy (CGE) reported overall survival rates of 92.3% at 1 year and 52% at 2 years, with two patients developing grade 3 pneumonitis and one developing grade 3 esophagitis (Hatayama et al. 2015).

The first randomized trial comparing proton versus photon chemoradiotherapy for locally advanced NSCLC was conducted by investigators from MDACC and MGH. This trial included stage IIB–IV (oligometastatic) NSCLC treated to 74 Gy (CGE) and had a Bayesian design assessing rates of local failure or grade 3 pneumonitis at 12 months. All patients had IMRT and passive scattering proton therapy plans generated, and patients were only randomized if both plans met predefined organ-at-risk constraints. Due to dosimetric differences, as well as proton insurance denials, 272 patients were enrolled to randomize just 149 patients. There was no significant difference in the rate of grade ≥3 radiation pneumonitis or local failure. The trial did, however, demonstrate a sharp learning curve with proton therapy, with the grade ≥3 radiation pneumonitis and local failure rate at 12 months of 31.0% for patients enrolled before the study midpoint versus only 13.1% for patients enrolled after the midpoint, and a notable zero patients developing grade ≥3 pneumonitis in the proton therapy arm after the study midpoint (Liao et al. 2018). These findings confirm the need to conduct rigorous trials of advanced modalities, and NRG Oncology RTOG 1308 is currently underway (Giaddui et al. 2016). That study, a phase III randomized trial comparing proton versus photon chemoradiotherapy to 70 Gy (CGE) for inoperable locally advanced NSCLC, is assessing overall survival, along with major cardiac toxicities (grade ≥2) and lymphocyte reduction (grade ≥4 lymphopenia).

More recent nonrandomized reports assessing survival outcomes following proton therapy for locally advanced NSCLC have been encouraging. A National Cancer Database study of 140,383 NSCLC patients treated with thoracic radiation showed that on multivariate analysis the 99% treated with photon therapy had an increased risk of death relative to the 1% treated with proton therapy (hazard ratio 1.46, $p < 0.001$). Among stage II–III NSCLC patients, the 5-year overall survival rate was 15% with photons versus 22% with protons ($p = 0.01$), and this survival benefit widened on propensity score matching (14% vs. 23%, $p = 0.024$) (Higgins et al. 2017). A prospective study of 47 patients with unresectable stage III NSCLC who were treated with concurrent chemotherapy and proton therapy to 70 Gy (CGE) to the primary lesion and 66 Gy (CGE) to lymph nodes using adaptive planning reported a mean number of 2.5 replanning sessions (range 1–4) performed based on the results of QA verification scans. The 2-year rates of overall survival, PFS, and local control were 77%, 43%, and 84%, respectively. No grade ≥3 pneumonitis was seen, and there was no significant deterioration in the quality-of-life scores after 24 months other than alopecia (Iwata et al. 2021).

While hypofractionated photon therapy delivered with concurrent chemotherapy for locally advanced NSCLC is often thought to result in prohibitive toxicities, with 3 of 21 patients dying from treatment complications in the CALGB 31102 trial reported in 2018 (Urbanic et al. 2018) and 7 of 92 patients dying from treatment complications in a cohort from the University of Warmia and Mazury, Poland, study reported in 2020 (Glinski et al. 2020), proton therapy may more safely allow for hypofractionation. This has the advantage of increasing the biological effective dose that has the potential to improve tumor control and survival while increasing patient convenience, improving access to proton therapy, and reducing costs of therapy. The Proton Collaborative Group conducted LUN005 multicenter phase I–II trial of hypofractionated proton therapy with concurrent chemotherapy for stage II–III NSCLC. Proton therapy was delivered to 60 Gy (CGE) in progressively higher doses per fraction, from 2.5 to 3.0 to 3.53 to 4 Gy (CGE) per fractions. Among 18 patients assessed, no maximum tolerated dose was identified, and no high-grade toxicities related to proton therapy were identified (Hoppe et al. 2020).

Proton therapy may also be particularly beneficial when delivered before or after surgery as part of trimodality therapy for locally advanced NSCLC. In the first report of adjuvant proton therapy by investigators from the University of Pennsylvania, 28 patients achieved excellent early local recurrence-free survival at 1 year (94%), with only one patient developing a grade 3 pneumonitis and two patients developing grade 3 esophagitis (Remick et al. 2017). In a recent retrospective report by investigators from MDACC, 61 proton postoperative patients were compared to 75 IMRT postoperative patients treated from 2003 to 2016. Median overall survival was 76 months for proton patients and 46 months for IMRT patients. Proton-treated patients had lower doses to critical normal tissues, and that led to a better toxicity profile, with fewer grade ≥2 pneumonitis (4.9% vs. 17.3%, $p = 0.104$), grade ≥2 esophagitis (23.0% vs. 60.0%, $p = 0.024$), and cardiac toxicities (4.9% vs. 14.7%, $p = 0.090$), as well as an overall lower total toxicity burden (grade ≥2 pneumonitis, cardiac, or esophageal toxicity) (odds ratio 0.35; 95% CI, 0.15–0.83; $p = 0.017$) (Boyce-Fappiano et al. 2021).

While most of the above reports to date have employed passive scattering proton therapy, the increasing use of pencil beam scanning proton therapy may further improve the therapeutic ratio of proton therapy. In a recent nonrandomized comparison of two prospective cohorts of 139 patients with stage II–IIIB and limited stage IV (solitary brain metastasis) NSCLC treated with concurrent chemotherapy and passive scattering ($n = 86$) or IMPT ($n = 53$), IMPT had lower mean lung (13.0 Gy vs. 16.0 Gy, $p < 0.001$), heart (6.6 Gy vs. 10.7 Gy, $p = 0.004$), and esophagus (21.8 Gy vs. 27.4 Gy, $p = 0.005$) doses, which allowed IMPT patients to have lower rates of grade ≥3 pulmonary (2% vs. 17%, $p = 0.005$) and cardiac (0% vs. 11%, $p = 0.01$) toxicities, as well as fewer overall grade ≥4 toxicities (0% vs. 7%). Patients receiving IMPT also had a trend toward longer median overall survival (36.2 months vs. 23.9 months, $p = 0.09$) (Gjyshi et al. 2021).

7 Reirradiation

Locoregional failure within the first 2 years of therapy can occur in as many as 30–50% of locally advanced NSCLC patients, with 25% having isolated locoregional recurrences (Curran et al. 2011; Bradley et al. 2015; Albain et al. 2009). Achieving local control in these patients is critical given that local control directly impacts overall survival in this patient population (Auperin et al. 2010; Machtay et al. 2012). However, the management of these recurrences in the setting of prior radiotherapy is challenging. Options for management most commonly include surgery, systemic therapy, and reirradiation (Vyfhuis et al. 2018). Surgery is often challenging due to the need to operate in a previously irradiated surgical bed, and with nodal metastases surgery alone is often not adequate to maximize the chance of sustained long-term control. Historically, many of these patients have been managed with chemotherapy alone, but while this modality has the potential to improve survival, it generally does not provide an option to cure patients who still have disease that is localized. Immunotherapy is increasingly being considered in these patients, although only a minority of patients will respond. As such, a second course of radiotherapy can often provide the best chance of cure in patients with locoregional recurrences.

Reirradiation of thoracic malignancies has the advantages of being an effective treatment modality to palliate symptoms, providing durable local control and in some cases achieving prolonged survival or even cure (Fischer-Valuck et al. 2020). Thoracic reirradiation, however, is often challenging given concerns for excessive toxicities, presenting a common barrier to the safe delivery of a definitive dose of reirradiation to 60 Gy.

Protons provide an opportunity for reirradiation in the thorax when there would otherwise be few radiotherapy options (Simone et al. 2020). The lack of exit dose with proton therapy may allow for complete sparing of structures that have already been exposed to a level of radiation reaching their maximum dose tolerance from the prior radiotherapy course. Namely, proton therapy can significantly decrease doses in the reirradiation setting to the spinal cord, previously unirradiated lung, heart, and esophagus. In fact, IMPT was shown to significantly reduce dose to normal tissues for reirradiation compared with all other external beam radiation therapy modalities (Troost et al. 2020). With lower organs-at-risk doses, proton therapy also offers the potential for escalation of reirradiation dose, which may be particularly important for relatively radioresistant recurrent NSCLC.

Investigators from MDACC reported on their experience using proton reirradiation. They demonstrated the feasibility and efficacy of definitive-dose reirradiation in a cohort of 31 patients with intrathoracic recurrent NSCLC (McAvoy et al. 2013). In a larger retrospective cohort of 102 patients re-treated with either IMRT or passive scattering proton therapy in a variety of doses per fraction to a median EQD2 reirradiation dose of 60.48 Gy (CGE), median overall survival was 14.7 months, and only 17% of patients had any acute grade ≥3 toxicity (7% esophageal, 10% pulmonary). This report also demonstrated that higher reirradiation dose independently predicted for overall survival (hazard ratio = 0.246; 95% CI, 0.075–0.86; $p = 0.021$) (McAvoy et al. 2014).

In a University of Pennsylvania-led multicenter prospective trial of 57 patients with recurrent NSCLC re-treated with proton therapy to a median reirradiation dose of 66.6 Gy, reported toxicities were notable, with grade 3 or higher toxicities (acute or late) occurring in 42% of patients, with four patients developing grade 4 and six patients developing grade 5 toxicities. Factors associated with toxicities included high volume of central region overlap, high doses to the esophagus, high doses to the heart, and receipt of concurrent chemotherapy. Despite these significant toxicities, survival was impressive, with a median survival of 14.9 months from the completion of reirradiation, 16.8 months from reirradiation start, and nearly 2 years from the time of locoregional recurrence (Chao et al. 2017).

In a cohort of 79 patients with locoregional lung cancer recurrences reirradiated at eight institutions with proton therapy to a median dose of 60 Gy (CGE) on the Proton Collaborative Group (PCG) prospective database, the median survival was 15.2 months. Acute and late grade 3 toxicities occurred in 6% and 1%, respectively, and three patients died after PBT from possible radiation toxicity (Badiyan et al. 2019).

The largest report of IMPT reirradiation to date was a series of 27 patients treated with definitive doses of thoracic reirradiation to a median of 66 Gy (CGE). The median overall survival for the cohort was 18.0 months, and reirradiation was well tolerated, with only 7% of patients developing a grade 3 pulmonary toxicity and no patients developing a grade 4 or 5 toxicity (Ho et al. 2018).

8 Small Cell Lung Cancer

While data on the use of proton therapy for small cell lung cancer are much more limited than for NSCLC, proton therapy may be particularly beneficial in minimizing toxicities for limited-stage small cell patients (Verma et al. 2018) who often have a heavier smoking history and greater comorbidity index than their NSCLC counterparts and who may receive twice-daily irradiation and its resulting risk of significant esophagitis (Turrisi et al. 1999). A small cohort from the University of Florida demonstrated the feasibility and dosimetric superiority of proton therapy for small cell lung cancer (Colaco et al. 2013). The first prospective study assessing the use of proton therapy for limited-stage small cell lung cancer was reported by the University of Pennsylvania investigators (Rwigema et al. 2017). Among their 30-patient cohort, protons allowed for significant dose reductions to the lungs, heart, and spinal cord relative to backup IMRT plans, which allowed for a toxicity profile that was much more favorable than modern photon historical controls (Faivre-Finn et al. 2017). In fact, only one patient each developed grade ≥3 esophagitis and grade ≥3 pneumonitis. Survival outcomes were comparable to outcomes reported with photon therapy, with a median overall survival of 28.2 months (Rwigema et al. 2017).

9 Conclusions

Proton therapy has an increasingly well-demonstrated role in the treatment of both early-stage and locally advanced NSCLC. Proton therapy has well-established dosimetric superiority to photon therapy in reducing irradiation dose to normal critical thoracic structures, which can lead to fewer toxicities and better preservation of patient quality of life. Proton therapy also has the potential to more safely deliver dose escalation, more adequately treat bulky tumors adjacent to critical structures, and improve the therapeutic ratio of trimodality therapy. Reirradiation may allow for durable disease control and even offer a new chance of cure following locoregional recurrence after prior radiotherapy in select patients. Proton therapy has emerging roles in the treatment of small cell lung cancer and other thoracic malignancies. Early-stage NSCLC lesions that are central/ultra-central or greater than 5 cm might benefit most from proton therapy. Locally advanced NSCLC patients with bulky primary tumors, contralateral mediastinal or hilar lymph node metastases, or preexisting lung disease might benefit most from proton therapy. Pencil beam scanning proton therapy offers dosimetric benefits over passive scattering proton therapy, and early data suggest that these dosimetric benefits can be translated to toxicity reductions and potentially even survival benefits from pencil beam scanning and IMPT. Experience, however, matters when delivering proton therapy, and significant care must be taken to account for uncertainties in treatment and to account for and mitigate intrafractional organ motion. Prospective comparative trials are needed to definitively quantify the benefit of proton therapy and to identify which subsets of patients can most benefit from this advanced modality, and NRG Oncology RTOG 1308 is actively accruing. While early in vitro data suggest a potential immunogenic advantage for proton therapy (Gameiro et al. 2016), additional data on the combination of proton therapy with immunotherapy are needed. Additionally, the role of proton therapy for oligometastatic and oligoprogressive NSCLC should be further explored.

Conflict of Interest None.

Funding None.

References

Albain KS, Swann RS, Rusch VW et al (2009) Radiotherapy plus chemotherapy with or without surgical resection for stage III non-small-cell lung cancer: a phase III randomised controlled trial. Lancet 374(9687):379–386

Auperin A, Le Pechoux C, Rolland E et al (2010) Meta-analysis of concomitant versus sequential radiochemotherapy in locally advanced non-small-cell lung cancer. J Clin Oncol 28(13):2181–2190

Badiyan SN, Rutenberg MS, Hoppe BS et al (2019) Clinical outcomes of patients with recurrent lung cancer reirradiated with proton therapy on the Proton Collaborative Group and University of Florida Proton Therapy Institute Prospective Registry studies. Pract Radiat Oncol 9(4):280–288

Ball D, Mai GT, Vinod S, et al; TROG 09.02 CHISEL investigators (2019) Stereotactic ablative radiotherapy versus standard radiotherapy in stage 1 non-small-cell lung cancer (TROG 09.02 CHISEL): a phase 3, open-label, randomised controlled trial. Lancet Oncol 20(4):494–503

Baumann BC, Mitra N, Harton JG et al (2019) Comparative effectiveness of proton vs photon therapy as part of concurrent chemoradiotherapy for locally advanced cancer. JAMA Oncol 6(2):237–246

Boyce-Fappiano D, Nguyen QN, Chapman BV et al (2021) Single institution experience of proton and photon-based postoperative radiation therapy for non-small-cell lung cancer. Clin Lung Cancer 22(5):e745–e755. [PMID 33707003]

Bradley JD, Paulus R, Komaki R et al (2015) Standard-dose versus high-dose conformal radiotherapy with concurrent and consolidation carboplatin plus paclitaxel with or without cetuximab for patients with stage IIIA or IIIB non-small-cell lung cancer (RTOG 0617): a randomised, two-by-two factorial phase 3 study. Lancet Oncol 16:187–199

Bush DA, Slater JD, Bonnet R et al (1999) Proton-beam radiotherapy for early-stage lung cancer. Chest 116:1313–1319

Bush DA, Slater JD, Shin BB et al (2004) Hypofractionated proton beam radiotherapy for stage I lung cancer. Chest 126:1198–1203

Bush DA, Cheek G, Zaheer S et al (2013) High-dose hypofractionated proton beam radiation therapy is safe and effective for central and peripheral early-stage non-small cell lung cancer: results of a 12-year experience at Loma Linda University Medical Center. Int J Radiat Oncol Biol Phys 86(5):964–948

Chang JY, Zhang X, Wang X et al (2006) Significant reduction of normal tissue dose by proton radiotherapy compared with three-dimensional conformal or intensity-modulated radiation therapy in stage I or stage III non-small-cell lung cancer. Int J Radiat Oncol Biol Phys 65:1087–1096

Chang JY, Komaki R, Lu C et al (2011) Phase 2 study of high-dose proton therapy with concurrent chemotherapy for unresectable stage III nonsmall cell lung cancer. Cancer 117:4707–4713

Chang JY, Senan S, Paul MA et al (2015) Stereotactic ablative radiotherapy versus lobectomy for operable stage I non-small-cell lung cancer: a pooled analysis of two randomised trials. Lancet Oncol 16(6):630–637

Chang JY, Jabbour SK, De Ruysscher D et al (2016a) Consensus statement on proton therapy in early-stage and locally advanced non-small cell lung cancer. Int J Radiat Oncol Biol Phys 95(1):505–516

Chang JY, Senan S, Paul MA et al (2016b) Stereotactic ablative radiotherapy versus lobectomy for operable stage I non-small-cell lung cancer: a pooled analysis of two randomised trials. Lancet Oncol 16:630–637

Chang JY, Zhang X, Knopf A et al (2017a) Consensus guidelines for implementing pencil-beam scanning proton therapy for thoracic malignancies on behalf of the PTCOG Thoracic and Lymphoma Subcommittee. Int J Radiat Oncol Biol Phys 99(1):41–50

Chang JY, Zhang W, Komaki R et al (2017b) Long-term outcome of phase I/II prospective study of dose-escalated proton therapy for early-stage non-small cell lung cancer. Radiother Oncol 122:274–280

Chang JY, Verma V, Li M et al (2017c) Proton beam radiotherapy and concurrent chemotherapy for unresectable stage III non-small cell lung cancer: final results of a phase 2 study. JAMA Oncol 3(8):e172032

Chao HH, Berman AT, Simone CB II et al (2017) Multi-institutional prospective study of reirradiation with proton beam radiotherapy for locoregionally recurrent non-small cell lung cancer. J Thorac Oncol 12(2):281–292

Chi A, Chen H, Wen S et al (2017) Comparison of particle beam therapy and stereotactic body radiotherapy for early stage non-small cell lung cancer: a systematic review and hypothesis-generating meta-analysis. Radiother Oncol 123:346–354

Choi JI, Simone CB II (2019) Stereotactic body radiation therapy versus surgery for early stage non-small cell lung cancer: clearing a path through an evolving treatment landscape. J Thorac Dis 11(Suppl 9):S1360–S1365

Colaco RJ, Huh S, Nichols RC et al (2013) Dosimetric rationale and early experience at UFPTI of thoracic proton therapy and chemotherapy in limited-stage small cell lung cancer. Acta Oncol 52(3):506–513

Curran WJ Jr, Paulus R, Langer CJ, Komaki R, Lee JS, Hauser S, Movsas B, Wasserman T, Rosenthal SA, Gore E, Machtay M, Sause W, Cox JD (2011) Sequential vs. concurrent chemoradiation for stage III non-small-cell lung cancer: randomized phase III trial RTOG 9410. J Natl Cancer Inst 103(19):1452–1460

Dess RT, Sun Y, Matuszak MM et al (2017) Cardiac events after radiation therapy: combined analysis of prospective multicenter trials for locally advanced non-small-cell lung cancer. J Clin Oncol 35:1395–1402

Diwanji TP, Mohindra P, Vyfhuis M et al (2017) Advances in radiotherapy techniques and delivery for non-small cell lung cancer: benefits of intensity-modulated radiation therapy, proton therapy, and stereotactic body radiation therapy. Transl Lung Cancer Res 6(2):131–147

Dowdell S, Grassberger C, Sharp G, Paganetti H (2016) Fractionated lung IMPT treatments: sensitivity to setup uncertainties and motion effects based on single-field homogeneity. Technol Cancer Res Treat 15(5):689–696

Edelman MJ, Hu C, Le QT et al (2017) Randomized phase II study of preoperative chemoradiotherapy ± panitumumab followed by consolidation chemotherapy in potentially operable locally advanced (stage IIIa, N2+) non-small cell lung Cancer: NRG Oncology RTOG 0839. J Thorac Oncol 12(9):1413–1420

Faivre-Finn C, Snee M, Ashcroft L et al (2017) Concurrent once-daily versus twice-daily chemoradiotherapy in patients with limited-stage small-cell lung cancer (CONVERT): an open-label, phase 3, randomised, superiority trial. Lancet Oncol 18(8):1116–1125

Fischer-Valuck BW, Robinson CG, Simone CB II et al (2020) Challenges in re-irradiation in the thorax: managing patients with locally recurrent non-small cell lung cancer. Semin Radiat Oncol 30(3):223–231

Gameiro SR, Malamas AS, Bernstein MB et al (2016) Tumor cells surviving exposure to proton or photon radiation share a common immunogenic modulation signature, rendering them more sensitive to T cell-mediated killing. Int J Radiat Oncol Biol Phys 95:120–130

Gerweck LE, Kozin SV (1999) Relative biological effectiveness of proton beams in clinical therapy. Radiother Oncol 50(2):135–142

Giaddui T, Chen W, Yu J et al (2016) Establishing the feasibility of the dosimetric compliance criteria of RTOG 1308: phase III randomized trial comparing overall survival after photon versus proton radiochemotherapy for inoperable stage II-IIIB NSCLC. Radiat Oncol 11:66

Gjyshi O, Xu T, Elhammali A et al (2021) Toxicity and survival after intensity-modulated proton therapy versus passive scattering proton therapy for NSCLC. J Thorac Oncol 16(2):269–277

Glinski K, Socha J, Wasilewska-Tesluk E, Komosinska K, Kepka L (2020) Accelerated hypofractionated radiotherapy with concurrent full dose chemotherapy for locally advanced non-small cell lung cancer: a phase I/II study. Radiother Oncol 148:174–180

Gomez DR, Tang C, Zhang J et al (2019) Local consolidative therapy vs. maintenance therapy or observation for patients with oligometastatic non-small-cell lung cancer: long-term results of a multi-institutional, phase II, randomized study. J Clin Oncol 37(18):1558–1565

Hata M, Tokuuye K, Kagei K et al (2007) Hypofractionated high-dose proton beam therapy for stage I non-small-cell lung cancer: preliminary results of a phase I/II clinical study. Int J Radiat Oncol Biol Phys 68:786–793

Hatayama Y, Nakamura T, Suzuki M et al (2015) Preliminary results of proton-beam therapy for stage III non-small-cell lung cancer. Curr Oncol 22:370–375

Higgins KA, O'Connell K, Liu Y et al (2017) National cancer database analysis of proton versus photon radiation therapy in non-small cell lung cancer. Int J Radiat Oncol Biol Phys 97(1):128–137

Ho JC, Nguyen QN, Li H et al (2018) Reirradiation of thoracic cancers with intensity modulated proton therapy. Pract Radiat Oncol 8(1):58–65

Hoppe BS, Michalski JM, Mendenhall NP et al (2014) Comparative effectiveness study of patient-reported outcomes after proton therapy or intensity-modulated radiotherapy for prostate cancer. Cancer 120:1076–1082

Hoppe BS, Henderson R, Pham D et al (2016) A phase 2 trial of concurrent chemotherapy and proton therapy for stage III non-small cell lung cancer: results and reflections following early closure of a single-institution study. Int J Radiat Oncol Biol Phys 95:517–522

Hoppe BS, Nichols RC, Flampouri S et al (2020) Hypofractionated proton therapy with concurrent chemotherapy for locally advanced non-small cell lung cancer: a phase 1 trial from the University of Florida and Proton Collaborative Group. Int J Radiat Oncol Biol Phys 107(3):455–461

Iwata H, Murakami M, Demizu Y et al (2010) High-dose proton therapy and carbon-ion therapy for stage I non-small cell lung cancer. Cancer 116:2476–2485

Iwata H, Demizu Y, Fujii O et al (2013) Long-term outcome of proton therapy and carbon-ion therapy for large (T2a-T2bN0M0) non-small-cell lung cancer. J Thorac Oncol 8:726–735

Iwata H, Akita K, Yamaba Y et al (2021) Concurrent chemo-proton therapy using adaptive planning for unresectable stage 3 non-small cell lung cancer: a phase 2 study. Int J Radiat Oncol Biol Phys 109(5):1359–1367

Kahalley LS, Peterson R, Ris MD et al (2020) Superior intellectual outcomes after proton radiotherapy compared with photon radiotherapy for pediatric medulloblastoma. J Clin Oncol 38(5):454–461

Kanemoto A, Okumura T, Ishikawa H et al (2014) Outcomes and prognostic factors for recurrence after high-dose proton beam therapy for centrally and peripherally located stage I non-small-cell lung cancer. Clin Lung Cancer 15:e7–e12

Kang M, Huang S, Solberg TD et al (2017) A study of the beam-specific interplay effect in proton pencil beam scanning delivery in lung cancer. Acta Oncol 56(4):531–540

Kesarwala AH, Ko CJ, Ning H et al (2015) Intensity-modulated proton therapy for elective nodal irradiation and involved-field radiation in the definitive treatment of locally advanced non-small-cell lung cancer: a dosimetric study. Clin Lung Cancer 16(3):237–244

Levin WP, Kooy H, Loeffler JS et al (2005) Proton beam therapy. Br J Cancer 93:849–854

Liao Z, Lee JJ, Komaki R et al (2018) Bayesian adaptive randomization trial of passive scattering proton therapy and intensity-modulated photon radiotherapy for locally advanced non-small-cell lung cancer. J Clin Oncol 36(18):1813–1822

Lin L, Kang M, Huang S et al (2015) Beam specific planning target volumes incorporating 4DCT for pencil beam scanning proton therapy of thoracic tumors. J Appl Clin Med Phys 16:281–292

Lin SH, Merrell KW, Shen J et al (2017a) Multi-institutional analysis of radiation modality use and postoperative outcomes of neoadjuvant chemoradiation for esophageal cancer. Radiother Oncol 123(3):376–381

Lin L, Souris K, Kang M et al (2017b) Evaluation of motion mitigation using abdominal compression in the clinical implementation of pencil beam scanning proton therapy of liver tumors. Med Phys 44(2):703–712

Lin SH, Hobbs BP, Verma V et al (2020) Randomized phase IIB trial of proton beam therapy versus intensity-modulated radiation therapy for locally advanced esophageal cancer. J Clin Oncol 38(14):1569–1579

Liu H, Chang JY (2011) Proton therapy in clinical practice. Chin J Cancer 30:315–326

Lomax AJ (2008) Intensity modulated proton therapy and its sensitivity to treatment uncertainties 1: the potential effects of calculational uncertainties. Phys Med Biol 53(4):1027–1042

Macdonald OK, Kruse JJ, Miller JM et al (2009) Proton beam radiotherapy versus three-dimensional conformal stereotactic body radiotherapy in primary peripheral, early-stage non-small-cell lung carcinoma: a comparative dosimetric analysis. Int J Radiat Oncol 75:950–958

Machtay M, Bae K, Movsas B et al (2012) Higher biologically effective dose of radiotherapy is associated with improved outcomes for locally advanced non-small cell lung carcinoma treated with chemoradiation: an analysis of the radiation therapy oncology group. Int J Radiat Oncol Biol Phys 82(1):425–434

Makita C, Nakamura T, Takada A et al (2015) High-dose proton beam therapy for stage I non-small cell lung cancer: clinical outcomes and prognostic factors. Acta Oncol 54:307–314

McAvoy SA, Ciura KT, Rineer JM et al (2013) Feasibility of proton beam therapy for reirradiation of locoregionally recurrent non-small cell lung cancer. Radiother Oncol 109(1):38–44

McAvoy S, Ciura K, Wei C et al (2014) Definitive reirradiation for locoregionally recurrent non-small cell lung cancer with proton beam therapy or intensity modulated radiation therapy: predictors of high-grade toxicity and survival outcomes. Int J Radiat Oncol Biol Phys 90(4):819–827

Molitoris JK, Diwanji T, Snider JW III et al (2018) Advances in the use of motion management and image guidance in radiation therapy treatment for lung cancer. J Thorac Dis 10(Suppl 21):S2437–S2450

Molitoris JK, Diwanji T, Snider JW III et al (2019) Optimizing immobilization, margins, and imaging for lung stereotactic body radiation therapy. Transl Lung Cancer Res 8(1):24–31

Nakayama H, Sugahara S, Tokita M et al (2010) Proton beam therapy for patients with medically inoperable stage I non-small-cell lung cancer at the University of Tsukuba. Int J Radiat Oncol Biol Phys 78:467–471

Nakayama H, Satoh H, Sugahara S et al (2011) Proton beam therapy of stage II and III non-small-cell lung cancer. Int J Radiat Oncol Biol Phys 81:979–984

Nantavithya C, Gomez DR, Wei X et al (2018) Phase 2 study of stereotactic body radiation therapy and stereotactic body proton therapy for high-risk, medically inoperable, early-stage non-small cell lung cancer. Int J Radiat Oncol Biol Phys 101(3):558–563

National Comprehensive Cancer Network (2021) Non-small cell lung cancer version 4.2021. www.nccn.org. Accessed May 2021

Nguyen QN, Ly NB, Komaki R et al (2015) Long-term outcomes after proton therapy, with concurrent chemotherapy, for stage II-III inoperable non-small cell lung cancer. Radiother Oncol 115:367–372

Nichols RC, Huh S, Henderson R et al (2011) Proton radiation therapy offers reduced normal lung and bone marrow exposure for patients receiving dose-escalated radiation therapy for unresectable stage III non-small-cell lung cancer: a dosimetric study. Clin Lung Cancer 12:252–257

Nihei K, Ogino T, Ishikura S et al (2006) High-dose proton beam therapy for stage I non-small-cell lung cancer. Int J Radiat Oncol Biol Phys 65:107–111

Onishi H, Araki T, Shirato H et al (2004) Stereotactic hypofractionated high-dose irradiation for stage I non-small cell lung carcinoma: clinical outcomes in 245 subjects in a Japanese multiinstitutional study. Cancer 101:1623–1631

Oshiro Y, Okumura T, Kurishima K et al (2014) High-dose concurrent chemo-proton therapy for stage III NSCLC: preliminary results of a Phase II study. J Radiat Res 55(5):959–965

Patel SH, Wang Z, Wong WW et al (2014) Charged particle therapy versus photon therapy for paranasal sinus and nasal cavity malignant diseases: a systematic review and meta-analysis. Lancet Oncol 15(9):1027–1038

Perez CA, Stanley K, Grundy G et al (1982) Impact of irradiation technique and tumor extent in tumor control and survival of patients with unresectable non-oat cell carcinoma of the lung: report by the Radiation Therapy Oncology Group. Cancer 50:1091–1099

Poulsen PR, Eley J, Langner U et al (2018) Efficient interplay effect mitigation for proton pencil beam scanning by spot-adapted layered repainting evenly spread out over the full breathing cycle. Int J Radiat Oncol Biol Phys 100:226–234

Remick JS, Schonewolf C, Gabriel P et al (2017) First clinical report of proton beam therapy for postoperative radiotherapy for non-small-cell lung cancer. Clin Lung Cancer 18(4):364–371

Robinson CG, Patel AP, Bradley JD et al (2015) Postoperative radiotherapy for pathologic N2 non-small-cell lung cancer treated with adjuvant chemotherapy: a review of the National Cancer Data Base. J Clin Oncol 33(8):870–876

Roelofs E, Engelsman M, Rasch C, et al.; ROCOCO Consortium (2012) Results of a multicentric in silico clinical trial (ROCOCO): comparing radiotherapy with photons and protons for non-small cell lung cancer. J Thorac Oncol 7:165–176

Romesser PB, Cahlon O, Scher E et al (2016) Proton beam radiation therapy results in significantly reduced toxicity compared with intensity-modulated radiation therapy for head and neck tumors that require ipsilateral radiation. Radiother Oncol 118(2):286–292

Rwigema JM, Verma V, Lin L et al (2017) Prospective study of proton-beam radiation therapy for limited-stage small cell lung cancer. Cancer 123(21):4244–4251

Sanford NN, Pursley J, Noe B et al (2019) Protons versus photons for unresectable hepatocellular carcinoma: liver decompensation and overall survival. Int J Radiat Oncol Biol Phys 105(1):64–72

Sejpal S, Komaki R, Tsao A et al (2011) Early findings on toxicity of proton beam therapy with concurrent chemotherapy for nonsmall cell lung cancer. Cancer 117:3004–3013

Senthi S, Haasbeek CJA, Slotman BJ et al (2013) Outcomes of stereotactic ablative radiotherapy for central lung tumours: a systematic review. Radiother Oncol 106:276–282

Shan J, Yang Y, Schild SE et al (2020) Intensity-modulated proton therapy (IMPT) interplay effect evaluation of asymmetric breathing with simultaneous uncertainty considerations in patients with non-small cell lung cancer. Med Phys 47(11):5428–5440

Simone CB II (2017) Thoracic radiation normal tissue injury. Semin Radiat Oncol 27(4):370–377

Simone CB II, Dorsey JF (2015) Additional data in the debate on stage I non-small cell lung cancer: surgery versus stereotactic ablative radiotherapy. Ann Transl Med 3:172

Simone CB II, Jones JA (2013) Palliative care for patients with locally advanced and metastatic non-small cell lung cancer. Ann Palliat Med 2(4):178–188

Simone CB II, Rengan R (2014) The use of proton therapy in the treatment of lung cancers. Cancer J 20(6):427–432

Simone CB II, Burri SH, Heinzerling JH (2015) Novel radiotherapy approaches for lung cancer: combining radiation therapy with targeted and immunotherapies. Transl Lung Cancer Res 4(5):545–552

Simone CB II, Plastaras JP, Jabbour SK et al (2020) Proton reirradiation: expert recommendations for reducing toxicities and offering new chances of cure in patients with challenging recurrence malignancies. Semin Radiat Oncol 30(3):253–261

Speirs CK, Dewees TA, Rehman S et al (2016) Heart dose is an independent dosimetric predictor of overall survival in locally advanced non-small cell lung cancer. J Thorac Oncol 12:293–301

Stuschke M, Kaiser A, Pöttgen C et al (2012) Potentials of robust intensity modulated scanning proton plans for locally advanced lung cancer in comparison to intensity modulated photon plans. Radiother Oncol 104(1):45–51

Terasawa T, Dvorak T, Ip S et al (2009) Systematic review: charged-particle radiation therapy for cancer. Ann Intern Med 151:556–565

Timmerman R, McGarry R, Yiannoutsos C et al (2006) Excessive toxicity when treating central tumors in a phase II study of stereotactic body radiation therapy for medically inoperable early-stage lung cancer. J Clin Oncol 24:4833–4839

Troost EGC, Wink KCJ, Roelofs E et al (2020) Photons or protons for reirradiation in (non-)small cell lung cancer: Results of the multicentric ROCOCO *in silico* study. Br J Radiol 93(1107):20190879

Turrisi AT III, Kim K, Blum R et al (1999) Twice-daily compared with once-daily thoracic radiotherapy in limited small-cell lung cancer treated concurrently with cisplatin and etoposide. N Engl J Med 340(4):265–271

Urbanic JJ, Wang X, Bogart JA et al (2018) Phase 1 study of accelerated hypofractionated radiation therapy with concurrent chemotherapy for stage III non-small cell lung cancer: CALGB 31102 (Alliance). Int J Radiat Oncol Biol Phys 101(1):177–185

Veiga C, Janssens G, Teng CL et al (2016) First clinical investigation of cone beam computed tomography and deformable registration for adaptive proton therapy for lung cancer. Int J Radiat Oncol Biol Phys 95(1):549–559

Verma V, Simone CB II, Werner-Wasik M (2017a) Acute and late toxicities of concurrent chemoradiotherapy for locally-advanced non-small cell lung cancer. Cancers (Basel) 9(9):120

Verma V, Rwigema JM, Malyapa RS et al (2017b) Systematic assessment of clinical outcomes and toxicities of proton radiotherapy for reirradiation. Radiother Oncol 125(1):21–30

Verma V, Shostrom VK, Kumar SS et al (2017c) Multi-institutional experience of stereotactic body radiotherapy for large (≥5 centimeters) non-small cell lung tumors. Cancer 123(4):688–696

Verma V, Choi JI, Simone CB II (2018) Proton therapy for small cell lung cancer. Transl Lung Cancer Res 7(2):134–140

Videtic GMM, Donington J, Giuliani M et al (2017) Stereotactic body radiation therapy for early-stage non-small cell lung cancer: executive summary of an ASTRO evidence-based guideline. Pract Radiat Oncol 7(5):295–301

Vyfhuis MAL, Rice S, Remick J et al (2018) Reirradiation for locoregionally recurrent non-small cell lung cancer. J Thorac Dis 10(Suppl 21):S2522–S2536

Wang C, Nakayama H, Sugahara S et al (2009) Comparisons of dose-volume histograms for proton-beam versus 3-D conformal X-ray therapy in patients with stage I non-small cell lung cancer. Strahlenther Onkol 185:231–234

Wang J, Wei C, Tucker SL et al (2013) Predictors of postoperative complications after trimodality therapy for esophageal cancer. Int J Radiat Oncol Biol Phys 86:885–891

Westover KD, Seco J, Adams JA et al (2012) Proton SBRT for medically inoperable stage I NSCLC. J Thorac Oncol 7(6):1021–1025

Wink KCJ, Roelofs E, Simone CB II et al (2018) Photons, protons or carbon ions for stage I non-small cell lung cancer—results of the multicentric ROCOCO in silico study. Radiother Oncol 128(1):139–146

Xiang M, Chang DT, Pollom EL (2020) Second cancer risk after primary cancer treatment with three-dimensional conformal, intensity-modulated, or proton beam radiation therapy. Cancer 126(15):3560–3568

Zhou J, Yang B, Wang X et al (2018) Comparison of the effectiveness of radiotherapy with photons and particles for chordoma after surgery: a meta-analysis. World Neurosurg 117:46–53

Heavy Particles in Non-small Cell Lung Cancer: Carbon Ions

S. Tubin, P. Fossati, S. Mori, E. Hug, and T. Kamada

Contents

1 Introduction 1075
2 Physical and Radiobiological Properties of Carbon Ions 1076
3 Preclinical Research in CIRT 1079
4 Treatment Planning 1082
5 Clinical Outcomes of CIRT 1084
References 1087

1 Introduction

Lung cancer is the leading cause of cancer deaths in the developed countries. Despite the tremendous efforts in non-small cell lung cancer (NSCLC) research and significant improvements in patient care within the last decade, the 5-year overall survival rate remains poor, resulting in 68% for patients with stage IB disease and less than 10% for those with stage IVA–IVB disease (Goldstraw et al. 2016). Although different types of treatment for patients with NSCLC are currently available, surgery represents the treatment of choice for resectable disease in operable patients. However, considering the fact that the median age at diagnosis of NSCLC is around 72 years, and that over 85% of NSCLC patients are current or ex-smokers, and thus highly affected by important multi-comorbidities, surgery may not be an optimal treatment for all. An estimated surgical resection rate for NSCLC is variable among different countries ranging from 10% to 37% (Free et al. 2007; Koyi et al. 2002; Dillman et al. 2009; Little et al. 2005; de Cos et al. 2008). For patients being inoperable, or those having an unresectable NSCLC, the conventional radiotherapy historically represented an alternative treatment opportunity offering the 5-year survival rate of only 15–30% (Jeremic et al. 2002; Sibley 1998), which was pretty inferior compared to those achieved with surgery (Naruke et al. 2001; Mountain 1997). With the technological advances in radiation oncology in terms of high degree of treatment accuracy and dose delivery, the stereotactic body radiotherapy (SBRT)/stereotactic ablative radiotherapy (SABR) became the standard of care for peripheral, medically inoperable early-stage NSCLC (esNSCLC), offering the safe treatment with high local control rates exceeding 90% if the biological effective dose (BED) is higher than 100 Gy ($BED^{10} \geq 100$ Gy) (Zheng et al. 2014). However, less evidence are available to allow for recom-

S. Tubin (✉) · P. Fossati · S. Mori · E. Hug
MedAustron Ion Therapy Center,
Wiener Neustadt, Austria
e-mail: Slavisa.Tubin@medaustron.at

T. Kamada
Hospital of the National Institute of Radiological Sciences, National Institutes for Quantum and Radiological Science and Technology, Chiba, Japan

mendations to be made for central ("no fly zone"-tumors, within 2 cm from proximal bronchial tree) and ultracentral NSCLC (within 1 cm from proximal bronchial tree), which are considered to be unsafe targets. Thus, the 2-year freedom from severe toxicity was reported to be 83% for peripheral tumors, compared to only 54% for those centrally located (Timmerman et al. 2006). Furthermore, it has been previously established that the risk of grade ≥3 radiation-induced pneumonitis is meaningfully higher in patients affected by chronic pulmonary diseases (Kim et al. 2019). Thus, radiation-induced toxicity represents a main worry in radiation oncology, driving the treatment outcomes. From the other hand, curative radiotherapy requires high radiation dose that, especially in the centrally located NSCLC, exceeds the tolerance of surrounding organs at risk (OARs). Carbon ions radiotherapy (CIRT) due to their particularly favorable dose-depth profile and higher biological effectiveness compared to photons may allow for a reduction in radiation dose delivered to OARs and increase in radiation dose delivered to the tumor. These proprieties may be translated into clinical advantages for NSCLC patients affected by limited pulmonary reserve, whose tumors are located in close proximity of OARs.

The rational for the use of CIRT in treatment of NSCLC is related but not limited to the following capabilities: reduced dose to the OARs, safer delivery of higher radiation dose, and dose escalation to the tumor, especially if close to the critical OARs, which may translate to the improved therapeutic ratio because of the reduced toxicity, improved local tumor control and survival. This is possible thanks to their inverted dose-depth profile which, compared to photons, is determined by the charge and mass of carbon ions, and therefore finite range, resulting in much lower entrance dose proximal to the tumor, nearly full energy deposition within the Bragg peak corresponding to tumor site, and almost no exit dose deposition to the tissues distal to the tumor. Additionally, a very high amount of energy that will be deposited at the end of carbon ion's range forming the Bragg peak determines high-density ionization events giving to CIRT pretty higher radiobiological effectiveness (RBE) compared to the photons (Kanai et al. 1997). Therefore, due to better dose distribution and higher RBE compared to photon radiotherapy, CIRT is very appropriate for centrally located NSCLC surrounded by critical structures, those "very peripheral" close to the chest wall or brachial plexus, multiple lung lesions, or in-field recurrences following prior irradiation.

Considering that the first radiotherapy hospital dedicated for carbon ion treatments, the National Institute of Radiological Sciences (NIRS) in Chiba, Japan, has been established in mid-90 s, CIRT represents a relatively young radiotherapy concept whose biophysical advantages are still subject of continuous research. Since its conception in 1994 at NIRS, the effectiveness and safety of CIRT have been assessed through very large number of preclinical and clinical studies (Mohamad et al. 2018). Following the completion of the early preclinical experiments, the first phase I/II clinical trials with CIRT for stage I NSCLC were initiated in October 1994 (Kanai et al. 1999). The evidence created since then, and especially in the last decade, supports the remarkable therapeutic potential of carbon ions, and will be the subject of discussion in the following paragraphs.

2 Physical and Radiobiological Properties of Carbon Ions

Carbon ions are positively charged particles and as such deposit their energy interacting with matter in three main ways: (1) they interact with electrons (mainly electrons of the outer molecular orbitals) and cause direct ionizations, (2) they interact with nuclei with elastic Coulomb scattering, and (3) they interact with nuclei with inelastic nuclear interactions.

The first interaction is responsible for the characteristics depth dose profile of positively charged particle. Each ion loses only a limited amount of energy in any ionization event. In sheer contrast to photons, there is very little attenuation of the particle beam. Each particle, interacting and loosing energy, slows down and this changes its probability to further interact. In particular, the probability to cause ionization increases when particles slow down and this results in the well-known Bragg peak.

As can be seen in Fig. 1, carbon ion beams deposit a low and almost constant dose in the entrance path, a steep dose peak at the end of the range, and a low-dose tail after the peak. The position of the peak can be determined varying the initial energy.

In the second kind of interaction, carbon ions are deviated by the electric field of nuclei in the patient tissues. This results in a change of direction and therefore in a loss of sharpness of the lateral penumbra.

Carbon ions have a mass that is comparable with that of most nuclei in the patient body. Therefore their angular deflection is much smaller than for lighter particles (e.g., protons) and carbon beams maintain their lateral sharpness also in depth.

The third kind of interaction results in a change in the nuclear structure of the incident carbon nucleus and/or of the nuclei in the patient body. It is a complex phenomenon that depends on the exact composition of the tissues. As a result of these nuclear interactions, gamma photons, neutrons, and nuclear species lighter than C12 are created (all species with $Z = 1–5$), these nuclear fragments have a residual range which is higher than that of the original carbon ion and are responsible for the distal fragmentation tail in the depth dose profile. Nuclear interactions are important not only because they produce fragments but also because they cause a loss of the primary particles. Particles heavier than carbon may be of interest for specific applications (e.g., very large target volumes); however, heavier ions produce more inelastic nuclear interaction which lead to loss of primary and this ultimately limits the possibility to use very heavy ions in a clinical setting.

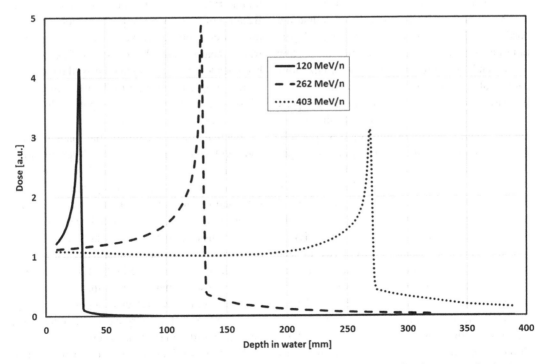

Fig. 1 Depth dose profile of carbon ions beam in water (each dose profile is normalized to the entrance dose)

From the clinical point of view, carbon ion physical properties can be considered very similar to those of protons. The sharper lateral penumbra can result in a better conformity, as compared to protons, especially for deep targets of complex shape; on the other hand, the distal fragmentation tail is a disadvantage and can result in higher integral dose.

The main reason why carbon ions are used in the clinic is however their potential radiobiological advantage.

The depth dose profile of photons is related to the beam attenuation. When a single photon deposits its energy, it is lost. High dose is delivered in the superficial layers because many photons interact there. Fewer photons penetrate to the deeper layers and deposit their energy there. When a photon causes an ionization, it is the first time that it interacts with the patient body. The quality of ionizations caused in depth is not different to that of those caused superficially (at least as a first approximation and disregarding the changes in photon beam spectrum, which however has minimal impact on radiobiological endpoints). On the contrary, each heavy charged particle penetrates until its end of range, where the Bragg peak is located (except of course the particle lost because of fragmentation). Each particle changes its physical properties as it slow downs and therefore the quality of ionizations caused along the particle's path changes. The increased dose deposition in the Bragg peak region is due to an increase in the density of ionization events. Density of ionization is typically described by the amount of energy deposited per unit of length along the particle path and it is called Linear Energy Transfer or LET. The LET of photons (and neutrons) is constant. The LET of particles increases toward the end of their path. From the biological point of view, the LET is linked to the mean distance between two ionization events. When this mean distance is comparable with the DNA double helix diameter, the radiobiological properties of the beam change dramatically. It is common to refer to beams which cause this dense ionization as "high LET." Photons are low LET radiation, and fast neutrons are high LET radiation. Particle therapy is neither low nor high LET. LET of particles change along the beam path. However protons reach a high LET that corresponds to dense ionization only in the very distal portion of their depth dose profile, where the absorbed dose is already low and they are commonly considered low LET. Carbon ions reach a LET correspondent to dense ionization approximately in the proximal part of the Bragg peak. Therefore carbon ions deposit in the entrance plateau a low dose with low LET and in the Bragg peak a high dose with high LET. Carbon ions are synthetically described as high LET; however, this has to be understood as "high LET in the Bragg peak."

Nuclear fragments produced because of inelastic nuclear interaction are typically low LET particles. They deposit a low dose with low LET and therefore their contribution is not extremely relevant.

High LET can produce complex clustered DNA damages that are more difficult to repair. The majority of the effects of high LET are due to direct damage and are not mediated by free radicals. A single high LET particle can produce lethal damage. Damage repair capability plays a minor role in determining the final effects. Because of these two last phenomenon, cell killing dose–response curve deviates marginally from linearity and the effect of fractionation becomes less relevant. In synthesis, the radiobiological properties of high LET differ from those of low LET and high LET is potentially more effective in killing tumor cells.

In a real clinical treatment, the shape position and depth of the target are given. Typically multiple beams with different incidence are used. Each portion of the patient body (both in the target volumes and in the organs at risk) is ultimately exposed to a mixed field composed of carbon ions of different energy and of fragments. Schematically we can consider that each voxel in the patient receives some high LET dose deposited by slow primary carbon that are stopping there and some low LET dose deposited by fragments and by fast primary carbon that are going through in order to stop elsewhere.

The high LET component of carbon ion is, as said, more effective in killing cells. The same absorbed physical dose is producing more cell killing. This increase cell killing is typically described in comparison with a reference radiation, and for historical reasons, the reference radiation employed is always photons.

The ratio between the dose of photons and the dose of carbon ions that produce the same cell killing is called the Relative Biological Effectiveness or RBE.

$$\text{RBE} = \frac{D_{\text{ref}}}{D_{\text{test}}}$$

The RBE depends on the biological endpoints selected. Its order of magnitude is however of great interest. The high LET portion of a carbon ion has typically a RBE between 3 and 4 as compared to photons.

RBE can be determined precisely for in experimental endpoints with well-defined beam qualities. In the clinical settings, the basic radiobiological properties of tumors and patients tissue are both variable and unknown. Moreover the complexity of the mixed field of particle is such that it is basically impossible to obtain experimental data for all the possible scenarios.

Following the ICRU recommendation (ICRU 2016), in the clinical settings, carbon ions radiotherapy is prescribed, optimized, recorded, and reported in terms of RBE weighted dose. The RBE is calculated voxel by voxel using a complex radiobiological model that accounts for the overall properties of the mixed field of particles. In this way, voxels that receive a significant part of high LET dose will have a lower total physical absorbed dose. Two models are used in clinical practice. All carbon ion centers in Japan use the Kanai semi empirical/ modified MKM (Microdosimetric Kinetic Model) (Kanai et al. 2006; Inaniwa et al. 2015). This model focuses on the radiation quality in small domains (i.e., volumes of 5 μm diameter). The RBE is calculated according to dose and to the distribution of a measurable physical quantity: the lineal energy. The lineal energy is indirectly related to the ionization density but can be directly measured. The modified MKM model ultimately calculates RBE in terms of lineal energy spectra.

In European and Chinese centers, another model is employed: the LEM (Local Effect Model) (Krämer and Scholz 2000; Molinelli et al. 2016).

This model goes deeper in the very small and describes the dose distribution in the nanometer scale. The LEM model calculates the RBE in terms of LET spectra. On the one hand, LEM is potentially closer to the biologically relevant quantity of ionization density as compared to MKM, on the other hand, the LET spectra cannot be measured directly so the model is more of a black box.

In practice, the theoretical differences of these models are not extremely relevant for clinical practice. It is more important to acknowledge that, not only because of the different model but especially because of their practical implementation, RBE weighted doses cannot be converted at par values between the two systems. Therefore, extreme caution must be exerted when comparing published clinical results and when designing future studies (Molinelli et al. 2016; Fossati et al. 2012).

3 Preclinical Research in CIRT

Biological and physical potential of carbon ions over the photons have attracted lot of attention in the field of preclinical research. Several in vitro and in vivo studies have been conducted with the aim of assessing whether the aforementioned advantages of carbon ion radiotherapy (CIRT) have the potential to improve the radiotherapy outcomes and therefore to justify the construction of expensive CIRT facilities. Although the findings of performed studies in CIRT are definitely promising, the cost-effectiveness of building the CIRT facilities remains under discussion having its pros and cons. Returning to research, much effort has been put into observing the effects that high-LET carbon ions can exert on killing of tumor cells, especially hypoxic, radioresistant ones, immunogenic cell death, tumor invasiveness, migration, and metastatic spread.

Although many questions still need to be answered in that regarding, the available data are convincing making a good basis for translational research.

Tumor hypoxia is a major factor responsible for radioresistance, consequently leading to poor radiotherapy outcomes and prognosis in NSCLC (Eschmann et al. 2005; Vera et al. 2017). Since radiotherapy manifests its therapeutic efficacy by the formation of reactive oxygen species (ROS) following ionization of water in irradiated tissue, the lack of oxygen will significantly affect the radiotherapy killing of tumor cells (Quintiliani 1979). This "oxygen effect" is known as *the oxygen enhancement ratio (OER)* which represents the ratio of radiation doses necessary to achieve the same biological effect in terms of cells killing under hypoxic and normoxic conditions (Gray 1961). It is well known that for low energy transfer radiations (LET), like photons, OER corresponds to about 3, meaning that up to three times higher radiation dose is required to kill hypoxic tumor cells in respect to normoxic cells (Hall and Giaccia 2006). However, if the high-LET radiation is going to be used, like carbon ions, OER starts to reduce with LET above 100 keV/μm, reaching unity at high dose averaged LET-values of ~500 keV/μm (Furusawa et al. 2000). Thus, the hypoxia affects in minor measure tumor cell killing by carbon ions than by the photons. Klein et al. investigated effects of photon and carbon ion irradiation on tumor cell radiosensitivity under hypoxic conditions in NSCLC (Klein et al. 2017). Two human NSCLC cell lines, A549 and H1437, were irradiated with photons and carbon ions under hypoxia (1% O_2) and normoxia (21% O_2), and clonogenic survival was assessed. No significant oxygen effect was found following carbon ion irradiation, which was not the case with photon irradiation. Subtil et al. analyzed the effects of hypoxia-inducible factor (HIF)-1 signaling following carbon ion and photon irradiation in a human NSCLC model (Subtil et al. 2014). Following irradiation of A549 and H1299 cell lines, photons induced HIF-1α and target genes in oxygenated cells (1.6-fold; $P < 0.05$), with subsequent increased tumor angiogenesis (1.7-fold; $P < 0.05$). On the other hand, CIRT substantially diminished HIF-1α levels (8.9-fold; $P < 0.01$) and significantly delayed tumor growth ($P < 0.01$). Further research is required in order to confirm these findings, especially in a context of translational oncology research.

Very intriguing subject of research in modern radiation oncology represents *immunogenic cell death (ICD)*. ICD is a kind of cell death that triggers an immune antitumor response. ICD is characterized by the cell-surface expression of *damage associated molecular patterns (DAMPs)*, that as an "eat me" signal initiates phagocytosis of dying cancer cells (Garg et al. 2015). *Calreticulin (CRT)* is one of the most widely assessed DAMPs, accounting for the cell-biomarker for ICD (Obeid et al. 2007). It has been shown that radiotherapy is able of inducing ICD (Panaretakis et al. 2009), which in an ideal case may lead to a dramatic radiation-induced systemic antitumor immune response observable as a regression of an unirradiated, distant tumor lesion following irradiation of another tumor lesion (Demaria and Formenti 2013). This phenomenon is known as the abscopal effect. Huang et al. assessed the impact of CIRT on immune response in terms of *ICD* using four types of cancer cells, including A549 NSCLC cells (Huang et al. 2019). A549, U251MG glioma-cells, Tca8113 tongue squamous carcinoma cells, and CNE-2 nasopharyngeal carcinoma cells were exposed to photon-, proton- or carbon ion irradiation with 2, 4, and 10 Gy, and the cell-surface CRT level was analyzed by flow cytometry. Although all three types of radiation increased CRT exposure in all tumor cell lines, carbon ions exerted significantly stronger effects on CRT cell-surface expression than proton and photon radiation, which were equally effective. Furthermore, the same author performed similar study under normoxic and hypoxic conditions aimed to compare the effects of photons, protons, and carbon ions on the immune response, in terms of CRT, and programmed cell death ligand 1 (PDL1) expression (Huang et al. 2020). Again, four human tumor cell lines were irradiated with 4 Gy and the expression of CRT and PDL1 was detected 48 h after irradiation, and the median fluorescence intensities were compared by flow cytometry. Although all types of radiation inhibited significantly the colony formation of tumor cells under normoxia, the efficacy of photon and proton radiation, but not of carbon ion, was impaired under hypoxia. Under normoxia, CIRT enhanced CRT and PDL-1 expression compared to photon and proton radiation. However, under hypoxia, the CRT and PDL-1 expression levels were significantly upregulated at baseline, and radiation could not increase the expression further. Ohkubo et al. showed in the in vivo mouse experiments that CIRT upregulated membrane-associated immunogenic molecules (Ohkubo et al. 2010). They assessed the anti-metastatic lung efficacy of CIRT and immunotherapy by use of an in vivo murine model. Squamous cell carcinoma (NR-S1) cells were irradiated with 6 Gy single dose of carbon ions after being inoculated in the legs of C3H/HeSlc mice. Thirty-six hours after irradiation, α-galactosylceramide-pulsed dendritic cells were injected into the leg tumor. The untreated mice presented with 168 ± 53.8 metastatic nodules in the lungs, while the mice that have been treated presented with 2.6 ± 1.9 ($P = 0.009$) 2 weeks following irradiation. Furthermore, immunohistochemistry showed that *intracellular adhesion molecule 1* increased while the expression of S100A8 in lung tissue decreased only in the group treated with a combination of carbon ions and dendritic cells. More of exciting data on this topic can be found elsewhere (Shimokawa et al. 2016; Matsunaga et al. 2010).

The stage of the disease is the most important factor determining prognosis of cancer patients, where the metastatic disease dissemination usually represents the main cause of death (Mehlen and Puisieux 2006; Hanahan et al. 2011). Metastatic progression is a multi-step complex process beginning with loss of cellular polarity and adhesion followed by acquisition of motility and invasiveness with subsequent spread throughout the body (Fujita et al. 2015; Gandalovičová et al. 2016). For a successful metastasis, the migration and plasticity of cancer cells are required. In other words, metastatic progression involves evolution of well differentiated and organized cancer architecture to a migratory and invasive phenotype. Interestingly, accumulating evidence suggest that radiotherapy is able to affect the early metastatic process by hindering or even promoting it. Thus, it has been shown that low LET photon radiation may "improve" the plasticity of cancer cells leading to enhanced metastatic dissemination (Moncharmont et al. 2014). Several preclinical studies reported on this unfavorable aspect of photon radiation in lung but also pancreatic, sarcoma, glioma, head & neck, colon, liver, cervical, or prostate cancer cell lines (Fujita et al. 2011; Qian et al. 2002; Wild-Bode et al. 2001; Furmanova-Hollenstein et al. 2013; Ghosh et al. 2014; Kawamoto et al. 2012; Su et al. 2012; Yan et al. 2013; Pickhard et al. 2011; Cheng et al. 2006; Chang et al. 2013). On the contrary, due to a high LET, characterized by very dense ionization of traversed matter, CIRT is able of damaging subcellular organelles involved in early metastatic process, significantly affecting tumor cell ability to metastasize. Indeed, Akino et al. investigated the effects of CIRT on NSCLC cell proliferation, migration, and invasion. Two cell lines, A549 (lung adenocarcinoma) and EBC-1 (lung squamous cell carcinoma), were exposed to 4-MV X-ray and 290 MeV/nucleon carbon ion beam, respectively (Akino et al. 2009). Interestingly, X-ray increased cell proliferation at 0.5 Gy and by high-dose reduced migration and invasion of A549 cells. However, CIRT did not enhance proliferation, and it reduced the migration and invasion of both A549 and EBC-1 cells more effectively than X-ray. A very elegant in vivo experiment has been performed by Sato et al. who established a novel mouse model for assessing the tumor growth, metastatic potential, and radiosensitivity following repeated photon irradiation and CIRT (Sato et al. 2018). For that purpose, radioresistant NR-S1 squamous cell carcinoma cells arising from buccal mucosa were used, because of their ability to easily form metastatic nodules on the lung surface. After being inoculated into the right hind leg of C3H/He mouse, the tumors were treated with 30 or 15 Gy of photon or C-ion irradiation, respectively. The treated NR-S1 tumors were then transplanted into intact C3H/He mice 2 weeks following irradiation, and the regrown tumors were then again irradiated 2 weeks after the transplantation. This process was repeated six times, and tumor volume was measured. The photon irradiation promoted 2- to 3-fold tumor growth rate, lung metastasis and tumor microvessel formation, and 1.5- to 15-fold expression of angiogenic and metastatic genes in regrown tumors. The repeated CIRT did however not alter these characteristics. Similar findings in terms of suppression of the cancer metastatic potential by CIRT have been reported even for many other tumor cell lines (Takahashi et al. 2003; Ogata et al. 2005; Goetze et al. 2007; Rieken et al. 2012). It remains, however, to be seen whether these results can be reproduced in clinical practice in terms of prevention and control of the metastatic process.

4 Treatment Planning

Treatment planning of CIRT is a much more complex process compared to photon beam therapy, especially if dealing with moving targets. In order to benefit from the biophysical advantages of CIRT, maximal setup precision and high accuracy of tumor targeting and dose delivery are required. Generally, radiotherapy, especially the particle beam therapy of lung cancer is associated with substantial uncertainties related to the target movement, particle range uncertainties or anatomical changes (Kubiak 2016). The management of respiratory tumor motion occupies a special place in the CIRT planning process (Mori et al. 2018; Mohamad et al. 2018). Even a minor deviation from the planned dose delivery in terms of setup errors may have a much greater effect on the CIRT-dose distribution than is the case with photons, resulting in significant target underdosing with subsequent healthy tissue-overdosing (Karger et al. 2003). The reason for that is a very sharp distal dose fall off at the end of the Bragg peak, like previously discussed. Therefore, mitigation of such motion effects on treatment delivery is the main goal of the treatment planning, dealing with the management of interfractional and intrafractional motion. One of the major problems to face with in a CIRT treatment planning is a so-called interplay effect representing the deviation of the delivered from the planned radiation dose due to the motion between the tumor position and beam position (Dowdell et al. 2013). Treatment delivery technique, *passive beam scattering* or *active scanning*, respectively, affects the impact that tumor motion exerts on dose distribution (Mohamad et al. 2018; St James et al. 2018). In a case of conventional passive scattering, the monoenergetic beam is shaped by the passive collimators and compensators to be conformal with the tumor volume. More details on the passive scattering technique can be found elsewhere (Krämer et al. 2000). By the active scanning technique, a very narrow pencil beam delivers in an isoenergy "layer by layer," or slice by slice-fashion proper radiation dose to the "spots"-very small tumor segments, till the whole target volume will receive the planned dose (Haberer et al. 1993). Gesellschaft für Schwerionenforschung mbh (GSI) settled the hybrid scanning system with a pencil beam. Despite the fact that active scanning technique may offer an improved dose distribution that is more conformal, especially for irregular target shapes nearby critical structures, in a case of targets in motion that precision represents a "double sword" that may result in treatment failure. Several authors reported on inconsistency between beam scanning and target motion determining a very high sensitivity of active scanning technique to the target movement (Pedroni et al. 2004; Jäkel et al. 2007; Matsufuji et al. 2007; Mori et al. 2014a), compared to the passive beam scattering irradiation, which induced blurred dose distribution due to the motion. This is certainly of concern, considering that this kind of discrepancy may lead to an unwanted target-underdose with subsequent OAR-overdose, resulting in treatment failure and significant side effects. Additionally, since the stopping power of the traversed matter is given by tissue density within the beam path (for example, in order from the surface: skin, fat tissue, muscles, bones, and lung tissue) which determines the range of carbon ions, even the minor changes in tissue density during organs respiratory motion may significantly affect the CIRT delivery (Bert and

Durante 2011). Even a lesser skin shape changes (skin folds) due to a different patient positioning might be relevant. Finally, the anatomical changes during the treatment (for example, increase in the pleural effusion within the beam path, or tumor shrinkage) lead to the changes in tissue density affecting in that way the dose delivery in terms of particle range uncertainty. All these factors that do not significantly affect the success of the photon radiation treatment delivery are solid fragments integrated in the CIRT treatment planning.

Generally, in order to improve the CIRT-dose distribution, the *3D robust optimization* is performed to fine-tune the beam spot position and weight, or to advance the positional robustness by considering the worst-case scenario out of the various setup error scenarios, whereby the patient setup error is translated to a 3D-shift of the planning CT (Fredriksson et al. 2011). In a case of the organ motion, 3D robust optimization is integrated by the time-factor using a 4DCT dataset, an extended treatment planning being known as the *4D robust optimization* (Kanai et al. 2020). In such a case, the dose distribution will be calculated separately for each respiratory phase of 4DCT datasets in order to assess the internal motion scenario. Thus, an optimal CIRT treatment planning by NSCLC requires the 4D robust treatment plan optimization that needs to cover the evaluation of the worst-case scenario, internal motion scenarios, and setup error scenarios together.

Although it has a large clinical implication, positron emission tomography (PET) has been adopted also in the particle therapy treatment planning. The major concern in modern particle therapy planning remains the particle range uncertainty that is affected by several factors, most frequently represented by anatomical changes during the treatment (tumor response or progression, change in pleural effusion volume, atelectasis, etc.), imaging artifacts, an inappropriate conversion of the Hounsfield units into a particle stopping power, etc. All these and other factors can affect the particle range, or the total path length traversed by a charged particle before it will stop and deposit all its energy. Therefore, an appropriate particle range verification by treatment planning system proposed one plays the most important link in the treatment planning chain. Although several methods have been proposed for that purpose (Parodi and Polf 2018), the particle therapy positron emission tomography (PT-PET) has been proven and largely accepted to be appropriate for routine operation during patient treatments (Fiorina et al. 2018). A method is based on the nuclear reactions between the particles and the nuclei within the patient body whereby PT-PET measures positron emitter activity distribution along the beam path which will be compared to the predicted-calculated for the individual treatment plan. Thus, by improving the particle range verification, PT-PET might ideally allow for the reduction of the range-PTV margins further increasing the potential that particles may exert. More details on the use of PT-PET can be found elsewhere (Horst et al. 2019; Hofmann et al. 2019).

The effects of organ motion on dose delivery can be mitigated in different ways. Several strategies have been developed and successfully employed improving the radiotherapy outcomes in treatment of the thoracic and abdominal malignancies. These include the use of large margins covering the full range of motion (Ezhil et al. 2009), devices for limiting thoracic-abdominal respiration (Mampuya et al. 2014), respiratory restriction via breath-hold technique (Murphy et al. 2002), respiratory gating (Vedam et al. 2001), real-time dynamic tumor-tracking (Ceberg et al. 2010) and couching technique (Neicu et al. 2006). One of the most frequently used strategies to compensate for organ motion in the photon treatment planning is the addition of the geometrical margin in order to create the *internal target volume* (ITV). However, in CIRT treatment planning, the intrafractional organ motion causes deviations in the range of carbon ions which cannot fully be compensated by the conventional ITV-concept. Therefore, in CIRT, the *range-adapted ITV* is required and used for treatment planning (Knopf et al. 2013). More details on advances in motion management strategies can be found elsewhere (Minohara et al. 2000; Molitoris et al. 2018). Initially at

NIRS, respiratory gating was used for target motion management prior to scanning irradiation (Minohara et al. 2000). Although approximately half of the patients actually gained benefit from respiratory gating management, still this technology alone was showing the weaknesses (Mohamad et al. 2018). Due to a substantial interplay effect using scanned beams, significant deviations in dose distribution within the target have been observed indicating that respiratory gating was insufficient for motion management in scanning CIRT, if PTV was designed not considered range variations (Furukawa et al. 2017). Therefore, NIRS developed a combined approach adding to gating a fast phase-controlled rescanning, and range adapted-ITV based treatment planning, technology that allows fast re-irradiation of each point in the tumor multiple times within the respective gating window to average spot-spot doses, as a result, hot/cold spots could be suppressed (Mori et al. 2014b). Currently, Mori developed the real-time markerless respiratory-gated approach using deep learning networks in image processing (Mori 2017). The system that can track the tumor in real time using X-ray fluoroscopy without the fiducial markers can be applied on lung and liver treatments (Karube et al. 2016; Mori et al. 2016) and has been commissioned in 2019 (Mori et al. 2019). The feasibility study assessing the use of respiration-gated fast-rescanning CIRT has been recently published with the promising results (Ebner et al. 2017).

Within the last decade, CIRT technology has undergone significant advances that substantially improved CIRT performance, and this process continues very dynamically further to evolve (Kim et al. 2020). The current research and development trend, encompassing fast pencil beam scanning, a respiratory phase-controlled rescanning method for compensation of the interplay effects, superconducting rotating gantry or accurate beam modeling for the treatment planning system will further improve efficiency, robustness, and accuracy of CIRT for best patient-oriented care.

5 Clinical Outcomes of CIRT

In general, the extent of disease and the volume of the chest those require irradiation are important when considering the indication of radiation therapy for NSCLC. The same applies when considering the indication of CIRT for NSCLC. However, CIRT, which has a much better spatial dose distribution and biological effect than ordinary radiotherapy, makes it possible to safely perform radical treatment for high-risk cases like patients with poor lung function in a shorter period of time. Dosimetric studies showed an improved dose distribution with CIRT compared to photon radiotherapy for NSCLC in terms of lower OAR doses but more homogenous target coverage, potentially consenting for hypofractionation without increasing toxicity (Kubo et al. 2016). All clinical data on CIRT for NSCLC come from Japan.

Since October 1994, Japan has been conducting clinical trials of curative CIRT for NSCLC. The subjects are early-stage and locally advanced cases. Especially for early-stage case that occurs in the periphery of the lung field, a curative treatment could be established at the shortest once a day. In particular, recently, the indication has been expanded to early-stage NSCLC associated with interstitial pneumonia, and excellent treatment results have been obtained. Locally advanced NSCLC can be treated in about 4 weeks by combining mediastinal irradiation. The results of CIRT of NSCLC in the locally advanced case are also quite promising without concomitant chemotherapy. In the last 5 years, more than 500 patients with NSCLC have been treated with radical CIRT in Japan.

Regarding *the stage I peripheral NSCLC*, two dose-escalation studies were conducted from 1994 to 1999 at the NIRS. The initial study was using 18 fractions over 6 weeks, and then followed by the 9 fractions over 3 weeks. Initial study using 18 fractions demonstrated quite safe nature of carbon ion beam (the total dose was reached 90 Gy (RBE) without severe side effects). The next dose searching study using 3 weeks regimen was conducted, and it revealed that

72 Gy (RBE) in 9 fractions over 3 weeks was the most appropriate dose (Miyamoto et al. 2003). A phase II fixed dose study using 72 Gy (RBE) in 9 fractions over 3 weeks was conducted on 50 patients during the period of 1999 to 2000. With the median follow-up of 59.2 months, the 5-year local control (LC) rate and overall survival (OS) rate were 94.7% and 50%, respectively. Late grade 3 pulmonary radiographic reactions were observed in 15 patients and 10 grade 3 skin reactions were experienced in this study (Miyamoto et al. 2007a). Just after this study, from 2000 to 2003, another phase II trial using the total dose of 52.8 Gy (RBE) for stage IA and 60 Gy (RBE) for stage IIB in four fractions over 1 week was conducted on 79 patients. With the median follow-up of 38.6 months, the 5-year LC rate and OS rate were 90% and 45%, respectively. No late grade 3 or higher reactions were observed in the study (Miyamoto et al. 2007b). Also, the Gunma University Heavy Ion Medical Center in Japan performed in the time-period June 2010–March 2015, a phase II study assessing the efficacy and safety of hypofractionated CIRT in patients with stage I peripheral NSCLC (Saitoh et al. 2019). Thirty-seven patients with T1 and T2a tumors were treated with 52.8 Gy (RBE) and 60 Gy (RBE) in four fractions over 1 week, respectively. With an overall follow-up time of 56.3 months, and 62.2 months in the surviving patients, the actuarial LC rates of 91.2% and 88.1%, and OS rates of 91.9% and 74.9% were achieved after 2 and 5 years, respectively. Since there was no differences found between the T1 and T2a tumors in the 5-year LC rate (90.9% vs 86.7%, $P = 0.75$), T1 tumors showed better actuarial 5-year OS rates compared to T2a tumors: 80% vs. 66.7%. Finally, among the patients with T1 tumors there were no any ≥grade II toxicity, while two patients with T2a tumors experienced ≥grade 2 lung toxicity.

Interestingly, several authors reported on the prognostic value of the 18F-fluorodeoxyglucose (FDG) positron emission tomography/computer tomography (PET/CT) by early-stage NSCLC patients treated with CIRT. It is known that 18F-FDG PET/CT plays an important role in diagnose, staging, and treatment planning of NSCLC (Gallamini et al. 2014), but in addition it also offers a significant prognostic value in terms of the parameters like maximum standardized uptake value (SUVmax), metabolic tumor volume (MTV), and total lesion glycolysis (TLG) (Satoh et al. 2014). Shirai et al. assessed a pretreatment prognostic value of *maximum standardized uptake value (SUVmax)* among 45 patients with T1a-b and T2a NSCLC, treated with CIRT at a dose of 52.8 Gy (RBE) and 60.0 Gy (RBE), respectively, in four fractions (Shirai et al. 2017). For the analysis of the SUVmax predictive value, all patients were selected in two groups based on the mean NSCLC-SUVmax corresponding to 5.5: higher (≥5.5) and lower (<5.5) SUVmax groups. With the median follow-up time of 28.9 months, the 2-year LC, PFS, and OS rates were 93, 78, and 89%, respectively. Considering the SUVmax, those patients from the higher SUVmax group presented a significantly worse 2-years PFS and OS (61% and 76% ($P = 0.01$)) compared with the lower SUVmax group (89% and 96% ($P = 0.01$)), respectively. SUVmax has not predicted for the LC rate. Additionally, Shrestha et al. assessed the prognostic significance of volumetric FDG PET/CT parameters in CIRT for stage I NSCLC (Shrestha et al. 2020). They found that MTV predicted OS (HR 4.83, 95% CI 1.21–19.27, $P < 0.03$) and PFS (HR 5.3, CI 1.32–21.35, $P < 0.02$), independently. Its prognostic significance was highly reproducible, reliable, and even superior to tumor size in the OS and PFS, which has significant clinical implications, offering a possibility for selection of more aggressive stage I NSCLC types that might benefit from more aggressive treatments.

Based on the promising results of initial trials, NIRS decided to conducted a single-fraction phase I/II study that ends treatment in a day. A dose of 28 Gy (RBE) was employed as a starting dose, and then the dose was increased by 2 Gy (RBE). A total of 218 patients were enrolled in the study, the total dose was increased up to 50 Gy (RBE), and clinical trial was completed. With the median follow-up of 57.8 months, the 5-year LC rate and OS rate of all cases were 72.7% and 49.4%, respectively. In 20 patients treated with the dose of 48 to 50 Gy (RBE), the 5-year LC rate and OS were 95% and 69.2%, respectively. No late grade 3 or higher reactions were observed, and only 2% grade 2 toxicities were experienced in the single-fraction trial (Yamamoto et al. 2017). Few years later, Ono et al. published a long-term results of single-fraction CIRT for NSCLC (Ono et al. 2020). Fifty-seven patients with histologically confirmed stage T1-2N0M0 NSCLC, treated between June 2011 and April 2016 with 50 Gy (RBE) single-fraction CIRT were included. With the median follow-up time of 61 months (range: 6–97 months), the 3- and 5-year OS rates were 91.2% and 81.7%, while the 3- and 5-year LC rates were 96.4% and 91.8%, respectively. In addition to an excellent long-term OS and LC rate, no cases of ≥grade 2 pneumonitis were recorded, suggesting that single-fraction CIRT could be the treatment of choice for early-stage NSCLC in inoperable patients.

It is known that treatment of **NSCLC associated with interstitial lung disease (ILD)** is difficult. It is often experienced that no curative treatment is available for lung cancer with severe ILD. Between 2004 and 2014, 29 patients diagnosed with NSCLC and ILD were treated with CIRT. No patient was eligible for curative surgery or conventional radiotherapy secondary to ILD. With the median follow-up of 22.8 months, single-grade symptomatic progression (grade 2–3) was observed in 4 patients, while 1 patient experienced two-grade progression. Two patients experienced radiation-induced acute exacerbation. LC at 3 years was 63.3% (72.2% for stage I disease); OS at 3 years was 46.3% (57.2% for stage I disease). Radiation pneumonitis post-treatment progression correlated with dosimetric factors of the lungs (V5, V10) and a low pretreatment serum surfactant protein-D. CIRT could be useful as a low-risk, curative option for NSCLC patients with ILD, a population that is typically ineligible for conventional therapy. The DVH analysis showed that minimizing the low-dose region is important for reducing the risk of severe RP (Nakajima et al. 2017).

NIRS reported the treatment results of 141 cases of **locally advanced NSCLC (stage II, III)** who received CIRT between 1995 and 2015. The median age at the time of treatment was 75 years (range 40–88), of which T1: 21, T2: 57, T3: 43, T4: 20, N0: 51, N1: 45, N2: 40, N3: 5. The clinical stage was 2A: 34, 2B: 42, 3A: 45, 3B: 20 cases. There were 62 adenocarcinoma, 60 squamous cell carcinoma, 8 large cell carcinoma, and 11 others. The median dose was 72.0 Gy (RBE) (range 54.0–76.0). No patient received concurrent chemotherapy. Median follow-up periods were 29.3 (range 1.6–207.7) and 40.0 (range 10.7–207.7) months for all patients and survivors, respectively. Two-year LC, progression free survival, and OS rates were 80.3%, 40.2%, and 58.7%, respectively. There were 1 grade 4 mediastinal hemorrhage and 6 grade 3 pulmonary toxicities. Of these 141 patients, 32 were 80 years or older (median 82, range 80–88). With median follow-up of 22.4 months, the 2-year LC and OS were 83.5% and 68.0%, respectively. Only 1 patient experienced grade 3 radiation pneumonitis. Multivariate analysis showed adenocarcinoma and N2/3 classification as significant poor prognosticators of progression free survival. CIRT is an effective treatment with acceptable toxicity for locally advanced NSCLC, especially for elderly, age over 80 years, or patients with severe comorbidities who cannot be treated with surgery or chemo-radiotherapy (Hayashi et al. 2019, 2021; Anzai et al. 2020).

Very recently, the first study assessing the potential benefits of **CIRT compared to SBRT for early-stage NSCLC** has been published. Miyasaka et al. reported on a retrospective, single-institutional, and contemporaneous comparison study, which determined the differences in treatment outcomes between CIRT and SBRT in the management of early-stage NSCLC (Miyasaka et al. 2021). These propensity score-adjusted analyses showed improved treatment outcomes in favor of CIRT being the 3-year OS and LC rates 80.1% versus 71.6% ($P = 0.0077$) and 87.7% versus 79.1% ($P = 0.037$), respectively.

Potential advantages of **CIRT** have also been explored in patients affected by lung recurrences in terms of **lung re-irradiation**. Hayashi et al. reported in 2018 on the toxicity and efficacy of re-irradiation with CIRT. Ninety-five patients previously treated with CIRT were submitted between 2006 and 2016 to re-CIRT because of locoregionally recurrent, metastatic, or secondary lung tumors (Hayashi et al. 2018). Although the initial treatment was quite aggressive considering the hypofractionated regimens performed in 1–16 fractions with the median total dose of 52.8 Gy (RBE), the re-irradiation with CIRT has been given as in 12–16 fractions hypofractionated treatment with the median dose of 66.0 Gy (RBE). With the median follow-up time of 18 months, one patient experienced each of the following: grade 3 radiation pneumonitis and chest pain, grade 4 radiation pneumonitis, and grade 5 bronchopleural fistula. The 2-year LC and OS rates were 54.0% and 61.9%, respectively. Thus, re-CIRT can be offered as a fairly safe and moderately effective treatment option to the previously irradiated patients with recurrent primary or secondary lung cancer.

Although CIRT showed a very promising treatment outcomes in NSCLC, there are no to date, however, randomized controlled trials reporting on the long-term effectiveness and safety related to the use of CIRT and so it remains to be considered as an experimental treatment due to the lack of high-quality clinical research.

References

Akino Y, Teshima T, Kihara A, Kodera-Suzumoto Y, Inaoka M, Higashiyama S, Furusawa Y, Matsuura N (2009) Carbon-ion beam irradiation effectively suppresses migration and invasion of human non-small-cell lung cancer cells. Int J Radiat Oncol Biol Phys 75(2):475–481. https://doi.org/10.1016/j.ijrobp.2008.12.090

Anzai M, Yamamoto N, Hayashi K, Nakajima M, Nomoto A, Ogawa K, Tsuji H (2020) Safety and efficacy of carbon-ion radiotherapy alone for stage III non-small cell lung cancer. Anticancer Res 40(1):379–386. https://doi.org/10.21873/anticanres

Bert C, Durante M (2011) Motion in radiotherapy: particle therapy. Phys Med Biol 56(16):R113–R144. https://doi.org/10.1088/0031-9155/56/16/R01. Epub 2011 Jul 20

Ceberg S, Falk M, Af Rosenschöld PM et al (2010) Tumor-tracking radiotherapy of moving targets; verification using 3D polymer gel, 2D ion-chamber array and biplanar diode array. J Phys Conf Ser 250:012051

Chang L, Graham PH, Hao J, Ni J, Bucci J, Cozzi PJ et al (2013) Acquisition of epithelial-mesenchymal transition and cancer stem cell phenotypes is associated with activation of the PI3K/Akt/mTOR pathway in prostate cancer radioresistance. Cell Death Dis 4:e875

Cheng JC, Chou CH, Kuo ML, Hsieh CY (2006) Radiation-enhanced hepatocellular carcinoma cell invasion with MMP-9 expression throughPI3K/Akt/NF-kappa B signal transduction pathway. Oncogene 25:7009–7018

de Cos JS, Miravet L, Abal J et al (2008) Lung cancer survival in Spain and prognostic factors: a prospective, multiregional study. Lung Cancer 59:246–254

Demaria S, Formenti S (2013) Radiotherapy effects on anti-tumor immunity: implications for cancer treatment. Front Oncol 3:128. https://doi.org/10.3389/fonc.2013.00128

Dillman RO, Zusman DR, McClure SE (2009) Surgical resection and long-term survival for octogenarians who undergo surgery for non-small-cell lung cancer. Clin Lung Cancer 10:130–134

Dowdell S, Grassberger C, Sharp GC, Paganetti H (2013) Interplay effects in proton scanning for lung: a 4D Monte Carlo study assessing the impact of tumor and beam delivery parameters. Phys Med Biol 58(12):4137–4156. https://doi.org/10.1088/0031-9155/58/12/4137. Epub 2013 May 20

Ebner DK, Tsuji H, Yasuda S, Yamamoto N, Mori S, Kamada T (2017) Respiration-gated fast-rescanning carbon-ion radiotherapy. Jpn J Clin Oncol 47(1):80–83. https://doi.org/10.1093/jjco/hyw144. Epub 2016 Sep 27

Eschmann SM, Paulsen F, Reimold M et al (2005) Prognostic impact of hypoxia imaging with 18F-misonidazole PET in non-small cell lung cancer and head and neck cancer before radiotherapy. J Nucl Med 46:253–260

Ezhil M, Vedam S, Balter P et al (2009) Determination of patient-specific internal gross tumor volumes for lung cancer using four-dimensional computed tomography. Radiat Oncol 4:4

Fiorina E, Ferrero V, Pennazio F et al (2018) Monte Carlo simulation tool for online treatment monitoring in hadron therapy with in-beam PET: a patient study. Phys Med 51:71–80. https://doi.org/10.1016/j.ejmp.2018.05.002

Fossati P, Molinelli S, Matsufuji N et al (2012) Dose prescription in carbon ion radiotherapy: a planning study to compare NIRS and LEM approaches with a clinically-oriented strategy. Phys Med Biol 57(22):7543–7554. https://doi.org/10.1088/0031-9155/57/22/7543

Fredriksson A, Forsgren A, Hårdemark B (2011) Minimax optimization for handling range and setup uncertainties in proton therapy. Med Phys 38(3):1672–1684. https://doi.org/10.1118/1.3556559

Free CM, Ellis M, Beggs D et al (2007) Lung cancer outcomes at a UK cancer unit between 1998-2001. Lung Cancer 57:222–228

Fujita M, Otsuka Y, Yamada S, Iwakawa M, Imai T (2011) X-ray irradiation and Rho-kinase inhibitor additively induce invasiveness of the cells of the pancreatic cancer line, MIAPaCa-2, which exhibits mesenchymal and amoeboid motility. Cancer Sci 102:792–798

Fujita M, Yamadab S, Imaia T (2015) Irradiation induces diverse changes in invasive potential in cancer cell lines. Semin Cancer Biol 35:45–52. https://doi.org/10.1016/j.semcancer.2015.09.003

Furmanova-Hollenstein P, Broggini-Tenzer A, Eggel M, Millard AL, Pruschy M (2013) The microtubule stabilizer patupilone counteracts ionizing radiation-induced matrix metalloproteinase activity and tumor cell invasion. Radiat Oncol 8:105

Furukawa T, Hara Y, Mizushima K, Saotome N, Tansho R, Saraya Y, Inaniwa T, Mori S, Iwata Y, Shirai T et al (2017) Development of NIRS pencil beam scanning system for carbon ion radiotherapy. Nucl Instrum Methods Phys Res B 406:361–367

Furusawa Y, Fukutsu K, Aoki M et al (2000) Inactivation of aerobic and hypoxic cells from three different cell lines by accelerated (3)He-, (12)C- and (20)Ne-ion beams. Radiat Res 154(5):485–496. https://doi.org/10.1667/0033-7587(2000)154[0485:ioaahc]2.0.co;2

Gallamini A, Zwarthoed C, Borra A (2014) Positron emission tomography (PET) in oncology. Cancers (Basel) 6(4):1821–1889. https://doi.org/10.3390/cancers6041821

Gandalovičová A, Vomastek T, Rosel D, Brábek J (2016) Cell polarity signaling in the plasticity of cancer cell invasiveness. Oncotarget 7(18):25022–25049. https://doi.org/10.18632/oncotarget.7214

Garg AD, Dudek-Peric A, Romano E et al (2015) Immunogenic cell death. Int J Dev Biol 59:131–140. https://doi.org/10.1387/ijdb.150061pa

Ghosh S, Kumar A, Tripathi RP, Chandna S (2014) Connexin-43 regulatesp38-mediated cell migration and invasion induced selectively in tumour cells by low doses of gamma-radiation in an ERK-1/2-independent manner. Carcinogenesis 35:383–395

Goetze K, Scholz M, Taucher-Scholz G, Mueller-Klieser W (2007) The impact of conventional and heavy ion irradiation on tumor cell migration in vitro. Int J Radiat Biol 83(11–12):889–896. https://doi.org/10.1080/09553000701753826

Goldstraw P, Chansky K, Crowley J et al (2016) The IASLC lung cancer staging project: proposals for revision of the TNM stage groupings in the forthcoming (eighth) edition of the TNM classification for lung cancer. J Thorac Oncol 11:39–51

Gray LH (1961) Radiobiologic basis of oxygen as a modifying factor in radiation therapy. Am J Roentgenol Radium Ther Nucl Med 85:803–815

Haberer T, Becher W, Schardt D, Kraft G (1993) Magnetic scanning system for heavy ion therapy. Nucl Instrum Methods Phys Res A 330:296–305

Hall E, Giaccia A (2006) Radiobiology for the radiologist, 6th edn. Lippincott Williams & Wilkins, Philadelphia

Hanahan D, Weinberg RA, Adams JM et al (2011) Hallmarks of cancer: the next generation. Cell 144:646–674

Hayashi K, Yamamoto N, Karube M, Nakajima M, Tsuji H, Ogawa K, Kamada T (2018) Feasibility of carbon-ion radiotherapy for re-irradiation of locoregionally recurrent, metastatic, or secondary lung tumors. Cancer Sci 109(5):1562–1569. https://doi.org/10.1111/cas.13555

Hayashi K, Yamamoto N, Nakajima M, Nomoto A, Tsuji H, Ogawa K, Kamada T (2019) Clinical outcomes of CIRT for locally advanced NSCLC. Cancer Sci 110(2):734–741

Hayashi K, Yamamoto N, Nakajima M, Nomoto A, Ishikawa H, Ogawa K, Tsuji H (2021) Carbon-ion radiotherapy for octogenarians with locally advanced non-small-cell lung cancer. Jpn J Radiol 39:703. https://doi.org/10.1007/s11604-021-01101-z

Hofmann T, Pinto M, Mohammadi A et al (2019) Dose reconstruction from PET images in carbon ion therapy: a deconvolution approach. Phys Med Biol 64(2):025011. https://doi.org/10.1088/1361-6560/aaf676

Horst F, Adi W, Aricò G et al (2019) Measurement of PET isotope production cross sections for protons and carbon ions on carbon and oxygen targets for applications in particle therapy range verification. Phys Med Biol 64(20):205012. https://doi.org/10.1088/1361-6560/ab4511

Huang Y, Dong Y, Zhao J, Zhang L, Kong L, Lu JJ (2019) Comparison of the effects of photon, proton and carbon-ion radiation on the ecto-calreticulin exposure in various tumor cell lines. Ann Transl Med 7(20):542. https://doi.org/10.21037/atm.2019.09.128

Huang Y, Huang Q, Zhao J, Dong Y, Zhang L, Fang X, Sun P, Kong L, Lu JJ (2020) The impacts of different types of radiation on the CRT and PDL1 expression in tumor cells under normoxia and hypoxia. Front Oncol 10:1610. https://doi.org/10.3389/fonc.2020.01610

ICRU (2016) ICRU Report 93. J ICRU2 16(1–2):3–211. https://academic.oup.com/jicru/issue/16/1-2

Inaniwa T, Kanematsu N, Matsufuji N et al (2015) Reformulation of a clinical-dose system for carbon-ion radiotherapy treatment planning at the National Institute of Radiological Sciences, Japan. Phys Med Biol 60(8):3271–3286. https://doi.org/10.1088/0031-9155/60/8/3271

Jäkel O, Schulz-Ertner D, Debus J (2007) Specifying carbon ion doses for radiotherapy: the Heidelberg approach. J Radiat Res 48(Suppl A):A87–A95. https://doi.org/10.1269/jrr.48.a87

Jeremic B, Classen J, Bamberg M (2002) Radiotherapy alone technically operable, medically inoperable, early-stage (I/II) non-small-cell lung cancer. Int J Radiat Oncol Biol Phys 54:119–130

Kanai T, Furusawa Y, Fukutsu K et al (1997) Irradiation of mixed beam and design of spread out Bragg peak for heavy-ion radiotherapy. Radiat Res 147:78–85

Kanai T, Endo M, Minohara S, Miyahara N, Koyamaito H, Tomura H, Matsufuji N, Futami Y, Fukumura A, Hiraoka T, Furusawa Y, Ando K, Suzuki M, Soga F, Kawachi K (1999) Biophysical characteristics of HIMAC clinical irradiation system for heavy-ion radiation therapy. Int J Radiat Oncol Biol Phys 44(1):201–210. https://doi.org/10.1016/s0360-3016(98)00544-6

Kanai T, Matsufuji N, Miyamoto T et al (2006) Examination of GyE system for HIMAC carbon therapy. Int J Radiat Oncol 64(2):650–656. https://doi.org/10.1016/j.ijrobp.2005.09.043

Kanai T, Paz A, Furuichi W, Liu CS, He P, Mori S (2020) Four-dimensional carbon-ion pencil beam treatment planning comparison between robust optimization and range-adapted internal target volume for respiratory-gated liver and lung treatment. Phys Med 80:277–287. https://doi.org/10.1016/j.ejmp.2020.11.009

Karger CP, Schulz-Ertner D, Didinger BH, Debus J, Jäkel O (2003) Influence of setup errors on spinal cord dose and treatment plan quality for cervical spine tumours: a phantom study for photon IMRT and heavy charged particle radiotherapy. Phys Med Biol 48(19):3171–3189. https://doi.org/10.1088/0031-9155/48/19/006

Karube M, Mori S, Tsuji H, Yamamoto N, Nakajima M, Nakagawa K, Kamada T (2016) Carbon-ion pencil beam scanning for thoracic treatment—initiation report and dose metrics evaluation. J Radiat Res 57:576–581

Kawamoto A, Yokoe T, Tanaka K, Saigusa S, Toiyama Y, Yasuda H et al (2012) Radiation induces epithelial-mesenchymal transition in colorectal cancer cells. Oncol Rep 27:51–57

Kim H, Yoo H, Pyo H et al (2019) Impact of underlying pulmonary diseases on treatment outcomes in early-stage non-small cell lung cancer treated with definitive radiotherapy. Int J Chron Obstruct Pulmon Dis 14:2273–2281

Kim J, Park JM, Wu H (2020) Carbon ion therapy: a review of an advanced technology. Progress Med Phys 31:71–80. https://doi.org/10.14316/pmp.2020.31.3.71

Klein C, Dokic I, Mairani A et al (2017) Overcoming hypoxia-induced tumor radioresistance in non-small cell lung cancer by targeting DNA-dependent protein kinase in combination with carbon ion irradiation. Radiat Oncol 12:208. https://doi.org/10.1186/s13014-017-0939-0

Knopf AC, Boye D, Lomax A, Mori S (2013) Adequate margin definition for scanned particle therapy in the incidence of intrafractional motion. Phys Med Biol 58:6079–6094

Koyi H, Hillerdal G, Brandén E (2002) A prospective study of a total material of lung cancer from a county in Sweden 1997-1999: gender, symptoms, type, stage, and smoking habits. Lung Cancer 36:9–14

Krämer M, Scholz M (2000) Treatment planning for heavy-ion radiotherapy: calculation and optimization of biologically effective dose. Phys Med Biol 45(11):3319–3330. https://doi.org/10.1088/0031-9155/45/11/314

Krämer M, Jäkel O, Haberer T, Kraft G, Schardt D, Weber U (2000) Treatment planning for heavy-ion radiotherapy: physical beam model and dose optimization. Phys Med Biol 45(11):3299–3317. https://doi.org/10.1088/0031-9155/45/11/313

Kubiak T (2016) Particle therapy of moving targets-the strategies for tumour motion monitoring and moving targets irradiation. Br J Radiol 89(1066):20150275. https://doi.org/10.1259/bjr.20150275. Epub 2016 Jul 19

Kubo N, Saitoh JI, Shimada H, Shirai K, Kawamura H, Ohno T et al (2016) Dosimetric comparison of carbon ion and X-ray radiotherapy for stage IIIA non-small cell lung cancer. J Radiat Res 57:548–554. https://doi.org/10.1093/jrr/rrw041

Little AG, Rusch VW, Bonner JA et al (2005) Patterns of surgical care of lung cancer patients. Ann Thorac Surg 80:2051–2056; discussion 2056

Mampuya WA, Matsuo Y, Ueki N et al (2014) The impact of abdominal compression on outcome in patients treated with stereotactic body radiotherapy for primary lung cancer. J Radiat Res 55(5):934–939

Matsufuji N, Kanai T, Kanematsu N, Miyamoto T, Baba M, Kamada T, Kato H, Yamada S, Mizoe JE, Tsujii H (2007) Specification of carbon ion dose at the National Institute of Radiological Sciences (NIRS). J Radiat Res 48(Suppl A):A81–A86. https://doi.org/10.1269/jrr.48.a81

Matsunaga A, Ueda Y, Yamada S, Harada Y, Shimada H, Hasegawa M, Tsujii H, Ochiai T, Yonemitsu Y (2010) Carbon-ion beam treatment induces systemic antitumor immunity against murine squamous cell carcinoma. Cancer 116(15):3740–3748. https://doi.org/10.1002/cncr.25134

Mehlen P, Puisieux A (2006) Metastasis: a question of life or death. Nat Rev Cancer 6:449–458

Minohara S, Kanai T, Endo M, Noda K, Kanazawa M (2000) Respiratory gated irradiation system for heavy-ion radiotherapy. Int J Radiat Oncol Biol Phys 47:1097–1103

Miyamoto T, Yamamoto N, Nishimura H, Koto M, Tsujii H, Mizoe J, Kamada T, Kato H, Yamada S, Morita S, Yoshikawa K, Kandatsu S, Fujisawa T (2003) Carbon ion radiotherapy for stage I non-small cell lung cancer. Radiother Oncol 66:127–140

Miyamoto T, Baba M, Yamamoto N, Koto M, Sugawara T, Yashiro T, Kadono K, Ezawa H, Tsujii H, Mizoe J, Kamada T, Kato H, Yamada S, Morita S, Yoshikawa K, Kandatsu S, Fujisawa T (2007a) Curative treatment of stage I non-small-cell lung cancer with carbon ion beams using a hypofractionated regimen. Int J Radiat Oncol Biol Phys 67(3):750–758

Miyamoto T, Baba M, Sugane T, Nakajima M, Yashiro T, Kagei K, Hirasawa N, Sugawara T, Yamamoto N, Koto M, Ezawa H, Kadono K, Tsujii H, Mizoe J, Yoshikawa K, Kandatsu S, Fujisawa T (2007b) Carbon ion radiotherapy for stage I non-small-cell lung cancer using a regimen of four fractions during 1 week. J Thorac Oncol 2(10):916–926

Miyasaka Y, Komatsu S, Abe T, Kubo N, Okano N, Shibuya K, Shirai K, Kawamura H, Saitoh JI, Ebara T, Ohno T (2021) Comparison of oncologic outcomes between carbon ion radiotherapy and stereotactic body radiotherapy for early-stage non-small cell lung cancer. Cancers (Basel) 13(2):176. https://doi.org/10.3390/cancers13020176

Mohamad O, Makishima H, Kamada T (2018) Evolution of carbon ion radiotherapy at the National Institute of Radiological Sciences in Japan. Cancers (Basel) 10(3):66. https://doi.org/10.3390/cancers10030066

Molinelli S, Magro G, Mairani A et al (2016) Dose prescription in carbon ion radiotherapy: how to compare two different RBE-weighted dose calculation systems. Radiother Oncol 120(2):307–312. https://doi.org/10.1016/j.radonc.2016.05.031

Molitoris JK, Diwanji T, Snider JW 3rd, Mossahebi S, Samanta S, Badiyan SN, Simone CB 2nd, Mohindra P (2018) Advances in the use of motion management and image guidance in radiation therapy treatment for lung cancer. J Thorac Dis 10(Suppl 21):S2437–S2450. https://doi.org/10.21037/jtd.2018.01.155

Moncharmont C, Levy A, Guy JB, Falk AT, Guilbert M, Trone JC et al (2014) Radiation-enhanced cell migration/invasion process: a review. Crit RevOncol Hematol 92:133–142

Mori S (2017) Deep architecture neural network-based real-time image processing for image-guided radiotherapy. Phys Med 40:79–87. https://doi.org/10.1016/j.ejmp.2017.07.013. Epub 2017 Jul 23

Mori S, Zenklusen S, Inaniwa T, Furukawa T, Imada H, Shirai T, Noda K, Yasuda S (2014a) Conformity and robustness of gated rescanned carbon ion pencil beam scanning of liver tumors at NIRS. Radiother Oncol 111(3):431–436. https://doi.org/10.1016/j.radonc.2014.03.009. Epub 2014 Apr 28

Mori S, Inaniwa T, Miki K, Shirai T, Noda K (2014b) Implementation of a target volume design function for intrafractional range variation in a particle beam treatment planning system. Br J Radiol 87:20140233

Mori S, Karube M, Shirai T, Tajiri M, Takekoshi T, Miki K, Shiraishi Y, Tanimoto K, Shibayama K, Yasuda S et al (2016) Carbon-ion pencil beam scanning treatment with gated markerless tumor tracking: an analysis of positional accuracy. Int J Radiat Oncol Biol Phys 95:258–266

Mori S, Knopf AC, Umegaki K (2018) Motion management in particle therapy. Med Phys 45(11):e994–e1010. https://doi.org/10.1002/mp.12679

Mori S, Sakata Y, Hirai R, Furuichi W, Shimabukuro K, Kohno R, Koom WS, Kasai S, Okaya K, Iseki Y (2019) Commissioning of a fluoroscopic-based real-time markerless tumor tracking system in a superconducting rotating gantry for carbon-ion pencil beam scanning treatment. Med Phys 46(4):1561–1574. https://doi.org/10.1002/mp.13403

Mountain CF (1997) Revisions in the international system for staging lung cancer. Chest 111:1710–1717

Murphy MJ, Martin D, Whyte R, Hai J, Ozhasoglu C, Le QT (2002) The effectiveness of breath-holding to stabilize lung and pancreas tumors during radiosurgery. Int J Radiat Oncol Biol Phys 53(2):475–482

Nakajima M, Yamamoto N, Hayashi K, Karube M, Ebner D, Takahashi W, Anzai M, Tsushima K, Tada Y, Tatsumi K, Miyamoto T, Tsuji H, Fujisawa T, Kamada T (2017) Carbon-ion radiotherapy for non-small cell lung cancer with interstitial lung disease: a retrospective analysis. Radiat Oncol 12(1):144

Naruke T, Tsuchiya R, Kondo H et al (2001) Prognosis and survival after resection for bronchogenic carcinoma based on the 1997 TNM-staging classification: the Japanese experience. Ann Thorac Surg 71:1759–1764

Neicu T, Berbeco R, Wolfgang J, Jiang SB (2006) Synchronized moving aperture radiation therapy (SMART): improvement of breathing pattern reproducibility using respiratory coaching. Phys Med Biol 51:617–636

Obeid M, Tesniere A, Ghiringhelli F et al (2007) Calreticulin exposure dictates the immunogenicity of cancer cell death. Nat Med 13:54–61. https://doi.org/10.1038/nm1523

Ogata T, Teshima T, Kagawa K, Hishikawa Y, Takahashi Y, Kawaguchi A, Suzumoto Y, Nojima K, Furusawa Y, Matsuura N (2005) Particle irradiation suppresses metastatic potential of cancer cells. Cancer Res 65(1):113–120

Ohkubo Y, Iwakawa M, Seino K, Nakawatari M, Wada H, Kamijuku H, Nakamura E, Nakano T, Imai T (2010) Combining carbon ion radiotherapy and local injection of α-galactosyl ceramide-pulsed dendritic cells inhibits lung metastases in an in vivo murine model. Int J Radiat Oncol Biol Phys 78(5):1524–1531. https://doi.org/10.1016/j.ijrobp.2010.06.048

Ono T, Yamamoto N, Nomoto A, Nakajima M, Isozaki Y, Kasuya G, Ishikawa H, Nemoto K, Tsuji H (2020) Long term results of single-fraction carbon-ion radiotherapy for non-small cell lung cancer. Cancers (Basel) 13(1):112. https://doi.org/10.3390/cancers13010112

Panaretakis T, Kepp O, Brockmeier U et al (2009) Mechanisms of pre-apoptotic calreticulin exposure in immunogenic cell death. EMBO J 28:578–590. https://doi.org/10.1038/emboj.2009.1

Parodi K, Polf JC (2018) In vivo range verification in particle therapy. Med Phys 45:e1037–e1050

Pedroni E, Bearpark R, Böhringer T, Coray A, Duppich J, Forss S, George D, Grossmann M, Goitein G, Hilbes C, Jermann M, Lin S, Lomax A, Negrazus M, Schippers M, Kotle G (2004) The PSI gantry 2: a second generation proton scanning gantry. Z Med Phys 14(1):25–34. https://doi.org/10.1078/0939-3889-00194

Pickhard AC, Margraf J, Knopf A, Stark T, Piontek G, Beck C et al (2011) Inhibition of radiation induced migration of human head and neck squamous cell carcinoma cells by blocking of EGF receptor pathways. BMC Cancer 11:388

Qian LW, Mizumoto K, Urashima T et al (2002) Radiation-induced increase in invasive potential of human pancreatic cancer cells and its blockade by a matrix metalloproteinase inhibitor, CGS27023. Clin Cancer Res 8:1223–1227

Quintiliani M (1979) Modification of radiation sensitivity: the oxygen effect. Int J Radiat Oncol Biol Phys 5(7):1069–1076. https://doi.org/10.1016/0360-3016(79)90621-7

Rieken S, Habermehl D, Wuerth L, Brons S, Mohr A, Lindel K, Weber K, Haberer T, Debus J, Combs SE (2012) Carbon ion irradiation inhibits glioma cell migration through downregulation of integrin expression. Int J Radiat Oncol Biol Phys 83(1):394–399. https://doi.org/10.1016/j.ijrobp.2011.06.2004. Epub 2011 Nov 4

Saitoh JI, Shirai K, Mizukami T, Abe T, Ebara T, Ohno T, Minato K, Saito R, Yamada M, Nakano T (2019) Hypofractionated carbon-ion radiotherapy for stage I peripheral non small cell lung cancer (GUNMA0701): prospective phase II study. Cancer Med 8(15):6644–6650. https://doi.org/10.1002/cam4.2561

Sato K, Nitta N, Aoki I et al (2018) Repeated photon and C-ion irradiations in vivo have different impact on alteration of tumor characteristics. Sci Rep 8:1458. https://doi.org/10.1038/s41598-018-19422-x

Satoh Y, Onishi H, Nambu A, Araki T (2014) Volume-based parameters measured by using FDG PET/CT in patients with stage I NSCLC treated with stereotactic body radiation therapy: prognostic value. Radiology 270(1):275–281. https://doi.org/10.1148/radiol.13130652

Shimokawa T, Ma L, Ando K, Sato K, Imai T (2016) The future of combining carbon-ion radiotherapy with immunotherapy: evidence and progress in mouse models. Int J Part Ther 3(1):61–70. https://doi.org/10.14338/IJPT-15-00023.1. Epub 2016 Aug 29

Shirai K, Abe T, Saitoh JI, Mizukami T, Irie D, Takakusagi Y, Shiba S, Okano N, Ebara T, Ohno T, Nakano T (2017) Maximum standardized uptake value on FDG-PET predicts survival in stage I non-small cell lung cancer following carbon ion radiotherapy. Oncol Lett 13(6):4420–4426. https://doi.org/10.3892/ol.2017.5952

Shrestha S, Higuchi T, Shirai K et al (2020) Prognostic significance of semi-quantitative FDG-PET parameters in stage I non-small-cell lung cancer treated with carbon-ion radiotherapy. Eur J Nucl Med Mol Imaging 47:1220–1227. https://doi.org/10.1007/s00259-019-04585-0

Sibley GS (1998) Radiotherapy for patients with medically inoperable stage I non-small-cell lung cancer. Cancer 82:433–438

St James S, Grassberger C, Lu HM (2018) Considerations when treating lung cancer with passive scatter or active scanning proton therapy. Transl Lung Cancer Res. 7(2):210–215. https://doi.org/10.21037/tlcr.2018.04.01

Su WH, Chuang PC, Huang EY, Yang KD (2012) Radiation-induced increase in cell migration and metastatic potential of cervical cancer cells operates via the K-Ras pathway. Am J Pathol 180:862–871

Subtil FS, Wilhelm J, Bill V, Westholt N, Rudolph S, Fischer J, Scheel S, Seay U, Fournier C, Taucher-Scholz G, Scholz M, Seeger W, Engenhart-Cabillic R, Rose F, Dahm-Daphi J, Hänze J (2014) Carbon ion radiotherapy of human lung cancer attenuates HIF-1 signaling and acts with considerably enhanced therapeutic efficiency. FASEB J 28(3):1412–1421. https://doi.org/10.1096/fj.13-242230. Epub 2013 Dec 17

Takahashi Y, Teshima T, Kawaguchi N, Hamada Y, Mori S, Madachi A, Ikeda S, Mizuno H, Ogata T, Nojima K, Furusawa Y, Matsuura N (2003) Heavy ion irradiation inhibits in vitro angiogenesis even at sublethal dose. Cancer Res 63(14):4253–4257

Timmerman R, McGarry R, Yiannoutsos C et al (2006) Excessive toxicity when treating central tumors in a phase II study of stereotactic body radiation therapy for medically inoperable early-stage lung cancer. J Clin Oncol 24:4833–4839

Vedam SS, Keall PJ, Kini VR, Mohan R (2001) Determining parameters for respiration-gated radiotherapy. Med Phys 28:2139–2146

Vera P, Thureau S, Chaumet-Riffaud P et al (2017) Phase II study of a radiotherapy total dose increase in hypoxic lesions identified by 18F-misonidazole PET/CT in patients with non–small cell lung carcinoma (RTEP5 study). J Nucl Med 58:1045–1053

Wild-Bode C, Weller M, Rimber A, Dichigans J, Wick W (2001) Sublethal irradiation promotes migration and invasiveness of glioma cells: implications for radiotherapy of human glioblastoma. Cancer Res 61:2744–2750

Yamamoto N, Miyamoto T, Nakajima M, Karube M, Hayashi K, Tsuji H, Tsujii H, Kamada T, Fujisawa T (2017) A dose escalation clinical trial of single-fraction carbon ion radiotherapy for peripheral stage I non-small cell lung cancer. J Thorac Oncol 12(4):673–680

Yan S, Wang Y, Yang Q, Li X, Kong X, Zhang N et al (2013) Low-dose radiation-induced epithelial-mesenchymal transition through NF-kappaB in cervical cancer cells. Int J Oncol 42:1801–1806

Zheng X, Schipper M, Kidwell K et al (2014) Survival outcome after stereotactic body radiation therapy and surgery for stage I non-small cell lung cancer: a meta-analysis. Int J Radiat Oncol Biol Phys 90:603–611

The Role of Nanotechnology for Diagnostic and Therapy Strategies in Lung Cancer

Jessica E. Holder, Minnatallah Al-Yozbaki, and Cornelia M. Wilson

Contents

1 Introduction 1094
2 **Conventional Methods of Lung Cancer Detection** 1095
3 **Conventional Methods of Treating Lung Cancer** 1095
4 **Nanotechnology** 1096
5 **Nanoparticles** 1097
5.1 Liposomes 1097
5.2 Polymeric Nanoparticles 1099
5.3 Quantum Dots 1099
5.4 Gold Nanoparticles 1099
5.5 Dendrimers 1100
5.6 Carbon Nanotubes 1100
5.7 Magnetic Nanoparticles 1100
6 **Nanotechnology in the Detection of Lung Cancer** 1100
7 **Nanotechnology in the Treatment of Lung Cancer** 1101
8 **The Use of Nanoparticles in Radiation Oncology** 1104
9 **Conclusion** 1105
References 1105

J. E. Holder · M. Al-Yozbaki
School of Human and Life Sciences, Canterbury Christ Church University, Discovery Park, Sandwich, UK

C. M. Wilson (✉)
School of Human and Life Sciences, Canterbury Christ Church University, Discovery Park, Sandwich, UK

Department of Molecular and Clinical Cancer Medicine, Institute of Translation Medicine, University of Liverpool, Liverpool, UK

Novel Global Community Educational Foundation, Hebersham, NSW, Australia
e-mail: cornelia.wilson@canterbury.ac.uk

Abstract

Lung cancer is globally the second most common cancer accounting for millions of deaths each year in both men and women. Early diagnosis is still difficult due to the cancer growing silently in the lung resulting in late diagnosis and high mortality. In recent years, nanotechnology has been advancing the diagnosis and cancer therapy modalities. A number of nanotherapies based around nanoparticles (NPs) have been developed to treat ailments such as pain, infectious diseases, and cancer. Nano-based medicine is providing a pharmacokinetic and pharmacodynamic advantage over current chemotherapy such as bioavailability, intestinal absorption, solubility, and targeted delivery. The progress that has led to the development of emerging cancer therapies in the clinic for the treatment of lung cancer is reaching fruition. Herein, this chapter outlines the current developments in nanomedicine for lung cancer diagnosis and therapy using NPs including liposomes, polymeric NPs, quantum dots, gold NPs, dendrimers, carbon nanotubes, and magnetic NPs.

1 Introduction

Cancer is the leading cause of death in the United Kingdom with around 450 people dying from the disease each day (Cancer Research UK 2020a). Incidence rates have been increasing since the early 1990s; this is largely attributed to the growing aging population, and the number of cancer cases is predicted to rise by more than 40% by 2035 to around 514,000 new cases per year (Cancer Intelligence team 2019). Cancer research has generated an extensive array of knowledge, revealing cancer to be a vastly heterogenous disease involving dynamic changes in the genome that allow tumor growth and metastasis (Hanahan and Weinberg 2000; Hanahan and Weinberg 2011). Lung cancer accounts for approximately 1.8 million deaths each year, accounting for nearly a fifth of all cancer deaths (Bray et al. 2018). Lung cancer has one of the poorest survival outcomes compared with other cancers, with over two-thirds of patients being diagnosed at advanced stages when curative treatment is not feasible (Del Ciello et al. 2017). Most lung cancers present as asymptomatic in the first stages and do not show symptoms until they have metastasized. Common symptoms include a persistent cough, coughing up blood, chest pain, weight loss, and fatigue (The American Cancer Society medical and editorial content team 2019a; Beckles et al. 2003).

Dependent upon the histology of the cancer cells, lung cancer is classified as either non-small cell lung carcinoma (NSCLC) or small cell lung carcinoma (SCLC). NSCLC is the most common form of lung cancer, accounting for over 85% of all cases compared to 15% in SCLC. The major subtypes of NSCLC are squamous cell carcinoma, adenocarcinoma, and large cell carcinoma (Molina et al. 2008; Devesa et al. 2005; National Health Service 2019). NSCLC begins in various types of epithelial cells lining the lungs, whereas SCLC almost always begins in the bronchi (The American Cancer Society medical and editorial content team 2019b; Davis 2020). SCLC is a more aggressive form of lung cancer, and patients with this type of cancer tend to have a poor prognosis due to the rate at which it can metastasize as well as a high rate of relapse with many patients relapsing within a year (Matsui et al. 2006). Tobacco smoking is the greatest risk factor associated with lung cancer, with up to 90% of lung cancer attributed to smoking. However, other factors including exposure to occupational carcinogens such as asbestos, air pollution, and genetic and epigenetic changes are also major contributors to a person's risk of developing lung cancer (de Groot et al. 2018; Malhotra et al. 2016; Shah 2006). Although the predominant cause of both types of lung cancer is smoking, SCLC is more strongly linked to smoking than NSCLC. This includes second-hand tobacco smoke; a 30% increase in the risk of developing NSCLC is observed in those living with a smoker compared to 60% for SCLC (WebMD 2020; Kim et al. 2014). An increased frequency of all types of lung cancer is also seen in those who mine uranium, but again, the most common type is SCLC (Pesch et al. 2012).

Establishing the specific type of lung cancer that a patient has is vital for enhancing the responsiveness of that cancer to treatment. For example, establishing that a patient has squamous cell carcinoma is important when selecting agents used in chemotherapy as certain agents are less effective and more toxic when used to treat this type of cancer (Yu et al. 2016). This is an example of personalized medicine, where the treatment decisions are based on the histology of the cancer. Genetic characteristics of the tumor can also determine the treatment options available, such as epidermal growth factor (EGFR) tyrosine kinase inhibitors (TKIs) being used to treat tumors with EGFR mutations (Travis 2014). The stage at which lung cancer is diagnosed has a great impact on prognosis. For NSCLC, there are four stages (stages I–IV) and multiple substages. Stages are determined using the Tumor, Node, Metastasis (TNM) staging system, with larger tumors and those that have spread to the lymph nodes and distant organs being classified as a higher stage (Cancer Research UK 2020b; Heineman et al. 2017). SCLC is described as either limited disease (LD) or extensive disease

(ED). LD means the cancer is contained to a single area on one side of the chest, whereas in ED the cancer has spread beyond one area (Cancer Research UK 2020c). Approximately 80% of patients with NSCLC have stage III or IV when diagnosed, and around two-thirds of patients with SCLC have ED. Being diagnosed at the late stages of lung cancer limits the treatment options of patients as it can exclude them from surgical resection of the tumor corresponding with a poor prognosis (Markman 2020; Birring and Peake 2005; Cancer.Net Editorial Board 2019).

The poor prognosis for lung cancer highlights the vital need to develop new detection and treatment methods. Nanotechnology is a field that is being researched in various scientific disciplines and has the potential to lead to revolutionary advances in medicine, genomics, physics, and many other areas (Patil et al. 2008). In medicine, nanotechnology has many potential uses including new methods of detecting, diagnosing, and treating diseases such as lung cancer (Emerich and Thanos 2005). Such uses of nanotechnology are discussed in this chapter.

2 Conventional Methods of Lung Cancer Detection

Various techniques are available to diagnose and stage lung cancer. A chest radiograph is usually the first step in diagnosing lung cancer; it provides initial information but is unable to characterize or stage the disease (Woodman et al. 2021). Patients with suspected lung cancer will have a computed tomography (CT) scan to gather more information and determine if further investigation, such as a biopsy, is required. Those patients presenting with a metastatic disease, which has progressed outside the thorax, will have a biopsy sample taken from the safest and most accessible site (Navani et al. 2015). However, in patients whose disease is contained in the thorax, a biopsy is usually done by a bronchoscopy or guided using a CT scan. Positron emission tomography (PET) and further CT scanning can be used in staging of the disease. Invasive sampling of mediastinal lymph nodes may also be carried out depending on factors such as tumor positioning and size of lymph nodes (Silvestri et al. 2013).

Advances in molecular biology have allowed for more differentiation of lung cancer subtypes through detection of specific biomarkers such as activation mutations in genes including epidermal growth factor receptor (EGFR) and anaplastic lymphoma kinase (ALK). Several methods can be used to identify molecular markers such as immunohistochemistry (IHC), fluorescence in situ hybridization, as well as more sensitive techniques such as Sanger sequencing and mass spectrometry-based genotyping (Cryer and Thorley 2019). Cancer biomarkers provide essential information about how patients will respond to certain types of treatment, and this can greatly improve the efficacy of a patient's treatment plan.

At present, lung cancer diagnosis and staging can require many different procedures and take several weeks. During this time, patient's conditions may deteriorate, and this could cause them to be unfit for certain treatments by the time a treatment plan has been made. This highlights the importance for new imaging techniques that nanotechnology can offer.

3 Conventional Methods of Treating Lung Cancer

The methods used in treating lung cancer will depend upon the type of cancer presenting in the patient, the stage of the cancer, the size and position of the tumor, as well as the overall health of the patient (National Health Service 2019; National Health Surface 2019). In NSCLC, for those patients with stage I or II cancer, the main treatment is surgery. This may be a lobectomy (removal of part of the lung) or a pneumonectomy (removal of the whole lung), depending on the extent of the disease (Cancer Research UK 2019a). This may be followed by chemotherapy to decrease the chance of cancer recurrence and radiotherapy depending upon the success of surgery. Some patients with stage I and II NSCLC are not eligible for surgery; this is primarily due to impaired lung function, and the patient will instead have radiotherapy or chemoradiotherapy (Shirish et al. 2012). Generally, surgery alone is not able to treat stage III NSCLC. Instead, these patients are treated with combined modality therapy; this can include surgery to remove as much of the tumor as possible, followed by radiotherapy and chemotherapy (Willow 2020). Alternatively, immunotherapy and targeted cancer therapy may be used. Immunotherapy stimulates the patient's immune system to target the cancer; checkpoint inhibitors which target checkpoint proteins on immune cells are commonly used (The American Cancer Society medical and editorial content team 2020). Patients with NSCLC will commonly be tested for molecular abnormalities and may be suitable for targeted therapy such as anti-EGFR and anti-vascular endothelial growth factor (VEGF) antibodies (ESMO 2015; Mascaux et al. 2017). While the main aim of treatment for stages I–III NSCLC are to cure the disease, in stage IV the goal of the treatment is to manage symptoms and prolong the patient's life span (Socinski et al. 2013). Treatment for stage IV may incorporate therapies used in stages I–III as well as symptom control treatments such as cryotherapy and the use of an airway stent to help the patient's breathing.

SCLC is rarely treated with surgery since in most cases it has spread to other parts of the body at the time of diagnosis (National Health Surface 2019). In the small number of SCLC cases diagnosed in early stages of the disease, surgery may be possible, followed by chemotherapy or radiotherapy to reduce the risk of the cancer returning (Cancer Research UK 2019b). For LD SCLC, the main treatment is chemotherapy usually followed by radiotherapy; however, if the patient is healthy enough, they may have chemoradiotherapy. After treatment, if the cancer in the lung has stopped growing, patients may have radiotherapy to the head, called prophylactic cranial radiotherapy (PCR); this aims to kill any cancer cells that may have spread to the brain but are too small to be detected (Kurup and Hanna 2004). For ED SCLC, treatment is aimed at slowing the spread of the disease and managing symptoms. If the patient is healthy enough, they will undergo chemotherapy, and depending on the outcome of this, they may also have radiotherapy (PDQ® Adult Treatment Editorial Board 2020). As in LD, patients with ED SCLC may also have PCR, as well as undergo treatments to manage their symptoms. To date, there have been no approved targeted therapies for SCLC attributed to the fact that druggable mutations are rarely identified during sequencing in SCLC (Zhang and He 2013; Saito et al. 2018).

The rate of recurrence of lung cancer varies depending on the histological subtype and stage of the disease. In NSCLC, the rate is between 30 and 55%, with recurrence typically occurring within 5 years for earlier stages of the disease and decreasing to 2 years for stage IV (Sasaki et al. 2014; Uramoto and Tanaka 2014). In SCLC, around 70% of patients will experience recurrence, and this is usually within 2 years, with those with ED being more likely to relapse (Matsui et al. 2006; Asai et al. 2014). New treatments offered by nanotechnology may be able to reduce the rate of relapse currently seen in lung cancer.

Conventional treatment for lung cancer can result in surrounding healthy tissues being damaged and cause numerous adverse effects. Nanotechnology can offer new methods of drug delivery, which can target the drugs directly to cancer cells and therefore minimize damage to healthy cells (Sarkar et al. 2017).

4 Nanotechnology

Nanotechnology is the manipulation of matter on the molecular or atomic level. It is considered a multidisciplinary field of scientific research into different types of nanoparticles and applications of nanomaterials and nanodevices in various aspects of life (Poonia et al. 2017). Definitions of nanodevices typically feature the requirements that the device or its essential components are man-made and that it should be between 1 and 100 nm in size (Ferrari 2005).

Nanotechnology offers various tools which can aid in diagnosing, treating, and preventing cancer, such as new imaging agents, methods of delivering drugs directly to cancer cells, and agents which can monitor predicative molecular changes in precancerous cells allowing preventative action to be taken against metastasis (Baptista 2009). Frequently with cancers that are hard to detect such as lung, prostate, and ovarian cancer, patients are diagnosed at later stages of the disease when metastasis has occurred. When utilized in diagnostics, nanotechnology offers the chance to improve the detection of cancer and reduce the number of patients presenting with advanced-stage cancers. The properties of nanoparticles make them a promising tool in medicine. Their large surface area and ability to modify surfaces make them useful in cancer detection. For example, nanoparticles can be utilized to bind to receptors that are overexpressed in certain tumors and provide imaging information: this increases specificity and aims to improve cancer detection (Biju et al. 2008; Sajja et al. 2009).

Various nanoparticles are being investigated for their ability to target chemotherapy drugs to tumor cells. Physiochemical properties of nanoparticles such as small size and composition allow them to pass through challenging areas, such as the blood-brain barrier, and limit their uptake in healthy cells, thus improving efficacy and decreasing toxic side effects (Brigger et al. 2002). Nanoparticles can be made up of various materials, a number of which will be discussed.

5 Nanoparticles

Nanoparticles are made up of carbon, metal, metal oxides, or organic matter and can be engineered to various shapes, sizes, and compositions and with different surface chemistries (Wang and Wang 2014; Ealia and Saravanakumar 2017). These properties have allowed for several types of nanoparticles to be produced with novel biological applications (Fig. 1). The nanoparticles that will be discussed are solid lipid nanoparticles, liposomes, polymeric nanoparticles, gold nanoparticles, quantum dots, carbon nanotubes, dendrimers, and magnetic nanoparticles.

5.1 Liposomes

The first nanoparticle platform was liposomes, which were first described in 1965 as a model for intracellular membranes (Bangham 1993). Liposomes are small, spherical vesicles, with one or more phospholipid bilayers that are self-assembling and can be created from cholesterol and natural phospholipids (Akbarzadeh et al. 2013). Liposomes can be classified by their size and number of bilayers into multilamellar vesicles (MLV) and unilamellar vesicles. MLVs contain several bilayers and are between 500 and 5000 nm in size. Unilamellar vesicles have a single bilayer and are described as either large unilamellar vesicles (LUV) which are 200–800 nm or small unilamellar vesicles which are 100 nm or smaller (Periyasamy et al. 2012; Sharma and Sharma 1997). Liposomes can also be modified to produce additional properties. Immunoliposomes have antibodies attached to the membrane and allow them to target cells of interest. Long-circulating liposomes are coated within polymers, such as polyethylene glycol (PEG), to form a protective layer and achieve a longer circulation of the liposome and increase bioavailability (Torchilin 2005). Characteristics of liposomes such as their diverse compositions, ability to transport and protect various biomolecules, and the fact that they are highly biocompatible and biodegradable sparked interest in the medical field (Wang and Wang 2014; Torchilin 2005). Since their discovery, liposomes have been adapted for use in the clinic to enable trafficking of proteins, nucleic acids, and drugs. The advantages of liposomes as drug carriers are that they can protect drugs from degradation and target specific cells, limiting drug uptake in healthy cells and reducing adverse effects (Ahmed et al. 2019). In medicine, liposomes have been widely used in the treatment of parasitic diseases and infections and in anticancer therapies. Cancer cells can be targeted by liposomes using the unique properties they display such as increased acidity and vascularization and tumor-specific markers they display (Mo et al. 2012; Maeda et al. 2000; Yue and Dai 2018).

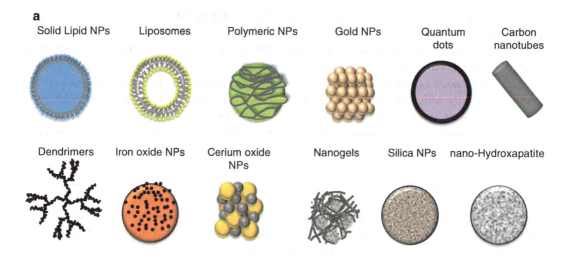

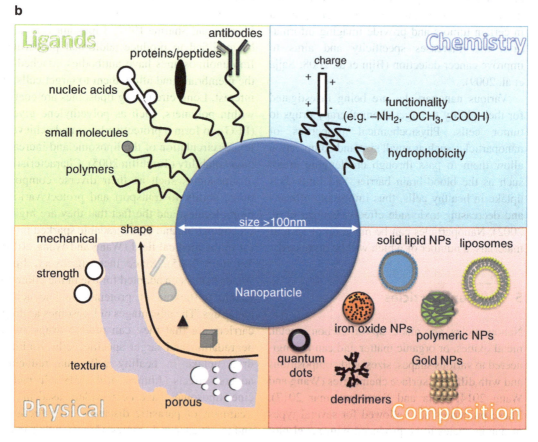

Fig. 1 Examples of nanoparticles. (**a**) Schematic representation of the structures of several nanoparticles. (**b**) Schematic of the properties of nanoparticles including composition, surface chemistry, target ligands, and physical properties. (Image reproduced with permission from Wilson et al. (2015))

5.2 Polymeric Nanoparticles

Polymeric NPs are colloidal particles within the size range of 1–1000 nm; they include nanospheres and nanocapsules (Zielińska et al. 2020). Nanospheres have a solid core surrounded by a polymer and a matrix structure into which molecules can be internalized or chemically attached to the surface (Kong 2016; Kondiah et al. 2018). Nanocapsules are a vesicular system with a solid shell and inner liquid core, with the molecules being confined to the inner cavity (Wawrzynczak et al. 2016). Polymeric NPs have many potential biomedical applications as their structures can be modified to allow them to deliver active components to specific sites and respond to physiological changes or external stimuli. The design of polymeric NPs will depend upon the therapeutic application, the site they are targeting, and how they will be administered (Elsabahy and Wooley 2012). As with liposomes, polymeric NPs have been investigated as potential drug carriers. They can localize the release of drugs to the therapeutic sites reducing the impact of the drug on healthy cells and potentially decreasing side effects (Owens and Peppas 2006). As well as this, polymeric NPs have a higher encapsulation efficiency and greater storage stability than liposomes (Andrade et al. 2011).

5.3 Quantum Dots

Quantum dots (QDs) were first created in the 1980s and are semiconducting, man-made nanocrystals measuring around 2–10 nm, which can transport electrons (Bhatia 2016). QDs have a semiconducting inorganic core, commonly cadmium selenide (CdSe), and an organic shell, typically zinc selenide (ZnS) (Jovin 2003). The size of QDs affects their excitation energy, and consequently they can be made to emit or absorb specific wavelengths of light by altering their size (Yin et al. 2019). The properties of QDs are also dependent upon their shape, composition, and structure (Nanowerk 2020). QDs have many applications such as solar cells, photodetectors, light-emitting diodes (LED), and medical imaging (Lutfullin et al. 2020). QDs producing near-infrared fluorescence (NIRF) have been developed more recently. NIRF light can penetrate tissues much deeper than visible light and, when used in vitro, can produce images with a high signal-to-background ratio (Weissleder 2006). The main drawback of using QDs in clinics is that they are made of potentially toxic metal atoms, which can cause cytotoxicity by increases in the colloidal effect and formation of photon-induced free radicals (Smith and Nie 2009). However, it has been reported that QDs can be tolerated in vivo when biocompatible surface coatings are used (Kirchner et al. 2005).

5.4 Gold Nanoparticles

Gold nanoparticles (AuNPs) are small gold particles, also known as colloidal gold when dispersed in water (Chen et al. 2014). AuNPs have historically been used for staining glass due to their optical properties; however, more recently, it has been researched for possible uses in biotechnology (Giljohann et al. 2010; Sigma Aldrich 2020). There are various subtypes of AuNPs that vary in size, shape, and physical properties; these include gold nanospheres, nanorods, nanoshells, and nanocages (Cai et al. 2008). Studies have shown that AuNPs have numerous advantages over other nanomaterials due to the highly optimized protocols allowing for the creation of AuNPs with unique properties (Sztandera et al. 2019). Several properties make AuNPs suitable for drug delivery; for example, they are inert, nontoxic, and biocompatible (Rana et al. 2012). AuNPs can also be used in diagnostics; when they bind to target surfaces, this can alter physiochemical properties of the AuNPs and produce detectable signal (Yeh et al. 2012).

5.5 Dendrimers

Dendrimers are branched, synthetic polymers with highly symmetric, layered architecture (Lee et al. 2005). They have a globular structure, which is divided into three sections: the core, the interior, and the periphery (Gitsov and Lin 2005). The branching units of dendrimers are described by generations, with the central branched core being generation 0 (G0) and the branches attached to this core being G1, increasing with additional branching points (Wolinsky and Grinstaff 2008). Several classes of dendrimers exist, varying in solubility, degradability, and biological activity; however, the most widely studied are polyamidoamine (PAMAM) and polypropylene imine (PPI) dendrimers (Gupta et al. 2010). Dendrimers' unique properties such as their size, controlled branched structure, and guest-host chemistry make them an attractive tool for drug delivery (Dhanikula and Hildgen 2007). Dendrimers can capture bioactive agents by encapsulation into their interior or by chemically attaching or absorbing them onto the dendrimer surface (Svenson and Tomalia 2005). Dendrimers also have potential uses in diagnostics and have been used as carriers for magnetic resonance imaging (MRI) contrast reagents as well as in photonic oxygen sensing (Kobayashi and Brechbiel 2003; Ziemer et al. 2005).

5.6 Carbon Nanotubes

Carbon nanotubes (CNTs) are cylindrical molecules made up of rolled-up sheets of graphene (Holban et al. 2016). Single-walled CNTs (SWCNTs) are CNTs consisting of a single rolled-up graphene sheet, which has a diameter of less than 1 nm. Multiwalled CNTs (MWCNTs) consist of several interlinked sheets of graphene and can have diameters of more than 100 nm (Berger 2021). CNTs have good thermal conductivity and mechanical strength and extremely low electrical resistance; as a result, CNTs have applications in several fields (Rahman et al. 2019). CNTs have been used as additives to various materials in electronics, optics, plastics, and other nanotechnology fields (He et al. 2013). CNTs also have biomedical applications, including artificial implants, cancer cell identification, and drug and gene delivery (Eatemadi et al. 2014).

5.7 Magnetic Nanoparticles

Magnetic nanoparticles (MNPs) are a class of nanoparticles that can be manipulated under the influences of an external magnetic field (Shahri 2019). Due to their multifunctional properties such as small size, superparamagnetism, and low toxicity, MNPs have attracted interest from a range of fields including biology, medicine, and physics (Majidi et al. 2016). In biological and biomedical applications, the MNPs are commonly composed of iron oxide NPs such as maghemite and magnetite, due to their biocompatibility and chemical stability (Rosenberger et al. 2015; Cabrera et al. 2008). Iron oxide MNPs have shown promise in imaging technology as drug vehicles and cancer therapy with several undergoing clinical trials as theranostic agents for human use (Gul et al. 2019).

6 Nanotechnology in the Detection of Lung Cancer

QDs show potential as a new class of fluorescent labels for use in biomedicine. Using QDs, it is possible to perform multicolor imaging with a single excitation source due to the broad absorption and narrow emission characteristics of the particles (Misra et al. 2010). QDs allow for improved sensitivity of molecular and cellular imaging as well as improved signal brightness and greater signal stability (Wang et al. 2008). A 2012 study demonstrated a new method of detecting micrometastases of lung cancer. QDs labeled with the biomarker Lunx and surfactant protein A antibody were used to identify circulating tumor cells in NSCLC patients (Wang et al. 2012). QDs have also been used in microarrays to detect potential miRNA NSCLC biomarkers. This detection method made miRNA profiling more efficient than RT-PCR and therefore demonstrates QDs' potential applications in lung cancer detection (Fan et al. 2016).

AuNPs are of interest in bioimaging and diagnostics and have been utilized as effective imaging labels and contrast agents (Choi et al. 2010). These NPs have better absorption and scattering bands than conventional dyes and are more biocompatible in human cells (Jain et al. 2006). AuNPs can absorb and scatter various wavelengths of light depending upon their shape and size (Kim et al. 2011). Colloidal gold has been used for tumor targeting using surface-enhanced Raman spectroscopy (SERS) as the detection method. Using antibodies, the AuNPs can recognize EGFR; this allowed for the detection of small tumors and produced a much clearer signal than NIRF-emitting QDs (Qian et al. 2008). Biosensors are devices that convert a biological response to a detectable signal, such as electrochemical or optical signals (Malekzad et al. 2017). These devices can be used to detect disease, pathogens, and drugs, while NPs can improve their sensitivity (Woodman et al. 2021). An AuNP biosensor was developed to allow lung cancer to be detected in an individual's breath. This biosensor used an array of chemiresistors based on AuNPs and recognition assays that can differentiate the breath of a lung cancer patient from a healthy control patient. This biosensor offers a detection method for lung cancer that is quick, safe to perform, and noninvasive (Peng et al. 2009).

Carbon nanotubes have also been utilized in a similar way. Using MWCNTs, a chemiresistive biosensor was created that detects for a lung cancer biomarker, hexanal in an individual's breath (Janfaza et al. 2019). SWNTs have an emission range which covers the biological tissue transparency window and therefore are suitable for biological imaging (Liu et al. 2009). An electrode sensor that monitors the electrophysical responses from cells was created using semiconducting SWNTs. Using a single sensor, the cellular response to various compounds was investigated, including nicotine. This elicited a larger response in SCLC cells than healthy cells due to the overexpression of nicotinic acetylcholine receptors in SCLC cells (Ta et al. 2014). This device offers the chance to distinguish between lung cancer cells and healthy cells quickly and easily.

Magnetic NPs have been of interest for use as a target-specific MRI contrast agent. Superparamagnetic iron oxide NPs (SPIONs) are commonly used. The paramagnetic properties of iron oxide result in strong contrast effects in MRIs (Bulte and Kraitchman 2004). To improve sensitivity and specificity when detecting metastasis of lung cancer, SPIONs have been used in MRI. The SPIONs are able to target human lung adenocarcinoma cells and could be used in lung cancer diagnosis (Wan et al. 2016). SPIONs have been shown to have high specificity and appear to be safe for use at imaging doses (Bulte and Kraitchman 2004; Korchinski et al. 2015). It has also been demonstrated that SPIONs can be imaged in the lungs using the emerging imaging technique, magnetic particle imaging (MPI). Using this technique, SPIONs were used to label aerosols inside the lung with high sensitivity, demonstrating a potential new imaging technique for lung cancer (Tay et al. 2018).

As discussed, most lung cancer patients are not diagnosed until the late stages of the disease. This highlights the importance of developing new rapid detection methods, which can be used to screen patients for lung cancer to allow it to be detected in its earliest stages.

7 Nanotechnology in the Treatment of Lung Cancer

Nanotechnology has allowed the development of functionalized NPs facilitating increased cellular uptake at the tumor site and enhanced delivery of drugs (Fig. 2). Liposomes are widely used in drug delivery and have been used clinically in cancer therapy to target tumor sites and minimize side effects of cancer therapy (Jurj et al. 2017). Doxorubicin (DOX) is a drug commonly used to treat various types of cancer; however, it poses a risk of cardiac damage which can lead to heart failure and death (Woodman et al. 2021; Cancer

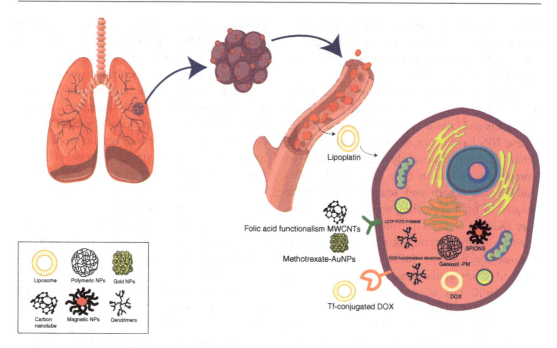

Fig. 2 Nanoparticle targeting to the tumor site for cancer therapy

Research UK 2020d). The use of liposomes as a drug delivery platform for DOX has shown enhanced accumulation in tumors compared with the free drug, as well as reduced cardiotoxicity and increased therapeutic efficacy in numerous experimental models (Gabizon et al. 2006). Two liposomal DOX formulations, Caelyx and Myocet, have received clinical approval for use in cancer treatment (Abraham et al. 2005). Transferrin (Tf), a glycoprotein involved in the absorption of iron, can be used for targeted therapy. Tf-conjugated DOX liposomes have been used in lung cancer models in rats and have showed increased absorption in lung cancer cells compared to healthy cells (Gaspar et al. 2012). Another chemotherapeutic treatment widely used in lung cancer is cisplatin. Cisplatin is shown to have a significant effect on the survival of patients with advanced lung cancer; however, its efficacy is limited by side effects such as nephrotoxicity, myelosuppression, and neurotoxicity (Barabas et al. 2008; Miyoshi et al. 2016). Lipoplatin is a liposomal formulation of cisplatin, which has been investigated for the treatment of several cancer types. Lipoplatin has been successful in multiple phase I, II, and III trials and has shown to be effective for treating NSCLC (Boulikas 2009). Lipoplatin is not detected by immune cells and therefore is able to circulate longer in body fluids, and it will extravasate preferentially into tumor sites due to leaky tumor vasculature (Fantini et al. 2011; Boulikas et al. 2005). Phase III studies of NSCLC treatment have shown lipoplatin to have lower neurotoxicity, nephrotoxicity, and myelotoxicity than cisplatin (Boulikas et al. 2007; Stathopoulos et al. 2010). One study also found that lipoplatin combined with paclitaxel (PTX) produced significantly higher response rates in patients with NSCLC compared to cisplatin with PTX (Stathopoulos et al. 2011). Despite these promising results, subsequent trials have been unable to demonstrate the superior efficacy of lipoplatin; this may be caused by suboptimum delivery to tumors as is seen in some clinical studies (Xu et al. 2018; Zahednezhad et al. 2020) (Table 1).

PTX is commonly used in the treatment of several cancers, including lung cancer. PTX is water insoluble, and therefore the lipid-based solvent Cremophor EL (CrEL) is used to encapsulate it. CrEL has been associated with side effects, including allergies and neuropathy, and alters the

Table 1 Formulations of NPs and active drugs that are clinically approved or undergoing clinical or preclinical trials for treatment of lung cancer

Product	Active drug	NP type	Clinical status	References
Abraxane	PTX	Albumin-bound combination	Approved for treatment of breast cancer, NSCLC, and pancreatic cancer	European Medicines Agency (2020), Gradishar (2006)
Genexol-PM	PTX	Polymeric	Approved for treatment of breast cancer and NSCLC in South Korea	Ahn et al. (2014)
Lipoplatin	Cisplatin	Liposome	Phase III clinical trials for treatment of NSCLC	Fantini et al. (2011)
Tf-conjugated DOX liposomes	DOX	Liposome	Preclinical trials for lung cancer treatment	Barabas et al. (2008)
MTX-conjugated gold nanocarriers	MTX	AuNPs	Preclinical trials for lung cancer treatment	Mandal (2021)
SWCNTs and graphene oxide with PTX	PXT	SWCNTs	Preclinical trials for lung cancer treatment	Guthi et al. (2010)

pharmacokinetic properties of PTX (Gelderblom et al. 2001). To reduce the effect of CrEL, novel polymeric NPs have been developed which can act as a vehicle for PTX. Genexol-PM is a polymeric NP formulation of PTX, which has been approved in South Korea for the treatment of breast cancer and NSCLC (Werner et al. 2013). The use of Genexol-PM allowed for higher doses of PTX to be delivered with lower toxicity compared to using CrEL with PTX (Ahn et al. 2014; Kim et al. 2004). For the treatment of NSCLC, Genexol-PM is given at a dose of 180 mg/m^2 once per week and up to 300 mg/m^2 every 3 weeks (Norouzi and Hardy 2021). One way to target PTX to tumor cells is by targeting EGFR often expressed in these cells. A small peptide AEYLR can recognize the overexpression of EGFR, and AEYLR conjugated to polymeric NPs could target drugs to cancer cells (Han et al. 2013, 2014).

Abraxane is an albumin-bound PTX formulation using a combination of different NPs, which has been approved by the FDA and the EMA for treatment of breast cancer, NSCLC, and pancreatic cancer (Drugs.com 2021; European Medicines Agency 2020). When administered, Abraxane binds to cell surface glycoprotein receptors (gp60) and interacts with an intracellular protein (caveolin-1) to form transcytotic vesicles. These vesicles cross the vascular endothelial cells to enter the tumor tissue (Gradishar 2006). Abraxane enables greater doses of PTX to be administered, with fewer side effects and decreased administration time, and eliminates the need for premedication (Bernabeu et al. 2017). For the treatment of NSCLC, Abraxane is administered at 100 mg/m^2 on days 1, 8, and 15 of a 21-day cycle; carboplatin is also administered on day 1 of each cycle (Abraxis BioScience LLC 2021). Several PTX nanoparticle formulations are in clinical trials for the treatment of various cancer types. For examples, NK 105 uses polymeric NPs to deliver PTX and is in phase III trials for the treatment of metastatic breast cancer and stomach cancer (Ma and Mumper 2013).

AuNPs have been used for the destruction of cancer cells by thermal ablation. When irradiated with laser pulses in the NIRF wavelength, AuNPs compromise the membrane integrity of surrounding cells and can be targeted to kill cancer cells using biomarkers such as EGFR and HER2 (Tong et al. 2007; Chen et al. 2007a). In one study, human breast cancer cells incubated with AuNPs were shown to undergo photothermally induced morbidity when exposed to NIRF light. Under the same conditions, cells not associated with AuNPs displayed no loss in viability (Hirsch et al. 2003). AuNPs can also be used for drug delivery to cancer cells. The chemotherapeutic agent methotrexate can be conjugated to AuNPs. This conjugate has been shown to suppress tumor growth in a mouse model of Lewis lung carcinoma, while an equal dose of the free drug had no effect (Chen et al. 2007b).

Dendrimers also have potential use in cancer therapeutics, and many studies are demonstrating their ability as anticancer drug delivery vehicles (Wolinsky and Grinstaff 2008). When used in drug delivery, dendrimers have been shown to preferentially accumulate in tumor cells and minimize toxicity in healthy cells (Mandal 2021). PEG can be conjugated with dendrimers to reduce toxicity and improve circulation time to achieve greater delivery to tumor sites (Thakur et al. 2015). One example of this is in DOX-functionalized dendrimer, which was prepared by PEGylation and used pH-sensitive hydrazone linkages to release DOX once inside tumor cells. In mouse models of colon cancer, when treated with the DOX-dendrimer, there was significantly higher uptake of DOX, and over 2 months there was total tumor regression and 100% survival. When treated with free DOX, there was a reduced uptake of DOX indicating that treatment was ineffective (Lee et al. 2006). Using a novel specific lung cancer-targeting peptide (LCTP; peptide sequence RCPLSHSLICY), a specific drug delivery vehicle for NSCLC chemotherapy was created. The LCTP was labeled with fluorescein isothiocyanate and conjugated with an acetylated PAMAM to form a drug delivery vehicle. This conjugate was found to be enriched in NSCLC cells compared with controls, suggesting that LCTP could successfully target this conjugate to tumor cells of NSCLC. Thus, this dendrimer may be a promising drug carrier for cancer treatment (Liu et al. 2010).

As with other NPs, CNTs have been studied for drug delivery to cancer cells. It has been reported that nonspherical NPs, such as CNTs, are retained in lymph nodes for longer than spherical NPs, and therefore multiple studies have used CNTs to target drugs to lymph node cancer cells (Elhissi et al. 2012). One study used folic acid-functionalized MWCNTs due to the overexpression of folic acid receptors seen in cancer cells. This CNT entrapped magnetic NPs containing cisplatin, and an external magnet was used to drag the MWNT to the lymph nodes. The CNT continually released cisplatin over several days and led to cancer cells' selective death (Yang et al. 2008). SWCNTs have been used with graphene oxide to potentiate the effect of PTX in the treatment of lung cancer. A study showed enhanced cell death in lung cancer cell lines by reactive oxygen species-dependent synergistic effect between CNTs and PTX (Arya et al. 2013).

MNPs have also been used as theranostic probes that can target drugs to lung cancer cells and track treatment through MRI at the same time. One example uses PNPs encoded with an LCTP that recognizes $\alpha_v\beta_6$ integrin on the surface of NSCLC cells. The PNPs encapsulate SPIONs and DOX for MRI tracking and drug delivery (Guthi et al. 2010). SPIONs can also be used for treating cancer through magnetic hyperthermia, a noninvasive therapy that uses heat to destroy cancer cells. When SPIONs are subjected to an alternating magnetic field, they generate heat which causes damage to the surrounding tissue. In mouse models of NSCLC, EGFR-targeted inhalable SPIONs resulted in increased accumulation of SPIONs in tumors and significant inhibition of lung tumor growth (Sadhukha et al. 2013).

Conventional methods used to treat lung cancer can damage healthy tissues, resulting in side effects, and are often unable to cure the disease at the later stages. Therefore, it is paramount to develop novel treatments for lung cancer which can target tumor cells to reduce adverse effects and improve the prognosis of lung cancer patients.

8 The Use of Nanoparticles in Radiation Oncology

Radiotherapy is used in more than half of all cases of cancer, and technological advancements have allowed patients to live longer and experience fewer side effects. However, despite these advancements, many patients will experience recurrence as some tumors are resistant to conventional radiotherapy (Scher et al. 2020). In recent years, there has been increasing interest in the use of NPs to enhance the efficacy of radiotherapy to reduce the rate of recurrence and minimize the effects on healthy tissue (Rancoule et al. 2016). As discussed, NPs have been used in cancer detection by improving imaging precision by targeting tumors and providing enhanced contrast effects. This technology can help localize radiotherapy to tumor sites and provide real-time information to evaluate tumor responses to the treatment (Wang and Tepper 2014). One example of this is zwitterionic gadolinium(III)-complexed dendrimer-entrapped AuNPs, created to enhance CT scans and MRI of lung cancer metastasis. In mouse models, this complex was able to target a_vb_3 integrin-expressing cancer cells and showed acceptable biocompatibility and effective imaging of lung cancer metastasis by CT scans and MRI (Liu et al. 2019). AuNPs can also potentially increase the efficacy of radiation oncology due to their high atomic number (Z). This makes them more likely to absorb photons and amplify the deposition of radiation within cancer cells; therefore, they are commonly used as dose enhancers for radiotherapy (Chen et al. 2020). Numerous studies have reported that AuNPs produce high local ionization in tumor tissue when radiation is applied, which shortens treatment time and reduces radiation doses. As a result, healthy tissues absorb less radiation, and therefore adverse effects are decreased (Babaei and Ganjalikhani 2014). Radiosensitizer AuNPs have been used in cell and animal models of various types of tumors (Abbasian et al. 2019; Kanavi et al. 2018; Cifter et al. 2015). In lung cancer cells, glucose-bound AuNPs in combination with megavoltage X-ray resulted in enhanced radiation effects by arresting the G2/M phase of the cell cycle and increasing apoptosis (Wang et al. 2013). This demonstrates the potential uses of NPs in radiation oncology—through targeted imaging and enhancing the effect of radiation in tumor cells.

9 Conclusion

Nanotechnology provides theranostic potential in the diagnosis and treatment of lung cancer. NPs are at the center of this technology, which have improved pharmacokinetic and pharmacodynamic profiles providing benefits to lung cancer patients. The properties of the NPs can be modified to improve the solubility and stability of drug formulations often at the crux of drug discovery. This allows NPs to be adapted by combining drugs and imaging molecules, facilitating diagnosis and therapy. Still, nanotechnology is not devoid of toxicities and requires advancements to improve outcome in clinical trials. The benefits of NPs provide a greater surface area bringing a higher dose of the drug to the tumor site. In addition, the NPs can be finely tuned through modification of their chemistry to precisely target the cancer. There are still some limitations of nanotechnology to overcome with much-needed research into improving production, drug formulation, pharmacokinetics, and tissue imaging. Nevertheless, nanotechnology has provided many therapeutic benefits to lung cancer patients, and future advancements in this area have great potential to treat lung cancer at the point of diagnosis.

References

Abbasian M et al (2019) Combination of gold nanoparticles with low-LET irradiation: an approach to enhance DNA DSB induction in HT29 colorectal cancer stem-like cells. J Cancer Res Clin Oncol 145(1):97–107

Abraham SA et al (2005) The liposomal formulation of doxorubicin. Methods Enzymol 391:71–97

Abraxis BioScience LLC (2021) Dosage & administration: abraxane + carboplatin. [cited 2021 07/02]. https://www.abraxanepro.com/advanced-non-small-cell-lung-cancer/dosing

Ahmed KS et al (2019) Liposome: composition, characterisation, preparation, and recent innovation in clinical applications. J Drug Target 27(7):742–761

Ahn HK et al (2014) A phase II trial of Cremophor EL-free paclitaxel (Genexol-PM) and gemcitabine in patients with advanced non-small cell lung cancer. Cancer Chemother Pharmacol 74(2):277–282

Akbarzadeh A et al (2013) Liposome: classification, preparation, and applications. Nanoscale Res Lett 8(1):102

Andrade F et al (2011) Nanocarriers for pulmonary administration of peptides and therapeutic proteins. Nanomedicine (Lond) 6(1):123–141

Arya N et al (2013) Combination of single walled carbon nanotubes/graphene oxide with paclitaxel: a reactive oxygen species mediated synergism for treatment of lung cancer. Nanoscale 5(7):2818–2829

Asai N et al (2014) Relapsed small cell lung cancer: treatment options and latest developments. Ther Adv Med Oncol 6(2):69–82

Babaei M, Ganjalikhani M (2014) A systematic review of gold nanoparticles as novel cancer therapeutics. J Nanomedicine 1:211–219

Bangham AD (1993) Liposomes: the Babraham connection. Chem Phys Lipids 64(1-3):275–285

Baptista P (2009) Cancer nanotechnology—prospects for cancer diagnostics and therapy. Curr Cancer Ther Rev 5(2):80–88

Barabas K et al (2008) Cisplatin: a review of toxicities and therapeutic applications. Vet Comp Oncol 6(1):1–18

Beckles MA et al (2003) Initial evaluation of the patient with lung cancer: symptoms, signs, laboratory tests, and paraneoplastic syndromes. Chest 123(1 Suppl):97S–104S

Berger M (2021) Carbon nanotubes—what they are, how they are made, what they are used for. [cited 2021 11/01]. https://www.nanowerk.com/nanotechnology/introduction/introduction_to_nanotechnology_22.php

Bernabeu E et al (2017) Paclitaxel: what has been done and the challenges remain ahead. Int J Pharm 526(1-2):474–495

Bhatia S (2016) Nanoparticles types, classification, characterization, fabrication methods and drug delivery applications. In: Natural polymer drug delivery systems. Springer, Cham, pp 33–93

Biju V et al (2008) Semiconductor quantum dots and metal nanoparticles: syntheses, optical properties, and biological applications. Anal Bioanal Chem 391(7):2469–2495

Birring SS, Peake MD (2005) Symptoms and the early diagnosis of lung cancer. Thorax 60(4):268–269

Boulikas T (2009) Clinical overview on Lipoplatin: a successful liposomal formulation of cisplatin. Expert Opin Investig Drugs 18(8):1197–1218

Boulikas T et al (2005) Systemic Lipoplatin infusion results in preferential tumor uptake in human studies. Anticancer Res 25(4):3031–3039

Boulikas T et al (2007) Lipoplatin plus gemcitabine versus cisplatin plus gemcitabine in NSCLC: preliminary results of a phase III trial. J Clin Oncol 25:18028–18028

Bray F et al (2018) Global cancer statistics 2018: GLOBOCAN estimates of incidence and mortality worldwide for 36 cancers in 185 countries. CA Cancer J Clin 68(6):394–424

Brigger I, Dubernet C, Couvreur P (2002) Nanoparticles in cancer therapy and diagnosis. Adv Drug Deliv Rev 54(5):631–651

Bulte JW, Kraitchman DL (2004) Iron oxide MR contrast agents for molecular and cellular imaging. NMR Biomed 17(7):484–499

Cabrera L et al (2008) Magnetite nanoparticles: electrochemical synthesis and characterization. Electrochim Acta 53:3436–3441

Cai W et al (2008) Applications of gold nanoparticles in cancer nanotechnology. Nanotechnol Sci Appl 1:17–32

Cancer Intelligence team (2019) Cancer in the UK. [cited 2020 08/11]. https://www.cancerresearchuk.org/sites/default/files/state_of_the_nation_april_2019.pdf

Cancer Research UK (2019a) Treatment for non-small cell lung cancer (NSCLC). [cited 2020 14/12]. https://www.cancerresearchuk.org/about-cancer/lung-cancer/treatment/non-small-cell-lung-cancer

Cancer Research UK (2019b) Treatment for small cell lung cancer (SCLC). [cited 15/12 2020]. https://www.cancerresearchuk.org/about-cancer/lung-cancer/treatment/small-cell-lung-cancer

Cancer Research UK (2020a) Cancer mortality for all cancers combined. [cited 2020 17/12]. https://www.cancerresearchuk.org/health-professional/cancer-statistics/mortality/all-cancers-combined

Cancer Research UK (2020b) TNM staging. [cited 2020 17/12]. https://www.cancerresearchuk.org/about-cancer/lung-cancer/stages-types-grades/tnm-staging

Cancer Research UK (2020c) Limited and extensive stage (small cell lung cancer). [cited 2020 17/12]. https://www.cancerresearchuk.org/about-cancer/lung-cancer/stages-types-grades/limited-extensive

Cancer Research UK (2020d) Doxorubicin. [cited 25/01 2021]. https://www.cancerresearchuk.org/about-cancer/cancer-in-general/treatment/cancer-drugs/drugs/doxorubicin

Cancer.Net Editorial Board (2019) Lung cancer—small cell: stages. [cited 2020 17/12]. https://www.cancer.net/cancer-types/lung-cancer-small-cell/stages#:~:text=About%201%20out%20of%203,stage%20disease%20when%20first%20diagnosed

Chen J et al (2007a) Immunogold nanocages with tailored optical properties for targeted photothermal destruction of cancer cells. Nano Lett 7(5):1318–1322

Chen YH et al (2007b) Methotrexate conjugated to gold nanoparticles inhibits tumor growth in a syngeneic lung tumor model. Mol Pharm 4(5):713–722

Chen X, Li Q, Wang X (2014) Gold nanostructures for bioimaging, drug delivery and therapeutics. In: Baltzer N, Copponnex T (eds) Precious metals for biomedical applications. Woodhead Publishing, pp 163–176

Chen Y et al (2020) Gold nanoparticles as radiosensitizers in cancer radiotherapy. Int J Nanomedicine 15:9407–9430

Choi YE, Kwak JW, Park JW (2010) Nanotechnology for early cancer detection. Sensors (Basel) 10(1):428–455

Cifter G et al (2015) Targeted radiotherapy enhancement during electronic brachytherapy of accelerated partial breast irradiation (APBI) using controlled release of gold nanoparticles. Phys Med 31(8):1070–1074

Cryer AM, Thorley AJ (2019) Nanotechnology in the diagnosis and treatment of lung cancer. Pharmacol Ther 198:189–205

Davis C (2020) Small cell lung cancer vs. non-small cell lung cancer. [cited 2020 16/11]. https://www.medicinenet.com/non-small_cell_lung_cancer_vs_small_cell/article.htm

de Groot PM et al (2018) The epidemiology of lung cancer. Transl Lung Cancer Res 7(3):220–233

Del Ciello A et al (2017) Missed lung cancer: when, where, and why? Diagn Interv Radiol 23(2):118–126

Devesa SS et al (2005) International lung cancer trends by histologic type: male:female differences diminishing and adenocarcinoma rates rising. Int J Cancer 117(2):294–299

Dhanikula RS, Hildgen P (2007) Influence of molecular architecture of polyether-co-polyester dendrimers on the encapsulation and release of methotrexate. Biomaterials 28(20):3140–3152

Drugs.com (2021) Abraxane FDA approval history. [cited 2021 06/02]. https://www.drugs.com/history/abraxane.html

Ealia S, Saravanakumar M (2017) A review on the classification, characterisation, synthesis of nanoparticles and their application. IOP Conf Ser Mater Sci Eng 263:032019

Eatemadi A et al (2014) Carbon nanotubes: properties, synthesis, purification, and medical applications. Nanoscale Res Lett 9(1):393

Elhissi AM et al (2012) Carbon nanotubes in cancer therapy and drug delivery. J Drug Deliv 2012:837327

Elsabahy M, Wooley KL (2012) Design of polymeric nanoparticles for biomedical delivery applications. Chem Soc Rev 41(7):2545–2561

Emerich D, Thanos C (2005) Nanotechnology and medicine. Expert Opin Biol Ther 3(4)

ESMO (2015) Personalised medicine at a glance: lung cancer. [cited 2020 15/12]. https://www.esmo.org/for-patients/personalised-medicine-explained/Lung-Cancer

European Medicines Agency (2020) Abraxane. [cited 2021 06/02]. https://www.ema.europa.eu/en/medicines/human/EPAR/abraxane

Fan L et al (2016) Identification of serum miRNAs by nano-quantum dots microarray as diagnostic biomarkers for early detection of non-small cell lung cancer. Tumour Biol 37(6):7777–7784

Fantini M et al (2011) Lipoplatin treatment in lung and breast cancer. Chemother Res Pract 2011:125192

Ferrari M (2005) Cancer nanotechnology: opportunities and challenges. Nat Rev Cancer 5(3):161–171

Gabizon AA, Shmeeda H, Zalipsky S (2006) Pros and cons of the liposome platform in cancer drug targeting. J Liposome Res 16(3):175–183

Gaspar MM et al (2012) Targeted delivery of transferrin-conjugated liposomes to an orthotopic model of lung cancer in nude rats. J Aerosol Med Pulm Drug Deliv 25(6):310–318

Gelderblom H et al (2001) Cremophor EL: the drawbacks and advantages of vehicle selection for drug formulation. Eur J Cancer 37(13):1590–1598

Giljohann DA et al (2010) Gold nanoparticles for biology and medicine. Angew Chem Int Ed Engl 49(19):3280–3294

Gitsov I, Lin C (2005) Dendrimers—nanoparticles with precisely engineered surfaces. Curr Org Chem 9:1025–1051

Gradishar WJ (2006) Albumin-bound paclitaxel: a next-generation taxane. Expert Opin Pharmacother 7(8):1041–1053

Gul S et al (2019) A comprehensive review of magnetic nanomaterials modern day theranostics. Front Mater 6:179

Gupta U et al (2010) Ligand anchored dendrimers based nanoconstructs for effective targeting to cancer cells. Int J Pharm 393(1-2):185–196

Guthi JS et al (2010) MRI-visible micellar nanomedicine for targeted drug delivery to lung cancer cells. Mol Pharm 7(1):32–40

Han CY et al (2013) A novel small peptide as an epidermal growth factor receptor targeting ligand for nanodelivery in vitro. Int J Nanomedicine 8:1541–1549

Han C et al (2014) Small peptide-modified nanostructured lipid carriers distribution and targeting to EGFR-overexpressing tumor in vivo. Artif Cells Nanomed Biotechnol 42(3):161–166

Hanahan D, Weinberg RA (2000) The hallmarks of cancer. Cell 100(1):57–70

Hanahan D, Weinberg RA (2011) Hallmarks of cancer: the next generation. Cell 144(5):646–674

He H et al (2013) Carbon nanotubes: applications in pharmacy and medicine. Biomed Res Int 2013:578290

Heineman DJ, Daniels JM, Schreurs WH (2017) Clinical staging of NSCLC: current evidence and implications for adjuvant chemotherapy. Ther Adv Med Oncol 9(9):599–609

Hirsch LR et al (2003) Nanoshell-mediated near-infrared thermal therapy of tumors under magnetic resonance guidance. Proc Natl Acad Sci U S A 100(23):13549–13554

Holban A, Grumezescu A, Andronescu E (2016) Inorganic nanoarchitectonics designed for drug delivery and anti-infective surfaces. In: Grumezescu A (ed) Surface chemistry of nanobiomaterials. William Andrew Publishing, pp 301–327

Jain PK et al (2006) Calculated absorption and scattering properties of gold nanoparticles of different size, shape, and composition: applications in biological imaging and biomedicine. J Phys Chem B 110(14):7238–7248

Janfaza S et al (2019) A selective chemiresistive sensor for the cancer-related volatile organic compound hexanal by using molecularly imprinted polymers and multiwalled carbon nanotubes. Mikrochim Acta 186(3):137

Jovin TM (2003) Quantum dots finally come of age. Nat Biotechnol 21(1):32–33

Jurj A et al (2017) The new era of nanotechnology, an alternative to change cancer treatment. Drug Des Devel Ther 11:2871–2890

Kanavi MR et al (2018) Gamma irradiation of ocular melanoma and lymphoma cells in the presence of gold nanoparticles: in vitro study. J Appl Clin Med Phys 19(3):268–275

Kim TY et al (2004) Phase I and pharmacokinetic study of Genexol-PM, a cremophor-free, polymeric micelle-formulated paclitaxel, in patients with advanced malignancies. Clin Cancer Res 10(11):3708–3716

Kim B, Tripp S, Wei A (2011) Tuning the optical properties of large gold nanoparticle arrays. Mater Res Soc Symp Proc 61:676

Kim CH et al (2014) Exposure to secondhand tobacco smoke and lung cancer by histological type: a pooled analysis of the International Lung Cancer Consortium (ILCCO). Int J Cancer 135(8):1918–1930

Kirchner C et al (2005) Cytotoxicity of colloidal CdSe and CdSe/ZnS nanoparticles. Nano Lett 5(2):331–338

Kobayashi H, Brechbiel MW (2003) Dendrimer-based macromolecular MRI contrast agents: characteristics and application. Mol Imaging 2(1):1–10

Kondiah P et al (2018) Nanocomposites for therapeutic application in multiple sclerosis. In: Inamuddin A, Asiri A (eds) Applications of nanocomposite materials in drug delivery. Woodhead Publishing, pp 391–408

Kong I (2016) Polymers with nano-encapsulated functional polymers. In: Thomas S, Shanks R, Chandrasekharakurup S (eds) Micro and nano technologies: design and applications of nanostructured polymer blends and nanocomposite systems. William Andrew Publishing, pp 125–154

Korchinski DJ et al (2015) Iron oxide as an MRI contrast agent for cell tracking. Magn Reson Insights 8(Suppl 1):15–29

Kurup A, Hanna NH (2004) Treatment of small cell lung cancer. Crit Rev Oncol Hematol 52(2):117–126

Lee CC et al (2005) Designing dendrimers for biological applications. Nat Biotechnol 23(12):1517–1526

Lee CC et al (2006) A single dose of doxorubicin-functionalized bow-tie dendrimer cures mice bearing C-26 colon carcinomas. Proc Natl Acad Sci U S A 103(45):16649–16654

Liu Z et al (2009) Carbon nanotubes in biology and medicine: in vitro and in vivo detection, imaging and drug delivery. Nano Res 2(2):85–120

Liu J et al (2010) Novel peptide-dendrimer conjugates as drug carriers for targeting nonsmall cell lung cancer. Int J Nanomedicine 6:59–69

Liu J et al (2019) Zwitterionic gadolinium(III)-complexed dendrimer-entrapped gold nanoparticles for enhanced computed tomography/magnetic resonance imaging of lung cancer metastasis. ACS Appl Mater Interfaces 11(17):15212–15221

Lutfullin M, Sinatra L, Bakr O (2020) Quantum dots for electronics and energy applications. [cited 2020 21/12/20]. https://www.sigmaaldrich.com/technical-documents/articles/materials-science/quantum-dots-noncadmium.html

Ma P, Mumper RJ (2013) Paclitaxel nano-delivery systems: a comprehensive review. J Nanomed Nanotechnol 4(2):1000164

Maeda H et al (2000) Tumor vascular permeability and the EPR effect in macromolecular therapeutics: a review. J Control Release 65(1-2):271–284

Majidi S et al (2016) Current methods for synthesis of magnetic nanoparticles. Artif Cells Nanomed Biotechnol 44(2):722–734

Malekzad H et al (2017) Noble metal nanoparticles in biosensors: recent studies and applications. Nanotechnol Rev 6(3):301–329

Malhotra J et al (2016) Risk factors for lung cancer worldwide. Eur Respir J 48(3):889–902

Mandal AK (2021) Dendrimers in targeted drug delivery applications: a review of diseases and cancer. Int J Polym Mater Polym Biomater 70(4):287–297

Markman M (2020) Lung cancer stages. [cited 2020 17/11/20]. https://www.cancercenter.com/cancer-types/lung-cancer/stages#:~:text=Stage%20IV%20non%2Dsmall%20cell,they%20are%20in%20stage%20IV

Mascaux C et al (2017) Personalised medicine for non-small cell lung cancer. Eur Respir Rev 26(146):170066

Matsui K et al (2006) Relapse of stage I small cell lung cancer ten or more years after the start of treatment. Jpn J Clin Oncol 36(7):457–461

Misra R, Acharya S, Sahoo SK (2010) Cancer nanotechnology: application of nanotechnology in cancer therapy. Drug Discov Today 15(19–20):842–850

Miyoshi T et al (2016) Risk factors associated with cisplatin-induced nephrotoxicity in patients with advanced lung cancer. Biol Pharm Bull 39(12):2009–2014

Mo R et al (2012) Multistage pH-responsive liposomes for mitochondrial-targeted anticancer drug delivery. Adv Mater 24(27):3659–3665

Molina JR et al (2008) Non-small cell lung cancer: epidemiology, risk factors, treatment, and survivorship. Mayo Clin Proc 83(5):584–594

Nanowerk (2020) What are quantum dots? [cited 2020 21/12]. https://www.nanowerk.com/what_are_quantum_dots.php#:~:text=Quantum%20dots%20(QDs)%20are%20man,cells%20and%20fluorescent%20biological%20labels

National Health Service (2019) Lung cancer. [cited 2020 16/11]. https://www.nhs.uk/conditions/lung-cancer/

National Health Surface (2019) Lung cancer—treatment. [cited 2020 14/12]. https://www.nhs.uk/conditions/lung-cancer/treatment/

Navani N et al (2015) Lung cancer diagnosis and staging with endobronchial ultrasound-guided transbronchial needle aspiration compared with conventional approaches: an open-label, pragmatic, randomised controlled trial. Lancet Respir Med 3(4):282–289

Norouzi M, Hardy P (2021) Clinical applications of nanomedicines in lung cancer treatment. Acta Biomater 121:134–142

Owens DE, Peppas NA (2006) Opsonization, biodistribution, and pharmacokinetics of polymeric nanoparticles. Int J Pharm 307(1):93–102

Patil M, Mehta DS, Guvva S (2008) Future impact of nanotechnology on medicine and dentistry. J Indian Soc Periodontol 12(2):34–40

PDQ® Adult Treatment Editorial Board (2020) Small cell lung cancer treatment. [cited 2020 17/12]. https://www.cancer.gov/types/lung/hp/small-cell-lung-treatment-pdq#_72

Peng G et al (2009) Diagnosing lung cancer in exhaled breath using gold nanoparticles. Nat Nanotechnol 4(10):669–673

Periyasamy P et al (2012) Nanomaterials for the local and targeted delivery of osteoarthritis drugs. J Nanomater 6:1–13

Pesch B et al (2012) NOTCH1, HIF1A and other cancer-related proteins in lung tissue from uranium miners—variation by occupational exposure and subtype of lung cancer. PLoS One 7(9):e45305

Poonia M et al (2017) Nanotechnology in oral cancer: a comprehensive review. J Oral Maxillofac Pathol 21(3):407–414

Qian X et al (2008) In vivo tumor targeting and spectroscopic detection with surface-enhanced Raman nanoparticle tags. Nat Biotechnol 26(1):83–90

Rahman G et al (2019) An overview of the recent progress in the synthesis and applications of carbon nanotubes. C 5:1–31

Rana S et al (2012) Monolayer coated gold nanoparticles for delivery applications. Adv Drug Deliv Rev 64(2):200–216

Rancoule C et al (2016) Nanoparticles in radiation oncology: from bench-side to bedside. Cancer Lett 375(2):256–262

Rosenberger I et al (2015) Targeted diagnostic magnetic nanoparticles for medical imaging of pancreatic cancer. J Control Release 214:76–84

Sadhukha T, Wiedmann TS, Panyam J (2013) Inhalable magnetic nanoparticles for targeted hyperthermia in lung cancer therapy. Biomaterials 34(21):5163–5171

Saito M et al (2018) Development of targeted therapy and immunotherapy for treatment of small cell lung cancer. Jpn J Clin Oncol 48(7):603–608

Sajja HK et al (2009) Development of multifunctional nanoparticles for targeted drug delivery and noninvasive imaging of therapeutic effect. Curr Drug Discov Technol 6(1):43–51

Sarkar S et al (2017) Advances and implications in nanotechnology for lung cancer management. Curr Drug Metab 18(1):30–38

Sasaki H et al (2014) Prognosis of recurrent non-small cell lung cancer following complete resection. Oncol Lett 7(4):1300–1304

Scher N et al (2020) Review of clinical applications of radiation-enhancing nanoparticles. Biotechnol Rep (Amst) 28:e00548

Shah P (2006) Clinical consideration in lung cancer. In: Desai SR (ed) Lung cancer. Cambridge University Press, Cambridge, pp 1–11

Shahri M (2019) Magnetic materials and magnetic nanocomposites for biomedical application. In: Henry D (ed) Harnessing nanoscale surface interactions. Elsevier, pp 77–95

Sharma A, Sharma U (1997) Liposomes in drug delivery: progress and limitations. Int J Pharm 154:123–140

Shirish G, Suresh R, Gregory K (2012) Treatment of lung cancer. Radiol Clin North Am 50(5):961–974

Sigma Aldrich (2020) Gold nanoparticles: properties and applications. [cited 2020 23/12]. https://www.sigmaaldrich.com/technical-documents/articles/materials-science/nanomaterials/gold-nanoparticles.html

Silvestri GA et al (2013) Methods for staging non-small cell lung cancer: diagnosis and management of lung cancer, 3rd ed: American College of Chest Physicians evidence-based clinical practice guidelines. Chest 143(5 Suppl):e211S–e250S

Smith AM, Nie S (2009) Next-generation quantum dots. Nat Biotechnol 27(8):732–733

Socinski MA et al (2013) Treatment of stage IV non-small cell lung cancer: diagnosis and management of lung cancer, 3rd ed: American College of Chest Physicians evidence-based clinical practice guidelines. Chest 143(5 Suppl):e341S–e368S

Stathopoulos GP et al (2010) Liposomal cisplatin combined with paclitaxel versus cisplatin and paclitaxel in non-small-cell lung cancer: a randomized phase III multicenter trial. Ann Oncol 21(11):2227–2232

Stathopoulos GP et al (2011) Comparison of liposomal cisplatin versus cisplatin in non-squamous cell non-small-cell lung cancer. Cancer Chemother Pharmacol 68(4):945–950

Svenson S, Tomalia DA (2005) Dendrimers in biomedical applications—reflections on the field. Adv Drug Deliv Rev 57(15):2106–2129

Sztandera K, Gorzkiewicz M, Klajnert-Maculewicz B (2019) Gold nanoparticles in cancer treatment. Mol Pharm 16(1):1–23

Ta VT et al (2014) Reusable floating-electrode sensor for the quantitative electrophysiological monitoring of a nonadherent cell. ACS Nano 8(3):2206–2213

Tay ZW et al (2018) In vivo tracking and quantification of inhaled aerosol using magnetic particle imaging towards inhaled therapeutic monitoring. Theranostics 8(13):3676–3687

Thakur S et al (2015) Impact of pegylation on biopharmaceutical properties of dendrimers. Polymer 59:67–92

The American Cancer Society medical and editorial content team (2019a) Signs and symptoms of lung cancer. [cited 2020 17/11]. https://www.cancer.org/cancer/lung-cancer/detection-diagnosis-staging/signs-symptoms.html

The American Cancer Society medical and editorial content team (2019b) What is lung cancer? [cited 2020 16/11]. https://www.cancer.org/cancer/lung-cancer/about/what-is.html

The American Cancer Society medical and editorial content team (2020) Immunotherapy for non-small cell lung cancer. [cited 2020 14/12]. https://www.cancer.org/cancer/lung-cancer/treating-non-small-cell/immunotherapy.html

Tong L et al (2007) Gold nanorods mediate tumor cell death by compromising membrane integrity. Adv Mater 19:3136–3141

Torchilin VP (2005) Recent advances with liposomes as pharmaceutical carriers. Nat Rev Drug Discov 4(2):145–160

Travis WD (2014) The 2015 WHO classification of lung tumors. Pathologe 35(Suppl 2):188

Uramoto H, Tanaka F (2014) Recurrence after surgery in patients with NSCLC. Transl Lung Cancer Res 3(4):242–249

Wan X et al (2016) The preliminary study of immune superparamagnetic iron oxide nanoparticles for the detection of lung cancer in magnetic resonance imaging. Carbohydr Res 419:33–40

Wang AZ, Tepper JE (2014) Nanotechnology in radiation oncology. J Clin Oncol 32(26):2879–2885

Wang EC, Wang AZ (2014) Nanoparticles and their applications in cell and molecular biology. Integr Biol (Camb) 6(1):9–26

Wang X et al (2008) Application of nanotechnology in cancer therapy and imaging. CA Cancer J Clin 58(2):97–110

Wang Y et al (2012) Detection of micrometastases in lung cancer with magnetic nanoparticles and quantum dots. Int J Nanomedicine 7:2315–2324

Wang C et al (2013) Enhancement of radiation effect and increase of apoptosis in lung cancer cells by thio-glucose-bound gold nanoparticles at megavoltage radiation energies. J Nanopart Res 15(5):1642

Wawrzynczak A, Feliczak-Guzik A, Nowak I (2016) Nanosunscreens: from nanoencapsulated to nanosized cosmetic active forms. In: Grumezescu A (ed) Nanobiomaterials in galenic formulations and cosmetics. William Andrew Publishing, pp 25–46

WebMD (2020) Small-cell lung cancer. [cited 2020 17/12]. https://www.webmd.com/lung-cancer/small-cell-lung-cancer#1

Weissleder R (2006) Molecular imaging in cancer. Science 312(5777):1168–1171

Werner ME et al (2013) Preclinical evaluation of Genexol-PM, a nanoparticle formulation of paclitaxel, as a novel radiosensitizer for the treatment of non-small cell lung cancer. Int J Radiat Oncol Biol Phys 86(3):463–468

Willow J (2020) Stage 3 lung cancer: prognosis, life expectancy, treatment, and more. [cited 2020 14/12]. https://www.healthline.com/health/lung-cancer/stage-3-symptoms-outlook#:~:text=Stage%203%20lung%20cancer%20treatment,not%20indicated%20for%20stage%203B

Wilson CM et al (2015) The ins and outs of nanoparticle technology in neurodegenerative diseases and cancer. Curr Drug Metab 16(8):609–632

Wolinsky JB, Grinstaff MW (2008) Therapeutic and diagnostic applications of dendrimers for cancer treatment. Adv Drug Deliv Rev 60(9):1037–1055

Woodman C et al (2021) Applications and strategies in nanodiagnosis and nanotherapy in lung cancer. Semin Cancer Biol 69:349–364

Xu B et al (2018) Meta-analysis of clinical trials comparing the efficacy and safety of liposomal cisplatin versus conventional nonliposomal cisplatin in non-small cell lung cancer (NSCLC) and squamous cell carcinoma of the head and neck (SCCHN). Medicine (Baltimore) 97(46):e13169

Yang F et al (2008) Magnetic lymphatic targeting drug delivery system using carbon nanotubes. Med Hypotheses 70(4):765–767

Yeh YC, Creran B, Rotello VM (2012) Gold nanoparticles: preparation, properties, and applications in bionanotechnology. Nanoscale 4(6):1871–1880

Yin Q et al (2019) Excitation-wavelength and size-dependent photo-darkening and photo-brightening of photoluminescence from PbS quantum dots in glasses. Opt Mater Express 9(2):504–515

Yu KH et al (2016) Predicting non-small cell lung cancer prognosis by fully automated microscopic pathology image features. Nat Commun 7:12474

Yue X, Dai Z (2018) Liposomal nanotechnology for cancer theranostics. Curr Med Chem 25(12):1397–1408

Zahednezhad F et al (2020) The latest advances of cisplatin liposomal formulations: essentials for preparation and analysis. Expert Opin Drug Deliv 17(4):523–541

Zhang Y, He J (2013) The development of targeted therapy in small cell lung cancer. J Thorac Dis 5(4):538–548

Zielińska A et al (2020) Polymeric nanoparticles: production, characterization, toxicology and ecotoxicology. Molecules 25(16):3731

Ziemer LS et al (2005) Oxygen distribution in murine tumors: characterization using oxygen-dependent quenching of phosphorescence. J Appl Physiol (1985) 98(4):1503–1510

Part XII

Clinical Research in Lung Cancer

Translational Research in Lung Cancer

Haoming Qiu, Michael A. Cummings, and Yuhchyau Chen

Contents

1 Introduction 1113
1.1 NIH Roadmap for Translational Medicine 1113

2 **Prognostic Molecular Markers of Lung Cancer** 1114
2.1 Ras Oncogenes/p21 1114
2.2 p53 Tumor Suppressor Gene 1115
2.3 Gene Expression Profiles 1116

3 **Predictive Tumor Markers and Molecular Targets of Non-small Cell Lung Cancer** 1116
3.1 Epidermal Growth Factor Receptor (EGFR) Proto-oncogenes: c-erbB-1 1116
3.2 EML4-ALK Translocation 1118
3.3 Programed Cell Death Ligand 1 (PD-L1) 1119
3.4 Markers of DNA Repair: ERCC1 and RRM1 1121

4 **Clinical Translational Radiation Investigations of Non-small Cell Lung Cancer** 1124
4.1 Radiotherapy and Immune Checkpoint Inhibition for NSCLC 1124
4.2 Pulsed Paclitaxel Chemoradiotherapy: A Model of Translational Investigation of Radiosensitization 1125

5 Summary 1127

References 1128

H. Qiu · M. A. Cummings · Y. Chen (✉)
Department of Radiation Oncology, James P. Wilmot Cancer Center, University of Rochester Medical Center, Rochester, NY, USA
e-mail: Yuhchyau_Chen@urmc.rochester.edu

1 Introduction

1.1 NIH Roadmap for Translational Medicine

For decades, the National Institutes of Health (NIH) has been funding basic biomedical research that aims to understand how living organisms work until the NIH Roadmap initiative (Fig. 1), with increased focus on the need to "translate" basic research more quickly into human studies and then into tests and treatments that can improve clinical practices for the benefit of patients (Westfall et al. 2007). Since then, translational research for lung cancer has undergone evolution with tremendous progress in discovering new molecular markers of lung cancer, some of which provide the prognosis of tumors expressing such markers, while others predict the treatment response to specific molecular targeted therapy toward tumor-specific mutations and toward immunotherapy. The predictive marker discoveries have changed the landscape of lung cancer treatment into progressively more personalized medicine. We summarize the progress in translational investigations of molecular markers of lung cancer with an emphasis on non-small cell lung cancer (NSCLC) and present examples of clinical trials that are built on information from translational investigations in the laboratory.

"Blue Highways" on the NIH Roadmap

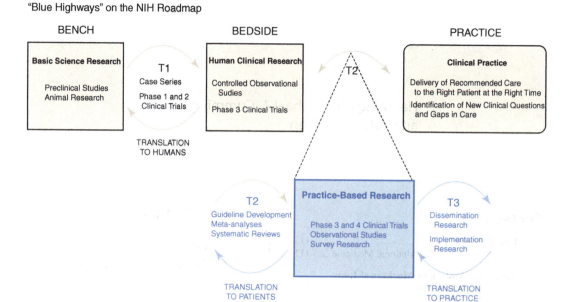

Fig. 1 The National Institutes of Health (NIH) Roadmap for Medical Research includes the traditional bench and bedside research (T1), the translational step (T2), and the new T2 and T3 steps. Historically, moving new medical discoveries into clinical practice (T2) has been haphazard, occurring largely through continuing medical education programs, pharmaceutical detailing, and guideline development. The expansion of the NIH Roadmap (blue part) includes an additional "practice-based research" and translational step (T3) to the incorporation of research discoveries into day-to-day clinical care. The research roadmap is a continuum, with overlap between sites of research and translational steps (Westfall et al. 2007, with permission)

2 Prognostic Molecular Markers of Lung Cancer

Numerous prognostic molecular markers for NSCLC have been investigated in recent decades, including EGFR, c-erB-2, c-erB-3, CD82, Ki-67, p120, p53, bcl-2, CD31 MIA-15-5, p21, p53, PCNA, Ki-67, p185[new] protein, RB protein, bcl-2 protein, H-ras-p21 protein, blood group A, K-ras, angiogenic marker factor viii, adhesion molecule CD-44, sialyl-Tn, blood group AMRP-1/CD9 gene, KA11/CD82, laminin receptor, FOS, JUN, ERBB1, cyclin A, TGF a, amphiregulin (AR), and others (Reviewed in Chen and Gandara 2006). Some markers were found to have prognostic values when investigated individually, but lost them when multiple factors were examined at the same time. Here, we summarize the two major prognostic molecular markers, K-ras and P53, as well as review the current state of prognostic gene signatures in NSCLC.

2.1 Ras Oncogenes/p21

The ras oncogene family encodes guanosine triphosphate-binding proteins with a 21 kd (p21) molecular weight. The proteins are localized at the inner surface of the cell membrane and are involved in the transduction of growth signals. There are three well-characterized members of the ras oncogene family: H-ras, K-ras, and N-ras (Barbacid 1987). The oncogenic potential of ras genes is triggered by point mutations occurring mainly in either codon 12, 13, or 61. A ras gene mutation is detected in 10–30% of NSCLC cases, and 80–90% of ras mutations occurred on codon 12 of the K-ras gene (Rodenhuis and Slebos 1992; Bos 1989; Slebos et al. 1990; Mitsudomi et al. 1991; Sugio et al. 1992). The mutations are frequently observed in smokers and are more frequent in adenocarcinoma than in squamous cell carcinoma (SCC) but absent in small cell lung cancer (SCLC) (Rodenhuis and Slebos 1992; Mitsudomi et al. 1991; Greatens et al. 1998; Brose et al. 2002; Riely et al. 2009). Several investigators have reported that ras mutations are a poor prognostic factor in NSCLC, and the absence of H-ras p21 expression was among the nine independent predictors for recurrence, while other researchers found no negative prognostic value to the K-ras mutation. Mascaux et al. (2005) performed a meta-analysis of more than 53 studies, which evaluated the K-ras mutation and outcomes in patients with NSCLC. They identified K-ras mutations or p21 overexpression by PCR assay as a negative prognostic factor for NSCLC (hazard ratio [HR] for death was 1.35; 95% confidence interval [CI], 1.16–1.56) and even worse HR for adenocarcinomas (HR 1.40; 95% CI, 1.18–1.65). Notably, investigations of ras using immunohistochemical stain (IHC) showed no prognostic values in the meta-analysis (HR 1.08; 95% CI, 0.86–1.34). The major criticism of such meta-analysis was that it was not based on prospectively designed studies, and the authors did not perform multivariate analyses to include other clinical prognostic variables such as tumor stage, performance status, and weight loss.

A large trial that prospectively assessed K-ras mutations was conducted as part of E3590 (Eastern Cooperative Oncology Group, Study No. 3590). Patients with stage II–IIIA NSCLC were randomized to receive postoperative radiation therapy or radiation therapy and chemotherapy (Schiller et al. 2001). The study found no correlation of overall survival (OS) or disease-free survival (DFS) with K-ras mutations. To date, attempts to directly target K-ras mutation for the treatment of NSCLC have not been successful, and efforts are focused on targeting pathways downstream to K-ras, such as MEK. In a randomized study, previously treated patients with K-ras mutations were randomized to chemotherapy or chemotherapy and a MEK inhibitor, selumetinib. The study showed a significantly increased overall response rate (ORR) of 37% vs. 0%, prolonged progression-free survival (PFS 5.3 months vs. 2.1 months), and a trend of increased OS (9.4 months vs. 5.2 months) (Janne et al. 2013).

2.2 p53 Tumor Suppressor Gene

p53 is a tumor suppressor gene (TSG) encoding a 53 kDa nuclear phosphoprotein with a transcriptional activator, which controls cell proliferation by regulating a G1-S checkpoint before DNA synthesis, through the cyclin-dependent kinase (CDK) pathway (Cordon-Cardo 1995). In response to DNA damage by ionizing radiation and a variety of chemical agents or carcinogens, p53 induces cells to repair damage or promote apoptosis (Yin et al. 1992; Hartwell 1992; Farmer et al. 1992). Mutations of the p53 gene are the most common findings in human cancer cells of all types (Greenblatt et al. 1994). The p53 gene is the most commonly mutated TSG in lung cancer, affecting 90% of SCLC and 50% of NSCLC (Mayne et al. 1999). Most mutations occur in evolutionarily conserved p53 exons 5–8. p53 mutations correlate with smoking, and most are of the type G to T transversions expected from tobacco smoke carcinogens.

More evidence linking smoking damage with p53 is that a major cigarette-smoke carcinogen known as benzopyrene selectively forms adducts at the p53 mutation hotspot (Kohno and Yokota 1999). The types of p53 mutations are varied and include missense, nonsense, and splicing abnormalities as well as larger deletions. The most common mutations are of the missense type, which often prolong the half-life of the p53 protein to several hours, leading to increased levels detectable by IHC, which can be used as a surrogate assay of p53.

The prognostic significance of p53 mutation/overexpression remains unclear as studies have showed conflicting findings. There are at least three published works on p53 meta-analysis. Mitsudomi et al. (2000) performed a meta-analysis of 43 articles. p53 alteration was detected either by overexpression of the protein (IHC) or as mutation by the DNA studies. They found that the incidence of p53 alteration in DNA studies was 37% (381/1031) and the incidence of protein overexpression was 48% (1725/3579). The incidence of p53 overexpression and mutation in adenocarcinoma (36% and 34%) was lower than that in SCC (54% and 52%). p53 alteration had a significant negative prognostic effect for adenocarcinomas but not for SCC. They concluded that p53 alteration either by protein overexpression or by DNA mutation was a significant marker of poor prognosis in patients with pulmonary adenocarcinoma. Steels et al. (2001) did a meta-analysis of 74 eligible papers. The studies were categorized by histology, disease stage, treatment, and laboratory technique. Combined hazard ratios suggested that an abnormal p53 status had an unfavorable impact on survival for all tumor stages (I–IV) and for both SCLC and adenocarcinoma. Huncharek et al. (2000) published a meta-analysis of eight studies investigating p53 mutations involving a total of 829 patients. They did not find p53 mutation as a prognostic marker in NSCLC and felt that selection bias, smoking history, race, geographic location, and socioeconomic status might have been the confounding factors. The prognostic value of p53 was examined in a prospective study by the abovementioned large trial of E3590 (Eastern Cooperative Oncology Group, Study No. 3590). This study did not find the correlation of OS or DFS with p53 protein expression and p53 mutation (Schiller et al. 2001).

2.3 Gene Expression Profiles

Gene expression profiling of resected lung tumors was made possible by microarray technologies and real-time reverse transcriptase-polymerase chain reaction (RT-PCR) analysis. Gene expression profiles have revealed the underlying heterogeneity of NSCLC classified by conventional histopathology, thus offering the possibility of molecular taxonomy (Bhattacharjee et al. 2001). Further, several studies have reported the prognostic value of discrete gene signatures in association with survival outcome for operable NSCLC. These gene expression profiles were generated from resected NSCLC with mostly stage I tumors. Prognostic gene signatures included 3–6 genes (Lau et al. 2007; Chen et al. 2007; Boutros et al. 2008), 20–64 genes (Guo et al. 2008; Lu et al. 2006; Sun et al. 2008), 125 genes (Larsen et al. 2007), and more than 2000 genes in the case of metagenes (Potti et al. 2006). All of these gene signatures have shown prognostic value for cancer survival independently or in combination with clinical factors. The largest gene signature set is the metagene, which is a collection of gene expression profiles that are computer generated and randomly assigned sets of 25–200 genes. The signatures contain 100 metagenes, which when combined include more than 2000 distinct genes. In theory, this large size allows for a predictive power for disease recurrence much greater than fewer numbers of genes. Initially, it was reported with an accuracy of 72–93% in different patient groups with stage IA NSCLC (Potti et al. 2006). However, the original report was retracted in March 2011 due to failure to reproduce results supporting the validation of the lung metagene model described in the article (Potti et al. 2011). Nonetheless, the prognostic value of global gene profiling remains an area of active research.

3 Predictive Tumor Markers and Molecular Targets of Non-small Cell Lung Cancer

3.1 Epidermal Growth Factor Receptor (EGFR) Proto-oncogenes: c-erbB-1

EGFR, also known as HER1 or erbB-1, is one of the four members of the erbB receptor tyrosine kinase family (Sharma et al. 2007). c-erB-1

(EGFR) is the proto-oncogene encoding the EGFR protein. In addition to erB-1, the erB family of tyrosine kinase receptor proteins also includes erb-B2 (HER2/neu), erb-B3, and erb-B4 (Franklin et al. 2002). Intracellular signaling is triggered by the binding of ligands, such as epidermal growth factor (EGF) resulting in the dimerization of EGFR molecules or heterodimerization with other closely related receptors, such as HER2/neu. Phosphorylation of the receptors through their tyrosine kinase domains leads to intracellular signal transduction and activation of proliferative signals and DNA synthesis (Yarden and Sliwkowski 2001; Jorissen et al. 2003; Kumar et al. 2008) (Fig. 2). In NSCLC, EGFR is more commonly overexpressed than HER2/neu and has been observed in 40–80% of cancer specimens (Franklin et al. 2002; Arteaga 2003; Berger et al. 1987). The prognostic value of EGFR overexpression analyzed by IHC stains and by FISH in lung cancer has been a controversial issue. Some reports indicated that EGFR overexpression was associated with a poor prognosis (Volm et al. 1992; Ohsaki et al. 2000; Cox et al. 2000), while others have shown no prognostic associations (Greatens et al. 1998; Rusch et al. 1997; Pfeiffer et al. 1996; Fontanini et al. 1998; D'Amico et al. 1999; Pastorino et al. 1997). Hirsch et al. (2003) reported analyses of the gene copy number of EGFR using the FISH technique as well as the protein expression using IHC stain and found that neither EGFR overexpression nor high gene copy number had any significant influence as an independent prognostic factor; thus, such information is not useful in routine practices (Ramalingham et al. 2011).

In contrast to the lack of prognostic and predictive value of protein overexpression and gene copy number, the somatic mutation of EGFR gene in the tyrosine kinase domain was found to be predictive for tumor response to treatments by EGFR-tyrosine kinase inhibitors (EGFR-TKIs).

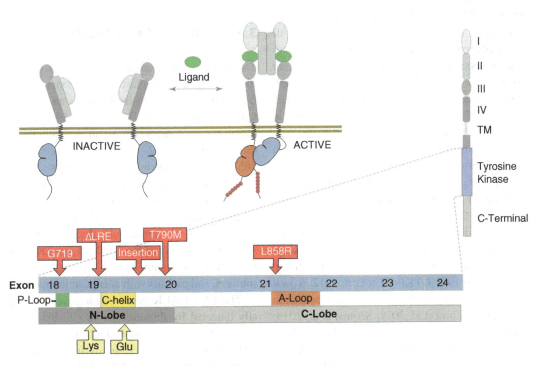

Fig. 2 Schematic presentation of EGFR activation. On extracellular ligand binding, the receptor dimerizes, allowing the cytoplasmic EGFR-TK to activate in a tail-to-head fashion. The locations of regions within EGFR-TK are indicated on the exon boundary map (Kumar et al. 2008, with permission)

Most patients with the mutations were women, nonsmokers, and those with bronchioloalveolar tumors (Kris et al. 2003; Fukuoka et al. 2003). EGFR mutations are present in approximately 10–15% of Caucasians and in nearly 30–50% of Asians, with the highest fraction of 57% in Japanese women (Sharma et al. 2007; Kosaka et al. 2004; Janne et al. 2005; Shigematsu et al. 2005; Han et al. 2005). Patients with EGFR mutations are highly responsive to EGFR-TKI treatments. The molecular basis for increased sensitivity to EGFR-TKI is due to somatic activating mutations in exons 18–21 of EGFR (commonly exon 19 deletions and L858R point mutation in exon 21) that encode the tyrosine kinase domain of the EGFR (Sharma et al. 2007). Mutations in exon 18 are known to confer sensitivity to EGFR-TKI, while exon 20 in-frame insertions are associated with resistance to treatment with TKI.

Several clinical trials have demonstrated EGFR-TKI superior to chemotherapy in ORR and PFS for stage IV NSCLC. The Iressa Pan-Asia Study (IPASS) was a landmark study reported by Mok et al. (2009). In this randomized phase III study of East Asia, patients had advanced pulmonary adenocarcinoma and nonsmokers or former light smokers would receive gefitinib vs. carboplatin plus paclitaxel chemotherapy. Twelve-month rate of PFS was 24.9% in gefitinib treatment arm and 6.7% in carboplatin/paclitaxel treatment arm. The median PFS of the gefitinib treatment arm was 6.5 months versus 1.5 months of the chemotherapy arm. The study showed superiority of gefitinib in the intention-to-treat population (HR 0.74; 95% CI: 0.65–0.85; $P < 0.001$). Other large randomized phase III studies conducted in Asia and Spain further confirmed the role of EGFR mutations as a major predictor of outcome to treatment by EGFR-TKIs (Han et al. 2012; Rosell et al. 2012; Mitsudomi et al. 2010; Maemondo et al. 2010; Zhou et al. 2011; Sequist et al. 2013; Wu et al. 2014). These studies led to the paradigm shift in using EGFR-TKIs as the first-line therapy in patients with advanced-stage NSCLC in the setting of known EGFR mutations.

For NSCLC with EGFR mutation at exon 19 deletion or L858 mutation in exon 21, both gefitinib and erlotinib have been the approved first-line and first-generation EGFR-TKI. Subsequently, second-generation EGFR-TKIs have been developed and include afatinib, dacomitinib, and neratinib. Patients responded to first- and second-generation EGFR-TKIs eventually would develop resistance at a median of 9–13 months (Suda et al. 2017). A further mutation in exon 20 of EGFR (T790M) contributes to approximately 50% of these resistant cases (Pao et al. 2005). Third-generation EGFR-TKIs were also developed, which include osimertinib, rociletinib (CO-1686), and olmutinib (HM61731). The ORRs of osimertinib, rociletinib, and olmutinib were 64%, 58%, and 29.2% in early clinical trials (Liao et al. 2015). Of note, osimertinib is the first global EFGR TKI approved for the treatment of NSCLC with EGFR T790M mutation.

3.2 EML4-ALK Translocation

The echinoderm microtubule-associated protein-like 4 (EML4)-anaplastic lymphoma kinase (ALK) fusion-type tyrosine kinase is an oncoprotein found in 4–7% of NSCLCs. The EML4-ALK fusion gene is generated by small inversion within the chromosome 2 short arm, encoding a 1059-amino-acid fusion protein. The N-terminal portion is identical to the human echinoderm microtubule-associated protein-like 4 (EML4) (Pollmann et al. 2006), and the C-terminal portion is the same as the intracellular domain of human ALK (Morris et al. 1994). The EML4-ALK translocation is most common in younger males, never-smokers, and patients with adenocarcinoma.

The EML4-ALK gene rearrangement is usually detected by fluorescence in situ hybridization (FISH) or immunohistochemistry. EML4 NSCLC occurs most commonly in clinical subgroups who share many of the clinical features of NSCLC likely to harbor EGFR mutation (Shaw et al. 2009). With rare exceptions, EML and EGFR mutations are mutually exclusive. EML translocation tends to occur in younger patients and those with locally advanced disease, while this relationship has not been reported for EGFR-mutant NSCLC (Inamura et al. 2009). EML4-ALK mutation responds to ALK inhibitors such as crizotinib, ceritinib, and alectinib. In a phase III study in patients with untreated advanced-stage NSCLC with ALK rearrangement treated with crizotinib versus chemotherapy, crizotinib had a significantly higher ORR (74% vs. 45%) and prolonged PFS (10.9 months vs. 7 months) (Solomon et al. 2014). At 46-month median follow-up interval, the median OS was not reached (NR) with crizotinib arm and was 47.5 months with chemotherapy (the study allows crossover). Survival probability at 4 years was 56.6% with crizotinib and 49.1% with chemotherapy (Solomon et al. 2018). In a phase III study of chemo-pretreated patients with advanced-stage ALK-rearranged NSCLC, crizotinib was superior to standard single-agent chemotherapy in terms of ORR (65% vs. 20%) and PFS (7.7 months vs. 3 months) (Shaw et al. 2013).

3.3 Programed Cell Death Ligand 1 (PD-L1)

In NSCLC, PD-L1 expression is a major predictive biomarker that is now routinely assessed to help direct the treatment for patients with metastatic NSCLC lacking a driver mutation such as EGFR or ALK (Hanna et al. 2020). PD-L1 is one of the two types of the ligand to programed cell death receptor 1 (PD-1). PD-1 is a type 1 transmembrane glycoprotein that belongs to the B7/CD28/CTLA-4 family of receptors (Patsoukis et al. 2020). PD-1 receptors are expressed at the surface of many cells of the adaptive and innate immune system including T cells, B cells, monocytes, NK T cells, and dendritic cells. Its ligands, PD-L1 or PD-L2, are expressed on the surface of tumor cells and antigen-presenting cells in the tumor microenvironment. Binding of the ligand to the PD-1 receptor recruits phosphatases such as SHP2 to the immune-receptor tyrosine-based switch motif in the PD-1 tail causing inhibition of T-cell receptor signaling and leads to decreased T-cell activation, proliferation, and survival (Sharpe and Pauken 2018). In normal hosts, the PD-1 pathway serves as a "checkpoint" to prevent autoimmune damage, especially in times of chronic inflammation. Tumor cells from a variety of malignancies including melanoma, lung, breast, renal, and others can co-opt this pathway by overexpressing PD-L1 on its surface. This results in the exhaustion and apoptosis of cytotoxic T cells and allows tumor cells to escape immune-mediated cell killing (Zak et al. 2017). Drugs preventing the binding of PD-L1 to PD-1 thereby upregulate immune-mediated tumor cell killing (Fig. 3).

PD-L1 expression in non-small cell lung cancer was studied in a pooled analysis of patients screened for eligibility in the KEYNOTE-001, -010, and -024 trials. Of the 4784 patients evaluable for PD-L1, 33% had tumor proportion scores (TPS) <1%, 38% had TPS of 1–49%, and 28% had TPS ≥50% (Aggarwal 2016). PD-L1 expression level is a predictive biomarker for the response to anti-PD-1/PD-L1 axis checkpoint inhibitor immunotherapy. The most commonly used drugs in this category include pembrolizumab and nivolumab, which are monoclonal antibodies that bind to and inhibit the PD-1 receptor, and atezolizumab and durvalumab, which are monoclonal antibodies against the PD-L1 ligand.

For tumors with high PD-L1 expression (>50% expression), immunotherapy monotherapy is the currently recommended treatment option. This is based on the results of the KEYNOTE-024 trial, which showed that for patients with high PD-L1 expression, pembrolizumab monotherapy was superior to platinum doublet chemotherapy with the median overall survival of 30 months vs. 14.2 months (Reck et al. 2016). Similar results from another randomized phase III study showed that for a

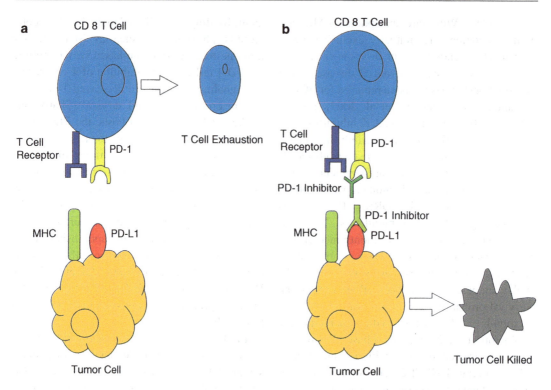

Fig. 3 A simplified schematic presentation of PD-1/PD-L1 axis and the effect of anti-PD-1 or anti-PD-L1 treatment. (**a**) Binding of tumor PD-L1 to the PD-1 receptor on T cells can induce T-cell anergy and can allow tumors to escape immune-mediated cytotoxicity. (**b**) Drug inhibition of the PD-1 receptor or PD-L1 ligand "removes the breaks" and upregulates immune-mediated cell killing

subset of patients with high PD-L1 expression, atezolizumab demonstrated improved overall survival compared with platinum chemotherapy (20 months vs. 13 months) (Herbst et al. 2020).

For patients with low PD-L1 expression (<50% expression), the standard of care is now platinum doublet chemotherapy plus immunotherapy for both squamous and nonsquamous histology. This is based on the KEYNOTE-189 trial, which showed that for patients with all levels of PD-L1 expression, pembrolizumab plus chemotherapy was superior to chemotherapy alone in 12-month OS (69% vs. 49%) (Gandhi et al. 2018). This improvement was seen in all subsets of patients; however, the greatest numerical benefit with immunotherapy was seen in patients with PD-L1 expression ≥1% versus those with <1%. Similar results were seen in another report, which showed an overall survival improvement with the addition of atezolizumab to chemotherapy (Socinski et al. 2018). For patients with squamous histology, the KEYNOTE-407 trial showed that in patients with all levels of PD-L1 expression, pembrolizumab plus chemotherapy was superior to chemotherapy alone in median OS (15.9 months vs. 11.3 months). While all patients benefited from the addition of pembrolizumab, PFS improvement was numerically greatest in those with higher PD-L1 expression (Paz-Ares et al. 2018).

3.3.1 BRAF Mutations

BRAF is a member of the RAF family of serine/threonine protein kinases that mediate tumorigenesis by phosphorylation of MEK and downstream ERK signaling pathway (Paik et al. 2011). BRAF-mutant NSCLC is observed in 2–4% of

NSCLC and is a heterogeneous disease. There are three functional classes of BRAF mutations: class I are V600-mutant kinase-activating dimers; class II are kinase-activating dimers; and class III are kinase-inactivating heterodimers. About 50% of BRAF mutations are BRAF V600E mutations, which are clinically less aggressive than classes II and III, and are more common in women and never-smokers (Dagogo-Jack et al. 2018; Paik et al. 2011; Chen et al. 2014; Brustugun et al. 2014). The BRAF V600E mutations respond to inhibitors dabrafenib and vemurafenib (Planchard et al. 2016).

3.3.2 ROS1 Rearrangement

ROS1 is a tyrosine kinase of the insulin receptor family. ROS1 translocation is seen in 2–3% of NSCLCs. ROS1 rearrangement occurs as a result of genetic translocations between the ROS1 gene with various fusion proteins, including CD74, syndecan 4 gene (SDC4), ezrin gene (EZR), tropomyosin 3 gene (TPM3), TRK-fused gene (TFG), zinc finger CCHC-type containing 8 gene (ZCCHC8), sarcolemma-associated protein gene (SLMAP), and myosin VC gene (MYO5C). All of these fusion partners preserved the tyrosine kinase domain of ROS1 (Park et al. 2018). Patients with ROS1 translocations tend to be younger, never-smokers with adenocarcinoma histological subtype, and often have wild-type EGFR and ALK receptor kinase gene. ROS1 mutation tumors have shown response to crizotinib and pemetrexed-based chemotherapy (Shaw et al. 2014).

3.3.3 RET Translocation

The RET proto-oncogene is a receptor kinase. The translocation between the RET gene and its various fusion partners CCDC6, KIF5B, NCOA4, and TRIM33 leads to abnormal expression and oligomerization of the chimeric kinase fusion proteins. The fusions lead to constitutively active oncogenesis. RET fusion has been identified in 1–2% of NSCLC (Takeuchi et al. 2012; Drilon et al. 2013) and is associated with increased risk of brain metastasis (Drilon et al. 2018). RET-positive NSCLC has a 64% response rate to selpercatinib (Drilon et al. 2020), and some patients respond to agents such as cabozantinib, vandetanib, sunitinib ponatinib, regorafenib, and lenvatinib.

3.3.4 MET Mutation

MET is a tyrosine kinase receptor. When activated, MET and its ligand hepatocyte growth factor (HGF) induce cell proliferation, survival invasion, motility, metastasis, and epithelial-to-mesenchyme transition (Feng et al. 2012). MET mutation can involve gene mutation, overexpression, gene amplification, and alternative splicing. MET overexpression is seen in 25–50% of NSCLC and MET amplification in 7%. Both MET and HGF are molecular targets for NSCLC treatment and respond to crizotinib, tivantinib, cabozantinib, and foretinib (Sadiq and Salgia 2013).

3.3.5 NTRK (Neurotrophic Tyrosine Kinase Receptor) Gene Fusions

The NTRK genes (NTRK1, NTRK2, NTRK3) encode tropomyosin receptor kinases (TRKs), which lead to differentiation and survival of central and peripheral nerve cells (Khotskaya et al. 2017; Vashnavi et al. 2015). NTRK gene translocations with other genes result in fusion proteins and constitutively activate tyrosine kinases (Vaishnavi et al. 2013). NTRK gene fusions are seen in about 0.2–3.3% of NSCLC and respond to entrectinib at about 70% rate, larotrectinib at about 72–85% rate, and to a lesser extent to taletrectinib, repotrectinib, and selitrectinib (Haratake and Seto 2020).

3.4 Markers of DNA Repair: ERCC1 and RRM1

The excision repair cross-complementation group 1 gene product (ERCC1) and the regulatory subunit of ribonucleotide reductase (RRM1) have been reported as being prognostic of outcome and predictors of therapeutic efficacy in patients with NSCLC. Both ERCC1 and RRM1 are critical to the nucleotide excision repair (NER) DNA repair pathway. Expression of these genes can both protect the host from the development or progression of cancer and protect tumors from the effects of chemotherapy. Low ERCC mRNA expression and low RRM1 mRNA expression have been correlated with improved survival in advanced NSCLC after treatment with cisplatin-based chemotherapy (Rosell et al. 2004; Simon et al. 2007; Bepler et al. 2008; Souglakos et al. 2008). Further, there is a strong correlation between mRNA expression levels of RRM1 and ERCC1 in NSCLC (Rosell et al. 2004; Simon et al. 2007).

3.4.1 ERCC1

The excision repair cross-complementation gene 1 (ERCC1) encodes a DNA repair protein and a member of the NER complex. In particular, the ERCC1 protein forms a heterodimer with xeroderma pigmentosum (XPF) group A protein and functions to create the 5' incision of damaged DNA. It is a highly conserved protein and plays a rate-limiting role in the NER pathway. ERCC1 polymorphisms have been implicated in carcinogenesis (Chen et al. 1998). However, ERCC1 function can also predict the capacity of tumor cells to repair after cytotoxic treatment, as NER is the primary mechanism for removing platinum-DNA adducts from the tumor DNA (Reed 1998). ERCC1 function and NER pathway have also been shown in vitro to explain the synergy between cisplatin and gemcitabine (Yang et al. 2000).

A retrospective study evaluated ERCC1 mRNA expression in 56 patients with advanced (stage IIIB or IV) NSCLC. These patients were treated with cisplatin and gemcitabine. The study demonstrated ERCC1 expression to be a significant predictor of OS, with ERCC1 low-expressing patients surviving 61.6 weeks as compared to 20.4 weeks in the ERCC1 high-expressing group, although improved tumor response to chemotherapy could not be shown (Lord et al. 2002). Subsequent retrospective studies using cisplatin and gemcitabine have confirmed that low ERCC expression is associated with better overall survival either singly (Ceppi et al. 2006; Hwang et al. 2008; Li et al. 2010) or in combination with low RRM1 expression (Rosell et al. 2004). Other studies, which have used other cisplatin-based therapies, have shown no increase in OS with low expression of ERCC1 (Booton et al. 2007; Fujii et al. 2008), although a differential tumor response was seen (Fujii et al. 2008).

The International Adjuvant Lung Cancer Trial, which randomized patients to receive cisplatin-based chemotherapy after a complete resection of stage I–III NSCLC, showed a small but statistically significant improvement in OS with the addition of chemotherapy (44.5% vs. 40.4% at 5 years) (Arriagada et al. 2004). However, when this study was retrospectively analyzed by ERCC1 protein expression, it was found that only patients with low ERCC1 expression derived benefit from the adjuvant cisplatin-based chemotherapy, while (Olaussen et al. 2006; Bepler et al. 2011).

The first prospective randomized clinical trial testing the concept of customized chemotherapy in NSCLC assessed the role of ERCC1 in treatment planning. The phase III study had 346 patients with stage IV NSCLC, and they were evaluated after being randomized to receive either docetaxel and cisplatin or a tailored regimen based on ERCC1 mRNA levels (docetaxel and cisplatin for low ERCC1 levels and docetaxel plus gemcitabine for higher ERCC1 levels). A significant improvement in the objective response rate was seen in the arm receiving the tailored treatment. However, there was no difference in DFS and OS in the study arms (Cobo et al. 2007).

3.4.2 RRM1

The ribonucleotide-diphosphate reductase M1 (RRM1) gene is the large regulatory subunit of ribonucleotide reductase, which catalyzes the production of deoxyribonucleotides from ribonucleotides preparatory to DNA synthesis during the S phase of the cell cycle. RRM1 is also essential for NER, as it provides the basis needed for restoration of the complementary DNA strand. RRM1 also plays a role in cell migration and metastases. The gene is encoded on 11p15.5 and is thought to be a TSG. In fact, RRM1 transgenic mice were significantly less likely to develop carcinogen-induced lung tumors (Gautam and

Bepler 2006). It is the dominant molecular determinant of gemcitabine efficacy.

A phase II study was performed in 53 patients with previously untreated NSCLC who were stratified in treatment based on real-time quantitative PCR mRNA levels of ERCC1 and RRM1. Treatments by different combinations of double-agent chemotherapy were based on low level vs. high level of ERCC1 and RRM1, showing feasibility of this approach (Simon et al. 2007).

In contrast with the expression in advanced-stage lung cancer, low RRM1 and ERCC1 expression appears to predict worse clinical outcomes in patients with earlier stage disease. A study of 187 patients with early-stage NSCLC who received no adjuvant therapy after surgery showed that RRM1 and ERCC1 were both determinants of survival (Zheng et al. 2007). This apparent paradox may be explained by the fact that intact DNA repair mechanisms in early-stage lung cancer may either prevent or compromise the gathering of further genomic mutations and progression of disease. Thus, both ERCC1 and RRM1 may predict patients with early-stage tumors that do not require further therapy and also inform appropriate chemotherapy for patients with more advanced cancers (Gazdar 2007).

3.4.3 hMSH2 and hMLH1

The human MutS homologue 2 (hMSH2) and human MutL homologue 1 (hMLH1) genes are key components in DNA mismatch repair processes for the recognition and replacement of erroneous base pairs. Mismatch repair reduces mutations at DNA replications, but is also thought to be involved as an adjunct to NER, with error-free repair of DNA interstrand cross-links (Wu et al. 2005). Dysfunction of these genes can lead to microsatellite instability or errors in replicating repeating DNA sequences. Clinically, mutations in these genes constitute hereditary nonpolyposis colorectal cancer type I (for MSH2) or type 2 (for MLH1), wherein patients carry a high risk for various gastrointestinal, genitourinary, and reproductive system cancers.

Certain polymorphisms in the hMSH2 gene have been shown to be associated with a decreased or increased risk of developing NSCLC (Jung et al. 2006; Hsu et al. 2007; Kim et al. 2010; Lo et al. 2011; Shih et al. 2010). In particular, decreased expression of the hMLH1 gene was seen more in SCLC, and decreased expression of the hMSH2 was more common in adenocarcinoma (Xinarianos et al. 2000).

In early-stage NSCLC, with no adjuvant therapy, MLH1 and MSH2 protein expression has not been shown to be prognostic (Cooper et al. 2008). However, hMLH1 gene inactivation (Xinarianos et al. 2000) and in general microsatellite instability (Woenckhaus et al. 2003) are associated with the risk of lymph node metastases. This indicates that mismatch repair defects can play a role in the development and progression of NSCLC.

The data is less clear, as in other DNA repair genes, as to whether inhibition of MSH2 correlates with improved survival in lung cancer patients requiring chemotherapy. A retrospective analysis of the International Adjuvant Lung Trial showed that patients with low MSH2 protein levels (about 38% of the whole) had trends toward improved survival and that no benefit was seen when MSH2 was high. Chemotherapy prolonged OS significantly for patients with tumors expressing low levels of both MSH2 and ERCC1 and also for low levels of MSH2 and P27 (a cell cycle protein) (Kamal et al. 2010). Another study of 179 patients did not show any association of hMLH1 or hMSH2 expression with disease outcomes in stage III NSCLC (Skarda et al. 2006). A third study showed improved survival for cases with low expression of hMLH1, but not hMSH2 (Scartozzi et al. 2006). Data to date indicates that decreased activity of the mismatch repair pathway can be associated with the development and progression of NSCLC. In more advanced disease, decreased activity in this pathway does not correlate robustly with an increased response to cytotoxic chemotherapy. This may indicate that although such cells may have a decreased ability to repair chemotherapy-induced defects, this is balanced by a mutagenic phenotype, allowing for phenotypic selection.

4 Clinical Translational Radiation Investigations of Non-small Cell Lung Cancer

Radiation tumoricidal effects are primarily from direct DNA double- and single-strand breaks or indirect DNA damages through reactive oxygen species. For this reason, translational research in radiotherapy traditionally has been focused on strategies that may enhance radiation tumoricidal effects through radiosensitization. However, much more has been discovered in recent years in radiation effects on the tumor microenvironment, which is now known to actively modulate the behavior and the outcome of cancer treatments. Various structures and cells exist in the tumor microenvironment including tumor-associated fibroblasts, vessels, extracellular matrix, immune cells, cytokines, and others. Radiation-induced changes in cytokines and immune cells in the tumor microenvironment can affect epithelial-mesenchymal transition and tumor metastasis, thus affecting cancer behavior (Arnold et al. 2018). We present examples of clinical translational investigations of radiation-immune modulation as well as a radiosensitization model of translational research for stage III NSCLC.

4.1 Radiotherapy and Immune Checkpoint Inhibition for NSCLC

Radiation interactions with the immune system have gained interests in the past decade (Dovedi et al. 2017). Radiation upregulates the MHC expression and novel peptide antigen expression of tumor cells (Reits et al. 2006), generates type I interferon (Deng et al. 2014b), and regulates macrophages, T cells, and NK cells to elicit immunogenic cell death (Ko et al. 2018). Radiation immunogenic cell death is associated with the release of damage-associated molecular patterns (DAMPs) that activate dendritic cells, present tumor antigens, and prime antigen-specific T cells in a dose-dependent manner (Golden et al. 2014). Preclinical investigations found that immunogenic cell death consisted of (1) cell surface translocation of calreticulin (Obeid et al. 2007), (2) extracellular release of high-mobility group protein box 1 (HMGB-1) (Yamazaki et al. 2014), and (3) extracellular release of adenosine-5′-triphosphate (ATP) (Rodriguez-Ruiz et al. 2019).

Cancer cell death as a result of radiation-induced immunogenic reaction has been described as creating an in situ vaccine (Formenti and Demaria 2009; Golden et al. 2020), based on the fact that radiation increases the immunogenicity of tumors. Such interaction is thought to be responsible for the "abscopal" effect of radiotherapy and has been investigated in preclinical animal tumor models (Dewan et al. 2009). While radiation abscopal effect historically has been a rare phenomenon, with the advent of immunotherapy targeting immune checkpoints for metastatic NSCLC and other cancer types, there have been more reports of clinical radiation abscopal effects in lung cancer (Ngwa et al. 2018; Demaria and Formenti 2020).

Preclinical investigations showed synergism of radiation and anti-PD-L1 treatment in promoting antitumor immunity in mice (Deng et al. 2014a). Radiation also induces the upregulation of PD-L1 receptor in various cancer types including lung cancer (Shen et al. 2017). The first clinical study supporting the interaction between radiation and PD-1/PD-L1 immune axis is the PACIFIC trial, which is a randomized phase III study for locally advanced NSCLC (Antonia et al. 2017; Antonia et al. 2018; Faivre-Finn et al. 2021). Seven hundred and thirteen patients with unresectable stage III NSCLC who have completed definitive thoracic radiotherapy (54–66 Gy) with concurrent chemotherapy without progression were enrolled in this trial. Patients were randomized (2:1) to receive a PD-L1 inhibitor durvalumab (10 mg/kg) vs. placebo every 2 weeks up to 12 months. The median PFS was 17.2 months vs. 5.6 months (HR 0.52), median OS 47.5 months vs. 29.1 months (HR 0.68), and ORR 28.4% vs. 16.0% ($P < 0.001$), all significantly in favor of the durvalumab arm. Grade 3 or 4 adverse events were higher with durvalumab 30.5% vs. 26.1%. The pneumonitis rate in the durvalumab was higher at 4.8% vs. 2.6%. A prespecified analysis using PD-L1 expression cutoff of 25% showed the PFS benefit with durvalumab in patients both above and below the cutoff threshold. An exploratory post hoc analysis using PD-L1 expression of 1% as cutoff showed that patients with ≥1% expression appeared to have greater benefit from durvalumab in unstratified hazard ratios for progression or death compared to those with <1%. The PACIFIC trial was the first clinical translational study showing that radiotherapy might have primed the host immune response in enhancing subsequent tumor immunogenic death to improve the cancer treatment outcome. A follow-up PACIFIC 4 trial is ongoing, which combines stereotactic body radiotherapy (SBRT) of large-dose, hypofractionated precision radiation with durvalumab vs. placebo for high-risk stage I NSCLC. A similar study combing SBRT and a PD-1 inhibitor, pembrolizumab, vs. placebo is also underway.

The synergy between SBRT and immunotherapy has been demonstrated in preclinical models in the potential to create the "abscopal effect," in which a local treatment such as SBRT may improve systemic tumor response to immunotherapy. This concept is being tested through many ongoing clinical trials for advanced-stage (III or IV) NSCLC combining local radiotherapy with PD-1 inhibitors nivolumab or pembrolizumab. Of note, a phase II pembrolizumab and radiotherapy trial randomized 76 patients with advanced or metastatic (stage IV) NSCLC to either pembrolizumab alone or pembrolizumab and SBRT to one lesion. Results showed significant improvement of ORR, PFS, and OS, although this did not meet a prespecified endpoint of clinical meaningfulness. The group that derived the greatest benefit from the addition of SBRT was those with PD-L1-negative tumors, suggesting that SBRT might be able to turn immunologically "cold" tumors "hot" (Theelen et al. 2019, 2020). There are other ongoing clinical trials combining local radiotherapy with immunotherapy for the treatment of mostly stage IV NSCLC and for early-stage NSCLC (Kordbacheh et al. 2018). The outcome of stage IV NSCLC studies may provide more clinical evidence of the abscopal effect of local radiotherapy.

4.2 Pulsed Paclitaxel Chemoradiotherapy: A Model of Translational Investigation of Radiosensitization

Locally advanced (stage III) NSCLC constitutes 20–30% of patients who present with NSCLC. Treatment of locally advanced stage III NSCLC remains a challenge to oncologists. Despite aggressive chemoradiation combination treatments, the outcome is quite poor with a high local chest tumor failure rate at approximately 50% and a high rate of distant metastasis at approximately 80% (Morton et al. 1991; Schaake-Koning et al. 1992; Mattson et al. 1988; Gandara et al. 1991; Marino et al. 1995; Arriagada et al. 1991; Sause et al. 2000; Curran et al. 2011; Furuse et al. 1999). The median OS using cisplatin-based chemoradiation is only 14–17 months from large randomized trials. Treatments for stage III NSCLC continue to be challenging in the attempt to improve chest tumor control and decrease distant metastasis. For this reason, various chemoradiotherapy combinations to enhance the chest tumor control for NSCLC have previously been tested (Chen and Okunieff 2004).

Due to the poor chest tumor control at conventional 60 Gy radiation dose, and due to the fact that almost all NSCLCs express EGFR, Radiation Therapy Oncology Group (RTOG) conducted a four-arm phase III randomized clinical trial (RTOG 0617) using concurrent chemotherapy (carboplatin/paclitaxel) with or without cetuximab (a monoclonal antibody to EGFR) in combination with two radiation doses 60 Gy vs. 74 Gy (Bradley et al. 2015). Findings of RTOG 0617 were surprisingly disappointing in that patients treated in the high-dose arm (74 Gy) had worse survival, and the addition of cetuximab to either 60 Gy or 74 Gy arm did not improve the outcome of OS or PFS. While there were no statistical differences in grade 3 or worse toxic effects between radiotherapy groups, the addition of cetuximab was associated with higher rates of grade 3 or worse toxic effects. Results of RTOG 0617 did not change the standard treatment of stage III NSCLC, yet the outcome of the aforementioned PACIFIC trial of chemoradiotherapy followed by durvalumab has now become the new standard of care for stage III NSCLC.

4.2.1 Preclinical Investigations of Pulsed Paclitaxel Radiosensitization of Lung Cancer Cell Lines

Here, we present a clinical translational investigation using pulsed, low-dose paclitaxel radiosensitization strategy to improve cancer control of stage III NSCLC (Chen et al. 2003; Lin et al. 2016), and we compare the outcomes among three randomized phase III clinical trials of RTOG 0617, PACIFIC trial, and pulsed paclitaxel chemoradiotherapy (Table 1).

Taxanes are the ideal radiation sensitizers due to the cell cycle effect in arresting cancer cells in the most sensitive phase of the cell cycle of G2/M (Sinclair and Morton 1966). Chen et al. (2001) conducted preclinical studies using lung cancer cell lines and investigated the effects of two taxanes: paclitaxel (Taxol) and docetaxel on radiosensitization. The preclinical data revealed the following: (1) after paclitaxel treatment, a minimum of 4 h was necessary for cell cycle progression to G2/M phase, the most radiosensitive phase of the cell cycle; (2) pulsed treatment of paclitaxel sustained G2/M cell cycle arrest; and (3) delaying radiation after taxane (paclitaxel or docetaxel) treatments led to better radiosensitizing effects than immediate radiation after drug treatments (Fig. 4) (Chen et al. 2001, 2003, 2011).

4.2.2 Translational Clinical Trial of Pulsed Paclitaxel Chemoradiotherapy

Based on preclinical information of the cell cycle and apoptotic effects of paclitaxel on lung cancer cell lines, a phase I/II clinical trial design applying concurrent pulsed low-dose, radiosensitizing paclitaxel and chest radiotherapy for stage III NSCLC was conducted. The experimental arm applied schedule-dependent paclitaxel delivered on alternating days (three times per week—M, W, F) at escalating low doses (15 mg/m^2, 20 mg/m^2, and 25 mg/m^2). Daily radiation was delayed for at least 4 h to allow for cell cycle progression of cancer cells into G2/M phase of the cell cycle, the most radiosensitive phase of the cell cycle. The pulsed low-dose paclitaxel schedule allowed for rapid clearance of drug from the plasma to minimize toxicity and yielded a 100% gross tumor ORR, a 3-year overall survival of 30%, and low rates of grade 3 or 4 toxicities (Chen et al. 2001, 2003, 2008). The kinetics of clinical tumor response was examined, and data showed that the bulk of the tumor shrinkage occurred within 4–6 weeks post-radiotherapy, and larger tumors shrunk faster (Zhang et al. 2008). A follow-up study was a multi-institutional randomized phase III trial comparing pulsed low-dose paclitaxel with weekly paclitaxel chemoradiotherapy for stage III NSCLC (Lin et al. 2016). The study enrolled approximately 70 patients in each arm. The outcome of the phase III clinical trial revealed much higher tumor ORR in the pulsed paclitaxel arm than the weekly paclitaxel arm (83.1% vs. 54.2%). Median PFS was significantly better in the pulsed paclitaxel arm (14.6 months vs. 9.4 months), but the median OS was not statistically different (32.6 months vs. 31.3 months). A summary of outcomes of these

Table 1 Median OS and PFS of three randomized phase III clinical trials for stage III NSCLC

Phase III trials (months)	RTOG 0617				PACIFIC		Taxol ChemoRT	
Treatment arms	60 Gy	74 Gy	Cxm	No Cxm	Durva	No Durva	3×/week	Weekly
Median OS	*28.7	20.3	25	24	*47.5	29.1	32.6	31.3
Median PFS	11.8	9.8	10.8	10.7	*17.2	5.6	*14.6	9.4

OS overall survival, *PFS* progression-free survival, *Cxm* cetuximab, *Durva* durvalumab
* P value reached statistical significance

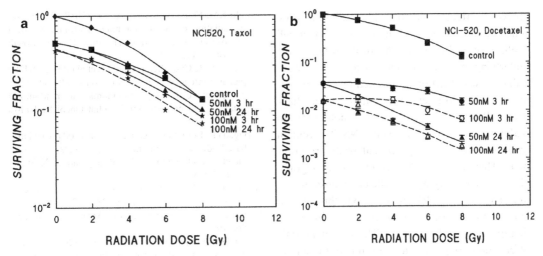

Fig. 4 Clonogenic survival curves of human lung cancer cell line NCI520. Cells were treated with either (**a**) paclitaxel (Taxol) or (**b**) docetaxel at two different drug concentrations (50 nM or 100 nM) for 3 h. After drug treatments, cells were either irradiated immediately or irradiated 24 h later. Radiation doses were 2, 4, 6, and 8 Gy vs. sham radiation (0 Gy). Both paclitaxel-treated cells and docetaxel-treated cells showed more cell death (steeper slopes) if radiation was delayed at 24 h, supporting better radiosensitizing effects by delaying radiation after drug treatments. For sham-irradiated cells (0 Gy), there were more cell death in the docetaxel (Y-axis of **b**) treated cultures than the paclitaxel (Y-axis of **a**) treated cultures, demonstrating more cytotoxic effects of docetaxel (Chen et al. 2001, 2011, with permission)

three randomized phase III clinical trials is shown in Table 1.

Outcomes of these phase III clinical trials employing various strategies with the attempt to improve chest tumor control and the OS revealed that high-dose RT to 74 Gy did not improve outcome and might be detrimental, while the addition of adjuvant durvalumab improved both the OS and PFS. The pulsed paclitaxel chemoradiation approach significantly improved the ORR of chest tumors, local tumor control, and PFS, but not the OS. Thus, an effective radiosensitizing regimen such as the pulsed paclitaxel approach may benefit from the addition of durvalumab to improve OS.

5 Summary

Translation research of NSCLC continues to evolve and has made breakthrough progress in recent decades. While efforts in defining molecular prognostic factors and molecular predictive markers continue, the approach of genomic analyses of tumors has yielded new molecular targets resulting in FDA approvals of many new drugs that are in practice changing molecular therapeutics selectively tailored to the tumor of individual patients with NSCLC. Tumor genomic analyses have identified several subtypes of NSCLC that can be treated with molecular targeted therapies mostly for stage IV NSCLC. However, the interaction between radiation and these new molecular targeted therapeutics for various new subtypes of NSCLC is largely unknown. These are potential translational research opportunities for radiation oncologist and biologists in the future.

Preclinical investigations in tumor-bearing mice suggested a radiation priming effect to enhance immunogenic cell death of tumors in that focal radiation interactions with immune system might exert systemic benefits, thus resulting in abscopal effects. To date, investigation in the interaction between radiotherapy and immune system remains an area of active research in lung cancer. While results of preclinical investigations support the combined treatment of hypofractionated radiotherapy and immunotherapy for abscopal effects, the optimal radiation dose schedule in promoting immunogenic cancer cell death is yet to be defined. More importantly, the underlying mechanism addressing why certain radiation dose fractionation schedule may be better than other dose schedules remains to be elucidated. Benefits of adding immunotherapy to SBRT treatment for early-stage NSCLC remain unknown until ongoing clinical trials are complete. There are, nonetheless, numerous ongoing clinical trials applying immune checkpoint inhibitors targeting the PD-1/PD-L1 axis through the combination of local radiotherapy with immunotherapy for stage IV NSCLC. These clinical trials offer unique opportunities to clinically examine radiation abscopal effects in NSCLC patients and may shed light on defining the optimal dose schedule of hypofractionated radiotherapy in inducing radiation immunogenic cell death.

The PACIFIC trial has set a new standard treatment for stage III NSCLC, but the failure of high-dose chest radiation of RTOG 0617 trial highlights the challenge of chest local therapy in improving chest tumor control and reducing distant cancer metastasis. Translational investigations to explore new ways to enhance radiation efficacy to improve chest local and regional tumor control will remain important as most stage III NSCLC tumors are large lesions with central mediastinal nodal metastasis, and thus not amenable to SBRT approach. Strategies that will improve chest tumor control without the radiation dose escalation plus adjuvant immunotherapy are anticipated to gain further improvement of cancer control of stage III NSCLC.

References

Aggarwal C (2016) Prevalence of PD-L1 expression in patients with non-small cell lung cancer screened for enrollment in KEYNOTE-001, -010, and -024. Ann Oncol 27:VVI363

Antonia SJ, Villegas A, Daniel D et al (2017) Durvalumab after chemoradiotherapy in stage III non-small-cell lung cancer. N Engl J Med 377:1919–1929

Antonia SJ, Villegas A, Daniel D et al (2018) Overall survival with durvalumab after chemoradiotherapy in stage III non-small-cell lung cancer. N Engl J Med 379:2342–2350

Arnold KM, Flynn NJ, Raben A et al (2018) The impact of radiation on the tumor microenvironment: effect of dose and fractionation schedules. Cancer Growth Metastasis 11:1–17

Arriagada R, le Chevalier T, Quoix E et al (1991) ASTRO plenary: effect of chemotherapy on locally advanced non-small cell lung carcinoma: a randomized study of 353 patients. Int J Radiat Oncol Biol Phys 20:1183–1190

Arriagada R, Bergman B, Dunant A et al (2004) Cisplatin-based adjuvant chemotherapy in patients with completely resected non-small-cell lung cancer. N Engl J Med 350:351–360

Arteaga CL (2003) ErbB-targeted therapeutic approaches in human cancer. Exp Cell Res 284:122–130

Barbacid M (1987) Ras genes. Annu Rev Biochem 56:779–827

Bepler G, Sommers KE, Cantor A et al (2008) Clinical efficacy and predictive molecular markers of neoadjuvant gemcitabine and pemetrexed in resectable non-small cell lung cancer. J Thorac Oncol 3:1112–1118

Bepler G, Olaussen KA, Vataire AL et al (2011) ERCC1 and RRM1 in the international adjuvant lung trial by automated quantitative in situ analysis. Am J Pathol 178:69–78

Berger MS, Gullick WJ, Greenfield C et al (1987) Epidermal growth factor receptors in lung tumours. J Pathol 152:297–307

Bhattacharjee A, Richards WG, Staunton J et al (2001) Classification of human lung carcinomas by mRNA expression profiling reveals distinct adenocarcinoma subclasses. Proc Natl Acad Sci U S A 98:13790–13795

Booton R, Ward T, Ashcroft L et al (2007) ERCC1 mRNA expression is not associated with response and survival after platinum-based chemotherapy regimens in advanced non-small cell lung cancer. J Thorac Oncol 2:902–906

Bos JL (1989) Ras oncogenes in human cancer: a review. Cancer Res 49:4682–4689

Boutros T, Chevet E, Metrakos P (2008) Mitogen-activated protein (MAP) kinase/MAP kinase phosphatase regulation: roles in cell growth, death, and cancer. Pharmacol Rev 60:261–310

Bradley JD, Paulus R, Komaki R et al (2015) Standard-dose versus high-dose conformal radiotherapy with concurrent and consolidation carboplatin plus paclitaxel with or without cetuximab for patients with stage IIIA or IIIB non-small-cell lung cancer (RTOG 0617): a randomized, two-by-two factorial phase 3 study. Lancet Oncol 16:187–199

Brose MS, Volpe P, Feldman M et al (2002) BRAF and RAS mutations in human lung cancer and melanoma. Cancer Res 62:6997–7000

Brustugun OT, Khattak AM, Tromborg AK et al (2014) BRAF-mutations in non-small cell lung cancer. Lung Cancer 84:36–38

Ceppi P, Volante M, Novello S et al (2006) ERCC1 and RRM1 gene expressions but not EGFR are predictive of shorter survival in advanced non-small-cell lung cancer treated with cisplatin and gemcitabine. Ann Oncol 17:1818–1825

Chen Y, Gandara D (2006) Molecular staging of non-small cell lung cancer. In: Syrigos KN, Nutting C, Roussos C (eds) Tumors of the chest: biology diagnosis and management. Springer, pp 159–176

Chen Y, Okunieff P (2004) Radiation and third generation chemotherapy. Hematol Oncol Clin N Am 18:55–80

Chen P, Wiencke J, Aldape K et al (1998) Association of an ERCC1 polymorphism with adult-onset glioma. Cancer Epidemiol Biomarkers Prev 9:843–847

Chen Y, Pandya K, Keng P et al (2001) Schedule dependent pulsed low-dose paclitaxel radiosensitization for thoracic malignancy. Am J Clin Oncol 24:432–437

Chen Y, Pandya K, Keng PC et al (2003) Phase I/II clinical trial using pulsed low-dose paclitaxel radiosensitization for thoracic malignancies: a therapeutic approach based on pre-clinical research of human lung cancer cells. Clin Cancer Res 9:969–975

Chen HY, Yu SL, Chen CH et al (2007) A five-gene signature and clinical outcome in non-small-cell lung cancer. N Engl J Med 356:11–20

Chen Y, Pandya K, Feins R et al (2008) Toxicity profile and pharmacokinetic study of a phase I low-dose schedule-dependent radiosensitizing paclitaxel chemoradiation regimen for inoperable non-small cell lung cancer (NSCLC). Int J Radiat Oncol Biol Phys 71:407–413

Chen Y, Pandya KJ, Hyrien O et al (2011) Preclinical and pilot clinical study of docetaxel chemoradiation for stage III non-small cell lung cancer. Int J Radiat Oncol Biol Phys 80:1358–1364

Chen D, Zhang LQ, Huang JF et al (2014) BRAF mutations in patients with non-small cell lung cancer: a systematic review and meta-analysis. PLoS One 9:e10135

Cobo M, Isla D, Massuti B et al (2007) Customizing cisplatin based on quantitative excision repair cross-complementing 1 mRNA expression: a phase III trial in non-small-cell lung cancer. J Clin Oncol 25:2747–2754

Cooper WA, Kohonen-Corish MR, Chan C et al (2008) Prognostic significance of DNA repair proteins MLH1, MSH2 and MGMT expression in non-small-cell lung cancer and precursor lesions. Histopathology 52:613–622

Cordon-Cardo C (1995) Mutations of cell cycle regulators. Biological and clinical implications for human neoplasia. Am J Pathol 147:545–560

Cox G, Jones JL, O'Byrne KJ (2000) Matrix metalloproteinase 9 and the epidermal growth factor signal pathway in operable non-small cell lung cancer. Clin Cancer Res 6:2349–2355

Curran WJ, Paulus R, Langer CJ et al (2011) Sequential vs. concurrent chemoradiation for stage III non-small cell lung cancer: randomized phase III trial RTOG 9410. J Natl Cancer Inst 103:1452–1460

D'Amico TA, Massey M, Herndon JE 2nd et al (1999) A biologic risk model for stage I lung cancer: immunohistochemical analysis of 408 patients with the use of ten molecular markers. J Thorac Cardiovasc Surg 117:736–743

Dagogo-Jack I, Martinez P, Yeap BY et al (2018) Impact of BRAF mutation class on disease characteristics and clinical outcomes in BRAF-mutant lung cancer. Clin Cancer Res 25:158–165

Demaria S, Formenti SC (2020) The abscopal effect 67 years later: from a side tory to center stage. Br J Radiol 93:20200042

Deng L, Liang H, Burnette B et al (2014a) Irradiation and anti-PD-L1 treatment synergistically promote antitumor immunity in mice. J Clin Invest 124: 687–695

Deng L, Liang H, Xu M et al (2014b) STING-dependent cytosolic DNA sensing promotes radiation-induced type I interferon-dependent antitumor immunity in immunogenic tumors. Immunity 41:843–852

Dewan MZ, Galloway AE, Kawashima N et al (2009) Fractionated but not single-dose radiotherapy induces an immune-mediated abscopal effect when combined with anti-CTLA-4 antibody. Clin Cancer Res 15:5379–5388

Dovedi SJ, Cheadle EJ, Popple AL et al (2017) Fractionated radiation therapy stimulates antitumor immunity mediated by both resident and infiltrating polyclonal T-Cell populations when combined with PD-1 blockade. Clin Cancer Res 23:5514–5526

Drilon A, Wang L, Hasanovic A et al (2013) Response to Cabozantinib in patients with RET fusion-positive lung adenocarcinomas. Cancer Discov 3: 630–635

Drilon A, Lin JJ, Filleron T et al (2018) Frequency of brain metastases and multikinase inhibitor outcomes in patients with RET-rearranged lung cancers. J Thorac Oncol 13:1595–1601

Drilon A, Oxnard GR, Tan DSW et al (2020) Efficacy of selpercatinib in RET fusion-positive non-small cell lung cancer. N Engl J Med 383:813–824

Faivre-Finn C, Vicente D, Kurata T et al (2021) Four-year survival with durvalumab after chemoradiotherapy in stage III NSCLC—an update from the PACIFIC trial. J Thorac Oncol 16(5):860–867

Farmer G, Bargonetti J, Zhu H et al (1992) Wild-type p53 activates transcription in vitro. Nature 358:83–86

Feng Y, Thiagarajan PS, Ma PC (2012) MET signaling: novel targeted inhibition and its clinical development in lung cancer. J Thorac Oncol 7:459–467

Fontanini G, De Laurentiis M, Vignati S et al (1998) Evaluation of epidermal growth factor-related growth factors and receptors and of neoangiogenesis in completely resected stage I-IIIA non-small-cell lung cancer: amphiregulin and microvessel count are independent prognostic indicators of survival. Clin Cancer Res 4:241–249

Formenti SC, Demaria S (2009) Systemic effects of local radiotherapy. Lancet Oncol 10:718–726

Franklin WA, Veve R, Hirsch FR et al (2002) Epidermal growth factor receptor family in lung cancer and pre-malignancy. Semin Oncol 29(1 Suppl 4):3–14

Fujii T, Toyooka S, Ichimura K et al (2008) ERCC1 protein expression predicts the response of cisplatin-based neoadjuvant chemotherapy in non-small-cell lung cancer. Lung Cancer 59:377–384

Fukuoka M, Yano S, Giaccone G et al (2003) Multi-institutional randomized phase II trial of gefitinib for previously treated patients with advanced non-small-cell lung cancer (The IDEAL 1 Trial). J Clin Oncol 21:2237–2246

Furuse K, Fukuoka M, Kawahara M et al (1999) Phase III study of concurrent versus sequential thoracic radiotherapy in combination with mitomycin, vindesine, and cisplatin in unresectable stage III non-small-cell lung cancer. J Clin Oncol 17:2692

Gandara DR, Valone FH, Perez EA et al (1991) Rapidly alternating radiotherapy and high dose cisplatin chemotherapy in stage IIIB non-small cell lung cancer. results of a Phase I/II study. Int J Radiat Oncol Biol Phys 20:1047–1052

Gandhi L, Rodriguez-Abreu D, Gadgeel S et al (2018) Pembrolizumab plus chemotherapy in metastatic non-small-cell lung cancer. N Engl J Med 378:2078–2092

Gautam A, Bepler G (2006) Suppression of lung tumor formation by the regulatory subunit of ribonucleotide reductase. Cancer Res 66:6497–6502

Gazdar AF (2007) DNA repair and survival in lung cancer—the two faces of Janus. N Engl J Med 356:771–773

Golden EB, Frances D, Pellicciotta I et al (2014) Radiation fosters dose-dependent and chemotherapy-induced immunogenic cell death. Oncoimmunology 3:e28518

Golden EB, Marciscano AE, Formenti SC (2020) Radiation therapy and the in situ vaccination approach. Int J Radiat Oncol Biol Phys 108:891–898

Greatens TM, Niehans GA, Rubins JB et al (1998) Do molecular markers predict survival in non-small-cell lung cancer? Am J Respir Crit Care Med 157:1093–1097

Greenblatt MS, Bennett WP, Hollstein M et al (1994) Mutations in the p53 tumor suppressor gene: clues to cancer etiology and molecular pathogenesis. Cancer Res 54:4855–4878

Guo NL, Wan YW, Tosun K et al (2008) Confirmation of gene expression-based prediction of survival in non-small cell lung cancer. Clin Cancer Res 14:8213–8220

Han SW, Kim TY, Hwang PG et al (2005) Predictive and prognostic impact of epidermal growth factor receptor mutation in non-small-cell lung cancer patients treated with gefitinib. J Clin Oncol 23:2493–2501

Han JY, Park K, Kim SW et al (2012) First-SIGNAL: first-line single-agent iressa versus gemcitabine and cisplatin trial in never-smokers with adenocarcinoma of the lung. J Clin Oncol 30:1122–1128

Hanna NH, Schneider BJ, Temin S et al (2020) Therapy for stage IV non-small-cell lung cancer without driver alterations: ASCO and OH (CCO) joint guideline update. J Clin Oncol 38:1608–1632

Haratake N, Seto T (2020) NTRK fusion-positive non-small-cell lung cancer: the diagnosis and targeted therapy. Clin Lung Cancer 22:1–5

Hartwell L (1992) Defects in a cell cycle checkpoint may be responsible for the genomic instability of cancer cells. Cell 71:543–546

Herbst RS, Giaccone G, de Marinis F et al (2020) Atezolizumab for first-line treatment of PD-L1-selected patients with NSCLC. N Engl J Med 383:1328–1339

Hirsch FR, Varella-Garcia M, Bunn PA Jr et al (2003) Epidermal growth factor receptor in non-small-cell lung carcinomas: correlation between gene copy number and protein expression and impact on prognosis. J Clin Oncol 21:3798–3807

Hsu HS, Lee IH, Hsu WH et al (2007) Polymorphism in the hMSH2 gene (gISV12-6T > C) is a prognostic factor in non-small cell lung cancer. Lung Cancer 58:123–130

Huncharek M, Kupelnick B, Geschwind JF et al (2000) Prognostic significance of p53 mutations in non-small cell lung cancer: a meta-analysis of 829 cases from eight published studies. Cancer Lett 153:219–226

Hwang IG, Ahn MJ, Park BB et al (2008) ERCC1 expression as a prognostic marker in N2(+) nonsmall-cell lung cancer patients treated with platinum-based neoadjuvant concurrent chemoradiotherapy. Cancer 113:1379–1386

Inamura K, Takeuchi K, Togashi Y et al (2009) EML4-ALK lung cancers are characterized by rare other mutations, a TTF-1 cell lineage, an acinar histology, and young onset. Mod Pathol 22:508–515

Janne PA, Engelman JA, Johnson BE (2005) Epidermal growth factor receptor mutations in non-small-cell lung cancer: implications for treatment and tumor biology. J Clin Oncol 23:3227–3234

Janne PA, Shaw AT, Pereira JR et al (2013) Selumetinib plus docetaxel for KRAS-mutant advanced non-small-cell lung cancer: a randomized, multicentre, placebo-controlled, phase 2 study. Lancet Oncol 14:38–47

Jorissen RN, Walker F, Pouliot N et al (2003) Epidermal growth factor receptor: mechanisms of activation and signaling. Exp Cell Res 284:31–53

Jung CY, Choi JE, Park JM et al (2006) Polymorphisms in the hMSH2 gene and the risk of primary lung cancer. Cancer Epidemiol Biomarkers Prev 15:762–768

Kamal NS, Soria JC, Mendiboure J et al (2010) MutS homologue 2 and the long-term benefit of adjuvant chemotherapy in lung cancer. Clin Cancer Res 16:1206–1215

Khotskaya YB, Holla VR, Farago AF et al (2017) Targeting TRK family proteins in cancer. Pharmacol Ther 173:58–66

Kim M, Kang HG, Lee SY et al (2010) Comprehensive analysis of DNA repair gene polymorphisms and survival in patients with early stage non-small-cell lung cancer. Cancer Sci 101:2436–2442

Ko EC, Raben D, Formenti SC (2018) The integration of radiotherapy with immunotherapy for the treatment of non-small cell lung cancer. Clin Cancer Res 24:5792–5806

Kohno T, Yokota J (1999) How many tumor suppressor genes are involved in human lung carcinogenesis? Carcinogenesis 20:1403

Kordbacheh T, Honeychurch J, Blackhall F et al (2018) Radiotherapy and anti-PD-1/PD-L1 combinations in lung cancer: building better translational research platforms. Ann Oncol 29:301–310

Kosaka T, Yatabe Y, Endoh H et al (2004) Mutations of the epidermal growth factor receptor gene in lung cancer: biological and clinical implications. Cancer Res 64:8919–8923

Kris MG, Natale RB, Herbst RS et al (2003) Efficacy of gefitinib, an inhibitor of the epidermal growth factor receptor tyrosine kinase, in symptomatic patients with non-small cell lung cancer: a randomized trial. JAMA 290:2149–2158

Kumar A, Petri ET, Halmos B et al (2008) Structure and clinical relevance of the epidermal growth factor receptor in human cancer. J Clin Oncol 26:1742–1751

Larsen JE, Pavey SJ, Bowman R et al (2007) Gene expression of lung squamous cell carcinoma reflects mode of lymph node involvement. Eur Respir J 30:21–25

Lau SK, Boutros PC, Pintilie M et al (2007) Three-gene prognostic classifier for early-stage non-small-cell lung cancer. J Clin Oncol 25:5562–5569

Li J, Li ZN, Yu LC et al (2010) Association of expression of MRP1, BCRP, LRP and ERCC1 with outcome of patients with locally advanced non-small cell lung cancer who received neoadjuvant chemotherapy. Lung Cancer 69:116–122

Liao BC, Lin CC, Yang JC (2015) Second and third-generation epidermal growth factor receptor tyrosine kinase inhibitors in advanced nonsmall cell lung cancer. Curr Opin Oncol 27:94–101

Lin H, Chen Y, Shi A et al (2016) Phase 3 randomized low-dose paclitaxel chemoradiotherapy study for locally advanced non-small cell lung cancer. Front Oncol 6:1–7

Lo YL, Hsiao CF, Jou YS et al (2011) Polymorphisms of MLH1 and MSH2 genes and the risk of lung cancer among never smokers. Lung Cancer 72:280–286

Lord RV, Brabender J, Gandara D et al (2002) Low ERCC1 expression correlates with prolonged survival after cisplatin plus gemcitabine chemotherapy in non-small cell lung cancer. Clin Cancer Res 8:2286–2291

Lu Y, Lemon W, Liu PY et al (2006) A gene expression signature predicts survival of patients with stage I non-small cell lung cancer. PLoS Med 3:e467

Maemondo M, Inoue A, Kobayashi K et al (2010) Gefitinib or chemotherapy for nonsmall-cell lung cancer with mutated EGFR. N Engl J Med 362:2380–2388

Marino P, Preatoni A, Cantoni A (1995) Randomized trials of radiotherapy alone versus combined chemotherapy and radiotherapy in stages IIIa and IIIb non-small cell lung cancer. A meta-analysis. Cancer 76:593–601

Mascaux C, Iannino N, Martin B et al (2005) The role of RAS oncogene in survival of patients with lung cancer: a systematic review of the literature with meta-analysis. Br J Cancer 92:131–139

Mattson K, Holsti LR, Holsti P et al (1988) Inoperable non-small cell lung cancer: radiation with or without chemotherapy. Eur J Cancer Clin Oncol 24:477–482

Mayne ST, Buenconsejo J, Janerich DT et al (1999) Familial cancer history and lung cancer risk in USA non-smoking men and women. Cancer Epidemiol Biomarkers Prev 8:1065

Mitsudomi T, Steinberg SM, Oie HK et al (1991) Ras gene mutations in non-small cell lung cancers are associated with shortened survival irrespective of treatment intent. Cancer Res 51:4999–5002

Mitsudomi T, Hamajima N, Ogawa M et al (2000) Prognostic significance of p53 alterations in patients with non-small cell lung cancer: a meta-analysis. Clin Cancer Res 6:4055–4063

Mitsudomi T, Morita S, Yatabe Y et al (2010) Gefitinib versus cisplatin plus docetaxel in patients with non-small-cell lung cancer harbouring mutations of the epidermal growth factor receptor (WJTOG3405): an open label, randomized phase 3 trial. Lancet Oncol 11:121–128

Mok TS, Wu YL, Thongprasert S et al (2009) Gefitinib or carboplatin-paclitaxel in pulmonary adenocarcinoma. N Engl J Med 361:947–957

Morris SW, Kirstein MN, Valentine MB et al (1994) Fusion of a kinase gene, ALK, to a nucleolar protein gene, NPM, in non-Hodgkin's lymphoma. Science 263:1281–1284

Morton RF, Jett JR, McGinnis WL et al (1991) Thoracic radiation therapy alone compared with combined chemoradiotherapy for locally unresectable non-small cell lung cancer. Ann Intern Med 115:681–686

Ngwa W, Irabor OC, Schoenfeld JD et al (2018) Using immunotherapy to boost the abscopal effect. Nat Rev Cancer 18:313–322

Obeid M, Tesniere A, Ghiringhelli F et al (2007) Calreticulin exposure dictates the immunogenicity of cancer cell death. Nat Med 13:54–61

Ohsaki Y, Tanno S, Fujita Y et al (2000) Epidermal growth factor receptor expression correlates with poor prognosis in non-small cell lung cancer patients with p53 overexpression. Oncol Rep 7:603–607

Olaussen KA, Dunant A, Fouret P et al (2006) DNA repair by ERCC1 in non-small-cell lung cancer and cisplatin-based adjuvant chemotherapy. N Engl J Med 355:983–991

Paik PK, Arcila ME, Fara M et al (2011) Clinical characteristics of patients with lung adenocarcinomas harboring BRAF mutations. J Clin Oncol 29:2046–2051

Pao W, Miller VA, Politi KA et al (2005) Acquired resistance of lung adenocarcinomas to gefitinib or erlotinib is associated with a second mutation in the EGFR kinase domain. PLoS Med 2:e73

Park S, Ahn B-C, Lim SW et al (2018) Characteristics and outcome of ROS1-positive non-small cell lung cancer patients in routine clinical practiced. J Thorac Oncol 123:1373–1382

Pastorino U, Andreola S, Tagliabue E et al (1997) Immunocytochemical markers in stage I lung cancer: relevance to prognosis. J Clin Oncol 15:2858–2865

Patsoukis N, Wang Q, Strauss L et al (2020) Revisiting the PD-1 pathway. Sci Adv 6:eabd2712

Paz-Ares L, Luft A, Vicente D et al (2018) Pembrolizumab plus chemotherapy for squamous non-small-cell lung cancer. N Engl J Med 379:2040–2051

Pfeiffer P, Clausen PP, Andersen K et al (1996) Lack of prognostic significance of epidermal growth factor receptor and the oncoprotein p185HER-2 in patients with systemically untreated non-small-cell lung cancer: an immunohistochemical study on cryosections. Br J Cancer 74:86–91

Planchard D, Kim TM, Maxieres J et al (2016) Dabrafenib in patients with BRAF (V600E)-positive advanced non-small cell lung cancer: a single-arm, multicentre, open-label, phase 2 trial. Lancet Oncol 17:642–650

Pollmann M, Parwaresch R, Adam-Klages S et al (2006) Human EML4, a novel member of the EMAP family, is essential for microtubule formation. Exp Cell Res 312:3241–3251

Potti A, Mukherjee S, Petersen R et al (2006) A genomic strategy to refine prognosis in early-stage non-small cell lung cancer. N Engl J Med 355:570–580

Potti A, Mukherjee S, Petersen R et al (2011) Retraction: a genomic strategy to refine prognosis in early-stage non-small cell lung cancer. N Engl J Med 364:1176

Ramalingham SS, Owonikoko TK, Khuri FR (2011) Lung cancer: new biological insights and recent therapeutic advances. CA Cancer J Clin 61:91–112

Reck M, Rodriguez-Abreu D, Robinson AG et al (2016) Pembrolizumab versus chemotherapy for PD-L1-positive non-small-cell lung cancer. N Engl J Med 375:1823–1833

Reed E (1998) Platinum-DNA adduct, nucleotide excision repair and platinum based anti-cancer chemotherapy. Cancer Treat Rev 24:331–344

Reits EA, Hodge JW, Herberts CA et al (2006) Radiation modulates the peptide repertoire, enhances MHC class I expression, and induces successful antitumor immunotherapy. J Exp Med 203:1259–1271

Riely GJ, Marks J, Pao W (2009) KRAS mutations in non-small cell lung cancer. Proc Am Thorac Soc 6:201–205

Rodenhuis S, Slebos RJ (1992) Clinical significance of ras oncogene activation in human lung cancer. Cancer Res 52:2665s–2669s

Rodriguez-Ruiz ME, Rodriguez I, Leaman O et al (2019) Immune mechanisms mediating abscopal effects in radioimmunotherapy. Pharmacol Ther 196:195–203

Rosell R, Danenberg KD, Alberola V et al (2004) Ribonucleotide reductase messenger RNA expression and survival in gemcitabine/cisplatin-treated advanced non-small cell lung cancer patients. Clin Cancer Res 10:1318–1325

Rosell R, Carcereny E, Gervais R et al (2012) Erlotinib versus standard chemotherapy as first-line treatment for European patients with advanced EGFR mutation-positive non-small-cell lung cancer (EURTAC): a multicentre, open-label, randomised phase 3 trial. Lancet Oncol 13:239–246

Rusch V, Klimstra D, Venkatraman E et al (1997) Overexpression of the epidermal growth factor receptor and its ligand transforming growth factor alpha is frequent in resectable non-small cell lung cancer but does not predict tumor progression. Clin Cancer Res 3:515–522

Sadiq AA, Salgia R (2013) MET as a possible target for non-small cell lung cancer. J Clin Oncol 31:1089–1096

Sause W, Kolesar P, Taylor S IV et al (2000) Final results of phase III trial in regionally advanced unresectable non-small cell lung cancer. Chest 117:358–364

Scartozzi M, Franciosi V, Campanini N et al (2006) Mismatch repair system (MMR) status correlates with response and survival in non-small cell lung cancer (NSCLC) patients. Lung Cancer 53:103–109

Schaake-Koning C, van den Bogaert W, Dalesio O et al (1992) Effects of concomitant cisplatin and radiotherapy on inoperable non-small cell lung cancer. N Engl J Med 326:524–530

Schiller JH, Adak S, Feins RH et al (2001) Lack of prognostic significance of p53 and K-RAS mutations in primary resected non- small-cell lung cancer on e4592: a laboratory ancillary study on an eastern cooperative oncology group prospective randomized trial of postoperative adjuvant therapy. J Clin Oncol 19:448–457

Sequist LV, Yang JC, Yamamoto N et al (2013) Phase III study of afatinib or cisplatin plus pemetrexed in patients with metastatic lung adenocarcinoma with EGFR mutations. J Clin Oncol 31:3327–3334

Sharma SV, Bell DW, Settleman J et al (2007) Epidermal growth factor receptor mutations in lung cancer. Nat Rev Cancer 7:169–181

Sharpe AH, Pauken KE (2018) The diverse functions of the PD1 inhibitory pathway. Nat Rev Immunol 18:153–167

Shaw AT, Yeap BY, Mino-Kenudson M et al (2009) Clinical features and outcome of patients with non-small-cell lung cancer who harbor EML4-ALK. J Clin Oncol 27:4247–4253

Shaw AT, Kim DW, Nakagawa K et al (2013) Crizotinib versus chemotherapy in advanced ALK-positive lung cancer. N Engl J Med 368:2385–2394

Shaw AT, Ou SH, Bang YJ et al (2014) Crizotinib in ROS1-rearranged non-small-cell lung cancer. N Engl J Med 371:1963–1971

Shen MJ, Xu LJ, Yang L et al (2017) Radiation alters PD-L1/NKG2D ligand levels in lung cancer cells and leads to immune escape from NK cell cytotoxicity via IL-6-MEK/Erk signaling pathway. Oncotarget 8:80506–80529

Shigematsu H, Lin L, Takahashi T et al (2005) Clinical and biological features associated with epidermal growth factor receptor gene mutations in lung cancers. J Natl Cancer Inst 97:339–346

Shih CM, Chen CY, Lee IH et al (2010) A polymorphism in the hMLH1 gene (-93G-->A) associated with lung cancer susceptibility and prognosis. Int J Mol Med 25:165–170

Simon G, Sharma A, Li X et al (2007) Feasibility and efficacy of molecular analysis-directed individualized therapy in advanced non-small-cell lung cancer. J Clin Oncol 25:2741–2746

Sinclair WK, Morton RA (1966) X-ray sensitivity during the cell generation cycle of cultured Chinese hamster cells. Radiat Res 29:450–474

Skarda J, Fridman E, Pevova P et al (2006) Prognostic value of hMLH1 and hMSH2 immunohistochemical expression in non-small cell lung cancer. A tissue microarray study. Biomed Pap Med Fac Univ Palacky Olomouc Czech Repub 150:255–259

Slebos RJ, Kibbelaar RE, Dalesio O et al (1990) K-ras oncogene activation as a prognostic marker in adenocarcinoma of the lung. N Engl J Med 323:561–565

Socinski MA, Jotte RM, Cappuzzo F et al (2018) Atezolizumab for first-line treatment of metastatic nonsquamous NSCLC. N Engl J Med 378:2288–2301

Solomon BJ, Mok T, Kim DW et al (2014) First-line crizotinib versus chemotherapy in ALK-positive lung cancer. N Engl J Med 371:2167–2177

Solomon BJ, Kim DW, Wu YL et al (2018) Final overall survival analysis from a study comparing first-line crizotinib versus chemotherapy in ALK-mutation-positive non-small-cell lung cancer. J Clin Oncol 36:2251–2258

Souglakos J, Boukovinas I, Taron M et al (2008) Ribonucleotide reductase subunits M1 and M2 mRNA expression levels and clinical outcome of lung adenocarcinoma patients treated with docetaxel/gemcitabine. Br J Cancer 98:1710–1715

Steels E, Paesmans M, Berghmans T et al (2001) Role of p53 as a prognostic factor for survival in lung cancer: a systematic review of the literature with a meta-analysis. Eur Respir J 18:705–719

Suda K, Bunn PA, Rivard CJ et al (2017) Primary double-strike therapy for cancers to overcome EGFR kinase inhibitor resistance: proposal from the Bench. J Thorac Oncol 12:27–35

Sugio K, Ishida T, Yokoyama H et al (1992) Ras gene mutations as a prognostic marker in adenocarcinoma of the human lung without lymph node metastasis. Cancer Res 52:2903–2906

Sun Z, Wigle DA, Yang P (2008) Non-overlapping and non-cell-type-specific gene expression signatures predict lung cancer survival. J Clin Oncol 26:877–883

Takeuchi K, Soda M, Togashi Y et al (2012) RET, ROS1 and ALK fusions in lung cancer. Nat Med 18:378–381

Theelen WSME, Peulen HMU, Lalezari F et al (2019) Effect of pembrolizumab after stereotactic body radiotherapy vs pembrolizumab alone on tumor response in patients with advanced non-small cell lung cancer: results of the PEMBRO-RT phase 2 randomized clinical trial. JAMA Oncol 5:1276–1282

Theelen WS, de Jong MC, Baas P (2020) Synergizing systemic responses by combining immunotherapy with radiotherapy in metastatic non-small cell lung cancer: the potential of the abscopal effect. Lung Cancer 142:106–113

Vaishnavi A, Capelletti M, Le AT et al (2013) Oncogenic and drug-sensitive NTRK1 rearrangements in lung cancer. Nat Med 19:1469–1472

Vashnavi A, Le AT, Doebele RC (2015) TRKing down an old oncogene in a new era of targeted therapy. Cancer Discov 5:25–34

Volm M, Efferth T, Mattern J (1992) Oncoprotein (c-myc, c-erbB1, c-erbB2, c-fos) and suppressor gene product (p53) expression in squamous cell carcinomas of the lung. Clinical and biological correlations Anticancer Res 12:11–20

Westfall JM, Mold J, Fagnan L (2007) Practice-based research-"Blue Highways" on the NIH roadmap. JAMA 297:403–406

Woenckhaus M, Stoehr R, Dietmaier W et al (2003) Microsatellite instability at chromosome 8p in non-small cell lung cancer is associated with lymph node metastasis. Int J Oncol 23(5):1357–1363

Wu Q, Christensen LA, Legerski RJ et al (2005) Mismatch repair participates in error-free processing of DNA interstrand crosslinks in human cells. EMBO Rep 6:551–557

Wu YL, Zhou C, Hu CP et al (2014) Afatinib versus cisplatin plus gemcitabine for first-line treatment of Asian patients with advanced non-small-cell lung cancer harbouring EGFR mutations (LUX-Lung 6): an open-label, randomised phase 3 trial. Lancet Oncol 15:213–222

Xinarianos G, Liloglou T, Prime W et al (2000) hMLH1 and hMSH2 expression correlates with allelic imbalance on chromosome 3p in non-small cell lung carcinomas. Cancer Res 60:4216–4221

Yamazaki T, Hannani D, Poirier-Colame V et al (2014) Defective immunogenic cell death of HMGB1-deficient tumors: compensatory therapy with TLR4 agonists. Cell Death Differ 21:69–78

Yang LY, Li L, Jiang H et al (2000) Expression of ERCC1 antisense RNA abrogates gemcitabine-mediated cytotoxic synergism with cisplatin in human colon tumor cells defective in mismatch repair but proficient in nucleotide excision repair. Clin Cancer Res 6:773–781

Yarden Y, Sliwkowski MX (2001) Untangling the ErbB signaling network. Nat Rev Mol Cell Biol 2:127–137

Yin Y, Tainsky MA, Bischoff FZ et al (1992) Wild-type p53 restores cell cycle control and inhibits gene amplification in cells with mutant p53 alleles. Cell 70:937–948

Zak KM, Grudnik P, Magiera K et al (2017) Structural biology of the immune checkpoint receptor PD-1 and its ligands PD-L1/PD-L2. Structure 25:1163–1174

Zhang H, Hyrien O, Pandya K et al (2008) Tumor response kinetics after schedule-dependent paclitaxel chemoradiation treatment for inoperable non-small cell lung cancer: a model for low-dose chemotherapy radiosensitization. J Thorac Oncol 3:563–568

Zheng Z, Chen T, Li X et al (2007) DNA synthesis and repair genes RRM1 and ERCC1 in lung cancer. N Engl J Med 356:800–808

Zhou C, Wu YL, Chen G et al (2011) Erlotinib versus chemotherapy as first-line treatment for patients with advanced EGFR mutation-positive non-small-cell lung cancer (OPTIMAL, CTONG-0802): a multicentre, open-label, randomised, phase 3 study. Lancet Oncol 12:735–742

Radiation Oncology of Lung Cancer: Why We Fail(ed) in Clinical Research?

Branislav Jeremić, Nenad Filipović, Slobodan Milisavljević, and Ivane Kiladze

Contents

1 Introduction 1135
2 General Aspects of Clinical Research 1136
3 Clinical Failures 1137
4 Controversial Issues 1139
5 Possible Solutions 1143
References 1143

Abstract

Clinical research in radiation oncology of lung cancer can bring important advances in the field of optimized treatment approaches in this disease. However, such a research has been a subject of many controversies, in particular in the light of lack of adequate number and quality of clinical trials which could have changed our standard policies. To address the comprehensive issue of clinical research in radiation oncology of lung cancer, several aspects will be considered: general aspects of clinical research generals, clinical failures, and some of existing, rather controversial issues identified. Finally, some of possible solutions for the current, grossly unfavorable, situation will be discussed.

B. Jeremić (✉)
School of Medicine, University of Kragujevac, Kragujevac, Serbia
e-mail: nebareje@gmail.com

N. Filipović
BioIRC, Center for Biomedical Engineering, Kragujevac, Serbia

S. Milisavljević
Department of Thoracic Surgery, University Clinical Center, Kragujevac, Serbia

I. Kiladze
Department of Clinical Oncology, Caucasus Medical Center, Tbilisi, Georgia

1 Introduction

Lung cancer is the major health problem worldwide, a consequence of its high morbidity and mortality, being the major cancer killer in both sexes. However, still existing dismal survival figures can also be attributed to a largely inadequate efforts to optimize prevention, screening, early diagnosis, treatment, and palliation efforts in this disease. In the treatment domain, radiation therapy (RT) remains one of the cornerstones of modern therapeutic endeavors due to its effectiveness in both curative and palliative setting, given either alone or in combination with surgery and/or chemotherapy (CHT) in the vast majority of patients.

Our efforts to optimize RT through various theoretical considerations, followed by initial steps in translational research, ending, finally in its practical application in daily clinic can only be rated as of rather low success. Not surprising, therefore, that improvements have been slow, incremental, and inadequate, having in mind that each year there is more than one million new lung cancer patients. Unfortunately, the vast majority of them either do not benefit from any of these "improvements" at all or do that only minimally. That is so irrespective of geography, race, or social status/income. This rather pessimistic view should be seen as nothing but a constant call to radiation oncologists worldwide to prioritize clinical research and produce more scientific data in one of the major battlegrounds in clinical research of oncology. It is so since clinical research is expected to bring important discoveries, do that continuously and help improve our ability to more successfully define the place and role of RT in the treatment of lung cancer than optimally implement RT in daily clinical practice.

To address the comprehensive issue of clinical research in radiation oncology of lung cancer, several aspects will be considered and possible solutions for the current, grossly unfavorable, situation will be discussed.

2 General Aspects of Clinical Research

If one tries to have a general, that is, more global, view on the issue of clinical research in Radiation Oncology (RO), one could start with the following questions: who does clinical research, how one does it and finally, when one does it? Starting with initial question, observation is that the vast majority of clinical trials in RO of lung cancer is mostly done within single-institutional setting, less within the group setting and even less within the intergroup setting. What, then can be expected from such exercise(s) but less patients enrolled per study of the lower level of strength of clinical evidence such studies can bring. This type of approach leads to inferior quality of clinical research and hampers implementation into a general clinical practice of RO of lung cancer. Similarly, when answering to a question how one does it, again, more phase I and II trials are observed and less phase III trials are performed. For example, one can take as an example of what two of the major groups (RTOG and EORTC) have done in the last several decades in the field of thoracic radiation therapy (TRT) in ED SCLC (Slotman et al. 2015; Gore et al. 2017). Even if we somehow limit this observation to the past 22 years since the publication of the pivotal study of Jeremic et al. (1999), the picture remains the same. While one may argue that this is an extreme case, reader is kindly asked to verify this observation with combined RT-CHT in, e.g., more prevalent Stage III NSCLC and these two group efforts. Finally, when one remains in the same time period (e.g., last three decade), but move to the domain of systemic therapy, it must be clearly observed that what have been, until recently, the driving force is more fashion and trend than the scientific idea. We have witnessed it in second, then the third generation of CHT agents, and "successfully" continued doing even in recent years. The vast majority of existing studies asked almost identical questions, with very similar study design, majority of which did not learn from predecessors' failures. How many times each of thoracic oncologists witnessed publication of a "novel" approach which was nothing but changing a regimen consisting of, e.g., 70 mg/sqm of paclitaxel given every week with 100 mg/sqm of cisplatin given every 3 weeks to a regimen consisting of 60 mg/sqm of paclitaxel given once a week with 50 mg/sqm of cisplatin given twice a week. One may even expect nothing less than that to happen in time with immunotherapy. Does this sound as "optimized" or to use a hype word of the last decades "personalized" medicine? Such research, speaking now with hindsight, brought no significant improvement in this field in the past, not to mention that thousands of patients have been exposed to meaningless clinical research that "misused" millions of Dollars and Euros worldwide. While situation with immunotherapy seems more optimistic, one should not forget that now organizations and societies approve such therapies, frequently offering only a couple of weeks of survival benefit, after a single prospective randomized clinical trial (PRCT). Designing and executing not only more PRCTs, but also more powerful (number of patients, statistical power) PRCTs to detect even smaller differences between standard and experimental arms, respectively, remain a quest one should not hesitate to join.

Another good example is the use of consolidation systemic therapy (CHT, targeted agents, immunotherapy) after initial concurrent RT/systemic therapy had been given. The issue of concern is evaluation of response after initial phase of treatment. Interestingly and quite disappointingly, many studies did not undertake such an effort. Even those who did, actually did not take it into account, i.e., continued with the consolidation systemic therapy even in patients with progressive disease (PD). Finally, even those who used it in non-PD patients did not make an effort to discriminate events occurring in three patient subgroups, those achieving a complete response (CR), partial response (PR), or stable disease (SD). This is an important issue due to large difference in tumor cells/burden existing after the initial concurrent RT/systemic part. It may have a substantial impact on appropriateness to continue with consolidation systemic therapy (e.g., CR-PR vs SD), type of consolidation drugs (same or switch), duration of treatment (in CR vs PR), to name but a few. Without this knowledge, many patients which received consolidation therapy and in the past and, unfortunately, many of the current ones on targeted and immunotherapy, received it without actually knowing have they been suitable candidates or not. While we wait for future trials in this setting to mandate evaluation of response and subsequent fate of various subgroups of patients undergoing it, radiation oncologists are encouraged to undertake retrospective analysis of previously published studies and gain basic information about this important issue.

3 Clinical Failures

The term "clinical failures" are used here to describe not failures as usually described in the literature (e.g., locoregional or distant) but our failures to scientifically observe important aspects during clinical studies performed in the past and to use then-gathered knowledge to optimize subsequent studies. In particular, this is referred to the time component to use gathered knowledge to optimize future attempts via clinical studies. These failures can broadly be separated into patient-related, tumor-related, and history of the disease-related.

Of patient-related observations, it was frequently observed that patients with performance status of less than 50% and/or those with pronounced weight loss (i.e. >5%) are experiencing more toxicity, having more treatment interruptions and/or dose reductions, all leading to poorer local control and ultimately, inferior survival. Hence, it may come as a surprise that although more recent studies tried as much as possible to exclude these patients from various dose-intensification trials, we do not have more clinical studies concentrating on those, rather unfavorable, prognostic group with only a few exemptions to this statement. Similarly, elderly have largely been neglected adequate access to clinical trials, possibly due to a fear that they could not tolerate intensive therapeutic interventions. While there are no firm data supporting this, rather nihilistic view, there are also not many prospective randomized clinical trials specifically addressing various aspects of treatments administered in the field of RO of lung cancer, where RT was given either alone or in combination with CHT. These observations may fall into a group of explanations of why we do not have more patients enrolled into clinical trials since the vast majority of clinical trials are continuously used to ask various questions about optimization via intensification of RT and/or CHT.

Of tumor-related factors, stage, histology, and location can be used to provide necessary framework for statements above. Stage III NSCLC is one of the focuses of clinical investigations in the field of lung cancer. Even with the most recent staging revision (Goldstraw et al. 2016; Rami-Porta et al. 2014), it still has 17 different T and N combinations. Even if we see the increase in possible combinations from previous 11 (Goldstraw et al. 2007) to currently existing 17 as big step forward, which it indeed is, we still continue using this, rather surgical, staging system. The big puzzle remains on why radiation oncologists do not embark on using more tumor volume-, rather than tumor size-driven staging system(s). This is especially so since we are living for, at least, the last 20 years, in an era of powerful computers which enabled easy 3D reconstruction of various volumes and, hence, fast computation of volumetrics. Fortunately, we do have data confirming the influence of tumor volumes on treatment outcome (Bradley et al. 2002; Basaki et al. 2006; Dehinge-Obeije et al. 2008; Werner-Wasik et al. 2008; Alexander et al. 2011; Lee et al. 2012). Importantly, these observations included both T and N component and their respective volumes. Regarding histology, it has been speculated for many years about more "local" character of the squamous cell carcinomas than other non-small cell carcinomas (e.g., adenocarcinoma, large cell carcinoma). If this is so, why then efforts have not been appropriately made towards optimization of our endeavors by using more local (e.g., RT dose escalation with/without radioenhancing administration of CHT) treatment options in this setting and, contrary to that, more/higher doses of CHT given with RT in adenocarcinomas and large cell carcinomas due to their presumably larger metastatic potential? Similarly, some observed more "local" character of peripheral lung cancers, especially early stage ones. Therefore, different approaches could have been explored in addressing these issues and helped gain insight about differences in both biological behavior of tumors located differently as well as design clinical trials addressing different therapeutic options tailored according to these characteristics. Additionally, observations from two studies (van Meerbeck et al. 2007; Sorenson et al. 2013) showed that histology may play an important role in decision-making process, acting as a predictor to a treatment success. In EORTC study (Van Meerbeck et al. 2007) squamous cell histology seemed superior, opposite to adenocarcinoma which had better prognosis in Scandinavian study (Sorenson et al. 2013), both studies being performed in Stage IIIA NSCLC. If the predictive analyses were performed, one could have learned about it and possibly reshape the design of subsequent group studies based on these findings.

Importance of patient-related and tumor-related factors and influence on treatment outcome could easily be seen in the case of Stage IIIA NSCLC. In spite of lacking evidence, many clinicians and groups and organizations still suggest the use of trimodality approach which employees neoadjuvant RT-CHT followed by surgery. In such case, patients are offered surgery after evaluation of the RT-CHT response and those deemed "eligible" (i.e., suitable) for surgery undergoing it. What still present as the major problem is that the decision-making process, which should take place and time during the multidisciplinary tumor (MDT) board meeting does not take into account predictive factors. They may preferentially point to neoadjuvant RT-CHT followed by surgery and not to exclusive RT-CHT in case such factors exist. But they do not. They have never been investigated as summarized several years ago (Jeremic et al. 2016). Besides this, another big problem lies in the fact that incorrect terminology had frequently been used. Many studies had used "predictive" to describe what a simple Cox proportional hazards model a.k.a. multivariate model (which identified prognostic, not predictive factors) identified as significant. Appropriate terminology must include a clear distinction between a *prognostic factor* being defined as clinical variable providing an information on the likely outcome in either an untreated patient or a patient treated with standard therapy. On the other side, a *predictive factor* is defined as clinical variable providing information on the likely survival benefit from treatment. These factors can be used to identify subgroups of patients most likely to benefit from a given therapy. In summary, *prognostic factor* defines the effects of patient- or tumor-related characteristics on the patient outcome, while *predictive factor* defines the effect of treatment on the tumor. An ideal setting for evaluating the prognostic and predictive significance of a clinical characteristic is PRCT with previously well known and widely accepted control group. If one determines that the survival benefit for patients treated with neoadjuvant RT-CHT followed by surgery as compared to those treated with exclusive concurrent RT-CHT differs by any of these characteristics, then the significance of a potential predictor is established (Clark et al. 2006; Clark 2008). Unfortunately, many studies claimed to have established one or more "predictors" in this setting, favoring trimodality approach, but they all have used, however, only a test for prognosticators, determining its independent influence on the treatment outcome.

Of other observations that could have easily changed our reality, by using them in clinic, events in locally advanced NSCLC and ED SCLC could nicely serve as supporting background. In locally advanced NSCLC, induction CHT followed by radical RT became one of the standard treatment options in the 1990s of the last century. In order to optimize it, various intensification attempts have been made, including administration of concurrent RT-CHT after induction CHT, including similar approaches with targeted agents and immunotherapy. What all of these studies clearly identified is insufficient local control obtained when one starts the treatment with induction systemic therapy, no matter how much you eventually intensify the second (concurrent) part of the combined treatment with either higher RT dose or more drugs/doses. El Sharouni et al. (2003) compared CT scans pre-and post-induction CHT, with emphasis on the time from the last induction CHT cycle to the time of RT treatment planning CT was actually done. They have measured an increase in gross tumor volumes (GTV) and subsequently define volume doubling times. During the waiting period (for the planning CT scan and start of RT), a total of 41% of all tumors became incurable, with the ratio of GTVs being in the range of 1.1–81.8! Tumor doubling times ranged 8.3–171 days, with the median of 29 days. When translated into a useful clinical language, these findings clearly showed that even if one may have thought (due to insufficient CT-based imaging) that response occurs (and that it matters), there is actually completely opposite situation: existing surviving tumor clonogens repopulates fast, leading tumors to regrow to the state of incurability. Various clinical studies reconfirmed that whatever you do after you start with CHT, failure is inevitable and comes fast. With this approach, only significantly more toxicity is observed (Vokes et al. 2002; Akerley et al. 2005; Socinski et al. 2008) also observed in when high dose 3D RT is used. Astonishing 12% mortality in the recent CALGB attempt (Socinski et al. 2008) to combine induction CHT with subsequent RT-CHT led to early stopping the trial.

4 Controversial Issues

They include a variety of issues having a significantly negative impact on clinical research in RO of lung cancer. Hospital/departmental workflow still seems to be one of the major problems in clinical research in the field of lung cancer worldwide. In particular, and what had been debated on conferences and meetings for a while, is the fact also observed in thoracic surgery and medical oncology and that is the following: institutions recruiting fewer patients are those whose participation adversely influences the study outcome. Recent publication of reanalysis of the RTOG0617 (Eaton et al. 2016) showed that to be the case. Participating institutions were categorized as low-volume centers or high-volume centers according to the number of patients accrued (≤ 3 vs. >3). Accrual for the former ($n = 195$) vs the latter ($n = 300$) ranged 1–3 vs. 4 1–8 patients. Treatment at high-volume centers was associated with statistically significantly longer overall survival (OS) and progression-free survival (PFS) (MST, 26.2 vs. 19.8 months; $p = 0.002$; median PFS: 11.4 vs. 9.7 months, $p = 0.04$). Impact of high-volume patients and, therefore, greater demands may have been the reason for high-volume centers to treat patients more often with intensity-modulated RT (54.0% vs. 39.5%, $p = 0\ 0.002$), with a likely consequence of having a lower esophageal dose (mean = 26.1 vs. 28.0 Gy, $p = 0.03$), and a lower heart dose (medianV5, $p = 0.006$; V50Gy, $p < 0.001$). Multivariate analysis reconfirmed these findings showing that high-volume center remained independent prognosticator of longer OS ($p = 0.03$). An important question this and similar analyses bring is what to do with it? Should one limit participation in PRCTs to centers with high-volume loads or not? If yes, that may seriously erode the whole concept of clinical research, but if no, again, what is to be done? More emphasis on training, especially in residents and young consultants? Or perhaps pre-trial site-specific education? Or even site-specific and group-oriented systematic (repeated at regular intervals) efforts? While some of these efforts are already underway, the results of RTOG0617 should not be repeated in the negative context and every effort should be made to take this issue into account before embarking on a PRCT.

Two additional issues could be connected with the question how one embarks (either the design or participation) to a PRCT? In the first example, which we can call an optimization process, the setting on dose and fractionation in limited disease small cell lung cancer (LD SCLC) will be discussed. Upon the publication of the data from the Intergroup study (Turrisi et al. 1999) showing that 45 Gy in 30 fractions in 15 treatment days in 3 weeks was superior to the RT of the same total dose given with one fraction a day (OD) for 5 weeks (25 fractions), many non-believers continued using OD RT with reasoning that 45 Gy given OD is simply not enough. Those more brave embarked on a study that tested the same BID regimen with high dose RT (66 Gy) given also with concurrent CHT (Faivre-Finn et al. 2017). While biologically effective dose (BED) in the intergroup study (Turrisi et al. 1999) was quite similar ($51.75Gy_{10}$ and $52.10\ Gy_{10}$, respectively) between the two arms, in the second case (Faivre-Finn et al. 2017) it was much higher for OD RT ($75.9Gy_{10}$). In spite of this attempt to explore dose response in LD SCLC, which can only be seen as a legitimate effort, lower dose of BID RT did not lead to inferior results when compared to high dose OD RT. These results questioned wisdom of optimization of our clinical and research efforts by having a "tubar" vision, or, in other words, revitalizing the "dead horse" (i.e., inferior option in the Intergroup study). Why, at the same time there were not more efforts to optimize the winning option, that of 45 Gy BID? Not a single attempt in the past 20 years, in spite of excellent results 54 Gy in 36 daily fractions in 18 treatment days in 3.5 days produced in the same setting (Jeremic et al. 1997)? Fortunately, we have just witnessed such an attempt in a fresh publication from Lancet Oncology (Grønberg et al. 2021). This study, including 22 centers showed that optimization process can be beneficial if on the right pathway. Norwegian group had compared previous standard (45 Gy BID) with the higher dose of the same BID pattern but to the total dose of 60 Gy. Higher dose produced significantly better OS and PFS but did not lead to more toxicity. In spite of the high number of patients enrolled in the two groups ($n = 170$), giving strong statistical power to the finding, authors concluded with rather modest words that 60 Gy BID could perhaps be considered as an alternative to other approaches.

Second issue is participation in a trial when one knows from the study design that RT characteristics are seemingly such that outcome would likely be inferior. Such is the case of adding RT to neoadjuvant CHT in a trimodality approach in patients with Stage IIIA/N2 NSCLC. Study design mandated RT is given as 45 Gy in 24 daily fractions concurrently with 2 cycles of CHT after which a few weeks were allowed as a treatment gap, at the end of which response evaluation was done. In patients with unsatisfactory response, those that remained inoperable, continuation of RT-CHT was mandated with RT of 16 Gy in 8 daily fractions (as per INT0139 study). This way, the specific and extremely unfavorable situation occurred. RT course effectively became a split course, known for decades to be inferior to a continuous course RT. Furthermore, this type of RT, split course was mandated to unfavorable, clearly poor-prognosis, patients since they remained inoperable. Whether participating radiation oncologists were aware of this situation is completely different question, but very few comments appeared as "constructive" criticism regarding this issue since the original publication. Hopefully, new generations of radiation oncologists would take this observation into account when considering participation in similar trials. This is especially so since both results of aforementioned INT0139 (Albain et al. 2009) and a series of prospective and retrospective studies (Sonett et al. 2004; Cerfolio et al. 2005; Daly et al. 2006; Suntharalingam et al. 2012; Allen et al. 2018; Donington et al. 2020) confirmed effectiveness of concurrent TRT-CHT given in both trimodality setting and as exclusive RT-CHT.

Some of the controversial issues are long-standing ones. While past experience on published data clearly identified policies of greater likelihood that positive study will be published than the negative one, recent years also witnessed that the results of even officially terminated studies, identified through clinicaltrials.gov website as such, never saw the light of the day. Importantly, the vast majority of such events occurred in drug-related studies. However, even positive studies, such as Scandinavian study comparing exclusive RT-CHT with trimodality surgical approach, presented at major scientific meeting (ASCO) (Sorensen et al. 2013) never reached readership of any journal since then. While the presentation and publication process is the internal matter of the study coordinators, PIs, and, frequently, industry, is there a way one would mandate full reporting of study results even if it is prematurely closed due to various reasons (e.g., poor accrual)? If so, we will then learn about exact data and details which may have led to such a fate and gather knowledge to be incorporated into a future studies design.

Another example shows how existing data never reach initial press/journal publication, or any subsequent one, in spite of tremendous importance and possibility of great policy shift. In case of meta-analysis on combined RT and CHT in locally advanced NSCLC (Aupérin et al. 2010), meta-analysts gathered almost 15 years ago and discussed all important aspects of three analyses which asked important questions about the timing of such a combination. An interesting aspect and potentially important clinical findings, that of age, were brought to the attention. In the analysis comparing induction CHT followed by RT versus RT alone, and mentioned in a slide presentation, increasing age proved to be an important and adverse factor of treatment outcome, suggesting that older patients should not be offered sequential combination, i.e., CHT followed by RT. Unfortunately, this finding never earned the place in full publication although it was clearly documented in full in a PhD thesis of main study statistician (Auperin 2010). Therefore, the opportunity to send the clear message to thoracic oncologists and patients that induction CHT followed by RT has a detrimental effect on older patients had been missed. Having known that the vast majority of lung cancer patients are not younger, but relatively older, that would seriously undermine position of CHT in this setting. Without going into speculation about the magnitude of the effect such finding would have on practicing thoracic oncologists, it, nevertheless, seems likely that thousands of patients continued to be exposed to inferior (efficacy, toxicity) treatment option over years.

Among controversial issues, some are personal in nature. We have all occasionally witnessed completely differing evidence-based versus expert-based opinions. Unfortunately, even some of the most prestigious institutions and groups/organizations all over the world suffer from this disease including also inherent specifics of medical profession and division between "big" specialities (e.g., surgery, internal medicine) and presumably "smaller" (e.g., radiation oncology). I am sure all of thoracic radiation oncologists occasionally witnessed unpleasant situations in daily clinic or during tumor board meetings where this had occurred. Collateral damage may well be our residents, who are primed with this type of really unacceptable behavior for which there should be only a zero tolerance. Extension to this is its soft version materialized in frequent existence (among radiation oncologists) of "non-believers" in evidence-based principles. Some people simply do not believe evidence they are presented with. Usually, this is not related to "constructive" (better said, productive) criticism, based on scientific merits, but rather finding excuses of how to interpret existing evidence. Even softer version of non-believing in existing evidence is seen in some of our colleagues who request always more evidence than is present and/or needed. Excuses goes from: (1) "this is only the first or second trial confirming that A is better than B", through (2) "logistics of our clinic prevent us of implementing this approach (e.g. BID fractionation)" to (3) "the statistical power of that particular study is not strong enough (too few patients)." Even in cases of existing meta-analyses and multiple large confirmatory trials there may be an obstacle to implement what is already proven. More than 15 years ago, (Langer et al. 2005) report on the CHT characteristics practiced in nonmetastatic lung cancer in the USA during the Patterns of Care Survey in 59 RT institutions. Informations have been sampled during a period 2000–2002. Only 6% of patients received BID RT in SCLC, only 22% received prophylactic cranial irradiation (PCI), and only 49% patients underwent CT-based treatment planning. Significantly more patients >70 years were treated at large nonacademic facilities compared with smaller nonacademic or academic institutions, surprising finding for non-treating institutions since a body of data exists on the effectiveness of RT in elderly or simply a finding underlining the lack of RT studies in this patient population. Some 5% patients with SCLC did not receive CHT, while 18% of stage I NSCLC patients receive RT-CHT and this percentage goes up to 34% for stage II NSCLC. Of additional importance is that 33% of locally advanced NSCLC receives only RT. Induction CHT was still widely practiced, while trend seemed to have favored consolidation CHT as well although no PRCT favoring it existed then. These examples are perfect show of practice of non-evidence-based medicine in lung cancer as they also nicely match observation from the choice of timing of RT-CHT in SCLC, choice of drugs, etc. They all fortify general impression that although combined RT and CHT are practiced by the majority of institutions in majority of locally advanced NSCLC and SCLC patients, there are still substantial variations in practice, most of which are not substantiated by the existing evidence. It remained unknown whether perhaps group affiliation of the sampled RT facilities influenced the practice, because it is likely to expect that academic and large nonacademic institutions/practicing physicians would feel some heat for non-recruiting patients into the juicy clinical studies investigating novel drugs or combinations. Another matter is how fast this can be observed in daily routine. It is hard completely to digest authors explanation that, e.g., LAMP study (Belani et al. 2005) widely influenced practice in the USA being published only as an abstract in the year 2002 (and had, therefore, only several months of its limited abstract life to exert influence on troublesome behavior of practicing physicians in this Patterns of Care Study, published in 2004) while, on the other side, RTOG 9410 (Curran Jr et al. 2000) did not exert such an influence, being published in the same way (abstract) in the year 2000! Speed of such an implementation is more than debatable.

To further extend this observation and make it more contemporary, one can turn to group and/organization-existing recommendations and guidelines. They sometimes suggest treatments that were never investigated and, therefore, without any scientific proof. One may take the example of the study where the drug atezolizumab has been used in ED SCLC and proven to be effective, (albeit of the magnitude of such proof!) prompting FDA to approve it in this setting. Interestingly, original study (Horn et al. 2018) allowed institution to use or not PCI, but TRT was not allowed. Most recent recommendations/guidelines from various parts of the world, however, allow TRT to be used in this setting of ED SCLC with Atezolizumab. While some thoracic oncologists jumped in that bandwagon fast and easy, there was very little discussion about such society/organization policies and consequences scientifically never tested, hence, unproven, treatments are recommended. Ultimately, who are radiation oncologists sitting in those committees approving non-existing therapies? Therapies for which we do not have even hints how they can act? Therapies that could do harm? Many questions remain unanswered in the atmosphere of pressure to adopt new and promising treatments, frequently obscured by non-existing data.

A number of controversial issues could also directly be connected with the clinical trial issues. While we have already mentioned that very few prospective phase III trials are produced (designed and executed) by radiation oncologists, another issue is that even those that are with clear outcomes and great potential for improving overall approach in lung cancer are frequently poorly implemented in practice. One good example is aforementioned BID trial in LD SCLC (Turrisi et al. 1999). Another good example may well be the so-called CHART (continuous hyperfractionated accelerated radiation therapy) which produced significant improvement in treatment outcome when compared to standard RT in inoperable NSCLC (Saunders et al. 1999). Due to its poor implementation, even in the UK, the National Health Service (NHS) there had to officially urge institutions to adopt such an approach. Also, as we mentioned above, some of the trials implemented in clinical practice are not those representing standards of treatment as various Patterns of Care Studies have shown (Movsas et al. 2003; Langer et al. 2005).

5 Possible Solutions

Possible solutions to overcome existing obstacles and improve our ability to undertake meaningful clinical research in RO of lung cancer could include improvements in education (both residents and staff radiation oncologists), identification of existing weaknesses in research domain which may present as obstruction to evidence-based oncology principles, fast implementation of proven clinical trials and meta-analyses, especially those favoring RT in lung cancer, necessary to produce more clinical trials by radiation oncologists, especially those which combine newest biological data of the disease with the latest technological capabilities of our profession, for which (all of the above) we actually need more patients. So, perhaps the very first step on our road towards improvement would be to leave the departmental premises and start both making our achievements more public to both general public and also to other medical professionals. One example, in the third decade of the twenty-first century, would include something that our colleagues medical oncologists already successfully adopted. Owing to rising webinars and podcasts, all done for the sake of faster promotion of various drugs, not only professional, but general oncology and non-professional audience is rapidly growing. By making various (here, meaning both patient and medical professionals!) target groups more aware of our capabilities, we may be able to successfully spread the word and recruit more patients for treatments and, hence, more of those suitable for clinical trials. Such trials should preferably combine biological and technological aspects of our profession in the field of lung cancer. Biological aspects such as irradiation-drug interactions could successfully be explored through translational research using mechanistic studies to enlighten the problem of irradiation-drug interactions. This is only if translational research is understood as "back and forth," from benchmark to bedside and back, aiming to continuously enrich our knowledge, performance capabilities and, ultimately, treatment results. Such clinical studies should ask simple questions, ask those questions important for radiation oncologists, being biology of the disease-driven and being at the same time, technology-adapted. This is the only way we, as a profession, could successfully integrate our capabilities and address burning questions in the field of lung cancer, a must for current and future generations of radiation oncologists involved in care of patients with lung cancer.

References

Akerley W, Herndon JE Jr, Lyss AP et al (2005) Induction paclitaxel/carboplatin followed by concurrent chemoradiation therapy for unresectable stage III non-small-cell lung cancer: a limited-access study–CALGB 9534. Clin Lung Cancer 7:47–53

Albain KS, Swann RS, Rusch VW et al (2009) Radiotherapy plus chemotherapy with or without surgical resection for stage III non-small-cell lung cancer: a phase III randomised controlled trial. Lancet 374:379–386

Alexander BM, Othus M, Caglar HB, Allen AM (2011) Tumor volume is a prognostic factor in non-small-cell lung cancer treated with chemoradiotherapy. Int J Radiat Oncol Biol Phys 79:1381–1387

Allen AM, Shochat T, Flex D et al (2018) High-dose radiotherapy as neoadjuvant treatment in non-small-cell lung cancer. Oncology 95:13–19

Auperin A (2010) Carcinomes broncho-pulmonaires non à petites cellules localement avancés: évaluation de la chimiothérapie associée à la radiothérapie par les méta-analyses sur données individuelles. Universite Paris XI, Faculte de Medecine Paris-Sud (These)

Aupérin A, Le Péchoux C, Rolland E et al (2010) Meta-analysis of concomitant versus sequential radiochemotherapy in locally advanced non-small-cell lung cancer. J Clin Oncol 28:2181–2190

Basaki K, Abe Y, Aoki M, Kondo H, Hatayama Y, Nakaji S (2006) Prognostic factors for survival in stage III non-small-cell lung cancer treated with definitive radiation therapy: impact of tumor volume. Int J Radiat Oncol Biol Phys 64:449–454

Belani CP, Choy H, Bonomi P et al (2005) Combined chemoradiotherapy regimens of paclitaxel and carboplatin for locally advanced non-small-cell lung cancer: a randomized phase II locally advanced multimodality protocol. J Clin Oncol 23:5883–5891

Bradley JD, Ieumwananonthachai N, Purdy JA et al (2002) Gross tumor volume, critical prognostic factor in patients treated with three-dimensional conformal radiation therapy for non-small-cell lung carcinoma. Int J Radiat Oncol Biol Phys 52:49–57

Cerfolio RJ, Bryant AS, Spencer SA, Bartolucci AA (2005) Pulmonary resection after high-dose and low-dose chest irradiation. Ann Thorac Surg 80:1224–1230

Clark GM (2008) Prognostic factors versus predictive factors: examples from a clinical trial of erlotinib. Mol Oncol 1:406–412

Clark GM, Zborowski DM, Culbertson JL et al (2006) Clinical utility of epidermal growth factor receptor expression for selecting patients with advanced non-small cell lung cancer for treatment with erlotinib. J Thorac Oncol 1:837–846

Curran WJ Jr, Scott C, Langer C, Komaki R, Lee JS, Hauser S (2000) Phase III comparison of sequential vs cancer (NSCLC): initial report of radiation therapy oncology group concurrent chemoradiation for pts with unresected stage III non small cell lung (RTOG 9410). Proc Am Soc Clin Oncol 19:484a. (Abstract 1891)

Daly BDT, Fernando HC, Ketchedjian A et al (2006) Pneumonectomy after high-dose radiation and concurrent chemotherapy for nonsmall cell lung cancer. Ann Thorac Surg 82:227–231

Dehing-Oberije C, De Ruysscher D, van der Weide H et al (2008) Tumor volume combined with number of positive lymph node stations is a more important prognostic factor than TNM stage for survival of non-small-cell lung cancer patients treated with (chemo)radiotherapy. Int J Radiat Oncol Biol Phys 70:1039–1044

Donington JS, Paulus R, Edelman MJ, for the NRG Oncology Lung Group et al (2020) Resection following concurrent chemotherapy and high-dose radiation for stage IIIA non–small cell lung cancer. J Thorac Cardiovasc Surg 160:1331–1345. e1

Eaton BR, Pugh SL, Bradley JD et al (2016) Institutional enrollment and survival among NSCLC patients receiving chemoradiation: NRG Oncology Radiation Therapy Oncology Group (RTOG) 0617. J Natl Cancer Inst 108:djw034

El Sharouni SY, Kal HB, Battermann JJ (2003) Accelerated regrowth of non-small cell lung tumors after induction chemotherapy. Br J Cancer 89: 2184–2189

Faivre-Finn C, Snee M, Ashcroft L, for the CONVERT Study Team et al (2017) Concurrent once-daily versus twice-daily chemoradiotherapy in patients with limited-stage small-cell lung cancer (CONVERT): an open-label, phase 3, randomised, superiority trial. Lancet Oncol 18:1116–1125

Goldstraw P, Crowley J, Chansky K, Giroux DJ, Groome PA (2007) The IASLC lung cancer staging project: proposals for the revision of the TNM stage groupings in the forthcoming (seventh) edition of the TNM classification of malignant tumours. J Thorac Oncol 2:706–714

Goldstraw P, Chansky K, Crowley J et al (2016) The IASLC lung cancer staging project: proposals for revision of the TNM stage groupings in the forthcoming (eighth) edition of the TNM classification for lung cancer. J Thorac Oncol 11:39–51

Gore EM, Hu C, Sun AY et al (2017) Randomized phase II study comparing prophylactic cranial irradiation alone to prophylactic cranial irradiation and consolidative extracranial irradiation for extensive-disease small cell lung cancer (ED SCLC): NRG Oncology RTOG 0937. J Thorac Oncol 12: 1561–1570

Grønberg BH, Killingberg KT, Fløtten Ø et al (2021) High-dose versus standard-dose twice-daily thoracic radiotherapy for patients with limited stage small-cell lung cancer: an open-label, randomised, phase 2 trial. Lancet Oncol 22:321–331

Horn L, Mansfield AS, Szczęsna A, IM power133 Study Group et al (2018) First-line Atezolizumab plus chemotherapy in extensive-stage small-cell lung cancer. N Engl J Med 379:2220–2229

Jeremic B, Shibamoto Y, Acimovic L, Milisavljevic S (1997) Initial versus delayed accelerated hyperfractionated radiation therapy and concurrent chemotherapy in limited small cell lung cancer. J Clin Oncol 15:893–900

Jeremic B, Shibamoto Y, Nikolic N, Milicic B, Milisavljevic S, Dagovic A, Aleksandrovic J, Radosavljevic-Asic G (1999) The role of radiation therapy in the combined modality treatment of patients with extensive disease small-cell lung cancer (ED SCLC): a randomized study. J Clin Oncol 17:2092–2099

Jeremic B, Casas F, Dubinsky P et al (2016) Surgery in stage IIIA nonsmall cell lung cancer: lack of predictive and prognostic factors identifying any patient subgroup benefiting from it. Clin Lung Cancer 17:107–112

Langer CJ, Moughan J, Movsas B et al (2005) Patterns of care survey (PCS) in lung cancer: how well does current U.S. practice with chemotherapy in the non-metastatic setting follow the literature. Lung Cancer 48:93–102

Lee P, Bazan JG, Lavori PW et al (2012) Metabolic tumor volume is an independent prognostic factor in patients treated definitively for non–small-cell lung cancer. Clin Lung Cancer 13:52–58

Movsas B, Moughan J, Komaki R et al (2003) Radiotherapy patterns of care study in lung carcinoma. J Clin Oncol 21:4553–4559

Rami-Porta R, Bolejack V, Giroux DJ, International Association for the Study of Lung Cancer Staging and Prognostic Factors Committee, Advisory Board Members and Participating Institutions et al (2014) The IASLC lung cancer staging project: the new database to inform the eighth edition of the TNM classification of lung cancer. J Thorac Oncol 9:1618–1624

Saunders M, Dische S, Barrett A, Harvey A, Griffiths G, Palmar M (1999) Continuous, hyperfractionated, accelerated radiotherapy (CHART) versus conventional radiotherapy in non-small cell lung cancer: mature data from the randomised multicentre trial. CHART steering committee. Radiother Oncol 52:137–148

Slotman BJ, Van Tinteren H, Praag JO et al (2015) Use of thoracic radiotherapy for extensive stage small-cell lung cancer: a phase 3 randomised controlled trial. Lancet 385:36–42

Socinski MA, Blackstock AW, Bogart JA (2008) Randomized phase II trial of induction chemotherapy followed by concurrent chemotherapy and dose-escalated thoracic conformal radiotherapy (74 Gy) in stage III non-small-cell lung cancer: CALGB 30105. J Clin Oncol 26:2457–2463

Sonett JR, Suntharalingam M, Edelman MJ et al (2004) Pulmonary resection after curative intent radiotherapy (>59 Gy) and concurrent chemotherapy in non-small-cell lung cancer. Ann Thorac Surg 78:1200–1205

Sorensen JB, Riska H, Ravn J et al (2013) Scandinavian phase III trial of neoadjuvant chemotherapy in NSCLC stages IB-IIIA/T3. J Clin Oncol 31(Suppl; abstr 7504)

Suntharalingam M, Paulus R, Edelman MJ et al (2012) Radiation therapy oncology group protocol 02-29: a phase II trial of neoadjuvant therapy with concurrent chemotherapy and full-dose radiation therapy followed by surgical resection and consolidative therapy for locally advanced nonsmall cell carcinoma of the lung. Int J Radiat Oncol 84:456–463

Turrisi AT 3rd, Kim K, Blum R (1999) Twice-daily compared with once-daily thoracic radiotherapy in limited small-cell lung cancer treated concurrently with cisplatin and etoposide. N Engl J Med 28:265–271

van Meerbeeck JP, Kramer GW, van Schil PE et al (2007) Randomized controlled trial of resection versus radiotherapy after induction chemotherapy in stage IIIA-N2 non-small-cell lung cancer. J Natl Cancer Inst 99:442–450

Vokes EE, Herndon JE 2nd, Crawford J (2002) Randomized phase II study of cisplatin with gemcitabine or paclitaxel or vinorelbine as induction chemotherapy followed by concomitant chemoradiotherapy for stage IIIB non small-cell lung cancer: cancer and leukemia group B study 9431. J Clin Oncol 20:4191–4198

Werner-Wasik M, Swann RS, Bradley J et al (2008) Increasing tumor volume is predictive of poor overall and progression-free survival: secondary analysis of the radiation therapy oncology group 93-11 phase I-II radiation dose-escalation study in patients with inoperable non-small-cell lung cancer. Int J Radiat Oncol Biol Phys 70:385–390

Randomized Clinical Trials: Pitfalls in Design, Analysis, Presentation, and Interpretation

Lawrence Kasherman, S. C. M. Lau, K. Karakasis, N. B. Leighl, and A. M. Oza

Contents

1 Introduction 1148
2 **The Anatomy of a Randomized Trial: Key Design Concepts and Elements** 1148
2.1 The Research Question 1149
2.2 Trial Design and Conduct 1150
2.3 Outcome Assessments 1152
2.4 Randomization Process 1153
2.5 Statistical Considerations 1153
3 **Ensuring Robust Data Analysis: Turning Chaos into Order** 1154
3.1 Interim Analyses 1155
3.2 Multiplicity 1155
4 **Presenting RCTs: Not All That Glitters Is Gold** 1155
4.1 Patient Enrollment and the CONSORT Diagram 1155
4.2 Comparison of Clinical Characteristics 1157
4.3 Efficacy Results 1157
4.4 Toxicity 1158
5 **Pitfalls in Interpretation: What Does It All Mean?** 1158
5.1 The Knowledge Gap 1158
5.2 Assessment of Study Endpoints and Interpretation of Statistical Analyses 1159
5.3 Clinical Significance 1161
5.4 Generalizability 1162
6 **Future of Clinical Studies** 1163
References 1163

L. Kasherman (✉)
Division of Medical Oncology and Hematology, Bras Family Drug Development Program, Princess Margaret Cancer Centre, University Health Network, University of Toronto, Toronto, ON, Canada

Department of Medical Oncology, Illawarra Cancer Care Centre, Wollongong, NSW, Australia

Concord Clinical School, Faculty of Medicine and Health, University of Sydney, Concord, NSW, Australia
e-mail: Lawrence.Kasherman@health.nsw.gov.au

S. C. M. Lau
Department of Medical Oncology, Princess Margaret Cancer Centre, University Health Network, University of Toronto, Toronto, ON, Canada

NYU Langone Health, Perlmutter Cancer Center, New York University, New York, NY, USA

K. Karakasis · A. M. Oza
Division of Medical Oncology and Hematology, Bras Family Drug Development Program, Princess Margaret Cancer Centre, University Health Network, University of Toronto, Toronto, ON, Canada

N. B. Leighl
Department of Medical Oncology, Princess Margaret Cancer Centre, University Health Network, University of Toronto, Toronto, ON, Canada

Abstract

Randomized controlled trials are one of the cornerstones of evidence-based medicine and have been widely employed to implement novel treatments into standard practice within all disciplines of medicine. Recently, there has been a monumental surge in novel oncology therapeutic development across various tumor sites, and with the urgency of rapid drug development, it has become increasingly important for clinicians to become familiar with research processes, analyses, and interpretation. This chapter will not dissect every aspect of randomized clinical trials, but instead highlight the core considerations taken and potential pitfalls of designing, analyzing, presenting, and interpreting these studies.

1 Introduction

In the current era of evidence-based medicine, randomized controlled trials (RCTs) are generally viewed as the gold standard (Hariton and Locascio 2018) for assessing the safety and efficacy of new therapeutic options across all disciplines of medicine, and in particular within the realm of oncology (Booth et al. 2008). Robustly designed, conducted, analyzed, and presented trials form the focal point behind the majority of federal governmental agency approvals (such as the U.S. Food and Drug Administration (FDA) and European Medicines Agency) of novel oncological therapeutics. Certainly, within the field of medical oncology in lung cancer, presentation of results and associated publications in peer-reviewed journals have led to more than 10 FDA drug approvals over the course of 2020 (The ASCO Post 2021), signifying the rapidity of scientific and therapeutic advancement within the field. These clinical breakthroughs, which perpetuate excitement and likely rapid drug implementation within the oncology clinician community, are likely to continue in the years to come as technological and scientific advances lead to novel biomarker and drug development. However, despite the rapidly evolving landscape of lung cancer therapeutics and anticipatory haste to report favorable results for those affected, it remains of utmost importance that preservation of integrity and quality assurance in unbiased research design and analysis is carried forth as an imperative for ethical equipoise. Although some biases in research are systematic and unavoidable, this needs to be accommodated for when reviewing the design of a randomized trial. Sources of bias, including selection, performance or reporting biases can clinically and statistically affect study results to a significant degree, and should be carefully examined to ensure robustness of data analysis and interpretation.

The World Health Organization (WHO) has developed the Good Clinical Research Practice (GCP) Principles, defining it as, *"a process that incorporates established ethical and scientific quality standards for the design, conduct, recording and reporting of clinical research involving the participation of human subjects. Compliance with GCP provides public assurance that the rights, safety, and well-being of research subjects are protected and respected, consistent with the principles enunciated in the Declaration of Helsinki and other internationally recognized ethical guidelines, and ensures the integrity of clinical research data* (Idänpään-Heikkilä 1994; World Health Organization 2005).". Although many of the principles refer to other issues such as trial conduct, data handling, privacy and ethics, unified standards around aspects of trial design, and reporting have been included as core concepts. This chapter will not be an instruction manual discussing the "how-to" of randomized clinical trials, but will instead be outlining crucial considerations concerning trial design, analysis, presentation, and interpretation and discuss examples of potential notable pitfalls within each domain particularly in the context of lung cancer therapeutics applicable across all disciplines in oncology research.

2 The Anatomy of a Randomized Trial: Key Design Concepts and Elements

The National Cancer Institute (NCI) defines a Randomized Clinical Trial as, "A study in which the participants are divided by chance into separate groups that compare different treatments or

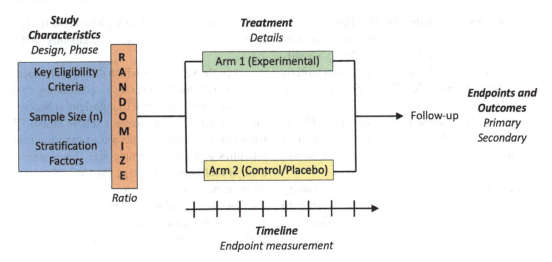

Fig. 1 Example schema template of a two-arm, randomized therapeutic clinical trial. The key study characteristics and population of interest are outlined on the left, with target sample size and stratification factors. Enrolled subjects are then randomized at a prespecified ratio, to receive either the experimental drug or the control drug. Patients are followed up for a duration of time with primary and secondary endpoints measured at certain timepoints

other interventions. Using chance to divide people into groups means that the groups will be similar and that the effects of the treatments they receive can be compared more fairly. At the time of the trial, it is not known which treatment is best (NCI 2021)." Although there is some variation with regard to trial design, such as number of study arms or study treatment phases, the key principles are maintained to minimize risk of bias affecting the overall results. Figure 1 outlines an example schema of a two-arm, randomized therapeutic trial. Several crucial components of randomized trial design are discussed in the section below.

2.1 The Research Question

At the core of every clinical trial, there is at least one primary question that is looking to be answered by this research, and along with that may be a number of research endpoints that are looking to be studied. Depending on the questions to be answered, statistical considerations (outlined later in this chapter) need to be tailored to employ the most feasible methods with the ultimate goal of meeting the aims and objectives. A few key definitions, which will be used frequently, are outlined below:

Aims: What is the proposed intention of the trial?

Objectives: What are the steps to be taken to achieve the research aim? Steps should be specific, measurable, achievable, realistic, and time-constrained (SMART).

Endpoints (NCI 2021): An event or outcome that can be measured objectively to determine whether the intervention being studied is beneficial. The endpoints of a clinical trial are usually included in the study objectives.

Surrogate endpoints (NCI 2021): An indicator or sign used in place of another to tell if a treatment works. They may be used instead of stronger indicators, such as longer survival or improved quality of life, because the results of the trial can be measured sooner, but do not always correlate well.

Progression-free survival (PFS): Time from randomization to disease progression or death from any cause. Usually measured in studies with metastatic disease.

Disease-free survival (DFS): Time from completion of primary treatment to disease progression or death from any cause without any signs or symptoms of that cancer. Also called relapse-free survival (RFS).

Overall survival (OS): Time from randomization to death from any cause.

- **Overall response rate (ORR):** Percentage of patients whose cancer shrinks or disappears after receiving treatment (NCI 2021). Usually measured using Response Evaluation Criteria In Solid Tumors (RECIST) criteria (Nishino et al. 2010).
- **Time to first subsequent therapy (TFST)** (Desai et al. 2019): Time from initiation of first-line treatment until the start of subsequent therapy or death.
- **Progression-free survival 2 (PFS2)** (Chowdhury et al. 2020): Time from randomization to objective tumor progression on next-line treatment or death from any cause.

When designing a randomized trial, the specific objectives and endpoints chosen are key to determining whether or not the original research question will not only be answered with robust statistical analysis, but also that a satisfactorily clinically meaningful result can be obtained.

2.2 Trial Design and Conduct

Once a specific research question with aims, objectives, and endpoints has been selected, the overall design of the trial needs to be considered, as this has significant implications on how the results are analyzed and interpreted upon study completion. Badly designed studies are more difficult to salvage than inadequately analyzed studies, as the data can simply be re-examined.

The overall study design is dependent on what phase of clinical trial is being conducted. Phase II randomized trials aim to assess the efficacy and toxicity profile of a novel treatment compared with standard treatment but utilize smaller sample sizes than phase III trials and often measure surrogate endpoints such as ORR or pathological complete response. They are conducted following successful completion of phase I clinical trials, where novel therapeutics are assessed for toxicity, optimal dosing, and scheduling (NCI 2021).

Phase III trials aim to compare efficacy of a novel treatment compared with standard treatments, with larger sample sizes. In most cases, they are only conducted once phase I and II trials have successfully met their endpoints (NCI 2021).

Given the velocity at which drug development is occurring within oncology, combining trial designs or using adaptive trial designs is becoming increasingly commonplace. Phase II and III trials can be flexibly combined to expedite trial timelines and reduce sample size, for example, using a multiarm, multistage (MAMS) design to allow comparison of multiple interventions or combinations against a single control arm. Moreover, the control arm can evolve over time as standard of care therapy changes (Parmar et al. 2017). An example of a successful MAMS trial includes the STAMPEDE phase II/III platform study in prostate cancer, with ten interventional arms and an evolving control arm (Fig. 2) (Carthon and Antonarakis 2016; James et al. 2017).

To ensure the focus of a study is specific to a particular population of interest, eligibility and exclusion criteria must be developed, with attention paid particularly to key patient, disease, and treatment-related factors. For example, a trial may specify that it will only enroll patients aged 18 years and over, with metastatic lung cancer that have progressed on first-line systemic therapy and have not previously received radiotherapy. When deciding upon criteria to list, it is important to remain broad enough to maximize recruitment, but also to include criteria specific enough to capture the patients for whom the research question is relevant. One common pitfall in recent clinical trials, particularly those involving immunotherapy or combination therapies is the exclusion of patients with Eastern Cooperative Oncology Group (ECOG) performance status 2 or greater, as it is thought that they are less likely to benefit. However, this becomes problematic as not only do these patients remain relatively understudied, but also that a significant proportion of patients with advanced cancers fall into this category and thus are not eligible to receive the drug as standard of care. Issues similar to the above for systemic therapy trials include those diagnosed with chronic hepatitis viral infections, human immunodeficiency virus infection, and

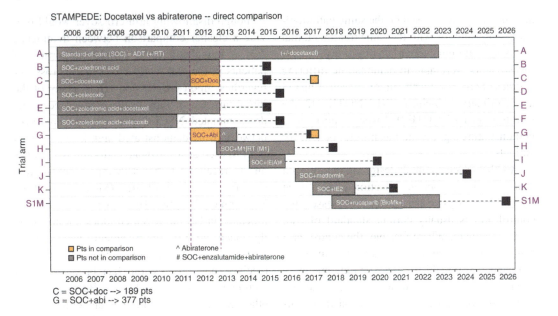

Fig. 2 STAMPEDE trial schema (taken from Stampedetrial.org) (Cancer Research UK 2021). Prime example of a multiarm, multistage (MAMS) design randomized clinical trial in metastatic prostate cancer (Sydes et al. 2018)

chronic immunocompromise such as those with prior organ transplantation.

A notable example of a practice-changing randomized trial with clear research aims and specific but relevant eligibility criteria is the KEYNOTE-024 trial, which was a phase III, open-label study which randomly assigned patients with previously untreated, advanced non-small cell lung cancer (NSCLC) with programmed death ligand 1 (PD-L1) expression on at least 50% of tumor cells without driver mutations to receive either pembrolizumab or platinum-based chemotherapy (Reck et al. 2016). The primary endpoint was PFS, and OS was a secondary endpoint.

The first publication of results in November 2016 demonstrated that of the 305 patients who were randomized, with a median follow-up of 11.2 months, the primary endpoint was met with a hazard ratio (HR) of 0.50 (95% confidence interval [CI]: 0.37 to 0.68; $p < 0.001$) suggesting a significant improvement in PFS with pembrolizumab. OS was also significantly improved in the pembrolizumab arm compared to the chemotherapy arm (HR 0.60; 95%CI: 0.41 to 0.89; $p = 0.005$). These results led to FDA approval for pembrolizumab monotherapy in the first-line setting for advanced NSCLC whose tumors expressed PD-L1 ≥ 50% (Drugs@FDA 2021). Subsequently, at the American Society of Clinical Oncology 2018 Annual Meeting, the results from the KEYNOTE-042 trial were presented (Lopes et al. 2018). This was also a phase III, open-label study which randomly assigned patients with previously untreated, advanced NSCLC to receive pembrolizumab or platinum-based chemotherapy, however patients only needed to have PD-L1 expression of 1% or greater to be eligible for recruitment. The primary endpoints for this trial were OS in those with PD-L1 ≥ 50%, PD-L1 ≥ 20%, and PD-L1 ≥ 1%. This trial also met its primary endpoints in all three PD-L1 sub-categories, with significant prolongation of OS with pembrolizumab as compared with chemotherapy. Interestingly, a post hoc exploratory subgroup analysis in light of prior KEYNOTE-024 results revealed that those with PD-L1 1–49% did not have significant OS benefit (HR 0.92; 95%CI: 0.77–1.11) whereas a larger degree of OS benefit was seen in PD-L1 ≥ 50% patients (HR 0.69; 95%CI: 0.56–0.85; $p = 0.003$) (Lopes et al. 2018). These two trials illustrate clearly that although they are focused on the same pathological disease subtype with the same treatment, that by using different biomarker eligibility criteria investigators were able to demonstrate differing degrees of efficacy. Furthermore, by selecting OS as the primary endpoint for KEYNOTE-042, the results from KEYNOTE-024 were confirmed as demonstrating significant, meaningful benefit for patients.

Another crucial point in designing randomized trials well is appropriate selection of treatment arms. When only two arms are being assessed, the control arm is usually current standard of care (SoC) treatment. Where feasible, the control arm can be placebo to allow the treatment arms to be as matched as possible to focus on outcome measurement and minimize differences in treatment administration, however this is not always ethically possible. However, clearly defining what SoC can be challenging, and ultimately when a control arm is not the current SoC, this has implications upon the validity of the overall trial results. For example, the POLO trial, published in 2019, was a phase III trial of patients with metastatic pancreatic cancer who carried a germline mutation in *BRCA1* or *BRCA2*, randomizing patients to receive either olaparib, a poly(adenosine diphosphate–ribose) polymerase (PARP) inhibitor, or placebo following completion of at least 16 weeks of first-line, platinum-based chemotherapy with no evidence of disease progression (Golan et al. 2019). The trial was reported to have met its primary endpoint of median PFS (7.4 months with olaparib versus 3.8 months with placebo; HR 0.53; 95%CI: 0.35–082; $p = 0.004$) although the trial was criticized for its choice of control arm, where continuous dosing of chemotherapy is the standard of care but patients instead received placebo alone upon cessation of prior chemotherapy. Consequently, the applicability of these trial results into standard treatment is uncertain, which reinforces that selection of treatment arms should be done purposefully.

One other major factor that has the potential to significantly impact survival outcomes is factoring in subsequent therapies on trial, and whether or not the control arm is allowed to crossover to experimental arm upon disease progression. Although disallowing arm crossover would provide a cleaner comparison between treatments, this is unrealistic as a certain proportion of patients in the real world will usually crossover regardless upon progression. Thus, many of the initial targeted therapy trials in advanced stage, driver-mutated NSCLC that allowed crossover between arms demonstrated significant benefits in PFS, used as a surrogate endpoint, but not OS due to receiving targeted therapies on progression from the control arm (Mok et al. 2009; Solomon et al. 2018). The lack of statistical significance in OS improvement does not necessarily mean no OS improvement, and survival post-progression, including number of lines received post-progression, has been shown to correlate with OS (Broglio and Berry 2009). In other cancers, other intermediate clinical endpoints have been examined as early indicators for OS benefit, for example TFST or PFS2, particularly when data is immature (González-Martín et al. 2019; Moore et al. 2018).

2.3 Outcome Assessments

When assessing outcomes for patients enrolled on RCTs, it is imperative that the method and timing are identical for all arms to reduce biased assessments, regardless of the timing of treatment cycles.

An issue that is not unique to randomized trials but is unique to oncology is the utility of central review to confirm oncological diagnoses or confirm progressive disease, where this assessment can be user dependent to an extent. This is clearly observed when rarer tumor histologies are being studied, confirmation of underlying histopathology can be useful by a central pathology center with experienced, subspecialized anatomical pathologists. An example where this can often be an issue is in gynecological malignancies. In the PORTEC-3 trial, which was a randomized, open-label phase III trial in patients with high-risk, resected endometrial cancer to receive either radiation alone or radiation concurrent with chemotherapy followed by adjuvant chemotherapy (de Boer et al. 2019). Upon reviewing the 1226 cases that were available from the Netherlands and the UK, in 43% of cases at least one pathology item changed after review, and in 102 patients (8%) this led to ineligibility for enrolment due to histological type, stromal involvement, or histological grade. These results emphasize the importance of ensuring enrolment of the correct patients onto study, to avoid inappropriate over- or undertreatment (de Boer et al. 2018).

Along the same vein, bias may also be introduced through inconsistent radiological assessments as an endpoint. Although OS is objective as it is represented as a timepoint, PFS and other endpoints that depend on imaging measurements are subject to inter-user variation especially in unblinded trials, despite the use of standardized criteria (RECIST). To help mitigate this, an increasing number of studies are using blinded independent central review (BICR), either in real-time or retrospectively, and including this as an endpoint in addition to imaging assessed by local investigators. This comparison assists in detecting whether any bias is present in investigator radiographic evaluations.

2.4 Randomization Process

Other aspects pertaining to randomized trial conduct, including blinding and allocation concealment, are generally well discussed in the literature and the majority of recent randomized trials tend to use standardized methods. Blinding of study participants and investigators, known as a "double-blind" study, can reduce the risk of selection bias in therapeutic trials; however, this is only ethical or possible when the treatment schedules and modalities in both arms are the same. For example, the FLAURA trial was able to be performed as a double-blind study as osimertinib and gefitinib are orally administered with daily dosing (Ramalingam et al. 2019). Conversely, the FLAURA2 trial, which is assessing osimertinib with or without platinum-based chemotherapy, cannot be blinded as those on the combination arm are receiving additional intravenous infusions without placebo control (U.S. National Library of Medicine 2021).

For both blinded and especially unblinded studies, known as "open-label," allocation concealment plays an even more crucial role to reduce selection bias. In studies where investigators are aware of which patients have been randomized to which treatments, it is important to reduce awareness (or increase randomness) of the allocation schedule by concealing the allocation sequence until the moment of assignment. Consequently, the methods of randomization are critical when considering the above. Key definitions are outlined below:

Unrestricted (simple) randomization: Patient allocation to one treatment group based upon a fixed probability, irrespective of prior allocations.
Stratified randomization: Patient allocation is stratified based upon nominated factors, such as age, sex, comorbidities.
Adaptive randomization: Patient allocation probability to a treatment arm is altered based upon prior allocations.
Permuted block randomization: Patient allocation based upon prespecified blocks with randomly ordered treatment assignments.
Minimization: Patient allocation to whichever arm minimizes imbalance in a set of baseline covariates.

Depending on how the trial is designed, for example, single site versus multicenter, different methods of randomization can affect risk of selection bias. Commonly, multicenter trials are stratified by recruiting site where separate randomization lists are kept at each site, thus when permuted block randomization is used, the risk of correctly guessing allocations is increased. In this situation, using minimization (without stratifying for site) would be a preferable method of decreasing risk of selection bias. All the above methods have associated pros and cons which should be taken into consideration when analyzing trials.

2.5 Statistical Considerations

Exploring the breadth of statistical methods and calculations employed across different randomized trial designs is beyond the scope of this chapter, but a clear grasp of the pivotal concepts is required to ensure a sound statistical model is developed.

One of the presumed aims of conducting a randomized trial is to recruit enough patients to sufficiently power the study to detect differences in the outcome of interest and to have confidence in extrapolating these results to the broader population. Key information required includes expected outcome rate in control arm; expected outcome rate in intervention arm(s); α, or the probability that a difference arises solely due to chance (type I error); and β, which is the probability that the study will *not* be able to find a significant difference if it is present (type II error; 1-β is also known as power). To maintain integrity of interpretation, endpoints and effect sizes *must* be prespecified to allow for accurate sample size estimations, particularly as the study needs to be adequately statistically powered and the proposed sample sizes should not be prohibitive to the study. Furthermore, estimated attrition should also be taken into consideration upon statistical design, as it is usually inevitable and reflective of real-world practice where patients dropout of studies or are lost to follow-up.

One of the contexts in which outcome assumptions and sample size calculations can vary is when study design is changed to a non-inferiority or equivalence design, rather than a superiority design. Within oncology therapeutic studies, non-inferiority studies are declining in popularity due to concerns about the arbitrary nature of defining a non-inferiority limit, in addition to requiring a much larger sample size than superiority studies to meet primary endpoints. Furthermore, although there is a high probability that non-inferiority studies are positive, it remains ethically questionable that if the trial was negative, patients enrolled on the investigational arm will have been receiving a drug *inferior* to the control.

3   Ensuring Robust Data Analysis: Turning Chaos into Order

Along the same vein as designing a clear statistical plan is ensuring robust, logical data analysis. At the data cutoff point, all outcome data collected should be checked for completeness and the percentages of missing data should be noted, as this will be factored into the impending data analysis.

Prior to trial commencement, the investigators will have prespecified whether analysis will use an intention-to-treat (ITT) or per-protocol (PP) analysis. The premise behind ITT analysis is that regardless of compliance or loss to follow-up, all participants will be analyzed according to the groups they were randomized to. This practice maintains sample size and study power and also preserves the purpose of participant randomization in that the groups will remain balanced for confounders or prognostic factors. By preserving sample size and the randomization process of the trial, ITT analyses tend to underestimate the outcome effect size (World Health Organization 2005).

Outside of trials, loss to follow-up or non-adherence is expected to an extent, thus when this occurs on trial it may be more reflective of real-world practice. Often, ITT and PP analyses are performed to reveal any significant differences, and in certain circumstances, such as in non-inferiority trials, the PP analysis is crucial to the outcome of the trial. Yet, when the dropout rates between arms are imbalanced, particularly due to reasons related to the study disease or intervention, this is known as "informative censoring" and may bias the study results.

One example of a large randomized trial is the SOLAR-1 study, which was a phase III, double-blinded study of patients with metastatic hormone-positive, HER2-negative breast cancer, with or without *PIK3CA* mutations, to receive fulvestrant plus oral alpelisib or oral placebo (André et al. 2019). The study recruited 572 patients, and primary endpoint was PFS in the *PIK3CA*-mutated cohort, and secondary endpoints included PFS in the non-mutated cohort and OS in both cohorts. After 20 months of follow-up, the study was published in 2019 having met its primary endpoint with a 5.3-month benefit in median PFS. However, it was noted that the intervention arm had significantly more treatment discontinuations (71 patients, 25%) compared with the control arm (12 patients, 4.2%) although patient-reported outcomes and quality of life were preserved (Ciruelos et al. 2021). Notably, OS did not demonstrate a statistically significant benefit even though the numerical difference was 8 months.

The discontinuation rate of greater than 20% in the intervention arm raises the question of whether the data remains unbiased; although if anything, had there been a lower dropout rate, the difference in effect size between the two arms would likely be even more pronounced. Nevertheless, when high discontinuation rates are present, the results are at risk of attrition bias leading to erroneous results, regardless of whether ITT analysis was performed. Methods to account for informative censoring include imputation techniques for missing data, or sensitivity analyses to account for different variables that may be causative for increased dropout.

3.1 Interim Analyses

When examining clinical trial design and data analysis, being aware of the number of secondary and interim analyses is an issue. The key principle is that all analyses should be *prespecified*, regardless of timing or number. Furthermore, the number of endpoints analyzed in a trial must also be prespecified, as this factors into the sample size calculations to ensure adequate power. The timing of interim analyses should ideally be decided upon prior to commencement of the study. They are usually overseen by a data monitoring committee, and decision regarding adjustments in trial design, sample size, and criteria for continuation or discontinuation. When interim analyses are performed more frequently, the α must be adjusted to account for increasing risk of type I error, and thus the value is lowered to reflect this.

3.2 Multiplicity

Similarly, when performing multiple subgroup analyses looking at secondary outcomes, the higher the number of analyses, the higher the chance of detecting a false-positive result, particularly if sampling is done from the same population repeatedly. This issue, also known as multiplicity, should be recognized and addressed prior to commencement of data analysis. Although simplification of study endpoints, summary statistics and composite endpoints can be used to mitigate this, trials in oncology often enroll a heterogeneous population with numerous subgroups of interest. Therefore, it is necessary to use statistical methods to adjust for multiplicity and nominate prespecified boundaries, which should be outlined in the study protocol and presented in the results. The aforementioned KEYNOTE-042 (Lopes et al. 2018; Mok et al. 2019) study had three sequential, co-primary endpoints using different biomarker cutoffs that sampled from overlapping patient populations, and also underwent two interim analyses. As a result, the α for each was adjusted accordingly and explicitly presented in the publication.

4 Presenting RCTs: Not All That Glitters Is Gold

The presentation of results in an oncology phase 3 RCT follows a common format: (1) presentation of patients who were enrolled in the study; (2) comparison of baseline clinical characteristics; (3) efficacy results; and (4) toxicity results. While going through the results that are being presented, it is important to keep going back to the research question to ensure that the appropriate endpoint measures are being used.

4.1 Patient Enrollment and the CONSORT Diagram

The CONSORT diagram (Fig. 3) is a diagram to show the flow of study patients through various stages of the trial. According to the CONSORT statement, each CONSORT diagram should include six elements: (1) number of patients assessed for eligibility, (2) number eligible, (3) number randomized, (4) number allocated to

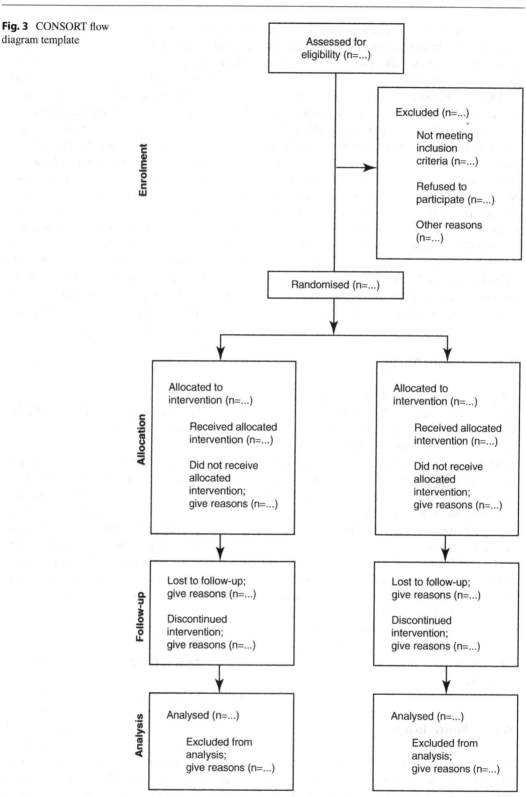

Fig. 3 CONSORT flow diagram template

each group, (5) number of patients who were lost to follow-up, and (6) number of patients included in the final analysis (Egger 2001).

4.2 Comparison of Clinical Characteristics

Characteristics of patients in the study are commonly presented in a table format to allow for easy comparison, commonly "Table 1" in most prospective phase 3 RCTs. This table gives the reader a quick summary of the type of patients that were included in the study. It is also important to examine the table for any differences between the groups that are being compared. The validity of study results in an RCT hinges on the fact that the only difference between the groups is the study intervention.

4.3 Efficacy Results

Common efficacy endpoints examined in a phase 3 RCT are overall response rates (ORR), progression-free survival (PFS), and overall survival (OS). Graphical figures often accompany the manuscript text in presenting efficacy results.

4.3.1 Visual Models of Tumor Response

Graphical presentation is most varied for response rates in clinical trials. In phase 3 RCTs, ORR is defined by RECIST or modified-RECIST, and expressed as percentages in the manuscript text or summarized in a table. Graphical figures are sometimes used in a phase 3 RCT. In contrast, response rates are of primary interest phase 1/2 studies as an early indicator of activity. Novel visual models such as waterfall plots, spider plots, and swimmers plot have emerged as ways to help with rapid interpretation of complex information. Their use has increased dramatically in recent years, appearing in abstracts, conference presentations, and manuscripts (Mercier et al. 2019; Shao et al. 2014; Chia et al. 2016; Kim and Prasad 2019). It is important to understand the limitations of these graphs.

Waterfall plots are ordered histograms that displays the maximal percentage of tumor reduction from baseline. Vertical bars are drawn for each patient across the x-axis and conventionally displayed from worst to best resulting in a downward flowing pattern—the waterfall (Mercier et al. 2019; Shao et al. 2014; Chia et al. 2016; Kim and Prasad 2019). It is important to remember that the maximal tumor shrinkage is not equivalent to the ORR determined by RECIST 1.1, which, requires a confirmatory scan at least 4 weeks later (Mercier et al. 2019; Shao et al. 2014; Chia et al. 2016; Kim and Prasad 2019). As a result, not every bar that falls below 30% corresponds to a RECIST defined response. Without a confirmatory scan, response rates on waterfall plots are highly subjected to interobserver variability and is an overrepresentation RECIST defined response rates (Mercier et al. 2019; Shao et al. 2014; Chia et al. 2016; Kim and Prasad 2019). The failed development of rociletinib is an excellent example of how this may be misleading. The initial phase 1 study of rociletinib, TIGER-X, reported a combined confirmed and unconfirmed response rate of 59%, leading to its designation as breakthrough therapy by the U.S. Food and Drug Administration (Sequist et al. 2016, 2015; Dhingra 2016). Unfortunately, as the data matured, response rates in the original cohort dropped to 45% and dropped even further to 28% with the addition of patients from the phase 2 TIGER-2 study (Sequist et al. 2016, 2015; Dhingra 2016). Rociletinib is no longer in development, and its failure is an important lesson on need for continued follow-up and mature data (Sequist et al. 2016; Dhingra 2016).

Spider plots introduces a time element in the visual illustration of response and is improvement over waterfall plots (Mercier et al. 2019). The percentage change in lesion diameter is plotted over time for each individual patient (Mercier et al. 2019; Chia et al. 2016). Spider plots have helped identify unique patterns of response, such as pseudoprogression, in patients receiving immunotherapy (Mercier et al. 2019; Chia et al. 2016). However, patients who progress or die early on trial may not have a subsequent scan to document tumor size, and determination of response using spider plots is an overestimation of treatment effect (Mercier et al. 2019; Chia et al. 2016). Visualization using spider plots is also challenging when there are large numbers of patients, especially when the lines cross.

Swimmer plots place greater emphasis on the duration of response (Chia et al. 2016). The *x*-axis represents time on treatment, and each patient is plotted as a horizontal bar. Various pieces of information such as the best response, time to response, and time to progression are incorporated into each bar/patient.

4.3.2 Graphical Display of Survival

Kaplan–Meier curves are the most common graphical method of displaying survival. The Kaplan–Meier model incorporates the concept of "censoring" in time-to-event calculations, where patients who are lost to follow-up are assumed to be noninformative and independent of survival (Chia et al. 2016). Graphically, the *y*-axis of a Kaplan–Meier is the probability of survival, and the *x*-axis is time. The probability of survival is 100% at the beginning of the study. The curve drops when an event (progression or death) takes place, and the height of the drop corresponds to the proportion of events divided by the number patients who are still known to be alive. Censored patients are illustrated by a tick mark on the curve (Chia et al. 2016). Kaplan–Meier curves help in visualization of treatment effects between groups in an RCT. They can also be compared for statistical significance using the log-rank test or cox proportional hazards model (Chia et al. 2016).

Forest plots are commonly included in RCTs to demonstrate the relative treatment effects of subgroups within the larger cohorts (Chia et al. 2016). The central line of a forest plot represents the null hypothesis, or the threshold at which no treatment effect is seen. The effect of each variable or subgroup is represented as a box, the point estimate, and a line that indicates the 95% confidence interval (Chia et al. 2016). If the 95% confidence interval does not cross the center, it indicates that subgroup variable influences treatment effect.

4.4 Toxicity

Reporting of treatment-related toxicities in oncology trials is standardized using Common Terminology Criteria for Adverse Events (CTCAE), which assigns a specific grade to each adverse event. In general, any grade 3 or higher adverse events are considered serious. Adverse events of interest are typically presented in a table format.

5 Pitfalls in Interpretation: What Does It All Mean?

Interpretation of RCT results must occur in the context of the pre-existing knowledge of the disease and should cover these areas: (1) Does the study question address a clinically relevant knowledge gap? (2) Is the study adequately designed and endpoints appropriately chosen to answer the clinical question? (3) Are the results clinically meaningful such that a change in clinical practice is warranted? (4) Are the results generalizable to a larger population?

In this section, we will delve deeper into issues of RCT interpretation using specific examples of RCTs performed in lung cancer. Many of the trials that we discuss here are drug therapy studies because of the sheer number of trials that have been published but also because the versatility of drug trial design helps illustrate the issues and controversies in interpreting studies. The principles of trial interpretation, however, remains the same across oncology disciplines.

5.1 The Knowledge Gap

Identifying the knowledge gap before delving into the specifics of a clinical trial will help with interpreting the results in context. With the speed at which trials are being performed and reported, the knowledge gap is constantly evolving. Take the space in first-line metastatic NSCLC, for example. There are more than ten RCTs that report on the use of immune checkpoint inhibitors in this setting (Reck et al. 2016; Mok et al. 2019; Gandhi et al. 2018; Paz-Ares et al. 2020a, 2021; Jotte et al. 2020; West et al. 2019; Socinski et al. 2018; Carbone et al. 2017; Hellmann et al. 2019; Sezer et al. 2021; Rizvi et al. 2020). The standard of care being compared in all these trials was platinum-based chemotherapy. It is reassuring that different RCTs report similar results.

5.2 Assessment of Study Endpoints and Interpretation of Statistical Analyses

The concepts of study design and clinical trial conduct were discussed above. The focus on this section is on assessing the appropriateness on study endpoints in prospective RCTs.

The goal of most cancer therapies is to prolong overall survival (OS). Measurement of OS may not be feasible or practical in all cases. Diseases with a long natural history, such as in hormone receptor positive breast cancer, may have a large number of patients who become lost to follow-up compromising the reliability of data over time. Waiting for OS data maturity may also cause delays in bringing effective therapies to patients with a terminal disease. As a result, surrogate endpoints are commonly reported. The predictive value of a surrogate endpoint is variable depending on the disease and types of therapy investigated. We will use specific examples of RCTs to illustrate some of the issues and controversies with different study endpoints below.

5.2.1 Early-Stage vs. Metastatic Disease: DFS and PFS

In early-stage disease, the use of DFS alone may not be sufficient in determining the effectiveness of adjuvant therapy. An improvement in DFS may only signify a delay in recurrence. This was the case in the CTONG study where adjuvant gefitinib in patients with resected *EGFR* mutant NSCLC had a DFS but not OS benefit (Wu et al. 2020a; Zhong et al. 2018). The similar OS further indicated that waiting to start gefitinib until disease recurrence was not detrimental to survival.

But does the degree of benefit matter? The ADAURA trial studied the use of adjuvant osimertinib in the same population (Wu et al. 2020b). At its first interim analysis, a dramatic improvement in DFS was reported (HR 0.17, 95%CI 0.11–0.26) (Wu et al. 2020b). As a result, the data safety and monitoring board recommended the trial to be stopped early (Wu et al. 2020b). Could this be the same scenario as with the CTONG study, where it only delays disease recurrence? Or is the magnitude of benefit so great that improvements in OS can be reasonably expected. Until the OS data becomes more mature, this remains one of the most controversial topics and highly debated topics in NSCLC.

In metastatic disease, PFS is considered an acceptable surrogate endpoint. PFS may also be a reasonable endpoint in locally advanced disease where high rates of disease recurrence are expected. For example, the PACIFIC study investigated the addition durvalumab after definitive chemoradiation in unresectable stage 3 NSCLC and found a significant improvement in PFS (Antonia et al. 2017). OS benefit was later confirmed (Antonia et al. 2018). As we will discuss below, it is prudent to report PFS and OS, even in the metastatic setting.

5.2.2 Metastatic Disease: PFS vs. OS

Specific considerations need to be given to PFS and OS endpoints within the clinical context of the disease, and its importance and context are dependent on disease setting and how they tie in with other endpoints such as patient-reported outcomes or quality of life to provide context.

In general, PFS is considered modestly predictive of OS in metastatic NSCLC. Studies demonstrating improvements in PFS and OS are straightforward to interpret and are often practice changing. For example, the KEYNOTE-189 and -407 studies of chemotherapy plus pembrolizumab improved PFS and OS over chemotherapy alone in nonsquamous and squamous NSCLC and quickly became the new standard of care (Gandhi et al. 2018; Paz-Ares et al. 2020a, 2018; Rodriguez-Abreu et al. 2020). There are instances of discordant PFS and OS results where OS is improved but not PFS. The OAK and

KEYNOTE-010 studies are good examples of these (Herbst et al. 2016; Rittmeyer et al. 2017). The dramatic OS but not PFS benefits of immune checkpoint blockade, as well as the tolerability of these agents, resulted in a rapid change in clinical practice. It is more challenging to interpret studies where a PFS but not OS benefit was seen, such as in the NEJ026 study of erlotinib without bevacizumab (Maemondo et al. 2020; Saito et al. 2019). Whether these results should change practice will depend on the degree of benefit in PFS as well as toxicity. We will elaborate further on clinically meaningful benefits in later sections of this chapter.

Relying on OS alone can be problematic. Data on OS can take a long time to mature, potentially delaying approvals of effective therapy. In diseases where the prognosis is short, such as in small cell lung cancer (SCLC), OS remains the most important endpoint. In contrast, OS may not the most appropriate outcome to report in first-line NSCLC studies. The ALEX study is a good example to illustrate this point. This study demonstrated PFS superiority of alectinib compared to crizotinib in *ALK*-positive NSCLC, establishing alectinib as the standard of care in 2017 (Mok et al. 2020; Peters et al. 2017). Since the natural disease course with treatment is long, data maturity for OS has still not been reached in 2020 (Mok et al. 2020; Peters et al. 2017). If OS were the only endpoint investigated, they would have been a significant delay in the approval and patient access to effective therapy.

OS may also be influenced by crossover and subsequent therapies. In the pivotal IPASS study, which established gefitinib as the gold standard in *EGFR* mutant NSCLC, OS were similar in the gefitinib and chemotherapy groups (HR 0.90, $p = 0.11$) (Mok et al. 2009; Fukuoka et al. 2011). If OS benefits were not seen despite significant PFS gains, then why did gefitinib become the standard of care? Fortunately, an explanation was found in the high rates of crossover. More than 60% of patients in the chemotherapy group subsequently received gefitinib (Mok et al. 2009; Fukuoka et al. 2011). Furthermore, the median OS of both groups were approximately 17–18 months, which was much longer than expected of historical controls receiving chemotherapy alone, supporting the overall effectiveness of gefitinib (Mok et al. 2009; Fukuoka et al. 2011).

5.2.3 Subgroup Analyses

In the era of precision medicine, subgroup analyses are often done to help understand differences in disease biology within NSCLC. Subgroup analyses may be prespecified, often when there is pre-existing evidence that a certain characteristic may behave differently or performed post hoc.

Results from subgroup analyses that are prespecified with an appropriate statistical plan are considered valid and provide vital information about disease biology. For example, in the phase 3 RCT comparing cisplatin in combination with pemetrexed or gemcitabine in advanced NSCLC, clear differences in pemetrexed activity were seen based on histology, even though it was found to be non-inferior in the overall cohort (Scagliotti et al. 2008). Subgroup analyses are not limited to clinical characteristics and in fact can be key in identifying predictive biomarkers. The IPASS study enrolled patients based on clinical characteristics (Asian, females, never smokers with adenocarcinomas) and explored the relevance of three potential biomarkers: *EGFR* mutations, *EGFR* gene copy number, and *EGFR* expression (Mok et al. 2009; Fukuoka et al. 2011). The final biomarker analysis confirmed that activating *EGFR* mutations were the key to determining efficacy of gefitinib and was a revolutionary step toward precision medicine (Mok et al. 2009; Fukuoka et al. 2011).

Post hoc analyses do not adjust for sample size and multiple testing and should be considered hypothesis generating. They remain useful in understanding disease biology and identify unmet needs future research. In the landmark studies of immune checkpoint inhibitors in previously treated NSCLC, it became apparent that *EGFR/ALK* mutant NSCLC do not respond, an effect that was seen across different studies of PD-1/PD-L1 inhibitor (Herbst et al. 2016; Rittmeyer et al. 2017; Borghaei et al. 2015). This led to the exclusion of EGFR/ALK mutations in subsequent first-line immunotherapy studies.

While the mechanisms remain elusive, the simple identification of this fact allows for a targeted approach in research and development. Post hoc analyses may also be requested by regulatory agencies. The European Medicines Agency requested a subgroup analysis of NSCLC patients with a PD-L1 expression of <1% treated with durvalumab in the PACIFIC study for regulatory decisions (Antonia et al. 2017, 2018; Paz-Ares et al. 2020b).

5.2.4 Statistical Considerations

It is crucial to evaluate the statistical results of a RCT using an intention-treat (ITT) analysis as it maintains the prognostic balance from randomization (Gupta 2011). A more detailed discussion of the concepts of ITT and per-protocol analyses can be found in an earlier section of this chapter.

Interim analysis is adaptive trial design that allows for presentation of what is learned during the course of a clinical study so that effective therapy may be given to patients in a timely fashion and to avoid harm in a futile study (Kumar and Chakraborty 2016). Interim analyses should be preplanned, and the statistical analyses adjusted accordingly in order to maintain the pre-specified type 1 error rate (Kumar and Chakraborty 2016). It is important to understand the limitations of a trial was terminated early. Particularly in those trials stopped early for benefit, systematic reviews have shown that the effect size is often an overestimate (Bassler 2010; Montori et al. 2005).

5.3 Clinical Significance

The next step in interpreting a clinical trial is to determine if the results are clinically meaningful necessitating a change in clinical practice. Statistical significance is a mathematical definition, used to determine the superior efficacy of one treatment over another. To fully understand the clinical significance of a new therapy, the magnitude of benefit, treatment-related toxicities, and quality of life are all important considerations.

5.3.1 Degree of Benefit

The p-value is simply the probability of falsely rejecting the null hypothesis and does not take into account the effect size of a treatment. To illustrate, we will use the OAK and REVEL studies as examples (Rittmeyer et al. 2017; Garon et al. 2014). The OAK trial randomized patients with NSCLC who progressed after platinum-based chemotherapy to atezolizumab or docetaxel. Survival with atezolizumab was superior with a median OS of 13.8 months vs. 9.6 months, $p = 0.0003$ (Rittmeyer et al. 2017). The REVEL study also studied NSCLC patients who progressed after first-line treatment with a platinum doublet. Patients who were randomized to docetaxel with ramucirumab had a superior median OS of 10.5 months compared to 9.1 months with docetaxel alone, $p = 0.02$ (Garon et al. 2014). Both trials demonstrated statistical significance but the absolute gains in survival were vastly different—4.2 months in OAK and 1.4 months in the REVEL study (Rittmeyer et al. 2017; Garon et al. 2014).

5.3.2 Toxicity

It is also important to consider the safety and toxicities that are associated with a new medication or intervention. By the time, an investigational treatment is being studied in a phase 3 RCT, a certain threshold of safety has been achieved but it is still important to characterize the toxicities in the context of current standard therapies. It is also not uncommon that rare toxicities seen in phase 1–2 studies become more apparent in phase 3 studies with a larger patient population. In RCTs involving oncology drugs, assessment of toxicity is standardized using the Common Terminology Criteria for Adverse Events (CTCAE).

In best case scenarios, the new intervention is both superior in efficacy and has a better side effect profile. The ALEX study comparing alectinib to standard crizotinib in *ALK*-positive NSCLC is an excellent example of this (Mok et al. 2020; Peters et al. 2017). Fortunately, this scenario is becoming more common with newer, more targeted therapies.

Clinical utility is harder to determine when the efficacy is superior, but the toxicities are worse.

We will use the development of second-generation irreversible *EGFR* inhibitors to illustrate this. Acquired resistance to *EGFR* TKIs led to the development of second-generation drugs and the idea that the upfront use of more potent second-generation *EGFR* inhibitors may delay the emergence of resistance. The ARCHER 1050 study was able to demonstrate this (Mok et al. 2018; Wu et al. 2017). Patients receiving upfront dacomitinib had a superior PFS and OS compared to gefitinib (Mok et al. 2018; Wu et al. 2017). Unfortunately, dacomitinib was poorly tolerated with a 50% incidence rate of grade ≥ 3 adverse events compared to 30% among those receiving gefitinib (Mok et al. 2018; Wu et al. 2017). This has led to controversy and debate on the clinical utility of this drug and given its poor tolerability, was never widely adopted into clinical practice.

5.3.3 Quality of Life

Standardized quality of life questionnaires can further assist in interpreting the clinical utility of a drug. It serves as a compound measure of the burden of symptoms from the underlying disease and treatment-related toxicities. In a highly symptomatic disease as NSCLC, effective treatment, despite the related side effects, can result in an overall improvement in quality of life. For example, PRO scores of patients receiving pembrolizumab plus chemotherapy in the KEYNOTE-189 study at 21-weeks were significantly better than those receiving chemotherapy alone despite higher rates of treatment-related toxicities (Gandhi et al. 2018; Rodriguez-Abreu et al. 2020; Garassino et al. 2020). These patient-reported outcomes (PROs) help address the question: Are the toxicities worth it? Quality of life endpoints are increasingly included in oncology RCTs and are accepted endpoints by regulatory agencies.

Although the accepted thresholds are different in curative-intent setting, quality of life measures are nevertheless important to consider. Take the practice-changing PACIFIC study for example (Antonia et al. 2017, 2018). The treatment course for patients with unresectable stage 3 NSCLC increase from 6 weeks to over 1 year with regular visits to the cancer center for treatment. Fortunately, durvalumab is well tolerated, and PROs were reassuringly maintained (Hui et al. 2019). In the highly debated ADAURA trial where data maturity in OS is awaited, maintenance of excellent PROs scores provides support for the use of adjuvant osimertinib (Wu et al. 2020b; Majem et al. 2021).

5.4 Generalizability

Assessment of generalizability requires careful examination of the inclusion and exclusion criteria used in the study. Are the results of a clinical trial applicable to real-world patients? We will discuss some of the common issues pertaining to generalizability in oncology trials.

Patient outcomes in clinical trials are generally better than in the real world. A common problem that partly explains this phenomenon is the exclusion of patients with an ECOG performance status of 2 or higher (Passaro et al. 2019). The ECOG performance status is a strong prognostic factor and fit patients generally perform better regardless of the therapy they receive (Passaro et al. 2019). Data on the appropriate management of these patients often come from post marketing analyses or single arm studies of patients with poor performance status (Passaro et al. 2019; Cheng et al. 2018; Gandara et al. 2017; Spigel et al. 2017).

Another common issue that limits generalizability of clinical trials is age. While most modern oncology trials no longer have an upper age limit in their exclusion criteria, older patients remain underrepresented in clinical trials. Older patients tend to have more underlying comorbidities and are more susceptible to complications and toxicities due to decreased organ reserve. They may also not receive the same degree of benefit from therapy. As an example, patients ≥ 70 years with resected colon cancer did not have any survival benefits with the addition of oxaliplatin to 5-FU as opposed to their younger counterparts (Tournigand et al. 2012). Fortunately, research in the field of geriatric oncology is rapidly advancing. Multiple scoring systems have been developed to help with clinical decision-making.

6 Future of Clinical Studies

The field of lung oncology is advancing rapidly with opportunities for novel clinical trial designs using Bayesian rather than frequentist statistics. Biomarker-directed basket or platform studies are increasingly used. For now, prospective RCTs remain the gold standard for assessing the safety and efficacy of new therapies against current best practices. A systematic approach to interpreting RCTs is a critical skill for all practicing clinicians.

References

André F, Ciruelos E, Rubovszky G et al (2019) Alpelisib for PIK3CA-mutated, hormone receptor–positive advanced breast cancer. N Engl J Med 380(20):1929–1940

Antonia SJ, Villegas A, Daniel D et al (2017) Durvalumab after chemoradiotherapy in stage III non–small-cell lung cancer. N Engl J Med 377(20):1919–1929

Antonia SJ, Villegas A, Daniel D et al (2018) Overall survival with durvalumab after chemoradiotherapy in stage III NSCLC. N Engl J Med 379(24):2342–2350

Bassler D (2010) Stopping randomized trials early for benefit and estimation of treatment effects systematic review and meta-regression analysis. JAMA 303(12):1180

Booth CM, Cescon DW, Wang L, Tannock IF, Krzyzanowska MK (2008) Evolution of the randomized controlled trial in oncology over three decades. J Clin Oncol 26(33):5458–5464

Borghaei H, Paz-Ares L, Horn L et al (2015) Nivolumab versus docetaxel in advanced nonsquamous non–small-cell lung cancer. N Engl J Med 373(17):1627–1639

Broglio KR, Berry DA (2009) Detecting an overall survival benefit that is derived from progression-free survival. J Natl Cancer Inst 101(23):1642–1649

Cancer Research UK. Information on STAMPEDE. http://www.stampedetrial.org/centres/information-on-stampede/. Accessed 21 Apr 2021

Carbone DP, Reck M, Paz-Ares L et al (2017) First-line nivolumab in stage IV or recurrent non–small-cell lung cancer. N Engl J Med 376(25):2415–2426

Carthon BC, Antonarakis ES (2016) The STAMPEDE trial: paradigm-changing data through innovative trial design. Transl Cancer Res 5(3 Suppl):S485–S490

Cheng Y, Zhou J, Lu S et al (2018) Phase II study of tepotinib + gefitinib (TEP+GEF) in MET-positive (MET+)/epidermal growth factor receptor (EGFR)-mutant (MT) non-small cell lung cancer (NSCLC). Ann Oncol 29:viii493

Chia PL, Gedye C, Boutros PC, Wheatley-Price P, John T (2016) Current and evolving methods to visualize biological data in cancer research. J Natl Cancer Inst 108(8):djw031

Chowdhury S, Mainwaring P, Zhang L et al (2020) Systematic review and meta-analysis of correlation of progression-free survival-2 and overall survival in solid tumors. Front Oncol 10:1349

Ciruelos EM, Rugo HS, Mayer IA et al (2021) Patient-reported outcomes in patients with PIK3CA-mutated hormone receptor–positive, human epidermal growth factor receptor 2–negative advanced breast cancer from SOLAR-1. J Clin Oncol. https://doi.org/10.1200/JCO.20.01139

de Boer SM, Wortman BG, Bosse T et al (2018) Clinical consequences of upfront pathology review in the randomised PORTEC-3 trial for high-risk endometrial cancer. Ann Oncol 29(2):424–430

de Boer SM, Powell ME, Mileshkin L et al (2019) Adjuvant chemoradiotherapy versus radiotherapy alone in women with high-risk endometrial cancer (PORTEC-3): patterns of recurrence and post-hoc survival analysis of a randomised phase 3 trial. Lancet Oncol 20(9):1273–1285

Desai K, Muston D, Adeboyeje G, Monberg MJ (2019) Association between time to first subsequent therapy (TFST) and overall survival (OS) in previously untreated patients with ovarian cancer (OC): a SEER Medicare database analysis. J Clin Oncol 37(15_Suppl):e17095

Dhingra K (2016) Rociletinib: has the TIGER lost a few of its stripes? Ann Oncol 27(6):1161–1164

Drugs@FDA. FDA-approved drugs. https://www.accessdata.fda.gov/scripts/cder/daf/. Accessed 18 Apr 2021

Egger M (2001) Value of flow diagrams in reports of randomized controlled trials. JAMA 285(15):1996

Fukuoka M, Wu Y-L, Thongprasert S et al (2011) Biomarker analyses and final overall survival results from a phase III, randomized, open-label, first-line study of gefitinib versus carboplatin/paclitaxel in clinically selected patients with advanced non–small-cell lung cancer in Asia (IPASS). J Clin Oncol 29(21):2866–2874

Gandara DR, Kowanetz M, Mok TSK et al (2017) Blood-based biomarkers for cancer immunotherapy: tumor mutational burden in blood (bTMB) is associated with improved atezolizumab (atezo) efficacy in 2L+ NSCLC (POPLAR and OAK). Ann Oncol 28(suppl_5):v460

Gandhi L, Rodríguez-Abreu D, Gadgeel S et al (2018) Pembrolizumab plus chemotherapy in metastatic non–small-cell lung cancer. N Engl J Med 378(22):2078–2092

Garassino MC, Gadgeel S, Esteban E et al (2020) Patient-reported outcomes following pembrolizumab or placebo plus pemetrexed and platinum in patients with previously untreated, metastatic, non-squamous non-small-cell lung cancer (KEYNOTE-189): a multicentre, double-blind, randomised, placebo-controlled. Lancet Oncol 21(3):387–397

Garon EB, Ciuleanu TE, Arrieta O et al (2014) Ramucirumab plus docetaxel versus placebo plus docetaxel for second-line treatment of stage IV non–small-cell lung cancer after disease progression on platinum-based therapy (REVEL): a multicentre, double-blind, randomised phase 3 trial. Lancet 384(9944):665–673

Golan T, Hammel P, Reni M et al (2019) Maintenance olaparib for germline BRCA-mutated metastatic pancreatic cancer. N Engl J Med 381(4):317–327

González-Martín A, Pothuri B, Vergote I et al (2019) Niraparib in patients with newly diagnosed advanced ovarian cancer. N Engl J Med 381(25):2391–2402

Gupta SK (2011) Intention-to-treat concept: a review. Perspect Clin Res 2(3):109–112

Hariton E, Locascio JJ (2018) Randomised controlled trials—the gold standard for effectiveness research: study design: randomised controlled trials. BJOG 125(13):1716–1716

Hellmann MD, Paz-Ares L, Bernabe Caro R et al (2019) Nivolumab plus ipilimumab in advanced non–small-cell lung cancer. N Engl J Med 381(21):2020–2031

Herbst RS, Baas P, Kim DW et al (2016) Pembrolizumab versus docetaxel for previously treated, PD-L1-positive, advanced non-small-cell lung cancer (KEYNOTE-010): a randomised controlled trial. Lancet 387(10027):1540–1550

Hui R, Özgüroğlu M, Villegas A et al (2019) Patient-reported outcomes with durvalumab after chemoradiotherapy in stage III, unresectable non-small-cell lung cancer (PACIFIC): a randomised, controlled, phase 3 study. Lancet Oncol 20(12):1670–1680

Idänpään-Heikkilä JE (1994) WHO guidelines for good clinical practice (GCP) for trials on pharmaceutical products: responsibilities of the investigator. Ann Med 26(2):89–94

James ND, de Bono JS, Spears MR et al (2017) Abiraterone for prostate cancer not previously treated with hormone therapy. N Engl J Med 377(4):338–351

Jotte R, Cappuzzo F, Vynnychenko I et al (2020) Atezolizumab in combination with carboplatin and nab-paclitaxel in advanced squamous NSCLC (IMpower131): results from a randomized phase III trial. J Thorac Oncol 15(8):1351–1360

Kim MS, Prasad V (2019) Assessment of accuracy of waterfall plot representations of response rates in cancer treatment published in medical journals. JAMA Netw Open 2(5):e193981

Kumar A, Chakraborty BS (2016) Interim analysis: a rational approach of decision making in clinical trial. J Adv Pharm Technol Res 7(4):118–122

Lopes G, Wu Y-L, Kudaba I et al (2018) Pembrolizumab (pembro) versus platinum-based chemotherapy (chemo) as first-line therapy for advanced/metastatic NSCLC with a PD-L1 tumor proportion score (TPS) ≥1%: open-label, phase 3 KEYNOTE-042 study. J Clin Oncol 36(18_Suppl):LBA4

Maemondo M, Fukuhara T, Saito H et al (2020) NEJ026: final overall survival analysis of bevacizumab plus erlotinib treatment for NSCLC patients harboring activating EGFR-mutations. J Clin Oncol 38(15_Suppl):9506

Majem M, Goldman J, John T et al (2021) OA06.03 patient-reported outcomes from ADAURA: osimertinib as adjuvant therapy in patients with resected EGFR mutated (EGFRm) NSCLC. J Thorac Oncol 16(3):S112–S113

Mercier F, Consalvo N, Frey N, Phipps A, Ribba B (2019) From waterfall plots to spaghetti plots in early oncology clinical development. Pharm Stat 18(5):526–532

Mok TS, Wu Y-L, Thongprasert S et al (2009) Gefitinib or carboplatin–paclitaxel in pulmonary adenocarcinoma. N Engl J Med 361(10):947–957

Mok TS, Cheng Y, Zhou X et al (2018) Improvement in overall survival in a randomized study that compared dacomitinib with gefitinib in patients with advanced non-small-cell lung cancer and EGFR-activating mutations. J Clin Oncol 36(22):2244–2250

Mok TSK, Wu Y-L, Kudaba I et al (2019) Pembrolizumab versus chemotherapy for previously untreated, PD-L1-expressing, locally advanced or metastatic non-small-cell lung cancer (KEYNOTE-042): a randomised, open-label, controlled, phase 3 trial. Lancet 393(10183):1819–1830

Mok T, Camidge DR, Gadgeel SM et al (2020) Updated overall survival and final progression-free survival data for patients with treatment-naive advanced ALK-positive non-small-cell lung cancer in the ALEX study. Ann Oncol 31(8):1056–1064

Montori VM, Devereaux PJ, Adhikari NKJ et al (2005) Randomized trials stopped early for benefit. JAMA 294(17):2203

Moore K, Colombo N, Scambia G et al (2018) Maintenance olaparib in patients with newly diagnosed advanced ovarian cancer. N Engl J Med 379(26):2495–2505

NCI dictionary of cancer terms. https://www.cancer.gov/publications/dictionaries/cancer-terms. Accessed 18 Apr 2021

Nishino M, Jagannathan JP, Ramaiya NH, Van den Abbeele AD (2010) Revised RECIST guideline version 1.1: what oncologists want to know and what radiologists need to know. Am J Roentgenol 195(2):281–289

Parmar MK, Sydes MR, Cafferty FH et al (2017) Testing many treatments within a single protocol over 10 years at MRC clinical trials unit at UCL: multi-arm, multistage platform, umbrella and basket protocols. Clin Trials 14(5):451–461

Passaro A, Spitaleri G, Gyawali B, De Marinis F (2019) Immunotherapy in non–small-cell lung cancer patients with performance status 2: clinical decision making with scant evidence. J Clin Oncol 37(22):1863–1867

Paz-Ares L, Luft A, Vicente D et al (2018) Pembrolizumab plus chemotherapy for squamous non–small-cell lung cancer. N Engl J Med 379(21):2040–2051

Paz-Ares L, Vicente D, Tafreshi A et al (2020a) A randomized, placebo-controlled trial of Pembrolizumab plus chemotherapy in patients with metastatic squamous NSCLC: protocol-specified final analysis of KEYNOTE-407. J Thorac Oncol 15(10):1657–1669

Paz-Ares L, Spira A, Raben D et al (2020b) Outcomes with durvalumab by tumour PD-L1 expression in unresectable, stage III non-small-cell lung cancer in the PACIFIC trial. Ann Oncol 31(6):798–806

Paz-Ares L, Ciuleanu T-E, Cobo M et al (2021) First-line nivolumab plus ipilimumab combined with two cycles of chemotherapy in patients with non-small-cell lung cancer (CheckMate 9LA): an international, randomised, open-label, phase 3 trial. Lancet Oncol 22(2):198–211

Peters S, Camidge DR, Shaw AT et al (2017) Alectinib versus crizotinib in untreated ALK-positive non–small-cell lung cancer. N Engl J Med 377(9):829–838

Ramalingam SS, Vansteenkiste J, Planchard D et al (2019) Overall survival with osimertinib in untreated, EGFR-mutated advanced NSCLC. N Engl J Med 382(1):41–50

Reck M, Rodríguez-Abreu D, Robinson AG et al (2016) Pembrolizumab versus chemotherapy for PD-L1–positive non–small-cell lung cancer. N Engl J Med 375(19):1823–1833

Rittmeyer A, Barlesi F, Waterkamp D et al (2017) Atezolizumab versus docetaxel in patients with previously treated non-small-cell lung cancer (OAK): a phase 3, open-label, multicentre randomised controlled trial. Lancet 389(10066):255–265

Rizvi NA, Cho BC, Reinmuth N et al (2020) Durvalumab with or without tremelimumab vs standard chemotherapy in first-line treatment of metastatic non–small cell lung cancer. JAMA Oncol 6(5):661

Rodriguez-Abreu D, Powell SF, Hochmair M et al (2020) Final analysis of KEYNOTE-189: pemetrexed-platinum chemotherapy (chemo) with or without pembrolizumab (pembro) in patients (pts) with previously untreated metastatic nonsquamous non-small cell lung cancer (NSCLC). J Clin Oncol 38(15_Suppl):9582

Saito H, Fukuhara T, Furuya N et al (2019) Erlotinib plus bevacizumab versus erlotinib alone in patients with EGFR-positive advanced non-squamous non–small-cell lung cancer (NEJ026): interim analysis of an open-label, randomised, multicentre, phase 3 trial. Lancet Oncol 20(5):625–635

Scagliotti GV, Parikh P, Von Pawel J et al (2008) Phase III study comparing cisplatin plus gemcitabine with cisplatin plus pemetrexed in chemotherapy-naive patients with advanced-stage non-small-cell lung cancer. J Clin Oncol 26(21):3543–3551

Sequist LV, Soria J-C, Goldman JW et al (2015) Rociletinib in EGFR-mutated non-small-cell lung cancer. N Engl J Med 372(18):1700–1709

Sequist LV, Soria J-C, Camidge DR (2016) Update to rociletinib data with the RECIST confirmed response rate. N Engl J Med 374(23):2296–2297

Sezer A, Kilickap S, Gümüş M et al (2021) Cemiplimab monotherapy for first-line treatment of advanced non-small-cell lung cancer with PD-L1 of at least 50%: a multicentre, open-label, global, phase 3, randomised, controlled trial. Lancet 397(10274):592–604

Shao T, Wang L, Templeton AJ et al (2014) Use and misuse of waterfall plots. J Natl Cancer Inst 106(12):dju331

Socinski MA, Jotte RM, Cappuzzo F et al (2018) Atezolizumab for first-line treatment of metastatic nonsquamous NSCLC. N Engl J Med 378(24):2288–2301

Solomon BJ, Kim DW, Wu YL et al (2018) Final overall survival analysis from a study comparing first-line crizotinib versus chemotherapy in ALK-mutation-positive non-small-cell lung cancer. J Clin Oncol 36(22):2251–2258

Spigel D, Schwartzberg L, Waterhouse D et al (2017) P3.02c-026 is nivolumab safe and effective in elderly and PS2 patients with non-small cell lung cancer (NSCLC)? Results of CheckMate 153. J Thorac Oncol 12(1):S1287–S1288

Sydes MR, Spears MR, Mason MD, et al (2018) Adding abiraterone or docetaxel to long-term hormone therapy for prostate cancer: directly randomised data from the STAMPEDE multi-arm, multi-stage platform protocol. Ann Oncol. 29(5):1235-1248. https://doi.org/10.1093/annonc/mdy072

The ASCO Post. 2020 FDA Approvals of drugs for cancer treatments. https://ascopost.com/issues/december-25-2020/2020-fda-approvals-of-drugs-for-cancer--treatment/. Accessed 18 Apr 2021

Tournigand C, André T, Bonnetain F et al (2012) Adjuvant therapy with fluorouracil and oxaliplatin in stage II and elderly patients (between ages 70 and 75 years) with colon cancer: subgroup analyses of the multicenter international study of oxaliplatin, fluorouracil, and leucovorin in the adjuvant Tre. J Clin Oncol 30(27):3353–3360

U.S. National Library of Medicine. A study of osimertinib with or without chemotherapy as 1st line treatment in patients with mutated epidermal growth factor receptor non-small cell lung cancer (FLAURA2). https://clinicaltrials.gov/ct2/show/NCT04035486. Accessed 18 Apr 2021

West H, McCleod M, Hussein M et al (2019) Atezolizumab in combination with carboplatin plus nab-paclitaxel chemotherapy compared with chemotherapy alone as first-line treatment for metastatic non-squamous non-small-cell lung cancer (IMpower130): a multicentre, randomised, open-label, phase 3 trial. Lancet Oncol 20(7):924–937

World Health Organization (2005) Handbook for good clinical research practice (GCP): guidance for implementation. World Health Organization, Geneva

Wu Y-L, Cheng Y, Zhou X et al (2017) Dacomitinib versus gefitinib as first-line treatment for patients with EGFR-mutation-positive non-small-cell lung cancer (ARCHER 1050): a randomised, open-label, phase 3 trial. Lancet Oncol 18(11):1454–1466

Wu Y-L, Zhong W, Wang Q et al (2020a) CTONG1104: adjuvant gefitinib versus chemotherapy for resected N1-N2 NSCLC with EGFR mutation—final overall survival analysis of the randomized phase III trial 1 analysis of the randomized phase III trial. J Clin Oncol 38(15_Suppl):9005

Wu Y-L, Tsuboi M, He J et al (2020b) Osimertinib in resected EGFR-mutated non–small-cell lung cancer. N Engl J Med 383(18):1711–1723

Zhong W-Z, Wang Q, Mao W-M et al (2018) Gefitinib versus vinorelbine plus cisplatin as adjuvant treatment for stage II–IIIA (N1–N2) EGFR-mutant NSCLC (ADJUVANT/CTONG1104): a randomised, open-label, phase 3 study. Lancet Oncol 19(1):139–148